Healthcare Delivery Reform and New Technologies:
Organizational Initiatives

Matthew Guah
Claflin University, USA

Medical Information Science
REFERENCE
MEDICAL INFORMATION SCIENCE REFERENCE
Hershey · New York

Director of Editorial Content: Kristin Klinger
Director of Book Publications: Julia Mosemann
Acquisitions Editor: Lindsay Johnston
Development Editor: Myla Harty
Typesetter: Milan Vracarich, Jr.
Production Editor: Jamie Snavely
Cover Design: Lisa Tosheff

Published in the United States of America by
Medical Information Science Reference (an imprint of IGI Global)
701 E. Chocolate Avenue
Hershey PA 17033
Tel: 717-533-8845
Fax: 717-533-8661
E-mail: cust@igi-global.com
Web site: http://www.igi-global.com

Library of Congress Cataloging-in-Publication Data

Healthcare delivery reform and new technologies : organizational initiatives /
Matthew Guah, editor.
p. cm.
Includes bibliographical references and index.
Summary: "This book contains cross-disciplinary research on strategic initiatives for healthcare reform that impact not only patients, but also organizations, healthcare providers, and policymakers"--Provided by publisher.
ISBN 978-1-60960-183-6 (hardcover) -- ISBN 978-1-60960-185-0 (ebook) 1. Health care reform--United States. 2. Medical informatics. I. Guah, Matthew W., 1963-
RA395.A3H4315 2011
362.1'0425--dc22
2010045830

British Cataloguing in Publication Data
A Cataloguing in Publication record for this book is available from the British Library.

Dedication

To my life-long sweetheart, Eve, and our especially lovely two boys, Michael and Matthew, all of UK, whose constant presence brings renewed motivations to all my work.

To all my brothers and sisters in Liberia, especially Emmanuel Guah, his wife and Philip JG Piah of Minnesota; the entire Waritay family, especially my delightful sister Miriama Daba of Philadelphia; and my special brother Michael Livesey and his family of Kingston-Upon-Thames.

Also to my recently re-established childhood friend Leon Deemi and his family of Dallas; not forgetting lovely Esther Deemi of Fortworth; as well as reliable Sarah Capps and her assiduous son Michael Mulbah, all of Houston.

Finally to my long-term family friends: George and Edna Brown and family of New Jersey, Matthew Kiamue and family of Philadelphia, as well as Massa Gray-Cassell and her charming and sweet-humoured daughter Edna Cassell, of Huntingdon Valley, Pennsylvania.

None of my publications would be possible without your thoughtfulness, love, kindness, affections and prayers.

Matthew Guah
Claflin University, USA

Table of Contents

Detailed Table of Contents

The evolution of healthcare in developed countries is subject to contrasting forces. The pressure to be innovative, technologically advanced in order to improve the quality of services has resulted in a significant increase in spending whilst at the same time governments are faced with budget constraints. Even though e-procurement initiatives can be seen as a solution to the latter, such initiatives have not been widely deployed and have not delivered the expected benefits so far. In this chapter, a case study of an e-procurement implementation of an Italian Local Healthcare Agency has been examined because of the comprehensive design of the e-procurement system, the differentiation of tools adopted and the multiple solutions already implemented. The aim of this work is to reconstruct, by following a knowledge management approach, the steps that have led to the introduction of e-procurement as a new operating practice, by redesigning supply purchasing, supply chain and logistic processes which take into consideration the interventions at the organisational level that are devised to support it.

Clinical trials are specific medical studies that use human subjects for the advancement of medicine. Evidence-based medicine requires the use of clinical trials to evaluate new treatments, devices, drugs, and modalities for the prevention and treatment of diseases. Clinical trials have not been particularly aggressive in their adoption of information technology (IT). In this analysis, we the authors examine the impact of electronic resources on the execution and management of clinical trials. Further, we the authors present a theoretical model showing the main areas of clinical trials that can be directly impacted by the adoption of electronic resources. The four areas identified are recruitment, data collection, process data management, and information dissemination.

This chapter attempts to elucidate the intricacies of primary health care delivery in Nigeria. Based on Decision Space concept which proposes that the tension between local and central government agents has an impact on the effectiveness of primary care delivery, the chapter shows that in the context of developing countries, this tension is marked by the absence of an effective regulatory and enforcement framework which results in a prominent informal decision space. Evidence for the study was gathered through an interpretive exploratory approach and therefore reflects an interpretation of interviewees' understanding. The findings show that the prominence of an informal decision space compromises the objectives of an information-based public health system. The chapter concludes that decentralisation in developing countries must have a coordinated top-down and bottom-up development component for it to be effective in improving the performance of primary health systems. One of the implications of the study is that researching decentralised healthcare delivery requires analytical models which are able to illuminate the complexities of local accountability in developing countries. The study also reveals the need to further research the dynamics of democratic decentralisation in developing countries as this goes beyond administrative structures but involve socio-cultural institutions.

This chapter argues that current techniques used in the domain of Information Systems is not adequate for establishing determinants of wireless technology in a clinical setting. Using data collected from India, this chapter conducted a first order regression modeling (factor analysis) and then a second order regression modeling (SEM) to establish the determinants of clinical influences as a result of using wireless technology in healthcare settings. As information systems professionals, the authors conducted a qualitative data collection to understand the domain prior to employing a quantitative technique, thus providing rigor as well as personal relevance. The outcomes of this study has clearly established that there are a number of influences such as the organizational factors in determining the technology acceptance and provides evidence that trivial factors such as perceived ease of use and perceived usefulness are no longer acceptable as the factors of technology acceptance.

Diabetes is one of the leading chronic diseases affecting Australians and is increasingly becoming a serious challenge and threat for both the quality of healthcare while increasing cost pressures on the Australian healthcare system. The goal of this study is to provide a transaction cost economics framework which can be used as a tool for high-level assessments of the economic viability of a pervasive technology solution developed by INET in the form of a wireless enabled mobile solution to facilitate superior diabetes self-management. In doing so, we prepare the inroads for proposing an approach for refined quantifiable assessments of a pervasive IT-enabled healthcare solution.

With the increasing shift in the population profile to the older demographic and rising healthcare costs, it is more critical for developed countries to deliver long-term and financially sustainable healthcare services, especially in the area of residential aged care. A consensus exists that innovations in the area of Wireless Sensor Networks (WSNs) are key enabling technologies for reaching this goal. The major focus of this article is WSN design considerations for ubiquitous wellness monitoring systems in residential aged care facilities. Major enabling technologies for building a pervasive WSN will be detailed, including descriptions on sensor design, wireless communication protocols and network topologies. Also examined are data processing methods and knowledge management tools to support the collection of sensor data and their subsequent analysis for health assessment. To introduce future healthcare reform in residential aged care, two aspects of wellness monitoring, vital signs and activities of daily living (ADL) monitoring, will be discussed.

A nursing home provides skilled nursing care and rehabilitation services to people with illnesses, injuries or functional disabilities, but most facilities serve the elderly. Nursing homes provide various services for different residents' needs, including daily care, assistance for the mentally disabled, and drug rehabilitation. The levels of care and quality of care provided by nursing homes have increased significantly over the past decade. The trend is toward continuous quality development and resident satisfaction; therefore, healthcare technology plays a significant role in nursing home operations. This article discusses general information about current nursing home conditions and systems in the United States and explores how technology and e-health help improve the nursing home development based on the present needs and trends. The authors also report on Thomasville Nursing Home, discussing current trends in nursing home technologies.

Pervasive healthcare is the field of application emerging from the combination of healthcare with pervasive computing, which is the computing paradigm that provides users with access to services in a transparent way, wherever they are and whichever their interacting device is. In this paper, a software infrastructure for pervasive healthcare is presented. Such an infrastructure aims at supporting medical practitioners with advanced pervasive access to medical data, which is also context-aware in the sense that the modality to fruit data depends on the device used by the operator and on his or her physical position within the environment. The paper also describes a service for high quality 3D rendering of medical volume data, which takes advantage of the software infrastructure to distribute the computational load upon the devices available in the environment in a completely transparent way to users.

During the past decade, many countries launched ambitious Electronic Health Record (EHR) programs with the objective to increase the quality of care while decreasing its cost. Pervasive healthcare aims itself at making healthcare information securely available anywhere and anytime, even in disconnected environments (e.g., at patient home). Current server-based EHR solutions badly tackle disconnected situations and fail in providing ultimate security guarantees for the patients. The solution proposed in this paper capitalizes on a new hardware device combining a secure microcontroller (similar to a smart card chip) with a large external Flash memory on a USB key form factor. Embedding the patient folder as well as a database system and a web server in such a device gives the opportunity to manage securely a healthcare folder in complete autonomy. This paper proposes also a new way of personalizing access control policies to meet patient's privacy concerns with minimal assistance of practitioners. While both proposals are orthogonal, their integration in the same infrastructure allows building trustworthy pervasive healthcare folders.

Preface

A book that combines healthcare and information and communication technology (ICT) usually turns out to be like viewing an old subject from a slightly different angle. The good thing about that is one or two new ideas often emerge and old ideas are seen in a new light. Most of the new ideas in this book and the new approach to old ideas are outlined in the Preface. The rest of the book might seem nonsensical at times if the Preface is not thoroughly read. From chapter 1 through Chapter 20, the reader is given different healthcare delivery reform initiatives, evidenced by all these contributions from around the globe.

HEALTHCARE REFORM MODELS

Although healthcare reform models came into existence in the early 1940s, their use did not become widespread until the middle of 1970s. The advent of computer-based healthcare reform models was in direct response to a series of very serious problems encountered by healthcare organizations, throughout the world, in the late 1990s—including increasing cost of maintaining an aging population by most western countries, double-digit inflation in various countries, increasing insurance bills, and increased government regulation (Teperi et al, 2009). These problems have placed enormous pressure on the administrators of healthcare organizations—and governments alike (Clegg & Shepherd, 2007). As it became increasingly apparent that manual reform strategies were not adequate to meet the increasing healthcare demands for future generation, ICT was considered for its extremely powerful tools, enabling healthcare administrators to cope more effectively with the many uncertainties (Wilson & Lankton, 2004).

After attending the AAA (American Accounting Association) annual meeting and AMCIS (American Conference on IS), I had the privilege of spending three weeks in the US—mainly visiting friends and family members—in Texas, PA, NJ and NY. Like most visitors to the US in the month of August 2009, I was fascinated by the healthcare reform debate as President Obama and his team tried to push through the 'Healthcare Reform Bill'. While this book is not particularly dedicated to the happenings around healthcare reform in the US, it is worth mentioning my observation here. Despite many waves of debate and piecemeal reforms, including millions spent on technology infrastructure, the U.S. health care system remains largely the same as it was decades ago. Critiques claim there is no convincing approach to changing the unsustainable trajectory of the system, much less to offsetting the rising costs of an aging population and new medical advances (Brennan, 2007; Scott et al, 2000). The Americans situation might have been significantly highlighted as the result of President Obama making healthcare his *number 1* agenda item. Nearly all countries in the developed world confront a similar challenge—finding the right way to create a well-resourced but sustainable system that provides healthcare and services of the highest quality for all. Notwithstanding the clear political differences, it is impossible to find credible opponents to the goal of providing 'universal health care' (Darzi, 2009). Every country is actively seeking a formula that suits it best in achieving this monumental goal.

The outcome of health care reform in Italy or Germany will no doubt be very different from those of USA or UK (Shaw et al, 2009). The NHS (national health service in UK) lies at the opposite end of the spectrum from the current U.S. system, in terms of both its structure (a tax-funded public program as opposed to mainly private, employment-based insurance) and the problems it faces (historically, a lack of resources and slow uptake of new treatments as opposed to bulging costs). In the late 1990s the UK had to confront reform on a scale as challenging as that being contemplated in the USA today (Solberg et al, 2007; Wanless, 2002).

In 1997, Britain had a new government, which then inherited a health care system that was chronically underfunded and suffering from a lack of capacity, with average waiting times of 18 months from referral to treatment. Funding for 1997 was £35 billion which has risen to £110 billion for 2010 (NAO, 2006). The result is waiting times are now as short as they've ever been — 10 years ago, patients waited approximately 18 months for treatment, and now they wait only a few weeks. Although both the causes of and responses to reform were very different from those on the opposite side of the Atlantic today, the NHS's experience can provide some valuable lessons to both Canada and the United States.

A key finding from my own research on the NHS is that it is important for physicians to be involved in both informing and leading change (Currie & Guah, 2007; Guah, 2008; Guah & Fink, 2008). Successive attempts at top-down regulation and reform in the UK damaged physicians' morale and bred distrust between physicians and all healthcare administrators—specifically politicians. Not having been central to the decision making, physicians subsequently didn't trust the proposals or fully understand the purpose of healthcare reform initiatives. On the contrary, who could disagree that if a physician understood what drives healthcare cost, he/she would have the *potential* to reduce those costs? One can assume that governments throughout the world have figured that out when it comes to paying for health care. Assuming therefore that President Obama's government wants to reduce costs, they would pay the providers less and take appropriate measures so all the other issues will go away. Applying a combination of reform initiatives to USA healthcare sector means this government would need have to address the below 5 issues--primarily:

- Technology for the Healthcare sector are double the costs other countries
- The emergency room usage has reached it's highest level
- 30% of medicare costs are for the last year of life
- 5% of the medicaid population uses up 50% of the resources
- admissions have gone up nationally 5% a year

ICT IN HEALTHCARE

Most members of the public find it refreshing to see politically naive, formerly unengaged Americans show up at town hall meetings (in the month of August 2009), asking questions and expressing personal opinions about a major government initiative. I was told this move to reform healthcare delivery process has motivated many—that would normally be at home watching television programme reruns—to participate in the political process. On several occasions, every major television channel was screening concerned citizens demonstrating their democratic rights by asking elected officials—including President Barrack Obama—tough questions and weighing in on what was missing from healthcare system. I couldn't stop myself thinking such feelings and desires far surpass what their 535 congressional representatives unilaterally decided was best for these citizens. Scientific mindset quickly noted that significant propaganda was also being spewed by many who appeared to have an agenda with certain degree of bias.

Notwithstanding, USA—along with most western countries—is experiencing an increasing aging population and a growing number of chronically ill people. This situation requires the national healthcare system that is not only prepared for higher future demands, but also equipped to face issues that could collapse an entire workforce (Constantinides & Barrett, 2006; Porter et al, 2009). The shift to a more consumer driven healthcare market is also impacting consumer expectations with regards to the quality and consistency of the care patients seeks (Badgett & Mulrow, 2005; Berwick, 2003; Davis, 2004). Moreover, patients facing a potentially life threatening disease are seeking the rapid responses from healthcare systems and operators and, including, better plans for treatments (Donaldson, 2008). On the other hand, the wide diffusion of wireless technologies along with the emerging of new devices and sensors are opening a new market of better and cheaper healthcare applications.

Within the last decade, we have seen Europe, Australia and now America show a new openness to changing healthcare systems that a number of people agree is broken. What is needed now is a clear strategy, by healthcare providers, that sets forth a comprehensive vision for the kind of health care system they want to achieve and a path for getting there. The central focus must be on increasing value for patients by efficiently achieving good outcomes, not merely *savings* money (Porter & Teisberg, 2006). Cost can truly be contained in health care by improving outcomes in a value-based system because achieving and maintaining good health is inherently less costly than dealing with poor health (Remler & Glied, 2006).

WHO SHOULD BENEFIT FROM THIS BOOK

Mr. William Beveridge, the founder of the NHS in 1942, has repeatedly been quoted as saying "a revolutionary moment in the world's history is a time for revolutions, not for patching". I'll interpret that in today's situation where the combination a global downturn sees us sitting on the time bomb of healthcare costs. There is no denying that healthcare in nearly all Western continents (including Canada, USA, Western Europe, and Australia) have reached such a moment. The publication of this book signifies that the matter is too important to be left to the politicians and policymakers. Our goal is to encourage—and even make it an urgent requirement—for all physicians to step up and lead the debate on healthcare reform initiatives.

This book includes original research articles, case studies from four different countries, all on the path of reforming their national healthcare delivery. It is concerned with the theory and practice of healthcare reform initiatives from around the globe. It attempts to outline a systematic approach to the policies, strategies and implementation of various healthcare reform initiatives as researched by our remarkable list of academic and industry researchers in the field.

I have a great pleasure in seeing this first in a series of books on international healthcare delivery reform initiatives published. I believe this book represents an important, but under-researched, topic. With new initiatives being declared every few months in this critical sector, keeping track on reforming healthcare delivery is an essential part of our tasks as academic researchers. I hope the fine contributions in this book will encourage the publication of more research in the area of healthcare reform. I appreciate the efforts of all my contributors and all reviewers for the International Journal Healthcare Delivery Reform Initiatives making this book a reality.

All these case studies in this issue provide brief literature reviews before presenting and interpreting their own research datasets. It is therefore our hope that this book, including 20 research articles, from 12 different countries (in Asia, Africa, Europe, America and Australia) all on the path of reforming their national healthcare delivery processes, would contribute to our understanding what reforming healthcare delivery process truly involves. I also hope this book will provide healthcare professionals, and academic researchers, with valuable information that is useful in the continuous search for successful reform to our healthcare delivery.

SPECIFIC HEALTHCARE REFORM INITIATIVES FROM AROUND THE WORLD

This section briefly describes each of the twenty-one cases presented in this book to examine the complex issue from different parts of the globe—including Africa, America, Asia and Europe—each give it different perspectives. In Chapter 1 Tommaso Federici and Andrea Resca offer insights related to the introduction of emerging technologies in a traditional sector. Their paper examines how the effectiveness of such initiative is influenced by factors such as large expenditures for a comprehensive design due to the need for different tools, the long-lasting experimentations and multiple solutions. Focusing on the dyadic level, the paper employs Lim's (2000) knowledge management approach to arrive at analytical results regarding the influence of incompleteness and asymmetry in the information sets involved in appropriately valuing e-procurement in an Italian local healthcare agency.

Chapter 2 is a contribution from Maricarmen Planas-Silva and Rhoda Joseph suggesting clinical trials to be a critical component of the advancement of medicine. It demonstrates an on-going reform initiative in the United States of America to prove that evidence based medical practices require the use of clinical trials to evaluate new treatments, devices, drugs and modalities for the prevention and treatment of diseases. As its subject the paper examines the use of and adoption of IT in clinical trials, especially within cancer treatment. It concludes by acknowledging that IT is not a panacea to clinical trials in the USA today mainly due to challenges in the areas of system interoperability and data security.

Chapter 3, by Adebusoye Anifalaje, takes the reader through the intricacies of primary healthcare delivery in Nigeria. The study examines the complex interaction of individual and contextual factors such as lack of value for process and knowledge depreciation in delivering healthcare provision benefits. After diagnosing the existing tension between local and central government agents and consequential impact on primary care delivery—in the context of developing countries—the paper argues the need for effective regulatory and enforcement framework.

Based on a decision space theory, the research findings include limitation in the actual roles of information within Nigeria's primary healthcare system, thus sabotaging the principles of a 'rational' public healthcare system. The study suggests implications for the complex decision making process in developing countries with regard to healthcare knowledge creation and opens up avenues for future research to validate the assumptions and results.

Chapter 4 is contributed by Raj Gururajan and uses both qualitative and quantitative data to derive outcomes of clinical usefulness as a driver of wireless technology for Indian healthcare.

The outcomes established that in addition to technology factor, clinical, administrative, and communication factors quite often play crucial role in determining the uptake of wireless technology for healthcare sector. Upon using PSL model to analyze a large set of data, the paper confirms that simply acquiring wireless technology would be insufficient to accomplish clinical usefulness and subsequently drive adoption and diffusion. It promotes the need to integrate wireless systems with process improvement and organizational change within Indian health service providers.

In Chapter 5, Blessing M. Maumbe, Meke Shivute and Vesper Owei examine the use of ICT in health service provision in Namibia in an attempt to contribute to the understanding of patterns to ICT use by both public and private health service providers and their patients. The study collects data from patients in the Khomas and Oshana regions in Namibia. IT identifies three main factor groupings (namely high technology, mobile technology and traditional technology). The paper provides insights for practice and for further research in signaling and incentives for a changing role of functional literacy and policy implications to healthcare delivery in Namibia.

Chapter 6, submitted by Gary Hackbarth and John McQuade, evaluated 31 Indoor Air Quality (IAQ) checklists using CATPAC for information completeness. They found that these sources differed in both the depth and breathe of information provided. The authors conclude that users of healthcare information may be underserved and that healthcare information providers might act in a more collaborative way to better balance the presentation of their information in terms of depth and breathe of presented content.

Chapter 7, by Robert Breas and Matthew Guah, is study on the need for readiness framework when implementing IS in healthcare institutions. They found that most systems in hospitals today concentrate on relatively simple coordination, resource allocation and documentation aspects of healthcare operations. Yet in practice, the adoption of new systems is still difficult and generally considered a very slow process. After interviewing large groups of healthcare actors, within a large teaching hospital in The Netherlands, they also identified a set of key bottlenecks in the IT adoption process. Their conclusions suggest that health care organizations should be better prepared in order to facilitate easier IT systems' adoption. They discuss the implications of these findings on our understanding of such things as clinical pathways, workflow management, and optimization of resource utilisation, clinical decision-making, staff training and quality improvement in healthcare delivery. They also propose a readiness framework as a prelude implementing new systems in this critical environment.

In Chapter 8, David Meinert and Dane Peterson, present their study that examined potential characteristics of physicians considered helpful in the identification of individuals that are most likely to pose a threat to the successful implementation of an EMR system in a multi-specialty clinic. The authors have provided a commentary, focusing on explanations of the results which demonstrated that older physicians and physicians with only minimal computer skills are more likely to have negative attitudes regarding EMR technology. The paper acknowledges that Medical specialists were most likely to have positive attitudes with respects to the use of EMR systems, while primary care physicians were most likely to have doubts regarding the purported benefits of EMR technology.

Chapter 9 is by Esko Alasaarela, Ravi Nemana, Steven DeMello, Nick S. Oliver and Masako Miyazaki, who present analysis of data from their international collaborative study that focused on the future of healthcare needs, technology requirements and solutions for effective use of wireless platform for health care delivery. The results help to clarify views on the incorporation of wireless platform for future health care delivery and personal health management. The paper contains key findings involving quality improvements and process enhancements as well as integration of personal health monitoring and suggestions that health promotion and illness prevention growth as a result of using mobile solutions. Like the Dutch study, this paper also proposes a framework that can be used in developing wireless health care solutions for managing diseases and related health problems.

Chapter 10 was submitted by Alalwany Hamid and Alshawi Sarmad, appraising the increasingly evolving research area of E-health. The authors list a number of characteristics necessary for the appropriate evaluation of E-health services and propose a criteria-based evaluation framework maximizing the full potential of ICT in healthcare delivery. They conclude that E-health evaluation framework improves our understanding of IS roles in healthcare and contributes to high quality healthcare services.

Chapter 11, by Ray Gururajan, Tiana Gurney and Abdul Hafeez-Baig, presents a study on wireless technology in Indian Healthcare. This qualitative research involving 200 completed surveys, contributes three major determinants for successful wireless technology in healthcare delivery: barriers, drivers and clinical inferences, along with several sub-components for each.

Nesaar Banderker and Jean-Paul Van Belle contribute chapter 12 with demonstration of how mobile technology is helping to improve the quality of healthcare delivery in South Africa despite the presence of resource constraints prevalent in all developing countries. Using qualitative research with thematic analysis the authors confirm a number of key adoption factors identified in prior research (namely job relevance, usefulness, perceived user resources and device characteristics) along with additional adoption factors (namely patient influence, support structures from national government and hospital administration, and unease in respect of malpractice legal suits).Chapter 13 is another USA contribution by Thomas Miller, Robert Morgan and Jennifer Wood. They review the use of tele-practice applications in rural community for clinical and educational purposes and propose a video teleconferencing model of healthcare for certain under-privileged populations. The paper also explains how professional consultation within teams may benefit rural educational systems. The authors outline mechanisms (processes) for successfully implementing their proposed model—Tele-health Intervention Project—for implementing a dimension of the public education campaign to reach underserved target groups in need of health and prevention education information across USA. They conclude that this model demonstrates the capability of reducing time and distance barriers in the provision of healthcare and education through tele-practice technology.

In Chapter 14 Torben Larsen explains how Integrated Homecare is combining efficacy with net savings to represent a prototype of integrated care with overlapping services for better clinical continuity in Denmark. The author includes frequent chronic conditions—such as stroke, heart failure, chronic obstructive pulmonary disease and mental disease—and exhibits parallel results to explain a common neuro-economic framework. Using a SWOT analysis of integrated homecare the paper emphasizes how various characteristics of integrated homecare can result to low-tech patient benefits, affordable by low and middle income countries, and low levels of trust across professions and settings. The paper also explains these two strategies recommended by European Union states:

Make a synthesis of existing and ongoing research as a health technology assessment (HTA) of IHC for multidisciplinary teamwork across the hospital and primary care interface; and Focus on dissemination by the formation of country specific multidisciplinary networks on IHC.

In Chapter 15 Esteban Pino, Dorothy Curtis, Thomas Stair and Lucila Ohno-Machado realized SMART, a pervasive health monitoring system for mass casualty emergencies and general ad hoc patient monitoring sites. The system prototype has been deployed in a hospital and evaluated over a period of eighteen months. As another remarkable result, authors demonstrated that the construction of real, effective and worthy pervasive systems can no longer be done without the cooperation of a multi-disciplinary team composed by computer science researchers and physicians that must work together.

Nilmini Wickramasinghe, Indrit Troshani, and Steve Goldberg, in Chapter 16 have focused their research on people suffering from diabetes, which is becoming one of the most serious threats for occidental life-style people. Authors have presented a solution that aims at facilitating the work of several healthcare stakeholders including government, healthcare providers that are looking for improved and measurable outcomes among diabetes patients. Specific benefits range from decreasing diabetes related complications to reducing the economic burden on the health system.

Leroy Chan, Branko Celler, James Zhang, and Nigel Lovell contributed Chapter 17 with focus on Wireless Sensor Networks design for ubiquitous wellness monitoring in residential aged care facilities. Authors have included brief descriptions on sensor design, wireless communication protocols and network topologies. They also have examined various data processing methods and knowledge management tools to support the collection of sensor data and their subsequent analysis for health assessment.

Shuyan Xie, Yang Xiao, and Hsiao-Hwa Chen have reported in Chapter 18 the current and future views of nursing home with specific interest for the United States. They have also examined the life of elder in a real nursing home, the Thomasville Nursing Home, in terms of the level of condition and management, residents' satisfactions and demands, government regulation and influence. They have also shown the ability of e-health technology to improve the quality of service in a nursing home to meet residents' needs.

In Chapter 19 Antonio Coronato, Luigi Gallo and Giuseppe De Pietro, have presented a pervasive infrastructure of services for smart medical environments. Such an infrastructure has been adopted to implement pervasive, seamless and context-aware access to medical data. The specific application has been focused on providing medical staff with high volume rendered data, which is a computing intense task and requires many computing resources. The approach proposed relies on a service e that is able to exploit even mobile computing resources to accomplish such a task in a transparent way for users.

The final contribution comes from Tristan Allard, Nicolas Anciaux, Luc Bouganim, Philippe Pucheral, and Romuald Thion, in Chapter 20, that concerns the realization of Electronic Health Records (HER) that must assure a high level of dependability and, particularly, of privacy. The proposed solution is based on the adoption of new hardware portable device, associating the security of a smart card to the storage capacity of a USB key, to give the control back to the patient over his medical history. The target is to complement a traditional EHR server with such a device in order to protect and share highly sensitive data among trusted parties and to provide a seamless access to the data even in disconnected mode.

FUTURE OF HEALTHCARE REFORM

We continue to be challenged by the need to find very efficient ways to reform healthcare delivery process that is both acceptable to the public and sustainable into the future? The above contributions have listed a number of efforts being undertaken. However, there still needs to be honest and reasonable organizing principles and realistic policy changes that could be adopted as part of a comprehensive reform initiative. Such initiatives should take into consideration that there are limited resources available to address pressing social problems, especially as we find healthcare providers more tightly squeezed—financially—in the current economic climate (Brown, 2001; Varkey et al, 2008). While healthcare delivery reform might not be possible without broadly expanding public programs or giving subsidies to healthcare providers, we must be careful not to exceed our ability to cover the additional cost.

A major reason for the growing number of people worldwide experiencing the lack of access to good healthcare facilities is the rising cost of healthcare. It should be considered mandatory for all healthcare plans—anywhere in the world—to contain an option that offers better value for all. Various mechanisms should also be available to help healthcare providers increase their actions to promote more effective competition among themselves.

The Internet age has helped our recognition that information is also a significant key to more informed decision-making in the healthcare (Devaraj & Kohli, 2000). When patients—and their carers—are faced with a choice of possible healthcare solutions, they need information that facilitates comparison. Governments from around the world should ensure the public has access to information on healthcare plans—along with choices that permit such comparisons without imposing excessive restrictions on what options may be offered to patients. This not only alleviates the greater challenge in developing reliable and accessible information about treatment alternatives, but also levels the quality of care different providers' offer to patients. Every patient involves in the healthcare process, generates enormous information—usually over a specified period—about healthcare and services, but much of that information is filed away and inaccessible.

The many cases above demonstrate that more health care does not necessarily mean that people will be healthier or live longer. An individual's state of health depends on many factors--genetic, lifestyle, occupational, environmental (Goossens et al, 2008). While greater access to healthcare information can help significantly, it is evidence show that policies and regulations (i.e. laws and regulations regarding compulsory seat belts and smoking bans in certain places) have done more to improve health in the society and longevity in particular nations than increasing the budgets for specific clinical services. Information systems that contribute to health promotion, for the purpose of avoiding disease outbreak, can also result into more return-on-investments—in terms of reducing the need for health spending—than policies to expand cost of treatment.

Privacy concerns, on the other hand, must be addressed and decisions must be made about who should have access to patient data and how such data can contribute to improved knowledge of both the effectiveness of alternative treatments and the performance evaluation of healthcare providers.

IMPLICATIONS & CONTRIBUTIONS

The preceding chapters recommend more studies of healthcare reform initiatives problems at a global context and through the integration of social, technical, and political perspectives. Overall, I am happy to have initiated a truly international journal making available the opportunity to bring together scholars adopting a variety of perspectives to examine the role of IT-led reform initiatives in the healthcare sector. This initial volume of a series containing various healthcare delivery reform initiatives research work makes a substantial contribution in enhancing our understanding of the complex challenges involved in reforming healthcare delivery. These chapters also open up a variety of avenues for research into healthcare reform initiatives and the role of information systems in improving the quality of healthcare delivery that I hope will spur further work in the general area of *Healthcare Information Management* as an important specialist area of academic study in business schools.

Nearly all chapters provide brief literature reviews before presenting and interpreting qualitative and/or quantitative research datasets. It is my hope that all of the papers in this volume provide healthcare professionals, and academic researchers, with valuable information that is useful in the continuous search for successful reform to our healthcare delivery processes.

Comprehensive reform will require simultaneous progress in all these areas because they are mutually reinforcing. For example, outcome measurement not only will improve insurance-market competition but also will drive the restructuring of care delivery. Delivery restructuring will be accelerated by bundled reimbursement. Electronic medical records will facilitate both delivery restructuring and outcome measurement. Moving ahead now on all these fronts is also important in order to align every stakeholder's interest with value, or reform will once again fail. However, a health care strategy, like any good strategy, involves a sequence of steps over time rather than an attempt to change everything at once. Road maps will be needed for rolling out changes in each area while giving the actors time to adjust.

Some new organizations (or combinations of existing ones) will be needed: a new independent body to oversee outcome measurement and reporting, a single entity to review and set healthcare reform standards, and possibly a third body to establish rules for bundled reimbursement. President Barack Obama has brought health care reform to the forefront of people's minds, not only in the US but also around the world. Repeatedly quoted statistics — on the numbers of uninsured Americans, for example, or the high, rapidly growing expenditures on health care — leave no room for ambiguity, and groups across the global political landscape in recognizing that health care systems are unsustainable in current forms. Quietly, we can safely assume that politicians and healthcare administrators—from around the world—are strategizing about healthcare reform in their respective domains.

The big question is whether any healthcare authority (be it American, British, Canadian, French, German, etc) is capable of moving beyond a reactive and piecemeal approach to a truly national health care strategy centered on value (Porter & Teisberg, 2006). This undertaking is complex, but the only real solution is to align everyone in the systemic thinking around a common goal: doing what's right for patients supported by the right type of IT, as discussed in this book.

REFERENCES

Badgett, R. & Mulrow, C. (2005). Annals of Internal Medicine (Editorial). *Using Information Technology to Transfer Knowledge: A Medical Institution Steps Up to the Plate 142*e (3)s 220-221.

Berwick, DM. (2003). Disseminating Innovations in Health Care. *Journal of the American Medical Association. 28*. (15), April 16, 2003.

Brennan, S. (2007). The biggest computer programme in the world ever! How's it going? *Journal of Information Technology*, 22, 202–211.

Brown, T. (2001) "Modernization or failure? *IT development projects in the UK public sectr". Financial Accountability and Managemen (7*:(4). 363-381.

Clegg & Shepherd (2007). The biggest computer programme in the world…ever!: time for a change in mindset? *Journal of Information Technologyl.22*, pp.212-221.

Constantinides, P. & Barrett, M. (2006). Large Scale ICT Innovation, Power, Organizational Change: The case of a regional health information netwo, ,.*The Journal of Applied Behavioral Science 42*, 76–90.

Currie, WL. & Guah, MW. (2007) A National Program For IT In The Organisational Field of Healthcare: A Example of Conflicting Institutional Logi, . *Journal of Information Technology*, , (3), 235-248.

Darzi A. (2009). A time for revolutions—the role of clinicians in health care reform. *New England Journal Medicinel.3*o.(6), e8.

Davis, K. (2004). Consumer-Directed Health Care: Will It Improve Health System Performance? *Health Services Research 29*1):),1219–34.

Devaraj, D. & Kohli, R. (2000). Information technology payoff in the health-care industry: a longitudinal study. Journal of Management Information Systlumessue (4), pp.41 – 67.

Donaldson, L. (2008). The challenge of quality and patient safety. *Journal of Royal Society of Mediclume 101*, pp.338-341.

Goossens, A., Bossuyt, Pand & de Haan, R.J. (2008). Physicians and Nurses Focus on Different Aspects of Guidelines When Deciding Whether to Adopt Them: An Application of Conjoint Analysis. *Medical Decision MakiolNo.* (1), pp.138-145.

Guah, M., and Fink, K. (2008) Cost of Controlling Modern Healthcare With Information Systems In: Learning from the Past & Charting the Future of the Discipline (Association for Information Systems): *Proceedings of the Fourteenth American Conference on Information Systems, Omnipress,* Madison 2008, 202-212.

Guah, MW. (2008). Case Study I: National Programme for IT. In M.W. Guah (Eds.), *Managing Very Large IT Projects in Businesses and Organizations,* (pp.209-242). Hershey, PA: IGI Global Press.

NAO (2006) *The National Programme for IT in the NHS.* 16 June, The Stationary Office, London.

Porter, M.E. & Teisberg, E.O. (2006). *Redefining Health Care: Creating Value-Based Competition on Rests*. MABoston: Harvard Business School Press.

Porter, ME, & Teisberg, EO. (2006). *Redefining health care: creating value-based competition on results.* Boston: Harvard Business School Press, 2006.

Porter, ME, Yasin, ZM, & Baron, JF. (2009). *Global health partner: obesity care*. Boston: Harvard Business School Publishing,.

Remler, D and & Glied, SA. (2006). How Much More Cost Sharing Will Health Savings Accounts Bring? *Health Affai 25(*4):),1070–78.

Scott, W.R., Ruef, M., MendP. and & Caronna, C. (2000). *Institutional Change and Healthcare Organitions,* . Chicago: University of Chicago Press.

Shaw, K., Cassel, CK., Black, C., & Levinson, W. (2009). Shared Medical Regulation in a Time of Increasing Calls for Accountability and Transparency: Comparison of Recertification in the United States, Canada, and the United Kingdom. *JA* 302: , 2008-2014

Solberg, LI., Klevan, DH. & Asche, SE. (2007). Crossing the Quality Chasm for Diabetes Care: The Power of One Physician, His Team, and Systems Thnking. *The Journal of the American Board of Family Mene 20,* No.(3), pp.299-306.

Varkey, P., HorA. and & Bennet, K.E. (2008). Innovation in Health Care: A Primer. American *Journal of Medical QuVol* Number (5), pp. 382-388.

Wanless, D. (2002) *Securing our Future Health: Taking A Long-Term View*. Final Report of an Independent Review of the long-term resource requirement for the NHS. www.hmtreasury.gov.uk/Consultations_and_Legislation/wanless/consult/wanless_final.cfm.

Wilson, E.V. & Lankton, N.K. (2004). Interdisciplinary Research and Publication Opportunities in Information Systems and Healthcare. *Communications of the Association for Information Sys, V14*, pp.332-343.

Chapter 1
Implementing E-Procurement in Public Healthcare:
The Knowledge Management Issue

Andrea Resca
Luiss "Guido Carli" University, Italy

Tommaso Federici
University of Tuscia, Italy

ABSTRACT

The evolution of public healthcare in developed countries is subject to contrasting forces. The pressure to be innovative and technologically advanced, in order to improve the quality of services, has resulted in a significant increase in spending, while governments are faced with budget constraints. Even though e-procurement initiatives can be seen as a solution for reducing expenditures, such initiatives have not been widely deployed and have not delivered the expected benefits so far. In this chapter, a case study of an e-procurement implementation of an Italian Local Healthcare Agency has been examined. This case is relevant because of the comprehensive design of the e-procurement system, the differentiation of tools adopted and the multiple solutions already implemented. The aim of this work is to analyze, adopting a knowledge management perspective, the steps that have led to the introduction of e-procurement as a new operating practice. The subsequent organisational interventions for redesigning purchasing activities, supply chain and logistic processes are then examined. Finally, main organizational issues at stake for a full deployment of e-procurement were taken into consideration.

INTRODUCTION

In large parts of Europe, the development of healthcare is subject to contrasting forces. On the one hand, there has been an explosion in spending and, at the same time, governments are faced with strict budget constraints. On the other hand, public healthcare is under pressure to be innovative, technologically advanced and to provide increasingly better quality of services.

DOI: 10.4018/978-1-60960-183-6.ch001

In this context, e-procurement can be seen as an instrument for providing solutions to the first issue of this dilemma. In the last decade, the European Commission issued two directives (2004/18/EC and 2004/17/ EC), according to the i2010 eGovernment Action Plan, with the aim of promoting e-procurement to achieve significant efficiency improvements – also in public healthcare – by reducing at the same time purchasing and administrative costs.

However, e-procurement initiatives in such area have not been widely deployed, and most of them have not so far, fully delivered the anticipated benefits. The main reason for the lack of tangible results is the traditional resistance of public institutions to IT-based process innovation and the complexity of healthcare procurement – in terms of the variety of goods, specificity, and of suppliers' numbers – that requires different supply processes and diverse competences.

In order to investigate this scenario in more detail, the case study of a large e-procurement implementation at an Italian public Local Healthcare Agency (LHA – Azienda Sanitaria Locale, ASL), considered one of the most advanced by the Central Procurement Agency (CONSIP), was explored. The same LHA has been recently awarded by the Italian Minister for Public Administration and Innovation as one of the Italy's 30 most innovative administrations, because of the later described e-Logistics introduction.

This case study is remarkable because of the comprehensive design of the e-procurement system, the differentiation in adopted tools, the robust testing (since 2000) and the multiple solutions already implemented and in process within the Agency. The decision to examine this case study is also due to the fact that the use of e-procurement tools is seen as only one aspect of a more profound reorganization of the entire supply process.

The interest of the present paper resides both on the relevance of the observed case and on its focus on the management of the complex transition process from a bureaucratic organizational structure, with fully paper-based procedures, to a more dynamic one, which is IT-based and paperless. In order to investigate these changes and the related managerial decisions, the knowledge management perspective was adopted, as knowledge seems to be one of the most critical success factors to be managed.

The purpose of this work is then to reconstruct - by performing interviews with some of the most representative players and examining documents and previous studies on this case - the managerial interventions that made this innovation possible and in particular how knowledge has been managed in this innovative programme. From this perspective, it was presumed that the introduction of e-procurement and the reorganization of purchasing, supply chain and logistical processes, had required diverse knowledge which has been investigated at the cognitive level, the organizational level and the social and institutional level of knowledge, proposed by Lam (2000).

Distinguishing between individual knowledge and knowledge related to a specific social context, this approach gives a comprehensive picture of the concept of knowledge. Furthermore, this perspective is helpful to examine the realities of Public Administrations (PAs) like LHAs, which are characterized by the importance of rules and procedures and by hierarchical organizational structures. Lam's extensive references to Mintzberg's classic studies (1979) is important in this point, as the organizational forms singled out by Mintzberg fit very well in the PA area, reinforcing the accurateness of this analysis.

RESEARCH STRATEGY

The research question of this work concerns the dissemination of innovation and primarily its adoption. The focus is on the ability of a specific organization to adopt an innovation and on the elements that facilitate or hamper such adoption. In other words, the issue is the impact, at an organizational level, that the introduction of innovation produces, and its possibility to be absorbed and managed.

At the basis of this investigation there is the concept of knowledge, as the element that characterizes an organization, both before the innovation introduction and after it. Therefore, a specific aspect to take into consideration is the meeting of established knowledge and the new one enabled by innovation.

The research strategy adopted to study the dynamics between established and new knowledge is based on a case study, which concerns innovation related to the introduction of a widespread e-procurement at the Local public Healthcare Agency of Viterbo. Because of its tendency towards innovation, as seen by the implementation of several e-procurement projects during a ten year period, the LHA of Viterbo can be considered as a suitable context for an explanatory case study (Yin, 2003). The analysis of such a case study provides answers which throw light on how and why innovation dissemination has taken place, on the basis of the organizational interventions that have been introduced.

The objective of this case study is also to throw light on the effects of these interventions in order to outline the dynamics at play by the introduction of e-procurement. These dynamics will be analysed looking at knowledge management approach by specifically adopting the Lam's model (2000). As it will be later detailed, this approach seems to be apt to investigate knowledge and its management alongside the innovation process.

Actually, Lam's perspective succeeds, to a certain degree, to highlight diverse types of knowledge which arise through the introduction of innovation. Therefore, using Yin's words (2003), it is possible to draw a pattern out of the connection between this perspective and the dynamics present in the case study.

In addition, as it is detailed below, the theoretical framework based on Lam's model leads to difficulty in interpreting the dissemination of adopting e-procurement and the suggestions in overcoming them. However, these results should not be generalized.

Regarding data collection, Federici's research (2005, 2006, 2009) informs the basis of this research project. Such works examine both the progression of the projects that have led e-procurement to the present state of the art, and the organizational changes introduced at the LHA of Viterbo. However, this is not only a bibliographic research, further internal documents were analyzed and semi-structured interviews conducted with some of the key representative managers in charge of procurement, both operating in the traditional and more innovative areas.

THEORETICAL FRAMEWORK

The issue of e-procurement in the public sector, which was once a scarcely discussed topic (Padhi & Mohapatra 2010, Hardy & Williams 2005, Somasundaram & Damsgaard 2005, Henriksen & Mahnke 2005, Ramanathan 2004, Devadoss et al. 2002), is a subject of increasing interest: in the last years several works (for a literature review, Kassim & Hussin 2010) were addressed to it, some of them dealing with the healthcare sector.

Studies on the e-procurement in this sector are mostly concerned with the analysis of the strategies (Panayiotis et al. 2010, Gonzalez et al. 2006, Zhenga et al. 2006), organizational preconditions and preparedness of the public bodies (Bof & Previtale, 2007, Wickramasinghe et al. 2005), process of introduction (Raffa & Esposito 2006) and even the sustainability of procurement (Walker et al. 2006).

Less frequent is research on the healthcare sector at a local operating level (Bof & Previtali 2007, Federici 2005, Federici 2006, Federici 2009, Federici & Resca 2007), where e-procurement solutions must be implemented, with impacts on the structures and the knowledge already existing within the organizations, which require different approaches.

Procurement Within the Healthcare Sector

Firstly, it is necessary to take into consideration that healthcare structures deliver critical and specialized services (vs. the rest of the PA): more than in other sectors, it is paramount to safeguard high quality standards for the purchasing of goods and services (and their impact on service quality), together with the economy and timeliness of purchases, the transparency of activities in an environment in which companies are subject to market competition and its governing principles. Healthcare spending for goods and services can be classified into three sections (Federici 2005):

- common for the whole PA, independent from the type of buying Administration (e.g.: phone services, office materials);
- common-but-differentiated, existing for all Administrations but highly differentiated through the buying sector (e.g. in the healthcare sector: maintenance and cleaning of hospital buildings);
- healthcare-specific, composed of drugs and medical devices (appliances and materials that, separately or jointly, are used in instances of injury, disease or surgical operation).

This diversity must be taken into account when devising innovative ways to manage procurement before choosing the most appropriate solutions, in order to improve quality and efficiency of supplies, whilst at the same time rationalizing and reducing spending. The large difference among the three spending categories indicated above and the availability of diverse electronic tools ask for a deep reflection on which solutions suit each type of good / service. This requires a segmented approach (Federici 2006).

Secondly, the term "procurement" is often used in a narrow sense, being associated with the sole purchasing phase, as can be seen in Panayioutou et al. (2004) or in Kim & Shunk (2004).

Consequently, the term "e-procurement" becomes a synonym for a class of electronic tool that directly link buyers and suppliers on the same network to make a deal. According to other studies (Ramanathan 2004, MacManus 2002), and with the typical operation of a healthcare agency, in this work "procurement" indicates a broader process, which begins with the need for a good or service and ends with its use and the payment for its supply. It involves:

purchase programming, the sourcing choice, the purchasing act, incoming material handling, warehouse logistics, inventory control and invoice processing.

An e-procurement system deals with the whole procurement process, and not just with its purchasing phase (Federici 2006). The term "e-procurement" here consistently indicates that organizational solutions supported by ICT-based tools, which allow electronic forms of procurement, are potentially more effective and efficient than traditional ones. Such solutions involve a more or less wide-reaching and thorough redesign process to take into account the entire life-time of a product or service.

E-procurement solutions include process redesign and the use of appropriate tools in two main areas, which have to be used in a complementary way to streamline the whole procurement process:

- *e-purchasing*, includes very different tools which allows the purchasing phase to be entirely managed, from finding a product to invoicing and payment, through online tenders (e-tendering) and the use of marketplaces and electronic catalogues (e-requisitioning), electronic invoice exchange and processing (e-invoice) and liquidation activity (e-payment);

- *e-logistics*: which aims to optimize the management of inventories (in healthcare structures: pharmacy and the supply office) and internal goods flows, based on Intranet/Extranet technologies, integrating Supply Chain Management (SCM) solutions, linking both internal and external players.

Knowledge Management: Lam's Perspective

The knowledge management approach and, especially, Lam's (2000) interpretation of it, considers three levels (the cognitive level, the organizational level and the societal-institutional level) that could outline the e-procurement phenomenon in a comprehensive manner. But the decision to turn to Lam's perspective is not only based on the relevance of this approach based on three levels, other authors did the same for investigating offshore software development (Nicholson & Sahay, 2004), innovation processes (Lemon & Sahota, 2004) or temporary organizations (Asheim, 2002). In particular, this methodological choice is validated by phenomena, such as innovation and temporary organizations, which distinguish the introduction of e-procurement at the LHA of Viterbo. Furthermore, as time passed by, Lam did not modify the approach here introduced but only some marginal aspects of it (Lam, 2002) as it can be considered a re-elaboration of her previous work (Lam, 1997).

The present issue is to build a bridge between an abstract concept like knowledge and an organizational process supported electronically, such as e-procurement in the healthcare sector. In other words, the question is how this process can be represented in terms of the concept of knowledge.

According to Lam's model, any organizational form, if seen through the lenses of the concept of knowledge, characterizes itself in terms of the three levels mentioned above. In particular, any individual, in a single or collective dimension, interacts with others on the basis of his/her background (the cognitive level of knowledge). The same individual operates in an organizational context with a low degree of autonomy, in the case of an organizational environment characterized by rigid procedures and routines, or a high degree of autonomy in case of an organizational environment loosely coupled (organizational level of knowledge).

Furthermore, he/she is part of a specific labour market that rewards some profiles, but not others; moreover he/she has formed a background on the basis of a particular educational or training institution (social-institutional level of knowledge).

Of course, these three levels overlap with each other and knowledge characterizing a specific organization is something unique that emerges from such an overlap. Nevertheless, Lam's approach leads to a wide-ranging perspective to investigate organizational life, and the introduction of an important innovation such as an e-procurement system.

To thoroughly examine Lam's work, it requires a detailed study of each level. The double entrance matrix is the methodological instrument used in order to analyse any level of knowledge. This matrix surveys relationships between two variables but in this case they are represented by dichotomies leading to a four cell matrix. For instance, the cognitive level is exemplified by the relationship between the ontological dimension of knowledge, presented in terms of the individual-collective dichotomy, and the epistemological dimension of knowledge, explicit-tacit dichotomy (see Figure 1). The same methodology has been used to examine the remaining two levels. So, each of the three levels of analysis generates a four cell matrix each with different content.

Opposing the explicit-tacit dichotomy and the individual-collective one at the cognitive level of knowledge, four categories emerge (Collins 1993, Blackler 1995):

Figure 1. Cognitive Level: Knowledge types (source: Lam 2000)

		Ontological Dimension	
		individual	**collective**
Epistemological Dimension	**explicit**	**Embrained** Knowledge *(abstract and theoretical)*	**Encoded** Knowledge *(information)*
	tacit	**Embodied** Knowledge *(action oriented)*	**Embedded** Knowledge *(values and beliefs sharing)*

- Embrained knowledge (individual-explicit) can be exemplified by what is learnt at school. It is abstract, theoretical and used to solve conceptual problems such as calculations and speculations;
- Embodied knowledge (individual-tacit) is based on practical experience. It does not depend on the activity of reasoning but on action alone. The "learning-by-doing" method represents this kind of knowledge and learning to ride a bicycle is a prime demonstration of it;
- Encoded knowledge (collective-explicit) is codified and stored into rules and procedures.
  Therefore, it is readily transmitted through language, signs and symbols (information). Scientific management principles, for example, are an attempt to codify workers' skills and 'know-how';
- Embedded knowledge (collective-tacit) represents the shared values and beliefs that define informal rules and norms of a specific social context which contributes to govern the interaction and communication among members of a society.

Lam's work looks for organizational forms that can support the type of knowledge mentioned above. In her understanding of this point, this result can be achieved by opposing 'knowledge agent' and 'standardization of knowledge and work' in the double enter matrix. 'Knowledge agent' is characterized by the individual-organization dichotomy and 'standardization of knowledge and work' by the dichotomy high-low. If the 'knowledge agent' is individual, there is the possibility to enjoy a certain degree of autonomy and subjects can develop their own know-how and practical problem-solving. If the 'knowledge agent' is the organization, the managerial hierarchy becomes the engine of organizational activities transforming individual knowledge in rules and procedures. A high 'standardization of knowledge and work' suggests a scenario in which each role is strictly coordinated with others in an environment characterized by hierarchical controls.

On the other hand, a low standardization outlines an organizational environment in which coordination is achieved via direct interaction and mutual adjustment and not on the basis of comprehensive design. The combination of these dichotomies results in four organizational ideal-types (see Figure 2):

- 'Professional bureaucracy' (embrained knowledge) experiences a reduced role at senior management level. Organizational activities are based on individual expertise which relates to specific professional bodies.

Figure 2. Organizational Level: Organizational forms (source: Lam 2000)

		Knowledge agent: **individual**	Knowledge agent: **organization**
Standardization of knowledge and work	**high**	Professional Bureaucracy	Machine Bureaucracy
	low	Adhocracy	J-form organization

Nevertheless, coordination and control are governed centrally through standardized and bureaucratic means. Hospitals are a typical example of this organizational form;

- in the 'machine bureaucracy' type (encoded knowledge), coordination and control are also centrally governed. Moreover, the entire organization is subject to a continuous process of formalization and codifi*cation of knowledge in which the top management tier is at the head of formulating strategies and directives;*
- the 'operating adhocracy' form (embodied knowledge) sees the loss of importance of the organizational chart and coordination and control is not based on rules and procedures.

In this instance, mutual adjustments among organizational actors prevail and activities are not managed vertically but left to the subjects' undertaking;

- the 'J form' (embedded knowledge) idealized characteristics in Japanese companies (Aoki 1988). Coordination is not loosely coupled as in adhocracies because of a strong corporate culture rather than hierarchical control. At the same time, horizontal coordination prevails giving rise to shared work experiences and joint problem solving amongst organizational members.

Lam maintains that knowledge outlined through organizational forms is not sufficient for investigating the entire knowledge configuration operating in organizations as they are part of a larger social context. Education and training systems (Maurice et al. 1986) and the nature of labour market organization (Marsden 1986) are the two elements believed to be able to enrich the understanding of knowledge at work in any organization leading, in this way, to the social and institutional level.

Labour market organization is interpreted according to the dichotomy occupation based labour market (OLM) and firm-based internal labour market (ILM). The former sketches a situation in which market forces govern personal careers and areas of learning. In the latter instance, expertise is internally controlled by firms causing a lower level of standardization and, thus, the difficulty of being governed by market forces. Regarding education and training systems, they can be studied according to the high or low degree of formalization and academic bias.

Again, a double entrance matrix can be built (see Figure 3): the opposition of ILM and OLM, in one dimension, and low and high degree of formalization and academic bias, in the other one, suggests four institutional configurations:

Figure 3. Social-Institutional Level: Education and Labour Market (source: Lam 2000)

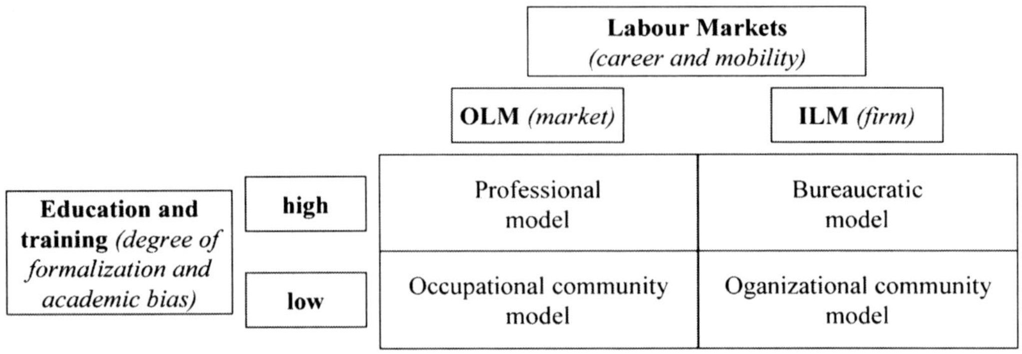

- the 'professional model' (embrained knowledge and 'professional bureaucracy') arises from a situation in which a high degree of formalization and academic bias, on the one hand, and OLM, on the other hand prevail. Here, certified expertise enables access into professional bodies and, on this basis, market forces can operate as personal careers are transparent and subject to continuous evaluation;
- in the 'bureaucratic model' (encoded knowledge and 'machine bureaucracy') there exists a high degree of formalization and academic bias. Expertise is far removed from problem-solving practices and is based upon a deductive method of reasoning. ILM characterizes this model as well and a narrow on-the-job training, in which careers are based on hierarchies of jobs with tiered boundaries, can contribute to establish a bureaucratic work model;
- even though the 'occupational community model' (embodied knowledge and 'operating adhocracy') characterizes itself because of OLM, inter-firm mobility is not based on certified expertise but on the 'know who' of member networks which consist of a cluster of interdependent occupations and firms. It is insides these communities that practical expertise and problem-solving can be maintained;
- the 'organizational community model' (embedded knowledge and 'J-form' organization) distinguishes itself because of a broad-based education and training system.

Learning by doing and problem-solving capabilities are encouraged to the detriment of abstract theoretical knowledge in a context in which team working is seen as an instrument for connecting different workforce layers. An ILM based on a broad on-the-job training and not linked to tiered boundaries but a common ranking system can contribute to build this community.

To sum up, a theoretical approach has been built up, with at its core the cognitive level, which constitutes the background for the organizational level that, in turn, constitutes the background for the societal-institutional level. The sum of these three levels (see Figure 4) enables a cumulative process of knowledge to be employed in organizational analysis.

Nevertheless, to represent a variable through a dichotomy has some limits: on the one hand, it streamlines the analysis of a phenomenon and, on the other hand, leads to a simplified representation of reality.

Figure 4. Knowledge, Organizations and Institutions: Three Interlocking Levels (source: Lam 2000)

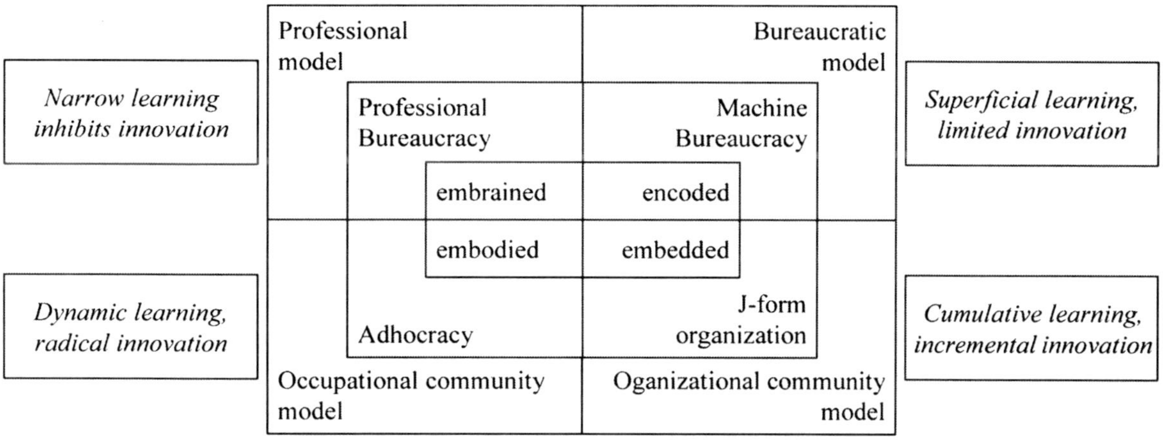

E-PROCUREMENT INTRODUCTION AT THE LHA OF VITERBO

Context and E-Procurement Experiences

The Viterbo's LHA– like similar organisations (Cicchetti 2004) – is divided into three distinct areas: hospital services, territory services, administration services. With about 3.200 administrative and healthcare employees, it provides healthcare to the province of Viterbo (859 hospital beds), with a production value of about 350 €m, which is determined according to the individual spending allocated for each citizen (a total of 297,686 people at the last population census, 2001).

With the aim of increasing efficiency and reducing the spending for goods and services procurement, Viterbo's LHA, since 2000, has conducted several experimental projects on e-procurement, in partnership with the Italian public as well private players (Federici 2005):

- the first initiative, in 2000, was a trial of a marketplace promoted by a private merchant: despite some positive results, this experiment ended prematurely, when the marketplace platform failed because of the low volume of transactions;
- in 2002 – when these tools were still under construction and not yet targeted to the healthcare sector – the LHA started to use the *Public Electronic Catalogue* of goods and services which could be purchased at pre-defined conditions established in the Framework Contracts previously negotiated by the Central Procurement Agency (CONSIP 2003) and the *Marketplace for the Public Administration* (MEPA), also created and managed by CONSIP (Viterbo's LHA was one of 20 Italian PAs to take an active part in the implementation of MEPA);
- in 2003 the first platform for e-tenders was tested, which was later dismissed because of its lack of functionality; recently it has been replaced by a new one, that manages a tender electronically, providing either a complete or partial solution (this latter leaves the offer evaluation off-line);
- the LHA also carried out two distinct projects on e-logistics, both of them were promoted by private companies and based on extensive outsourcing solutions supported by Extranet platforms. The first one (e-Logistics) involved central and departmental warehouse logistics for managing common goods and non specific devices used

routinely in hospital wards (e.g.: gauzes, disinfectants etc.). The second project (Operating room e-procurement) coupled the supply of specific medical devices used in operating rooms to their overall logistical management: its driver was the innovative 'intervention-based' concept of linking procurement to the surgical operations performed, instead of the traditional 'stock-based' approach to purely managing the inventory levels.

These pilot projects were all driven by the Procurement and Logistics (P&L) Department of the LHA. Results were remarkable, even though they were different in nature and dimension, also taking into consideration the obstacles met (technological, organizational and also normative), as in any innovation.

Post 2004, after these pilot projects were concluded, Viterbo's LHA launched an extensive programme. Its purpose was to innovate the end-to-end procurement process (as seen above), through the adoption of diverse solutions which were coherently linked to different and specific requirements. The first step was the implementation of multiple e-procurement solutions in two segments of the broad procurement process: namely the purchasing and invoicing phases.

At present, while traditional procurement procedures are still used, the state-of-art of the e-procurement at Viterbo's LHA is:

- the Marketplace for PA is frequently used to buy common goods, and also some non specific medical devices (such as gauzes and alcohol etc.), but not for large orders;
- the platform for e-tenders is sometime used, also for tenders over the EU threshold, but its application is limited because the specificity of some goods, the suppliers' unreadiness in some sector (on this issue, see also Bof & Previtali 2007) and the changes introduced by recent legislation;
- the full deployment in all hospitals of the Operating room e-procurement solution is currently ending;
- the implementation of the e-Logistics outsourcing solution for common goods and non specific devices, after some difficulties caused by the suppliers, was completed a few months ago.

Because the relevant results of this latter initiative, in terms of cost and time saving efficiency, which were analyzed in detail by Federici after the pilot phase (2005), and the great attention paid in assessing the outcomes, the LHA of Viterbo has been recently (May 2010) awarded by the Minister for Public Administration and Innovation at the end of the "Premiamo i risultati" ("Let's award results") contest, as one of the 30 Italian public administrations with the best innovation projects.

The case of Viterbo's LHA is remarkable because of the scale of the approach undertaken, the multiplicity of specialised solutions adopted, and the constant willingness towards process reengineering. The latter is highly significant when considering the vision held by managers in healthcare, who usually do not pair e-procurement adoption with process reengineering, as testified by Bof & Previtali's research (2007).

Managerial Interventions to Promote E-Procurement

Prior to starting the e-procurement introduction, the purchasing activities were divided among four Offices, on the basis of the typology of goods or services, as they are highly differentiated and specialized in healthcare. This requires the adoption of diverse procedures and connections to diverse suppliers. The subject of the four Offices is respectively: products (drugs, medical devices, consumables like paper and ink etc), general equipment (furniture, cars and elevators etc), electronic equipment (medical appliances and computers etc) and services..

The traditional purchasing Offices, which already existed before the e-procurement initiatives, were characterised by a knowledge oriented towards correctly applying the rigid external laws (settled by national or regional government, or by the EU) and procedures (determined by the same LHA), that regulate purchasing in a Public Administration. This sort of knowledge is strictly coded in rules and is shared within the Agency by means of official documents; for this reason, it can easily be transferred. Another important piece of knowledge concerns information about distinguishing characteristics of the product typology. To properly examine this issue, it is necessary to acquire more experience in the field, whilst the standard of education previously acquired for a position in this field had little or no relevance (actually, none of the interviewed Office supervisors had a degree). The training is entirely performed within the organization and the acquired expertise can only be used in the same Office. For this reason, career advancements and mobility are very limited.

Moreover, it is important to notice that, in this context, collaborations with purchasing Offices of similar structures (e.g.: others LHAs) are occasional, hampering the development of a professional network.

The four traditional Offices – each of them, as stated above, operates separately from the others – have an average a staff consisting of a supervisor and three clerks. Each role requires standardized tasks to be performed, which are typically: the sourcing of information about the product to be purchased (price, characteristics and suppliers), the writing, revising and issuing of the tender, support of the evaluation process and award notification. Despite knowledge being shared among staff in the same office, interchangeability is extremely difficult because of the tendency for staff to stay for long periods of time doing the same role. In this context the role of IT systems is to automate the traditional procedures, with office automation tools (word processing and occasionally spreadsheets) or legacy systems (accounting systems, to check fund availability and to reserve them). Consequently, a high IT literacy amongst personnel staff is not required to operate such systems.

The traditional purchasing Offices have a typical form of bureaucracy: because of their culture and organizational form, they are not very flexible and not so much disposed to change. Moreover, even though they are effective in managing their duties, their activity is not efficient, as the result of the above quoted research by Federici largely demonstrates.

As the General Manager of the LHA and the Director of P&L Dept explored new ways to gain efficiency and to produce savings (both in terms of cost and time), they promoted a programme to introduce e-procurement. Bearing in mind the diverse issues at stake, they considered the four Offices unfit to test this innovation and decided to set up a project team, composed of new resources.

The evaluation by the two managers of the LHA of Viterbo concurs with the results of research performed by Bof & Previtali (2007) which involved managers of Italian public healthcare bodies: the managers interviewed by the scholars found that those employees in charge of acquisition processes are low to medium skilled, and that, in order to overcome such obstacle, younger resources with a higher education and a higher IT literacy are necessary.

To achieve this, two young economic graduates were brought in to constitute the staff that jointly operated with other private or public partners involved in the above mentioned pilot projects. The above described scenario for the development of e-procurement is the result of a series of managerial decisions made by two senior managers, which was based on the assumption that the characteristics of the two sides – the traditional and the innovative – are quite different in terms of the knowledge requested, the means of operating, and staff profiles.

The work of this team was highly experimental (because this was one of the very first attempts at e-procurement in a healthcare sector), and adopted a trial-and-error approach, whereby knowledge increased through a learning- by-doing approach.

The level of education was quite high amongst those staff involved, nevertheless it was directly spent only in some parts of the work (such as analysis of the outcomes, auditing on costs ...). In addition, they were selected also because their high IT education (although they weren't IT experts) and their willingness to innovate, in comparison to workers in a traditional office environment. Low levels of willingness and resistance to re-align with new processes amongst the original administrative staff in public healthcare bodies (a typical outcome of bureaucratic structure) is a significant issue. Such issue is also highlighted in the work by Bof & Previtali (2007).

As parts of the constitutive platform for e-procurement, many diverse IT systems (office automation, marketplaces, platform for e-tenders, and e-logistics Extranet solutions etc.) were tested in real operations over a planned period of time. The aim of each test was to model a new organizational solution, in order to provide streamlined and effective process and to employ human resources in more value-added tasks.

The Team experienced a high level of individual autonomy in an environment where informal managerial controls have prevailed, the procurement sector to test has continuously changed jointly with the related IT and organizational solutions. Team members with time have increased their knowledge about the Agency structures, ways of operating, suppliers' characteristics, purchasing rules, and so on. But they conclude that they never perceived the initial lack of knowledge to be problematic, since they turned to an 'internal expert' on a specific topic, when they needed more detailed information in that field.

As regards the use of IT tools, they were trained in some of them, particularly the more structured ones, such as MEPA or e-tender platforms. Finally, they were used to collaborate with people operating on e-procurement in other LHAs and throughout the CONSIP (Central Procurement Agency), thus creating a professional network of e-procurement experts.

At the end of the testing phase, when it was decided to promote the widespread adoption of e-procurement, two more graduates were selected, and the former informal Team became a Unit called Innovative Projects (IP) devoted to the all e-procurement processing. This Unit was integrated with two other offices in charge of order and invoice processing, which had already moved to total paperless activity, and came under the coordination of the director of P&L Dept. Despite this formal change, the IP Unit used to work as a project team, with a high degree of delegation and informal controls.

Expertise was highly shared among the Unit workers, and they were fully interchangeable. They considered their knowledge easy to employ in a similar position in other administrations, but hardly worth it in other areas of the LHA. For this reason they judged their experience as exciting, but not so useful for career advancement (also because of Agency budget constraints).

The Unit in charge of e-procurement is continuing to differentiate itself from the traditional purchasing Offices, even if significant changes have taken place. Prior to these changes, the Unit was considered a separate entity for the designing and implementation of e-purchasing solutions. It differed from traditional Offices as it did not manage the sole purchasing phase but operated as a buyer (through on-line tenders or direct purchases performed using MEPA, a dedicated IT platform) and supervised the entire procurement process (including: supply chain and logistics) being directly linked to external providers, warehouses (for common goods and for medical devices and drugs) and internal departments who receive the supplied goods.

Now, three members of the IP Unit lead, respectively, three out of four of the traditional Offices.

This means that, on the one hand, the IP Unit has seen a decrease in its operative capacity but, on the other hand, the traditional Offices are experiencing a new leadership. This new leadership represents an important change as e-purchasing experiences are brought in. In fact, after being established, the IP Unit implemented projects to deliver new purchasing solutions, such as the e-Logistics project introduction, and the go-live phase of the Operating room e-procurement.

The decision to change the leadership of traditional Offices is seen by the P&L Dept. Director as a solution to fully substitute the traditional purchasing procedures with more innovative ones in all of their operations. The question is if this answer can, actually, mobilise new knowledge in order to allow the spread of e-purchasing at the P&L Dept. Level.

The transfer of personnel from the IP unit to the traditional Office does not represent a complete disbandment of such unit. Of course, it will no longer be in charge of the entire series of e-purchasing activities which have slowly, step by step, been assigned to it. Nevertheless, it is the intention of the P&L Dept. Director to maintain a unit which is able to manage innovative projects and experimental solutions. In some sense, the situation relates directly back to the old days when a small team was established in order to introduce the first steps of e-procurement.

KNOWLEDGE MANAGEMENT AT THE LHA ACCORDING TO LAM'S MODEL

As stated above, the objective is to study the introduction of e-procurement in the LHA using Lam's model. In other words, can this perspective interpret and evaluate the dynamics caused by this technological system in the organizational life of the Agency? In order to investigate these dynamics, the organizational setting at the LHA is investigated prior to the introduction of e-procurement.

The LHA is a typical PA and, if Lam's model is applied, this organization has a knowledge configuration which is characterized by the dominance of encoded knowledge. The reason for this is based on the prevalence of the collective- explicit dimension of knowledge at the cognitive level. Moving on to the organizational level, the 'machine bureaucracy' describes the organizational form which represents this administration and the 'bureaucratic model' outlines the social and institutional level with references to the labour market and the education and training system.

The analysis of the e-procurement narrative at the LHA is marked by a significant number of projects, and since 2000 a project instrument has been used in order to introduce such innovation.

The first question then concerns the impact of these projects. Here, it is important to notice that not only is the Agency under examination, but also a range of other actors – private IT vendors, public bodies like CNIPA (National Centre for the development of IT into the Public Administration) and CONSIP – were involved in these projects, thus affecting the knowledge configuration of the LHA.

These projects can be considered an organization in itself as, according to Daft (2003), organizations are: 1) social entities; 2) guided by objectives; 3) deliberately envisaged as coordinated and structured systems that 4) interact with an environment. E-procurement projects can surely be included in this definition. The issue is then to study if these organizational structures (pilot projects) share the same knowledge configuration as that of the LHA.

Starting with the cognitive level, in this instance encoded knowledge is of little importance.

The collective dimension, in particular, seems not appropriate to represent a context frequented by application vendors, Central Procurement Authority, university researchers, and an atypical administrative unit solely dedicated to the introduction of e-procurement (IP Unit). From this perspective the individual dimension of knowledge rather than the collective dimension seems to prevail. But the cognitive level also characterizes itself because of the explicit-tacit dichotomy. At first glance, the conditions for developing tacit knowledge do not seem to exist. However, this cannot be entirely ruled out as in specific contexts, this type of knowledge can be produced. In such conditions, embrained knowledge (individual-explicit) prevails.

Turning towards the organizational level, a 'professional bureaucracy' could represent organizational forms within e-procurement projects. This is because the 'knowledge agent' is the individual and his/her professionalism rather than the organization as in typical PAs.

Civil servants, engineers, lawyers, economists etc. with their specific expertise collaborate to manage pilot projects. 'Professional bureaucracies' also distinguish themselves, because of a high 'standardization of knowledge and work'.

The varied nature of actors participating in these projects renders it plausible control and coordination based on a high 'standardization of knowledge and work' although mutual adjustments and team working cannot be ruled out.

Taking into consideration the social and institutional level of knowledge, the 'professional model' emerges as the dominant model.

Members seem to be in the circle of the occupation-based market (OLM): professionals with a transparent and valuable career which is subject to market forces. Concerning education and training, a high degree of formalization and academic bias seem to emerge because of the disparate figures involved; even in this case, however, forms of learning-by-doing and team building are not a remote possibility.

The comparison between knowledge configuration of the LHA and innovative projects introduced to implement e-procurement systems highlights two diverse scenarios. The LHA distinguishes itself because of encoded knowledge, the 'machine bureaucracy' and the 'bureaucratic model'. Innovative projects distinguish themselves differently because of embrained knowledge, the 'professional bureaucracy' and the 'professional model'.

A further analytical step leads us to the reshaping of knowledge configuration of the LHA due to the introduction of e-procurement projects. From an analysis of this case study, it can be seen that only part of the LHA (the e-procurement Team that later will become the IP Unit) has been deeply involved in these projects. The IP Unit is a relative small Unit in comparison with the four Offices in charge of the traditional purchasing and logistical element, even though it was later been enlarged.

So, the point, now, is to investigate the impact of this Unit on the entire P&L Dept.

In order to examine this point, it is necessary to analyse the role of the IP Unit in the P&L Dept.

Interestingly, a dual role comes to the fore that of the agent in innovative projects and that of a unit in large bureaucracies like the LHA. This ambivalence is reflected in its specific knowledge configuration. A configuration in which, as time passes by, has developed embodied knowledge (individual-tacit): individual because of, as it has been stressed, the personal backgrounds of Unit members, and tacit because of the possibility of developing specific operational skills and know-how. Moving from the cognitive level to the organizational one, a situation arises in which the 'knowledge agent' becomes the individual member rather than the organization, and in such situations members are not subject to or bound by specific rules and procedures that would ordinarily affect the rest of the LHA.

As far as it concerns issues of coordination and control, mutual adjustment prevails suggesting a low 'standardization of knowledge and work'.

Therefore, the IP Unit turned to adhocracy as organizational form, rather than distinguishing itself because of the 'machine bureaucracy' as seen in the rest of the LHA.

Regarding the social and institutional level, it can be noticed the establishment of a low degree of formalization and academic bias, due to the importance of problem-solving and practical expertise, on the one hand, and of the occupation based labour market (OLM), on the other hand. Members of the IP Unit are not only employees of a large bureaucracy but are, at the same time, part of an inter-firm network formed by project partners. Therefore, it is the 'occupational community model' that defines the social-institutional level due to the connections established and the shared experiences of members.

Results of the cohabitation between the IP Unit and the P&L Dept. were taken into consideration, principally, in the previous section. However, drawing further conclusions, the organizational solution to constitute a specific unit like the IP one to introduce e-procurement can be considered successful, since the organizational forms like adhocracies lend themselves extremely well to innovative projects. Knowledge configuration mobilized in this way adapts itself in order to cooperate in a context where various actors exist. The good results reached by pilot projects bear witness to this fact. However, more problematic is the dissemination of innovation to the rest of the P&L Dept. Here, a knowledge configuration characterized by embodied knowledge, operating adhocracy and the 'occupational community model' is highly inadequate. This knowledge configuration responds to the idiosyncratic situations and tasks that exist in turbulent environments. On the other hand, this knowledge is inherently unstable. Consequently, the organizational chart loses its importance, roles are no longer designed in order to establish a comprehensive system and coordination and organizational members are no longer part of a general design that predetermines organizational objectives and the execution of task standards. The IP Unit can be considered, in some sense, isolated from the rest of the organization hampering the possibility of spreading an innovation like e-procurement to the entire P&L Dept.

The fact that IP Unit ex-members now in charge of three out of the four traditional Offices changes the working environment considerably. The importance of the IP Unit in the LHA decreases significantly, its influence becomes marginalised, and although it still governs the more experimental applications, it is far removed from the so called *business as usual* elements of the Agency.

Therefore, it is interesting to see what kind of knowledge characterises traditional Offices as a direct consequence of the influence of the new leaders that come from the IP Unit. At present, data is not yet available, due to the fact that at the moment of writing this chapter, the appointment of ex-IP Unit members had only just taken place. However, Lam's approach is useful to gain insights into the knowledge characteristics of the traditional Offices, as well as forming conclusions and points for further consideration.

CONCLUSION

To conclude, it is evident that the configuration of knowledge mobilized by the IP Unit is not entirely effective in supporting the introduction of e-procurement. This innovation is, on the one hand, extremely pervasive and complex to adopt but, on the other hand, the normal configuration of knowledge in PAs (such as the LHA) is able to support only superficial learning and limited innovation. Consequently, diverse dissemination solutions are required and the decision to assign the leading role to ex-members of the IP Unit in three traditional offices can be seen in this perspective.

From this perspective, we can question whether Lam's model is helpful to evaluate this type of intervention for extending e-procurement adoption. It is believed that knowledge configuration characterised by embedded knowledge, a 'J-form' organization and an 'organizational community model' could be a point of reference to follow. For example, as far as it concerns the organizational level, the 'knowledge agent' organization seems more appropriate than the individual one which exists in an adhocracy. Certainly, the traditional Offices are characterised by this organisational knowledge and it is not foreseeable that things will change in the future due to the fact that ex-members of the IP Unit acquired a leading position in these Offices.

It is expected that bureaucratic forms of control will continue to prevail, as the LHA is a large and established bureaucracy. But the organisational knowledge is characterised also by a level of standardisation of knowledge and work, and in this respect the experience acquired by ex-members of the IP Unit is decisive. The fact that mutual adjustment rather than any hierarchical integration constitutes the backbone of the IP Unit should prevent these Offices from moving in the direction of 'machine bureaucracy' where it prevails an organisational level of knowledge based on centralisation and on the role played by senior management.

Regarding the cognitive level, there is the risk that encoded knowledge, that one codified into roles and procedures, will continue to be prevalent. From this perspective, embodied knowledge acquired by ex-members of the IP Unit can lead to the development of tacit rather than explicit dimensions, and for this reason the risk can be mitigated.

Furthermore, using Lam's approach as point of reference, the role of ex-members of the IP Unit can create favourable conditions to transform the working environments of traditional Offices and, in particular, can have a positive influence on cross-functional teams. In other words, the specialisation and the lack of integration that characterised traditional Offices might be overcome due to the factor of integration played by the three new leaders. In fact, they are used, since their hiring, to work cooperatively and without differentiation among purchasing sectors. Then, this practice should now be transferred to the traditional Office.

Finally, regarding the social and institutional levels, the 'organisational community model' is an achievable objective. The experience gained in the IP Unit workplace represents a way to overcome the limitations regarding the high degree of formalisation and academic bias that typifies public administration careers, and the risk of excessive focus on the so-called 'on-the-job' training that tends to neglect practical experience and problem solving exercises.

ACKNOWLEDGMENT

The authors wish to acknowledge the correspondent persons of the LHA of Viterbo, whose willingness and contributions have been considerable and decisive for this research: Andrea Bianchini (Director of P&L Dept.), Silvia Dari and Tania Morano (in charge of IP Unit).

REFERENCES

Aoki, M. (1988). *Information, incentives and bargaining in the Japanese economy*. Cambridge, UK: Cambridge University Press. doi:10.1017/CBO9780511571701

Asheim, B. T. (2002). Temporary Organisations and Spatial Embeddedness of Learning and Knowledge Creation. *Geografiska Annaler. Series B, Human Geography*, *84*(2), 111–124. doi:10.1111/j.0435-3684.2002.00117.x

Blackler, F. (1995). Knowledge, knowledge work and organizations: an overview and interpretation. *Organization Studies*, *16*(6), 1021–1046. doi:10.1177/017084069501600605

Bof, F., & Previtali, P. (2007). Organisational Pre-Conditions for e-Procurement in Governments: the Italian Experience in the Public Health Care Sector. *The Electronic. Journal of E-Government*, *5*(1), 1–10.

Cicchetti, A. (2004). *La progettazione organizzativa*. Milano: FrancoAngeli.

Collins, H. M. (1993). The structure of knowledge. *Social Research*, *60*(1), 95–116.

CONSIP. (2003). *Il Programma di razionalizzazione della spesa per beni e servizi della Pubblica Amministrazione*. CONSIP Annual Report (*house journal*), Rome.

Daft, R. L. (2003). *Organization Theory and Design*. Chula Vista, CA: South-Western College Pub.

Devadoss, P. R., Pan, S. L., & Huang, J. C. (2002). Structurational Analysis of e-Government initiatives: a case study of SCO. *Decision Support Systems, 34*, 253–269. doi:10.1016/S0167-9236(02)00120-3

Federici, T. (2005). An Integrated Approach in Healthcare e-procurement: The Case-Study of the ASL of Viterbo. In Böhlen, M. et al. (eds.) *Proceedings of E-Government: Towards Electronic Democracy, TCGOV 2005* (LNAI 3416, p. 298). Berlin:Springer.

Federici, T. (2006). Public Healthcare: changes introduced when implementing e-procurement. In *Proceedings of the: Mediterranean Conference on Information Systems, MCIS 2006*. Venice, Italy, October 2006.

Federici, T. (2009). Introducing e-Procurement in a Local Healthcare Agency. In Scupola, A. (Ed.), *Cases on Managing E-services*. Hershey, PA, USA: Roskilde University, Denmark. Information Science Reference. doi:10.4018/978-1-60566-064-6.ch015

Federici, T., & Resca, A. (2007), Managing a widespread e-Procurement implementation in Public Healthcare. Proceedings of the *"Mediterranean Conference on Information Systems, MCIS 2007"*, Venice, Italy, 4-8 October.

González, M. E., Quesada, G., Urrutia, I., & Gavidia, V. (2006). Conceptual design of an e-health strategy for the Spanish health care system. *International Journal of Health Care Quality Assurance, 19*(2), 146–157. doi:10.1108/09526860610651681

Hardy, C., & Williams, S. P. (2005). Public eProcurement in Action: Policies, Practice and Technologies. In Böhlen, M. et al. (eds.) Proceedings of E-Government: Towards Electronic Democracy, TCGOV 2005 (LNAI 3416, p.286). Berlin: Springer.

Henriksen, H. Z., & Mahnke, V. (2005). E-Procurement Adoption in the Danish Public Sector. *Scandinavian Journal of Information Systems, 17*(2), 85–106.

Kassim, E. S., & Hussin, H. (2010). *Public E-procurement: A Research Synthesis, e-Education, e-Business, e-Management and e-Learning*. International Conference on, 150-154, 2010 International Conference on e-Education, e-Business, e-Management, IEEE.

Kim, J., & Shunk, D. L. (2004). Matching indirect procurement process with different B2B e-procurement systems. *Computers in Industry, 53*, 153–164. doi:10.1016/j.compind.2003.07.002

Lam, A. (1997). Embedded Firms, Embedded Knowledge: Problems of Collaboration and Knowledge Transfer in Global Cooperative Ventures. *Organization Studies, 18*(6), 973–996. doi:10.1177/017084069701800604

Lam, A. (2000). Tacit knowledge, organizational learning and societal institutions: an integrated framework. *Organization Studies, 21*(3), 487–513. doi:10.1177/0170840600213001

Lam, A. (2002). Alternative societal models of learning and innovation in the knowledge economy. *International Social Science Journal, 54*(171), 67–82. doi:10.1111/1468-2451.00360

Lemon, M., & Sahota, P. S. (2004). Organizational culture as a knowledge repository for increased innovative capacity. *Technovation, 24*(6), 483–498. doi:10.1016/S0166-4972(02)00102-5

MacManus, S. A. (2002). Understanding the Incremental Nature of E-procurement. Implementation at the State and Local levels. *Journal Public Procurement, 2*, 5–28.

Marsden, D. (1986). *The end of economic man*. New York: St. Martin's Press.

Maurice, M., Sellier, F., & Silvestre, J. J. (1986). *The social foundation of industrial power: a comparison of France and Germany*. Cambridge, MA: The MIT Press.

Mintzberg, H. (1979). *The structure of organizations*. Englewood Cliffs, NJ: Prentice Hall.

Nicholson, B & Sundeep Sahay. (2004). Embedded knowledge and offshore software development. *Information and Organization, 14*(4), 329–365. doi:10.1016/j.infoandorg.2004.05.001

Padhi, S.S. A1 & Mohapatra, P.K.J. (2010), Adoption of e-procurement in the government departments.*Electronic Government, an International Journal, 7*(1), 41-59.

Panayiotis, H. K., Kontogeorgisb, A., Stalidisc, G., & Kaggelidesd, K. (2010). Applying e-procurement system in the healthcare: the EPOS paradigm. *International Journal of Systems Science, 41*(3), 281–299. doi:10.1080/00207720903326878

Panayiotou, N. A., Gayialis, S. P., & Tatsiopoulos, I. P. (2004). An e-procurement system for governmental purchasing. *International Journal of Production Economics, 90*, 79–102. doi:10.1016/S0925-5273(03)00103-8

Raffa, L., & Esposito, G. (2006). The implementation of an e-reverse auction system in an Italian health care organization. *Journal of Public Procurement, 6*(1-3), 46–69.

Ramanathan, S. (2004) Diffusion of e-procurement in the public sector - revisiting centralization versus decentralization debates as a twist in the tale. In Leino T, Saarinen T, Klein S (eds). *Proceedings of the Twelfth European Conference on Information Systems*, 1546-1556. Turku, Finland:Turku School of Economics and Business Administration.

Somasundaram, R., & Damsgaard, J. (2005). Policy Recommendations for Electronic Public Procurement. *The Electronic. Journal of E-Government, 3*, 147–156.

Walker, H., Bakker, E., Knight, L., Gough, S., & McBain, D. (2006), Sustainable procurement in the English National Health Service: learning and practice. *Paper presented at the International Purchasing and Supply Education and Research Association*.San Diego, USA.

Wickramasinghe, N. S., Fadlalla, A. M. A., Geisler, E., & Schaffer, J. L. (2005). A framework for assessing e-health preparedness. *International Journal of Electronic Healthcare, 1*(3), 316–334. doi:10.1504/IJEH.2005.006478

Yin, R. K. (2003). *Case Study Research* (3rd ed.). Thousand Oaks, CA: Sage.

Zhenga, J., Bakkera, E., Knighta, L., Gilhespyb, H., Harlanda, C., & Walkera, H. (2006). A strategic case for e-adoption in healthcare supply chains. *International Journal of Information Management, 26*, 290–301. doi:10.1016/j.ijinfomgt.2006.03.010

Chapter 2
Perspectives on the Adoption of Electronic Resources for Use in Clinical Trials

Maricarmen D. Planas-Silva
Pennsylvania State University - Harrisburg, USA

Rhoda C. Joseph
Pennsylvania State University - Harrisburg, USA

ABSTRACT

Clinical trials are specific medical studies that use human subjects for the advancement of medicine. Evidence-based medicine requires the use of clinical trials to evaluate new treatments, devices, drugs, and modalities for the prevention and treatment of diseases. Clinical trials have not been particularly aggressive in their adoption of information technology (IT). In this analysis, we examine the impact of electronic resources on the execution and management of clinical trials. Further, we present a theoretical model showing the main areas of clinical trials that can be directly impacted by the adoption of electronic resources. The four areas identified are recruitment, data collection, process data management, and information dissemination.

INTRODUCTION

A clinical trial is a specific type of medical study utilizing human subjects to examine the development and progression of specific medical conditions under a specific intervention. The primary goal of clinical trials is to advance the prevention, diagnosis, and ultimate treatment of malignant illnesses (Markman, Petersen, and Montgomery, 2008). A clinical trial involves many stakeholders that participate and or facilitate in the development

DOI: 10.4018/978-1-60960-183-6.ch002

and execution of the study. Stakeholders include but are not limited to patients, participants, physician, nurses, clinical researchers, coordinators, contract research organizations (CROs), and the sponsors who provide the specific intervention and or economic resources needed for the execution, analysis, and completion of the clinical trial.

Clinical trials aim to provide benefits to the individuals that are afflicted with the specific disease. There are also added benefits to society and the medical profession with the advance of new medicines. Pharmaceutical companies have also seen record revenue generation by bringing new and innovative drugs to the market. However, clinical trials also encounter challenges associated with its administration and implementation. Information technology can be used as a tool to mitigate some of the data collection, data storage, and data processing issues inherent with the collection of large volumes of data.

Clinical trials are conducted in United States and around the world by different organizations such as the National Institutes of Health (NIH), pharmaceutical companies, biotechnology companies, universities, and other medical-related institutions that want to introduce a new product to the market. In the United States, the Food and Drug administration (FDA) is the unit of government that oversees and approves all new medical products for release into the market. For this reason, the FDA regulates how clinical trials are executed and to what extent electronic media and resources can be used. Bleicher (2003) has reviewed the history of technology in clinical trials and points out that the pharmaceutical industry has lagged significantly in the application of novel information technology (IT). The most recent empirical data indicates that an estimated 75% of clinical trails use mainly paper records for management of clinical trials (Alschuler, Kush, and Bain, 2004; Pavlovic and Miklavcic, 2007). In this study we present a theoretical model showing the main areas of clinical trials that can be directly impacted by the adoption of electronic resources. The four areas identified are recruitment, data collection, process data management, and information dissemination.

OVERVIEW OF CLINICAL TRIALS IN THE UNITED STATES

In order to bring a new drug to the market a pharmaceutical company needs to perform many clinical trials and spend millions of dollars. Further, clinical trials are done to determine the safety of a drug and compare effectiveness of different doses of the drug.

Clinical trials for testing a new treatment typically occur in three or four stages (typically listed as stages I through IV) (Houlton, 2004) and can range is cost from $500 million to more than $2 billion (Adams and Brantner, 2006). To understand how IT can impact or has impacted clinical trials, we first consider the different aspects of a typical clinical trial in cancer research. A novel cancer drug is first tested in phase I and phase II trials. If phase I trials and phase II trials are effective without safety issues, a phase III clinical trial is proposed and performed. Phase IV trials are conducted after FDA approval (i.e. post-marketing).

Phase III clinical trials determine the effectiveness and safety of the drug by using hundreds or thousand of subjects that are randomized in a blinded manner to either the treatment, or the control arm (placebo or standard treatment), where neither the patient nor the physician knows what group the patient is assigned to. In most cases, these studies involve many institutions or medical centers in the US and around the world. Thus, the use of IT for any of the stages of a clinical trial can greatly improve communications, increase data accuracy, reduce procedure times, and reduce associated costs. A Clinical Trial Protocol (CTP) explaining how the trial will be conducted is written and submitted to the respective authorities for approval. Clinical investigators are contacted to participate in the trial. Each clinical trial needs to recruit a specific number of subjects (cancer patients) that fit the eligible criteria.

In general, clinical investigators approach patients fitting the eligibility criteria to inquire about their interest in participating in a clinical study for a new investigational drug. The cancer patient agrees to participate in the clinical trial by signing an informed consent form. The patient is then randomized in a blind manner and treated according to the trial protocol, and followed for the length of the study. Many medical tests will be carried out before the patient starts the trial, during the trial, and even after the treatment has stopped. All the data on each patient must be collected and sent to the sponsor for data analysis.

The sponsor must ensure that the data quality is high and usually monitors each investigational site were clinical trials are conducted on a regular basis. High quality data is accurate, complete, consistent and timely (Haag, Baltzan and Phillips, 2006). At the end of the study, the sponsor analyzes the data to determine the effectiveness and safety of the drug. Then, the sponsor prepares the needed documents for the FDA containing the results of the clinical trials. The FDA evaluates all the data on the new drug and decides whether this novel drug can be approved for the market. For many years, most steps on a clinical trial used paper as source documents. In 1997, changes in FDA regulation allowed the use of electronic resources for documentation of clinical trials.

Federal Regulations

In March 1997, the FDA established guidelines (21 CFR part 11) for the use of electronic records and electronic signatures (FDA, 1997). In this regulation the FDA "set forth the criteria under which the agency considers electronic records, electronic signatures, and handwritten signatures executed to electronic records to be trustworthy, reliable, and generally equivalent to paper records and handwritten signatures executed on paper" (FDA, 1997). These guidelines support the use of electronic resources, in addition to the traditional paper-based formats for the management of data associated with clinical trials.

More recently, in May 2007, the FDA issued "Guidance for Industry: Computerized Systems Used in Clinical Investigations" (FDA, 2007). In this guidance, the FDA outlines principles to "... be used for computerized systems that contain any data that are relied on by an applicant in support of a marketing application, including computerized laboratory information management systems that capture analytical results of test conducted during a clinical trial" (FDA, 2007). This guidance establishes several recommendations for the use of computerized systems in different procedures related to clinical investigations such as standard operating procedures, source documentation and retention, internal security safeguards (limit access, audit trails and date/time stamps), external security safeguards and other system features (direct entry of data, data retrieval, dependability system documentation, system controls, change controls), and training of personnel (FDA, 2007). This is a great step forward to promote the use of IT in clinical trials.

CLINICAL TRIALS AND INFORMATION TECHNOLOGY (IT)

Data quality is an important issue in clinical trials since poor data quality can lead to approval of unsafe drugs or lack of approval for effective and safe drugs. For quality control, the FDA recommends the consistent use of clinical terminology and the need to alert users if data entered are outside of acceptable ranges (FDA, 2007). The FDA guidance also suggests avoiding program features that enter data as default (FDA, 2007). Effective systems for data collection quickly identify inconsistencies and allow problem resolution in a timely fashion. An IBM survey comparing electronic data collection (eDC) to paper data capture (as cited by Bleicher, 2003), showed that eDC reduces query costs from \$60 to \$10, and it also reduces the numbers of queries from 5-10 to 0.25-1.0, with the percentage of data requiring correction decreasing from 1-2% to 0.05-0.1%. Moreover, eDC drastically reduces the percentage of errors due to missing data from 48% to 0%, and also decreases the percentage of errors caused by inconsistent data from 35% to 5%. Thus, eDC has had a major positive impact on data collection for clinical trials.

In spite of the many benefits of using eDC, there are still many challenges to overcome. As already mentioned, some sponsors have built their own in-house system (legacy systems) to facilitate their clinical trials. Legacy systems are usually mainframe and batch processing applications that can contain duplicated data, and lack integrated user interfaces (Hess, 2005). When each sponsor requires proprietary software and hardware for their trial, clinical investigations can be constrained by a lack of systems interoperability (Adams, 2007). The web can provide an integrated platform to reduce some of the challenges associated with collection and sharing data from multiple, disparate systems. Many vendors such as Oracle, PhaseForward, and Compleware are important players that are providing systems that will help sponsors and CROs to conduct clinical trials using eDC.

Another important issue in eDC is the security of the data. Fortunately, web-based clinical trials if properly designed can be extremely secure using secure socket layer encryption and a clinical trial server isolated behind a firewall. The FDA recommends that access be limited to authorized individuals who log in using a password which must be periodically updated by the user (FDA, 2007). Another important component for the system according to FDA is the audit trail. This it the ability of the system to keep track of all changes made to the electronic records. Audit trials need to be computer-generated and time-stamped. For multi-national clinical trials that span different time zones there has to be a clear understanding of the time zone reference used (FDA, 2007). The ability to easily collect data about data (metadata) is another advantage of the use of eDC in clinical trials (Bleicher, 2003).

Adopting innovative IT to conduct and share data from clinical trials can accelerate the process of bringing novel and safe drugs to the market. As such, there are some components of the clinical trials enterprise in which the adoption of databases and electronic resources can critically impact.

THEORETICAL FRAMEWORK

Electronic resources refer to the use computer hardware, computer software, and telecommunications devices to capture, store and disseminate information. Electronic resources include, but are not limited to specific examples such as databases, data warehouses, and web-based applications. We use an analysis of the existing literature to develop a framework showing the four main areas of clinical trials that can be directly impacted by the use of electronic resources. The four main areas of impact that we identify are: patient recruitment, patient data collection, process data management, and dissemination of results.

Patient Recruitment

Online databases have changed the way patients are recruited for cancer and other clinical trials. Online databases have allowed patients to identify physicians conducting relevant trials and register to participate (Wei, Metz, Coyle et al., 2004). One major advantage of using databases for data collection on clinical trials is to ensure transparencies at multiple stages of the process (Houlton, 2004). The Health Insurance Portability and Accountability Act of 1996 (HIPAA) which is designed to protect the privacy of patient medical information, may have had an unintended negative effect on the recruitment of patients for clinical trials because of limitations on sharing information (Kleeman,

Table 1. Information fields for clinical trials database (extracted from www.clinicaltrials.gov)

DESCRIPTIVE	RECRUITMENT	ADMINISTRATIVE
1. Brief Title	1. Recruitment Status	1. NCT ID
2. Official Title	2. Enrollment	2. Organization ID
3. Brief Summary	3. Start Date	3. Secondary ID
4. Detailed Description	4. Completion Date	4. Study Sponsor
5. Study Phase	5. Eligibility Criteria	5. Collaborators
6. Study Type	6. Gender	6. Investigators
7. Study Design	7. Ages	7. Information Provided By
8. Primary Outcome Measure	8. Accepts Healthy Volunteers	8. Verification Date
9. Secondary Outcome Measure	9. Contacts	9. First Received Date
10. Condition	10. Location Countries	
11. Intervention		
12. Medline PMIDs		
13. Links		

2006). However, web-based applications can be an important facilitator for patient-driven clinical trial searches, and thus potentially limit challenges associated with to HIPAA regulations.

Past litigations against pharmaceutical companies argued that some companies have hidden information on the adverse side effects related to the use of the drugs during the clinical trials period (Benowitz, 2005; Turner, 2004). As a result of these problems entities such as medical journals, NIH, and U.S. Congress, require that all clinical trials be registered (Houlton, 2004). This registration requirement has given birth to web-based registries such as clinicaltrials.gov (Charatan, 2000) that contains information on over 53,590 trials across 154 countries. Cancer patients can search for information under a variety of options including cancer type, location of study, and organizational sponsor. Information fields for this database can be grouped into three main categories: descriptive, recruitment and administrative as summarized in Table 1.

More recently, the American Cancer Society has launched a registry for clinical trials to help patients identify a suitable clinical trial according to their disease (Anonymous, 2007). The emerging use of online databases is helping both patients and physicians with the recruitment stage of clinical trials.

Patient Data Collection

Another area where electronic resources are valuable to clinical trials is with the recording of patient data. Investments by healthcare organizations has resulted in the development of computer applications and medical informatics to facilitate patient care, communication between different healthcare workers, quality assurance, billing, reimbursements, and timely decision making (Fitzmaurice, Adams, and Eisenberg, 2002). Improvements in health care management have promoted the use of electronic means to facilitate clinical trials management. However, one challenge in the reform of healthcare management is the high variability in the ways that pharmaceutical companies use IT for clinical trials (Bleicher, 2003). The lack of standardized tools and methods can limit needed collaborations prior, during and after the implementation of clinical trials.

Multiple pieces of data are collected from each patient enrolled in a clinical trial. Several techniques have been used to collect general subject diary data or to fill the case report form (CRF). It is important also to understand that modern clinical trials involve additional aspects that were not included many years ago, such as collection of biological specimens (blood, tumor, saliva) concomitant with the intervention. These specimens are then used to develop better ways to predict those patients who will benefit from a specific treatment. These additional areas are considered as "translational research" and also need to be linked to the clinical trial database, which adds another level of complexity to the clinical trial enterprise (Adams, 2007).

A study published in 1998 identified the then new technology of faxes, scanners, optical readers, and the internet as accurate and reliable tools for data capture from clinical trials, even though expensive at the time (Lampe and Weiler, 1998). More recently, other authors have discussed the importance of remote data entry systems and electronic data collection eDC in clinical trials (Bleicher, 2003; Meadows, 2003). The advantages of these electronic means over the older paper-based format of entry are enormous. Instead of taking several months for the sponsor to receive paper data on each patient, now the speed of collection can be made in real-time thanks to web-enabled systems that capture data. This speed allows faster decision-making and better quality control of the data collected by the sponsor.

Process Data Management

Due to the confidential nature of clinical trial data, specific solutions that pharmaceutical companies use for their data management strategies are readily available to the public. However, Oracle indicates that "12 of the 12 pharmaceutical companies of Fortune Magazine's 2005 global top 500 run Oracle Applications" (Oracle, 2007) and "10 of the top 10 contract research organizations (CRO) run Oracle Applications" (Oracle, 2007). Thus, it is possible that many other pharmaceutical companies and biotech firms are using organization-wide databases and data warehousing products for their data management. Nevertheless, the data obtained from clinical trial needs to be analyzed using statistical software. Software that can be used to analyze clinical trial data is available from SAS (SAS 2007) and other vendors such as SPSS or Stata. Software for clinical trials should be compatible with the Operational Data Model (ODM) and Study Tabulation Data Model (SDTM) proposed by the Clinical Data Interchanges Standards Consortium (CDIS).

In the non-profit sector, the National Surgical Adjuvant Breast and Bowel Project (NASBP) developed a centralized data management system for cancer clinical trials they sponsor. This group has a centralized medical monitoring for all phase III clinical trials that incorporate data management, medical review, quality assurance, statistics, and IT (Soran, Nesbitt, Mamounas et al., 2006). Data management involves computerized edits and queries, data management metrics and training, internal quality reviews, delinquency listings, expectations reports, and protocol review (Soran et al., 2006). As in the case of industry, other non-profit institutions may have different procedures for their data management. Standardization of protocols may allow different institutions to share their data and results of clinical trials more frequently to foster synergy and avoid duplication of clinical trials.

Information Dissemination

Once clinical trials are completed the entire medical profession can potentially benefit from the dissemination of the results. The National Cancer Institute (NCI) has developed a database on clinical trial results that contains, in addition to most of the information contained in a clinical trial registry a statement on the results of the study. By visiting the website of pharmaceutical companies such as Glaxo-Smith-Kline (http://www.gsk.us.com) one can also find a registry of clinical trials and a database containing results of clinical trials for drugs that are currently on the market (http://ctr.gsk.co.uk/medicinelist.asp). The disseminated information about completed clinical trials typically consists of trial results in pdf format or links to articles published about the trial. Some information on clinical trial results also appears on the prescribing information for each drug.

In other companies such as Bristol-Myers-Squibb one can find two databases: a registry of all their clinical trials, including those for investigational drugs not yet in the market, and a database about the results of their clinical trials for drugs in the market (http://ctr.bms.com/ctd/start.do). Databases by pharmaceutical industries vary in their content and scope and may reflect variations in their legacy systems. Current developments in clinical trial standardization such as Clinical Data Interchange Standards Consortium (CDISC) can promote more standardized methods for sharing the results of clinical trials.

FUTURE DIRECTIONS AND IMPLICATIONS

The mission of CDISC is "to develop and support global, platform-independent data standards that enable information system interoperability to improve medical research and related areas of healthcare" (CDISC, 2007). CDISC "is an open, multidisciplinary, non-profit organization that has established worldwide industry standards to support the electronic acquisition, exchange, submission and archiving of clinical trials data and metadata for medical and biopharmaceutical product development" (CDISC, 2007). Recently, a team within the CDISC has produced a standard computable clinical trial protocol using the Biomedical Research Integrated Domain group (BRIDG) Model (Willoughby, Fridsma, Chatterjee et al., 2007). The BRIDG model is an informatics research platform to support clinical research (Willoughby et al., 2007). This model will be instrumental as a starting point for application development so that most or all steps of a clinical trail can be standardized, communicated to others and easily queried and exchanged between the different stakeholders involved in clinical trials.

In addition to the recent FDA guidance about computerized systems (see federal regulations), another important development in the application of IT to clinical trials is a formal collaboration between the FDA and NCI. Both organizations have agreed to create a product called Janus, which sets a standard for aggregation and exchange of clinical trials data (NCI and FDA, 2007). The Janus model will be compatible with the Cancer Biomedical Informatics Grid (caBIG™), a common infrastructure for sharing data tools and other resources among cancer researchers based on open source, open access, open development and federated (CaBig, 2007). The Janus project will help to streamline data management and potentially reduce the time required for the FDA to evaluate clinical trials. One goal of Janus is the implementation of a single integrated environment where information about clinical trials can be submitted electronically to the FDA. The FDA has also partnered with Duke University to modernize the way clinical trials are performed (FDA Initiatives, 2007).

There are key challenges associated with the implementation of more standardized products and the adoption of databases and electronic resources for clinical trials. The move towards standardized electronic resources is costly for larger pharmaceuticals companies that have invested many resources in developing their own models and legacy systems to conduct clinical trials (Bleicher, 2003). Stakeholders involved in clinical trials may also be comfortable with their current manual system and be reluctant to change. Pharmaceutical companies also are unwilling to release their confidential information due to the fierce competition in their industry (Turner, 2004). It can also be a daunting task to make all sponsors and stakeholders use the same system for all the steps of the clinical trials. Although this may not be feasible in the near future, it is possible that the FDA will require sponsors to use the Janus system once it is implemented.

An electronic solution for the clinical trial enterprise will need to integrate traditional clinical trial standards and biomedical research within each trial. Moreover, it will need to cover the different pre-clinical and clinical aspects of the value chain associated with clinical trials (Bleicher, 2003). Some patients may also have limited technology experience and an effective user-interface with components such as color screens, beeping prompts and feedback tools can reduce some inherent user challenges in an online environment (Schmier, Kane and Halpern, 2005). Ultimately some of the major challenges facing widespread adoption of electronic resources for clinical trials include: migration from legacy systems, lack of standardization, stakeholder participation, and user resistance to technology.

CONCLUSION

There are multiple ways in which electronic resources are beneficial to the implementation and execution of clinical trials. Firstly, well-designed user-interfaces can realize cost savings as well as improve efficiencies throughout the different stages of clinical trials data collection (Schmier et al., 2005). Secondly, online data searches can increase the level of participation of under-represented ethnic minorities, who traditional have a low rate of participation in cancer clinical trials (Markman et al., 2008). However, IT is not a panacea to clinical trials; system interoperability (Adams, 2007), and data security (Schmier et al., 2005) are important challenges that must be addressed. Effective use of IT can result in improved patient management and the early discontinuance of harmful and ineffective drugs. Electronic resources in clinical trials have seen a slow rate of adoption. However factors such as recent FDA guidance, mature and stable software vendors, and private sector initiatives can drive the adoption of electronic resources in clinical trials.

REFERENCES

Adams, C. P., & Brantner, V. V. (2006). Estimating the cost of new drug development: Is it really $802 million? *Health Affairs*, *25*(2), 420–428. doi:10.1377/hlthaff.25.2.420

Adams, M. R. (2007). Databases and the future of clinical trials in bladder cancer. *Urologic Oncology: Seminars and Original Investigations*, *25*, 330–332. doi:10.1016/j.urolonc.2007.05.003

Alschuler, L., Kush, R., & Bain, L. (2004). Improving Data Collection for Patient Care and Clinical Trials. *Science*, (March): 26.

Anonymous. (2007). TrialCheck(R) Cancer Clinical Trial Matching Interface to Debut on American Cancer Society Web Site, Retrieved on February 27, 2008 from *PR Newswire*, http://proquest.umi.com

Benowitz, S. (2005). Clinical Trial Transparency: Registries, Databases Raise Questions, Stir Debate. *Journal of the National Cancer Institute*, *97*(22), 1640–1641. doi:10.1093/jnci/dji421

Bleicher, P. (2003). Clinical trial technology: at the inflection point. *BIOSILICO*, *1*(15), 163–168. doi:10.1016/S1478-5382(03)02373-4

CaBig. (2007). Retrieved on November 26, 2007, from http://cabig.cancer.gov/connection/principles.asp

CDISC. (2007). Retrieved on November 23, 2007 from http://www.cdisc.org/about/index.html

Charatan, F. (2000). US launches new clinical trials database. *BMJ (Clinical Research Ed.)*, *320*(7236), 668. doi:10.1136/bmj.320.7236.668

FDA. (1997). 21 CFR Part 11: Electronic records; electronic signatures. Retrieved on November 20, 2007 from http://www.accessdata.fda.gov/scripts/cdrh/cfdocs/ cfcfr/CFRSearch.cfm?CFRPart=11

FDA. (2007). Guidance for Industry Computerized System Used in Clinical Investigations. Retrieved on November 20, 2007 from www.fda.gov/OHRMS/DOCKETS/98fr/04d-0440-gdl0002.pdf

Fitzmaurice, J. M., Adams, K., & Eisenberg, J. M. (2002). Three decades of research on computer applications in health care: Medical informatics support at the agency for healthcare research and quality. *Journal of the American Medical Informatics Association*, *9*(2), 144–160. doi:10.1197/jamia.M0867

Haag, S., Baltzan, P., & Phillips, A. (2006). *Business Driven Technology* (2nd ed.). McGraw-Hill.

Hess, H. M. (2005). Aligning technology and business: Applying patterns for legacy transformation. *IBM Systems Journal*, *44*(1), 25–45. doi:10.1147/sj.441.0025

Houlton, S. (2004). Time for Transparency. *Pharmaceutical Executive*, *24*(11), 40.

Initiatives, F. D. A. (2007). FDA and Duke Launch Public-Private Partnership to Modernize Clinical Trials. Retrieved on March 31, 2008 from http://www.fda.gov/oc/initiatives/criticalpath/partnership.html

Kleeman, E. (2006). Clinical trials face shortage of candidates. *Knight Ridder Tribune Business News, 1, October 2nd, RetrievedMarch5, 2008, from ABI/INFORM Dateline database. (Document ID: 1139651541).*

Lampe, A. J., & Weiler, J., M. (1998). Data capture from the sponsors' and investigators' perspectives: Balancing quality, speed, and cost. *Drug Information Journal*, *32*(4), 871–886.

Markman, M., Petersen, J., & Montgomery, R. (2008). An examination of the influence of patient race and ethnicity on expressed interest in learning about cancer clinical trials. *Journal of Cancer Research and Clinical Oncology*, *134*(1), 115–118. doi:10.1007/s00432-007-0263-4

Meadows, B. J. (2003). Eliciting Remote Data Entry System Requirements for the Collection of Cancer Clinical Trial Data. *Computers, Informatics, Nursing*, *21*(5), 234–240. doi:10.1097/00024665-200309000-00010

NCI and FDA. (2007). Memorandum of Understanding on Janus Study Data Repository. Retrieved on November 21, 2007, from http://www.fda.gov/OHRMS/DOCKETS/98fr/FDA-225-07-4301-mou0001.PDF

Oracle (2007). Retrieved on November 20, 2007, from http://www.oracle.com/industries/life_sciences/pharma.html.

Pavlovic, I., & Miklavcic, D. (2007). Web-Based Electronic Data Collection System to Support Electrochemotherapy Clinical Trial. *IEEE Transactions on Information Technology in Biomedicine*, *11*(2), 222–230. doi:10.1109/TITB.2006.879581

SAS. (2007). Retrieved on November 20, 2007, from http://www.sas.com/industry/ pharma/cdisc/.

Schmier, J. K., Kane, D. W., & Halpern, M. T. (2005). Practical applications of usability theory to electronic data collection for clinical trials. *Contemporary Clinical Trials*, *26*(3), 376–385. doi:10.1016/j.cct.2005.01.012

Soran, A., Nesbitt, L., & Mamounas, E. P. (2006). Centralized medical monitoring in phase III clinical trials: the National Surgical Adjuvant Breast and Bowel Project (NSABP) experience. *Clinical Trials*, *3*(5), 478–485. doi:10.1177/1740774506070747

Turner, E. H. (2004). A Taxpayer-Funded Clinical Trials Registry and Results Database. *PLoS Medicine*, *1*(3), 180–182. doi:10.1371/journal.pmed.0010060

Wei, S. J., Metz, J. M., & Coyle, C. (2004). Recruitment of Patients Into an Internet-Based Clinical Trials Database: The Experience of OncoLink and the National Colorectal Cancer Research Alliance. *Journal of Clinical Oncology*, *22*(23), 4730–4736. doi:10.1200/JCO.2004.07.103

Willoughby, C., Fridsma, D., & Chatterjee, L. (2007). A standard computable clinical trial protocol: The role of the BRIDG model. *Drug Information Journal*, *41*(3), 383–392.

This work was previously published in An International Journal of Healthcare Delivery Reform Initiatives, edited by Matthew W. Guah, pp. 16-24, copyright 2009 by IGI Publishing (an imprint of IGI Global).

Chapter 3
Decentralisation and Health Systems Performance in Developing Countries:
Impact of "Decision Space" on Primary Health Care Delivery in Nigeria

Adebusoye A. Anifalaje
London School of Economics and Political Science, UK

ABSTRACT

This article attempts to elucidate the intricacies of primary health care delivery in Nigeria. Among myriad complexities, the central proposition made herein is that the absence of an effective regulatory and enforcement framework in developing countries results in a prominent informal decision space. The findings show that the prominence of an informal decision space compromises the objectives of an information-based public health system. The article concludes that decentralisation in developing countries must have a coordinated top-down and bottom-up development component for it to be effective in improving the performance of primary health systems. One of the implications of the study is that researching decentralised healthcare delivery requires analytical models which are able to illuminate the complexities of local accountability in developing countries. The study also reveals the need to further research the dynamics of democratic decentralisation in developing countries as this goes beyond administrative structures but involve socio-cultural institutions.

INTRODUCTION

Health systems simply defined, are the foundational (i.e. institutional, political, legal, economic, technical and socio-cultural) arrangements through which health services are delivered to the population (Berman and Bossert 2000). There is a complex chain of interdependent factors which influence the performance of health systems. In developing countries where there are high

DOI: 10.4018/978-1-60960-183-6.ch003

mortality and morbidity rates, a multiplicity of stakeholders (i.e. rich nations, international donors, non-governmental organisations (NGOs), bilateral and multilateral agencies) employ different strategies to try and improve specific aspects of the health system (Okuonzi and Macrae 1995). These diverse and often uncoordinated interventions usually have a fragmentary effect on these systems (Buse and Watt 1996). In essence, the imperatives of international health policies and donor-aid practices have a tendency to weaken the capacity of national governments to independently formulate and implement policies which address the health needs of the population (Smith *et al.* 2008).

This article highlights the implications of decentralisation on the performance of health systems in Nigeria. By conceptualising decentralisation as a strategy for delivering health services through a primary health care system, the study is able to focus on the micro-level processes of the health system. The performance of a health system can therefore be investigated through the effectiveness of primary health care delivery. To study this phenomenon, decision space is adopted as an analytical tool (Bossert 1998). This framework conceptualises the multi-level dynamics of primary health decisions made by local government agents. Decision space illuminates the choices of local government actors and how these impact health system performance. It also frames the role of information in monitoring and evaluating the performance of health systems. There are three main reasons for adopting a local perspective of the decision space approach: firstly, primary health care services are the building blocks of general public health systems therefore we would expect a strong association between local and general public health systems performance; secondly, information systems are implemented with a view to aid planning and decision making at the local level. Consequently this focus provides an opportunity to go back one step to evaluate the intricacies of information practices (in a general sense) without reference to a particular health information systems project; lastly, local agents make health decisions out of a quagmire of often conflicting motivations and opposing evidence: this study will provide some insight into the possible factors that actually influence choices made regarding primary care delivery.

With decentralised health sectors, central governments through the Ministry of Health have a complex task of designing the framework through which local government agents can provide adequate health services (WHO 2000). Their challenges include developing the socio-economic, political, legal, administrative and institutional arrangements that will support the efficiency and effectiveness of primary care systems. The formal (and informal) authority afforded local government agents by the central government, combined with the discretions they exercise (both within and outside formal authority) make up their "decision space". The relationship between central and local government actors contributes formally and informally to the decisions made at the local level with consequences for the performance of primary health care systems.

The Decision space framework conceives the relational dynamics between the local and the central government through a principal-agent theory (Griffith 1966 and Rhodes 1986 in Bossert 1998) the central (or State) government as the principal and local governments as agents. It analyses the capacity of the principal to influence decisions made by local government agents in order to align them to the principal's objectives e.g. better performing health system. This being the case, the primary role of the Federal Ministry of Health for instance, would be to make adjustments to local agents' decision space in a way that would align their interests with national public health objectives. The central government can accomplish this by adopting a scheme of rewards and sanctions.

The framework tries to balance this top-down bias by suggesting the mutual influences of central and local government agents. The influence of local government agents is framed in terms of having direct and primary access to contextual knowledge and information which is required by central government agents. Information plays a crucial role in the study and analysis of health systems performance. Within the decision-space framework, local agents use information to evaluate the technical effectiveness of current primary care units and formulate appropriate operational intervention strategies. On the other hand, central government agents also employ this information to build a general public health picture as well as monitor the performance of local agents from a managerial perspective. However, the main thrust of the framework is geared towards the role of central government in aligning the interests of local government actors.

The main observation made in this study is that the decentralisation of health systems in developing countries operates predominantly through an informal decision space. This article therefore shows the consequences of this phenomenon on primary health care delivery. It further argues that this political dimension to analysing health systems performance is fundamental to understanding the challenges of health information system initiatives in developing countries. For these reasons it is important to conceptually explore and empirically investigate the impact of decision space on the delivery of primary health care. Consequently, the overall objective of this research project is to gain a better understanding of the implications of a decentralised health sector on the performance of the health system. To delimit the research focus and scope three questions are framed:

1. How does the decision space of local government actors impact primary health care?
2. In practice, what are the factors that shape, influence and determine the decision space?
3. To what extent does information drive health care decisions?

The empirical fieldwork for these questions was conducted in Nigeria. While agency-centred studies analyse the dynamics of the situated local contexts, they do not provide adequate tools to investigate the influence of the structures within which the agents exist and operate (some IS literature have tried to address this see Alvarez 2003). For instance, instead of studying the implementation or use of a specific information system, this study locates the problem domain within the socio-political dimension of health care delivery in Nigeria, providing a more robust platform for understanding the challenges of health information systems projects. This is because decision space approach serves as a multi-level contextual platform which incorporates the mutual influences of the macro and micro-level environment.

The main contribution of this article therefore is to illuminate the socio-political arrangements which affect the delivery of primary health care in Nigeria. Although focussing on the characteristics of local government agents, this study is able to reveal how the capacity of the State and Central governments impact on local agents' effectiveness in delivery primary health care. The study extends these findings to analyse the role information plays in local health systems and extrapolate to discuss the potential implications for the implementation and use of health information systems.

The rest of the article is presented in two broad sections. The first section is conceptual in nature including the literature review, conceptual framework and methodology. The second section details the empirical content of the study including the analysis and discussion and the research conclusions. A brief outline of implications for future research is also provided.

LITERATURE REVIEW

Health Care Delivery Strategies in Developing Countries

This section will provide the historical context of health delivery strategies in developing countries. Focussing on the challenges and complexities of primary health care, the literature shows the influences of global economic and political ideologies on national and local health care delivery policies.

Primary Health Care System

In the late 1970s, the international health community—comprising of World Health Organisation (WHO) member countries— turned its attention to the failing health systems of many developing countries. The central concern at the time was that majority of the population in poor countries lacked access to basic health care services and therefore suffered high rates of mortality and morbidity (Magnussen *et al.* 2004). An effort to address these failing systems was articulated in the WHO Alma Ata declaration (WHO 1978). The declaration conceived of health as a basic human right and sought to initiate programmes that will build sustainable health systems, with indiscriminate access for all, in developing countries. It proposed the primary health care (PHC) system as the principal means of achieving equitable health service delivery within and between countries (Starfield *et al.* 2005). By focussing on the community-level, health services are more accessible and interventions are likely to be more responsive to local needs as there is increased opportunity for effective local participation (Tarimo and Fowkes 1989). The argument is that there is increased accountability and improved health care service when policies and intervention strategies are formulated with the "users" in a way that aligns with their particular needs (Cornwall *et al.* 2000). With this system, greater emphasis is placed on health promotion and preventative strategies (Atkinson *et al.* 2005) rather than technologically sophisticated and curative bio-medical interventions (Bossert 1979). Cueto (2004) also suggested that PHC was introduced based on the implicit assumption that diseases in developing countries were contingent on socio-economic arrangements and therefore interventions required political will. As a result, the most important task was to mobilise the support of the international community to support the bottom-up approach of improving the performance of health systems. Under this arrangement therefore, the performance of health systems is dependent on the effectiveness and coordination of community-based health units.

By the mid 1980s, the vision of global health suffered several significant setbacks. Firstly, the objective to raise the minimum level of health in all poor countries of the world, was deemed too idealistic (Magnussen *et al.* 2004). Secondly, the proposed PHC system received little support because of the deeply institutionalised tertiary model and a reluctance of "experts and politicians in developed countries to accept the principle that communities should plan and implement their own healthcare services" (Hall and Taylor 2003: 17). Furthermore, with the decline of communism in the former Soviet Union, marketisation was gaining more ground as the appropriate economic ideology for modern society. Economic support for health projects was conditional on recipient countries adopting liberalisation policies. Hall and Taylor (2003) discuss the "failure" of PHC in light of these changes.

As an alternative approach, selective primary health care (SPHC) was adopted (Cueto 2004). In contrast to PHC, SPHC assumes that diseases in developing countries are a natural phenomenon which can be curtailed through economically-viable and technical interventions (Cueto 2004). This approach attempts to tackle major diseases especially those responsible for childhood mortality (Cueto 2004). The "success" of SPHC was attributed to three main factors: 1) its bias towards a market rationality; 2) specific goal of child health and 3) appeal to "rational" and technical interventions (Cueto 2004). While PHC is oriented towards improving general population health, SPHC is a vertical programme addressing specific diseases. The performance of SPHC is judged according to specific project objectives such as immunization coverage, disease control or eradication etc.

Decentralisation

Still driven by a techno-economic rationality, the 1990s was accentuated by a sustained interest in health sector reform. According to the Harvard School of Public Health, health reform is defined as:

sustained, purposeful and fundamental change" – "sustained" in the sense that it is not a "one shot" temporary effort that will not have enduring impacts; "purposeful" in the sense of emerging from a rational, planned and evidence-based process; and "fundamental" in the sense of addressing significant, strategic dimensions of health systems (Berman 1995).

With experiences of the 1980s showing that general health systems had been significantly weakened (Chatora and Tumusime 2004), organisational change, innovative sourcing of funds, increased market rationality, and customer-focussed health services were strategies (e.g. *The World Development Report 1993: Investing in Health*) (World Bank 1993) advocated as a means to achieving sustainable health reforms (Blaauw *et al.* 2003). Nonetheless, decentralisation emerges as a distinctive feature of these reforms albeit employed in shades and degrees (Jeppsson and Okuonzi 2000). Jeppsson & Okuonzi (2000) note for instance that Ugandan health decentralisation model shows power devolved to district levels as part of a wider political decentralisation agenda. On the other hand, they acknowledge that only the health service structure is decentralised in Zambia. Maintaining that useful lessons can be learnt from both approaches, they note that neither approach has been able to produce better health service delivery or improve poverty conditions.

There are often mistaken inferences made about decentralisation of public health service (which is a feature of primary health care) as a form of rolling back the state (Collins and Green 1994). So, based on this rationale, donor agencies fund specific health projects usually without much collaboration with national governments or consideration for the defined health priorities of recipient countries (Loewenson 1993, Okuonzi and Macrae 1995). The perception that developing countries lack requisite capacity e.g. in terms of adequate analytical skills for health policy formulation, is represented as a major obstacle to the effective collaboration necessary for health reform (Filmer *et al.* 1998, Jamison and Mosley 1991). The resultant coordination failure amongst diverse stakeholders (Buse and Watt 1996) precipitated a call for donors to invest in building aid recipients' capacity to develop appropriate health systems (Lee 1998). Besides, the sustainability of health systems in developing countries demand that governments take active responsibility in deciding the direction of public health intervention strategies. Initiatives like Sector-Wide Approaches (SWAp) were responses to the urgent call for the coordination of donor-funded projects and better collaboration with national governments (Peters and Chao 1998). The logic behind these programmes is that projects are based around commonalities of goals and strengthening of national capacity to fulfil its development objectives in terms of effective institutional arrangements and economic policies. There is an expectation that the outworking of a coordinated approach will also stimulate local participation, increase active engagement and provide stability necessary for long-term planning (Chilundo & Aanestad, 2003). However, effective collaboration between donors and recipient countries is made more difficult because it is contingent on trust and confidence in the capacity of recipient countries to manage their health systems. The perception that developing countries lack requisite capacity e.g. in terms of adequate analytical skills for health policy formulation constitutes a significant setback for SWAp (Filmer *et al.* 1998, Jamison and Mosley 1991). Tarimo and Fowkes (1989) identify four main challenges of compartmentalized approach to health reform in developing countries: 1) short-term mindedness in goal setting; 2) insufficient financial aid; 3) lack of appreciation of differences in local contexts; 4) implementation of vertical programmes as a matter of convenience as opposed to needs.

Economic Growth Approach

By the turn of the 21st century, it is widely stated that the problems of poverty and disease are neither technological nor a consequence of knowledge deficiency. However, from the mandate of the Millennium Development Goals, the challenge is perceived in terms of mustering enough political will and finance for a vision of global health. From an economic standpoint, the World Health Organisation (WHO) commission on *Macroeconomics and Health: Investing in health for economic development* report argues that investment in health is of paramount importance (WHO 2001). The main concern is to break the poverty cycle—which reinforces poor health—by boosting economic growth through significant "public investment" (Sachs *et al.* 2004: 122). Economic growth in turn has the capacity to increase productivity and consequently lower poverty (Sachs *et al.* 2004). The foundation of this strategy built on globalisation and depends to a very large extent on the provision of foreign aid. Although the effect of globalisation—in addition to effective institutional arrangements and adequate infrastructures—has been largely beneficial to health conditions, this link is drawn from an economic growth, trickle-down effect. As a result, there are required domestic conditions that must be present in order to reap the benefits. Therefore, foreign aid in itself is unlikely to produce the desired result if there are no frameworks established to guarantee that the finance will be used effectively towards development. However, for most developing countries, deregulation and liberalisation policies have not yielded growth or better health conditions (Cornia 2001).

While there is some agreement with the central proposition of the WHO r*eport on Macroeconomics and Health* that disease is a major player in engendering poverty and therefore investment in health is a key proponent in achieving economic development, there is a major contention regarding its approach. The main criticism of the report is the "reform for finance" approach which betrays a disposition towards the familiar structural adjustment programme (Waitzkin 2003). In this sense, it is argued that developing countries will be worse off while developed countries are able to exploit the opportunities created by these policies (Garrett 2007). The weakness of the WHO report can be linked to paying lip service to health as an end in its own right while actively pursuing an economic growth agenda (Waitzkin 2003).

In contrast to macro-level, top-down growth strategies, others argue that health crises in the developing countries have necessitated a change of strategy in delivering public health services by increasing community involvement and participation (Cornwall *et al.* 2000). The argument is that the bottom-up approach to development is related closely to the "health for all" policy while "new public management" health models detract from this goal (Gwatkin 2000). The realisation that there is increased accountability and improved health care system when policies and intervention strategies are formulated with the "users" (Cornwall 2000), constitutes a new wave of efforts that have started building which gives attention to the health of the poor as well as health inequalities (Gwatkin 2000).

There are observable evidence to suggest that much has to be understood about the complexity of this field because "[d]espite the emphasis placed during the last two decades on public delivery of comprehensive and equitable primary care to developing country populations, coverage remains far from universal and the quality often poor" (Mills *et al.* 2004). It is therefore still contended that PHC is "the only way to reach the poor and the vulnerable groups" (Masaiganah 2004).

Paradoxical Insight

While the decentralisation of the health sector is often implemented through a top-down process, its goal is to develop a bottom-up approach to improving health system performance (Atkinson 1995). As a consequence, health systems research has paid little attention to the socio-political arrangements of decentralisation at the local level (Atkinson et al. 2000, Smith 1997). There are two analytical insights which can be gained by examining this paradox from the local perspective. First, we can empirically investigate how this paradox impacts the extent to which local governments can effectively exercise authority in matters of health service delivery (Adeyemo 2005). Secondly, we can also critically analyse whether the real objective of the top-down process is to actually facilitate increased local decision making.

However, we are not just interested in the extent to which health systems are driven by the transfer of decision-making authority to the local level, but also the factors that affect the nature (or quality) of these decisions. There is a body of literature which attempts to tackle this issue and is based around themes such as rational health planning, evidence-based public health, information-centred health policy etc. The literature advocates a strong modernisation ethos through these concepts, providing equal impetus for technology-based health systems as necessary instruments for collecting, storing, analysing and disseminating health information (some examples of the debates: Dobrow *et al.* 2004, McMichael *et al.* 2005, Murray and Frenk 2001, Niessen *et al.* 2000).

Information and Health Systems in Developing Countries

There is a resonant consensus that effective health planning and interventions depend on accurate data (Green 1999). It is also accepted that relevant and reliable information forms the bedrock of any effective public health system (Stansfield 2005). The effective control or prevention of disease from an epidemiological perspective for instance, is dependent on accurate information regarding its prevalence and geographical distribution. The underperformance of health systems in developing countries have been attributed to the paucity of health information and lack of an information culture. As a result, there is underlying demand for a systematic process of collecting, storing, analysing and disseminating health data and it is to this end that arguments are made in favour of health information systems (HIS) (AbouZahr and Boerma 2005). Despite the relatively strong rationale for these systems, their implementation in developing countries has been shrouded in partial or complete "failure" (Heeks 2006, Littlejohns *et al.* 2003). To illuminate the challenges of information practices in developing countries, we can assess three dimensions of health information systems diffusion for improving health systems performance: 1) dataset consensus; 2) HIS integration; 3) HIS sustainability.

Dataset Consensus

It is argued that although the problem with health information systems in developing countries is the absence of complete and quality data, planning ahead on how data will be used and by whom, and under what circumstances and constraints have implications for future accessibility of data from health systems (McGrail and Black 2005). Accordingly, one of the key features of an information system at the primary health care level is an *essential data set, which may be defined as a set of the most important data elements, selected from all primary health care vertical programmes, that should be reported by health service providers on a routine basis, with the aim of being able to generate indicators that monitor the provision of health services in an integrated manner (Shaw 2005: 632)*

From the above definition, the striking advantage presented by establishing an essential data set is the relevance of the data for local level use. It is also clear that establishing an essential (or minimum) data set for health information would most likely be fraught with a lot of challenges. Some of the difficult questions to resolve would include how to determine the "most important data elements", according to what criteria, and primarily serving what (or whose) purpose (Bowker and Star 1999). We can infer from the fragmented nature of the health system in developing countries that achieving any consensus would be even more difficult because of the multiple stakeholders and interests represented. The alternative is for health workers to collect numerous data for different overlapping projects without regard to the duplication of efforts and wastage of already scarce resource. This alternative is increasingly unacceptable and ways are being sought to address the issue. Without belittling the complexity of this process Shaw (2005) provides a framework for developing this essential data set using the experience of an HIS project in South Africa as an illustration. There are roughly two sides to the framework.

Firstly, data collection is stratified according to information needs along a hierarchical structure. This process is organised such that each level (e.g. national, state and local government) collects data relevant to their needs but only returns relevant data to the upper levels. Secondly, this progresses as a bottom-up approach but a minimum national dataset is negotiated and directed from a top-down process (Shaw, 2005).

Integrating HIS

As previously mentioned, a major obstacle for primary health care is the proliferation of uncoordinated vertical programmes. This has a direct spill over effect on information systems projects. In developing countries, health information systems are largely designed as silos of compartmentalised systems (Braa 2000). Employing the concepts of "historicity and heterogeneity," Aanestad *et al.* (2005) provide an extensive analysis of the challenges inherent in integrating health information systems in developing countries. The problem of historicity relates to the influence of institutionalised systems (e.g. legacy systems), established approaches and dominant values which contend with the introduction of novel health information systems (for theoretical discussion, see Ciborra 2002, Ciborra and Associates 2000 on standards and information infrastructures). Heterogeneity on the other hand, reflects the impact of multiple donor agencies funding stand-alone vertical systems without consideration for the interdependencies that exist across health programmes (Chilundo and Aanestad 2004). Consequently, the integration of HIS goes beyond establishing standards like "minimum data sets" (Shaw 2005) or integrating different technological artefacts but by necessity includes the alignment of divergent actor orientations, goals and rationalities (Smith *et al.* 2008). Given the scale of the challenge, "coping" with some level of HIS fragmentation is arguably inevitable (Aanestad et al 2005).

HIS Sustainability

Embedded in the general idea of sustainability are the notions of self-sustenance and sufficiency but HIS sustainability focuses more on the capacity of "user organisations to identify and manage risks that threaten the long-term viability of the HIS, following the withdrawal of external support" (Kimaro and Nhampossa 2005: 276). Kimaro and Nhampossa (2005: 276-277) further propose factors that militate against the sustainability of HIS: "inadequate infrastructure and human resource capacity; inappropriate policies and strategies to manage the sustainability problem and fragmented donor policy." To mitigate these factors, they propose that HIS must become a part of the operational day-to-day fabric of the "institutions" using them i.e. they must become "institutionalised". Their central arguments are summed up as follows: 1) sustainable HIS, in addition to being institutionalised, must be designed and developed in a way that is easily adaptable to changing user needs and requirements; 2) the implementation of a new HIS embodies values that would demand the "cultivation and institutionalisation of a new kind of culture"; 3) "donors influence the processes of institutionalisation, and thus the sustainability of systems significantly."

An important perspective to HIS sustainability is the idea of scalability. This concept argues that health information systems must be dynamic and flexibly designed. Otherwise, rigidity to a specific level of the health care will limit its impact on general health systems, greatly diminish its acceptability and face oppositions to its institutionalisation. Therefore HIS must be have the capacity to be either scaled up (to national) or down (to local) according to the health information hierarchy of needs (for more discussion, see: Bergqvist *et al.* 2006, Braa *et al.* 2004, Mengiste and Nielsen 2006, Sahay and Walsham 2006)

A Case of Alignment

The HIS literature illuminate the rationale underpinning an information-based health system. The challenges to achieving consensus on data, integrating and sustaining HIS implementation initiatives can be understood from a different dimension by exploring the entrenchment of health systems in the political intrigue highlighted in the literature on health care delivery strategies in developing countries. The literature first shows a muddle of top-down versus bottom-up approach to health systems development. Therefore HIS implementation strategies although seeking to develop locally relevant systems, must navigate the politically-charged terrain of macro-level initiatives which have direct influence on the information gathered at the local level, how it is analysed, interpreted, used and disseminated. In the same breadth that the historicity of information systems resemble an infrastructure which has a direct influence on the introduction of new technologies, so does the history of primary health care delivery in developing countries impact innovative systems which may attempt to change the course of history. This is in the sense that central and local government agents in developing countries have developed motivations and capacities over the years. These represent their distinctive characteristics. Therefore any initiative to improve primary health care delivery through better information systems or any other tool will require an alignment of sorts which first and foremost appreciates the current and historical reality and culture and in collaborative dialogue allow a more effective system to evolve. There is an expectation that the outworking of these integrations will also stimulate local participation, increase active engagement and provide stability necessary for long-term planning *(Chilundo and Aanestad 2003)*.

The motivation of this research project is therefore driven by the question: "How can we understand the characteristics of the local context in order to appreciate the challenges of primary care delivery in developing countries?" This is discussed in the next section.

Research Question

This article proposes that HIS analyses although contextual, can be better illuminated through the framework of political dynamics intrinsic to health systems performance. Similarly, Smith *et al.* (2008) also argue that HIS implementation solely founded on "managerialist grounds would tend to be subverted by the reality of long-standing political structures" (Smith, *et al.* 2008). The political dimensions of primary care delivery are thus essential in the domain of health systems performance. Therefore the question of this study is, "*What are the implications of a decentralised health sector on the performance of the health system?*" As a broad question, it is delimited and made more concrete by asking three distinct but interrelated sub-questions:

1. How does the decision space of local government actors impact primary health care? This question attempts to deploy the decision space approach in understanding the implications of decentralisation on primary health care delivery. By critically adopting this approach, the study conceptually investigates the factors underpinning health systems performance at the primary care level. The question is important in framing how the decentralised health sector operates and the perceived influence of the principal on the decision space of local agents. Theoretically, this approach states that the principal (e.g. Central or State government) is able to align the activities of the agent (e.g. local government officials) to its objective through a scheme of rewards and sanctions. On the other hand, it also observes that agents wield considerable influence because they produce contextual information required by the principal. This question therefore illuminates how this tension impacts the primary health care system.
2. In practice, what are the factors that shape, influence and determine the decision space? This is a more contextual question aimed at finding out the diverse instruments, belief systems and ideologies that actually influence decisions at the local level. From an empirical angle, this question will assess and query the primacy of a formal decision space in the context of developing countries where there is significantly reduced capacity of the principal to either reward good performance or punish aberrant activities. This question will therefore attempt to draw out the prominence of an informal decision space.
3. To what extent does information drive health care decisions? This question problematises the linear conceptualisation linking information, health delivery strategy and outcome. The question is critical because the resultant informal decision space has far-reaching implications for the institutional, political and socio-cultural arrangements which influence decision making and health systems performance. The question therefore provides a more insightful study into the diverse role of information in primary health care delivery and health systems performance.

ANALYTICAL FRAMEWORK

While the conceptual framework is implicit in the research questions it is important to highlight its key features and how it will be used in this study.

Theoretical Context

Bossert (1998) developed the concept of decision space as part of a comprehensive framework to analyse the decentralisation of health systems in developing countries. In developing this analytical framework, it is noted that decentralisation is an instrumental means to achieving "equity, efficiency, quality and financial soundness" (this article refers to these goals generally as the objectives of better performing health systems) (Bossert

1998). The rationale underpinning such analytical tool was based on the claim that there was no adequate means of analysing three constitutive aspects of decentralisation:

(1) the amount of choice that is transferred from central institutions to institutions at the periphery of health systems, (2) what choices local officials make with their increased discretion and (3) what effect these choices have on the performance of the health system (Bossert 1998: 1513).

Bossert suggests that the principal-agent approach is possibly the most illuminating framework with which to analyse decentralisation. At the heart of the principal-agent approach is the conceptualisation of the relationship between the centre and the local. He maintains that there are policy implications for how the centre can influence decisions made at the local level in such a way that will increase the likelihood of better performing health systems.

Conceptual Tool

According to the principal-agent approach, decentralisation is understood from the perspective of the principal who uses various strategies to align the activities of the agent in achieving the principal's objectives. These include rewards, punishments and the monitoring of compliance through information returns. According to Bossert, the weakness of this approach is that it does not provide a way of identifying the "range of choice allowed by decentralisation" (pg. 1517). The decision space approach is essentially a modification of the principal-agent approach such that it incorporates this spectrum of choice devolved from the centre to the local levels.

There are three broadly defining aspects of the decision space approach: 1) *mapping the boundaries of the space;* 2) *conceptualising the consequence of decision space on local choice;* 3) *analysing the performance implications of the space.*

For the purposes of the questions posed in this study, the decision space approach will be adapted as an analytical framework in the following ways:

- *Mapping the decision space boundary:* contents of national policy documents regarding the role and responsibilities of local governments in primary health care delivery will be discussed at a general level in descriptive terms. Emphasis will be placed on empirically investigating the actual (i.e. informal) decision space boundaries of local officials in Nigeria and the relational dynamics between central (analytically including State government) and local government agencies. The nature of this informal decision space will also be analysed to draw implications on the level of contestation that exist between the two levels of government. Data will be collected to illuminate these dynamics and subsequent analysis would be guided by three propositions of the framework. 1) the decision space is created by legislative act; 2) informal decision space exists when there is ineffective enforcement of legislation; 3) decision space may be contested by local officials.
- *Decision space and local choice:* the issue of choice and decision space will be investigated along the lines of the following singular proposition: the impact that the decision space (formal and informal but concentrating more on the latter) has on the kinds of choices made by local officials.
- *Decision Space and performance implications: t*he study will look at the implications of the following three propositions of this framework (from the local actors' perspective) on primary care health systems performance in Nigeria: 1) incentives and sanctions used by the principal to align interests according to the characteristics of the agent;

2) health information as a monitoring tool: this proposition will analyse the response and perception of local agents to information as a performance management tool; 3) health information as a reflection of health systems performance: this proposition will investigate the opinions of local agents to information as a vital public health resource with implications for health systems performance.

METHODOLOGY

The methodology adopted by this study is by nature reflexive and located within the tradition of interpretive qualitative research (Walsham 1995, 2006). This approach has two basic characteristics – interpretation and reflection. Interpretation implies that the multiple perceptions provided by participants involved in the field situation are taken to represent 'reality' and that these perceptions are then interpreted by the researcher according to the adopted theories about the domain of study (Geertz 1973). The reflexivity mentioned here is in the spirit of what Scott (2000) defined as "lived methodology". Reflexivity is viewed as an essential part of the research process by stimulating critical reflection on taken-for-granted theories, accounts and interpretations (Walsham 1995, 2006). According to this approach, the empirical material is not bound to fit the framework of theoretical ideas, rather it allows research findings to inform and reshape analytical conceptions. At the same time, this approach allows a certain degree of flexibility in accommodating creative and innovative interpretations of decentralisation in the developing country context without prejudging their relevance to current understanding of health systems performance. While the research will involve studying the policy, institutional, structural and social context within which decentralisation is implemented, the focal unit of analysis will be the primary health care unit.

Research Method

Myers (1997), with specific reference to IS research, critically analyses the use of four possible qualitative research methods e.g. grounded theory, ethnography, action research and case study research. This next section justifies the appropriateness of a case study method for this research project.

Case Study Research

Case study as a research method is used to empirically investigate "a contemporary phenomenon within its real life context, especially when the boundaries between phenomenon and context are not clearly evident" (Yin 2003: 13). This article argues that according to Yin's (2003) criteria and definition, this research topic is best investigated using a case study method. Although in building the context of this study it is necessary to include historical and "processual" analysis (Pettigrew 1997), the principal focus of the investigation will concentrate on contemporary challenges of primary health care provision in Nigeria. From another perspective, case studies can also be employed for building new analytical frameworks (Eisenhardt 1989) for understanding the complexity of primary health care delivery.

This research employs a single-case design which gathers different perspectives within the Nigerian public health system but all these perspectives serve as a representative type of primary health care delivery (for example Shaw *et al.* 2007). These different perspectives are from different levels of the primary health care system. For instance, health information systems national consultant, State public health director, Community physician, Local family physician, general practitioner and Facility health care worker. These perspectives also have a wide geographic span ranging from East, West, North, South and Middle-belt.

The circumstance under which it would be suitable to conduct a single case study is when the case is either "critical," "unique," "typical," "revelatory" or "longitudinal," (Yin 2003:41-42). Accordingly, the choice of a single-case design is justifiable from the viewpoint of the case being representative i.e. "typical". The next section introduces a more concrete discussion of data collection methods including the unit of analysis and how these methodological considerations were translated in the fieldwork research.

Data Collection Methods

Interviews are arguably the most significant means of gathering qualitative data and semi-structured interviews the most widely used in information systems research (Myers and Newman 2007). Accordingly, the primary data collection method for this project was made up of five semi-structured telephone interviews of Nigerian primary care practitioners. This included: former state Director of Public Health, Permanent Secretary and current Head of Department of Community Medicine and Primary Care; Senior Registrar Family Medicine; and three primary care doctors. Information was also gleaned from personal communication with an health information system consultant in Nigeria.. Copious amounts of notes were taken during each interview after which they were word processed immediately. The main criteria for choosing interviewees were the depth of experience in their respective level of primary health care in Nigeria, the breadth of knowledge including levels of health care delivery and geographical location, understanding of the political dimension of delivering primary health care.

The substantive questions asked were related to the complexities of primary health care delivery in Nigeria. These questions were classified along the three sub-questions of the research project. The particular focus was on the experiences of local practitioners and their perspective regarding the influence of local and central government agents on the delivery of primary health care. Anecdotal or illustrative responses were encouraged especially where they provide a rich description of the situation.

To ensure reliability of data, evidence is triangulated from the different data sources to evaluate the congruence of opinions. Where there is a divergence of ideas, this is followed up by seeking clarity from the respondent after presenting the contrary view. In addition feedback was given to all interviewees to give them a chance to clarify the interpretations given by the researcher. Most of the interviewees were conducted over a couple of days which also gave room for reflection by both the respondent and the researcher.

The data is expected to serve as evidence in three main ways. First, the analysis and discussion should serve as a tool in persuading the audience of a more complex dynamic at work in delivering primary health care at the local level. Secondly, the evidence should be contextually rich enough to show that primary care delivery is not only technically challenging both also politically intricate.

Data Analysis and Discussion

In order to produce data that are more reflective of reality, data analysis will be conducted through the identified propositions of the conceptual framework and the researcher's informed intuition (Valsiner 2000). Under each proposition, themes from different data sources are highlighted, detailing the most recurring or significantly pronounced themes for the narrative analysis.

Understanding Decentralisation and Health Systems Performance in Nigeria

This section presents the findings from the field in an analytical way by adopting the framework propositions to discuss the evidence from the field. The analysis captures the main areas of input from all interviewees and represents the chain of recurring themes. Where this is not the case, a clear indication of the data source and the counter views are provided (interestingly, this only occurs in the discussion relating to the perceived quality and role of information in primary health care). An attempt is made to analyse these variations using the analytical framework and the researcher's understanding of the field.

Mapping the Decision Boundary

Decision Space: An Act of Legislation

Under the Nigerian *concurrent legislative list*, the constitution allows the provision of a decentralised health care system within the three tiers of government i.e. Federal, State and Local. General and specialist hospitals are principally assigned to the State and Federal government respectively and primary health care is provided by the local government. Having said this, the State and Federal government still provide technical assistance to the local government for instance on polio immunisation and rollback Malaria programme.

Primary health care is the first level of health care delivery service. It is community based therefore patients are only referred to general hospitals or specialist tertiary hospitals if this transfer is deemed necessary at the primary care level. There are three main delivery strategies: 1) health promotion including health education; 2) prevention of diseases (particularly communicable diseased) and immunisation programmes; and 3) provision of facilities for early diagnosis of diseases.

To deliver these functions, the primary care system comprises of health centres, clinics and posts. The health posts are the most remote, providing the most basic form of health care service. It typically operates as an outpatient facility. Health clinics mainly consist of maternity centres and dispensaries. They provide the treatment of minor diseases like malaria and diarrhoea. In the primary health system, health centres are the closest representation of hospitals. They provide extensive preventive health services including health promotion (e.g. environmental sanitation and education on personal hygiene). They also provide the diagnosis and treatment of diseases.

It is therefore constitutionally recognised that local government agents have the principal authority and responsibility for fulfilling these functions under the primary health care system. However, by legislation, the operations of the local government primary health care are directly supervised by the State Ministry of Health (SMOH) who is then accountable to the Federal Ministry of Health (FMOH). The local government reports to SMOH and these report annually and quarterly to the FMOH. One of the direct consequences of a weak accountability structure is presence of a considerably large informal decision space.

Informal Decision Space

In practice, there is no enforceable accountability structure at the local level. The oversight of the FMOH is across a wide distance therefore logistics are difficult for the FMOH which is based in the Capital, Abuja. There is also the issue of misplaced empathy and priority regarding the development of the health system in Nigeria. The FMOH gives an inordinate amount of attention to building hospitals and to curative medical approaches, even though this is not in concert with the national health policy. In effect, local government officials are not only autonomous but a significant proportion of their activities are carried out through an informal decision space.

In terms of proximity, the State has a better chance of being more effective in supervising PHC delivery because all medical officers from the local government meet monthly at the State level. Notwithstanding, the local health system is rife with general political apathy and instability. In theory, constituents can make complaints to the State regarding local government agents who do not deliver according to their terms of office. The State then calls the Local Government Chairman to account. If they can't defend their position then sanctions may be considered.

This is however highly unlikely. The SMOH does not have the capacity to either sanction or reward local government officials. The practical option is usually to appeal to their better judgement and sense of duty when they come together at the monthly meetings. In addition, downward accountability to local constituents does not really exist because of an endemic problem with the democratic process: voting is perceived as dangerous and so most people stay away instead of risking their lives. Therefore, local constituents have limited electoral power to call their public representatives to order because of the immature state of the democratic system.

The activities of local government agents are typified by self interest and excessive corruption. Even though there is a concerted effort by the federal government to curtail behaviours of corruption, the commissions set up to enforce this (i.e. National Anti-Corruption Commission and Economic and Financial Crimes Commission), are themselves perceived to be susceptible to corruption and are therefore ineffective. The ineffective enforcement of the formal decision space mapped out by legislation therefore produces a thriving informal decision space at the local level. Nigeria's primary health care system is perceived to be run by local officials who are not bound either by Federal or State health policy imperatives or legislation. There is therefore a different kind of contestation regarding the decision space afforded these local agents.

Decision Space Contested

Instead of local agents seeking a wider decision space, public health practitioners are seeking to extricate the functional delivery of PHC from the influence of politicians. Among other things, they argue that the bureaucratic bottleneck affects the effectiveness of the service provided. Some examples are that, requisitions are intolerably delayed before being fulfilled and immunisation exercises undertaken are not paid for in time. There is therefore a contention that health care delivery should not be run by government but possibly by health boards. This autonomy will include budget facilities and financial independence for public health practitioners.

Public health practitioners ascribe to the view that primary health care is a vital public health service with particular outreach to the poor. Their contention is not regarding the State provision of this service as a public good but its operational involvement. Therefore they protest that a lot more should be done to encourage initiatives such as the National Health Insurance Scheme because they are run by Health Maintenance Organisations and are therefore more accountable and scrutinised. In this case, Government should cater for the poor through a social security system but the primary health care service would still be provided by a third party.

As a summary, we observe that legislation allows the decentralisation of the health sector in Nigeria. However, the lack of an effective enforcement structure leads to a situation where the informal decision space is more prominent than the formal. Consequently, the exception becomes the rule and conceptually speaking, anomaly reigns. There is also a sense that the lack of enforcement is not primarily due to capability but the informal decision space thrives because the FMOH is not really interested in primary health but tertiary health care. Therefore, primary health care is invariably inefficient and the general health system essentially underperforming.

Decision Space and Local Choice

Local Choice Within an Informal Space

The choices made by local government officials have primarily been not to pay adequate attention to primary health care issues. Most of these officers are there for their own selfish reasons because the remuneration for holding this post has recently become more attractive and therefore people vie for these offices without an interest of the community at heart. This attitude affects the local delivery of health services adversely. Local government choices are based on politics and not need. Even those who would like to make a positive difference are constrained because as politicians the feel obliged to payback their election campaign sponsors who strongly influence the political agenda.

For instance, some of these choices translate into charging for immunisation which is meant to be provided free of charge. Another illustration is that the General Hospital which the State government says should be provided free health services at the point of delivery have become an operational farce. The only service which ends up being free is the initial consultation. The required drugs are invariably out of stock. This is because only a proportion of the allocation makes it to the hospital in the first place, the consignment that makes it most conveniently find its way to the nearest pharmacy where more money will be paid for it. When patients come for drugs, they are directed to the nearest pharmacy.

Some of the more substantive factors that influence local choice include the background of the local government chairman. Where this is a health background, there seems to be a better appreciation of PHC otherwise it is treated as least priority. Highly educated local government agents also contribute to the level of attention PHC receives. Other factors also depend on the agenda of influential personalities who may want to boast about their local government area and therefore lobby politicians for rapid health care development programmes in their area. The effect of these diverse influences can be seen where for instance there is a local government area with a population of five thousand being served by three health care centres while another population of seventy thousand does not have any health care centres.

Decision Space and Performance

In Nigeria, a large proportion of the community is rural (it is estimated that about three quarters of the population live in rural areas). This has serious implication for the health profile of the country. For instance, in spite of how sophisticated health service delivery is in the urban areas, this improvement only represents a significantly small proportion of the total population. Similarly, the lack of vital public infrastructures for health delivery in rural areas combined with the high level of poverty in these areas has resulted in the poor health status of the country as a whole. The primary health care service has a major role in determining the overall performance of the health system. However, PHCs in Nigeria are not efficient and there are significant difference between the extensive policy formulations at the centre and action at the local level. Even thought there are extensive policy directives on providing primary health care it is usually either ignored or not followed.

Incentives and Sanctions

To compound this issue, financial and non-financial incentives or sanctions are not applicable in the Nigerian context. In addition to the absence of an effective enforcement structure, the local government has an independent budget allocation and therefore the FMOH is not responsible for salaries of local PHC officials. The regime of incentives and sanctions are therefore too weak to bring about any substantial change in the local government's primary health care performance.

Nonetheless, the evaluation of health care delivery is conducted through the monitoring of health information.

Health Information as a Monitoring Tool

The local government sends required health information to the SMOH. These are received by career officers who normally should collate, analyse and verify the results but this is rarely done (if at all). Apart from the fact that there are very limited visits from the SMOH to verify data returns, when do visits do happen local governments are notified in advance, defeating the purpose of the exercise.

As an illustration, in one of the supposedly largest State hospitals serving a local government area, there have only been 3 visitations by the State Monitoring Teams and 1 visit by the federal government in the last 6 years. In fact, the purpose of the FG visit was to evaluate the feasibility of the hospital being a centre for AIDS treatment as supposed to monitoring the performance returns of the hospital.

In order to save face and not be found wanting, potentially damaging health data is often manipulated before being reported to the upper levels. For example there has been a programme of polio eradication every two months for the last one year where all children under five are supposed to be immunised however, polio is still widespread but the federal government does not report this. It is often said that anyone who knows anything about the health care system in Nigeria will not trust the health records.

Health Information as Health Systems Performance

The problems with reliable health records are much more nuanced as a component strategy of general public health. Information management is very crucial to primary health care in terms of health planning, disease monitoring and surveillance etc. There is a view from the Director of Public Health that primary health care in Nigeria has a good information management system. The argument is that prior to any intervention programme in a locality, a situational analysis is conducted to identity the main health problems and need. Therefore subsequent action is based on concrete and well studied information. From an operational management level, the State Primary Health Doctor's perception is also that health workers in the rural areas take data recording seriously. In addition, they are said to be meticulous in reporting the information they collect to the extent that some go out of their way to ensure accuracy. However, it is noted that there is another extreme set of workers who are unscrupulous regarding information collection. For example, an independent examiner on the programme for Polio eradication noted the "super-efficiency" with which certain health workers had administered the vaccinations and had logged all the information. On further investigated she realised that the vaccines had been disposed of and the time was spent meticulously cooking the log books.

Some other public health doctors (e.g. in the local government and private sector) however feel that many health workers don't appreciate data collection probably due to their level of education but still collect the data because it is mandatory. They admit that some errors in the data may suggest that health workers may not be as meticulous as community health physicians. Nonetheless, there is a view that it is highly unlikely that health workers would intentionally fabricate data especially since the data reported have to tally with other stakeholder data and reports (e.g. drug consignments).

There are two categories of data collation: the first is on disease surveillance and notification, the second is on monitoring and evaluation. A designated local primary care officer collects weekly disease surveillance data from primary health centres including some private establishments. These data focus on specific epidemic prone diseases like cholera. These data are sent to the SMOH epidemiologist who analyses the figures to see if an epidemic prevalence threshold has been broken. A monitoring and evaluation officer collects data from peripheral facilities monthly. These facilities ideally fill in the National Health Information Management System form everyday. Data collected include drugs dispensed, family planning, deliveries, treatments etc. Health data for the month are verified by the community health physician before being reported to the SMOH.

Generally, the reality of practice is that data reliability is not a priority in the primary health care system. As such there are no field surveys—conducted at either the local or state level—to verify the data reported. Data reliability is a major problem in Nigeria to the extent that there are even problems with the national census.

Assuming that records collected at the primary care level is mostly reliably. The data is rarely analysed and when analysed seldom lead to concrete action plans which will improve performance of the primary health care. There is therefore a substantial gap between information, policy and action. For example, when polio was reported at a local government area there was only one follow-up when there should have been a few.

Closely related to this is the fact that there is no feedback structure for local health practitioners to review the data submitted in light of a set performance target. There is a notion that the absence of feedback is partly due to the lack of appreciation of the effect it can have on performance at the ground level. Apart from the lack of appreciation, it is also suggested that local agents shy away from the additional cost of getting extra resources to fulfil this role.

There is evidence however to suggest that when the occasional feedback is given, it proves highly effective. For example, a feedback workshop on immunisation, which showed the performance level of a particular local government, motivated workers to try and bridge the gap between target and performance. This reaction is usually more accentuated when there is a comparison with other local government areas or states.

Empirical Findings and Framework Critique

Mapping the Decision Boundary

Nigeria has had a long-standing decentralised health system (Gupta *et al.* 2003). The framework helps to insightfully analyse the tensions that exist between the central and local agents in the delivery of primary health care. Furthermore, it gives clear indications regarding the objectives of a decentralised health system i.e. equity, efficiency, quality and financial soundness.

The decision space lens also helped illuminate the circumstances under which an informal decision space might be created e.g. lack of effective enforcement. In the context of the Nigerian health sector, this was clearly an issue which had unquestionable impact on the delivery of primary health care. The framework however, did not provide tools for understanding how to interpret a situation where the informal decision space is the norm rather than the anomaly and how to understand its potential impact on the performance of the health system (this would be discussed further in the conclusion). While there are definite decision boundaries for the delivery of primary health care at the local level, the peculiar nature of the informal decision space somewhat makes the discussion about the range of choice available to local agents irrelevant. The reality on the ground suggests that there are no effective structures to enforce formally defined choices at the local level. Choices made regarding primary health care are therefore practically autonomous. Consequently, the focus of this analytical framework on local agents contesting or negotiating for a wider decision space is not applicable. The contestation is however present in a more classic debate about the role of the State in providing public services (this theme would also be elaborated in the concluding sections).

Decision Space and Local Choice

While the original framework conceives the range of choices available to local agents in concrete terms (i.e. finance, human resource, facilities etc), this study adopts the notion of choice as an empirical object. That is, the effective and actual perception of choices applicable in the field. This is because, the PHC choices made at the local level in Nigeria are analysed through the perspective of an informal decision space. The analysis showed a prevalence of apathy towards health delivery and self-serving motivations. While it is evident that this has been detrimental to the primary care system in Nigeria, the framework highlighted that the particular characteristics of the local government in terms of motivations and capacity affects health systems performance. In the Nigerian context, there seemed to be an association between the local government agents' professional background (including level of education) and the delivery of primary health care. Suggesting that agent's with a medical background and high level of education are usually more motivated and capable of effectively delivering primary health care. The framework was therefore useful albeit through a slight modification of focus being more on the informal decision space.

Decision Space and Performance

The notion of control to achieve better health systems performance was not well developed in this framework. The analytical weight is predominantly skewed towards the principal i.e. central or state. The suggestions of an incentive or sanction strategy were not really useful in understanding health decentralisation and performance in the Nigerian context. This is partly because this section of the analytical tool is built on the assumptions of a formal decision space (which is by and large insignificant in practice). Nevertheless, the framework also indicates that the local agents also wield some influence over the principal because they generate and own contextual information needed by the principal. This provided a little more ammunition in understanding decision space and performance through the dimension of information. The study for instance was able to highlight how the local agents can manipulate data in order to cover up their poor performance. This analysis was also quite superficial because of the instrumental view of information portrayed in the framework.

In the concluding section, this article suggests how some concepts from the development and information systems literature might be able to provide a richer and more robust analytical approach to studying the link between local agent's decision space and performance.

To bring all the component parts of the study together, Figure 1 attempts to provide a brief snapshot of the links between the primary questions of this research project and its findings. This is done by operationalizing the research questions through specific analytical propositions and justifying the findings through exemplary evidence from the field.

CONCLUSION

In developing countries the study of decentralisation and health systems performance incorporates the analysis of an intricate web of agencies and institutional structures. This research project approached the problem domain from the perspective of tensions generated between the local level being agents and upper government levels (e.g. State and Federal) being principals. In particular, it investigated how the devolution of decision-making authority to local government agents (i.e. decision space) impact on the primary health care system. The following conclusions of this study navigate the subtle conceptual and empirical nuances of this problem domain.

Figure 1. Synthesising research questions, propositions and evidence

Analytical Proposition	Findings	Data Source: Evidence
Research Question: How does the decision space of local government actors impact primary health care?		
Decision Space: an act of legislation	**Local government actors provide PHC because Nigeria has a decentralised health system defined by legislation i.e. in the concurrent legislative list.**	Primary health care is provided by the local government, Secondary health by the State and Tertiary health care by the Federal government.
Incentives and Sanctions	**The informal decision space of local actors is detrimental to the delivery of primary health care in Nigeria because the State and Federal Government do not have the capacity to offer incentives or sanctions based on performance.**	**HIS Consultant:** "…at this stage the SMoH does not have teeth by which to either punish or reward LGAs that achieve or do not meet their targets"
Research Question: In practice, what are the factors that shape, influence and determine the decision space		
Informal Decision Space	**The absence of an effective enforcement structure resulted in an informal decision space**	**Director of Public Health:** "…level of corruption is abnormal… Motivation of agents is to satisfy themselves and line their pockets…"
Decision Space Contested	**Decision space not contested by local agents but by health practitioners**	**Senior Registrar Family Medicine** "Health care delivery should not be run by government. A lot more should be done to encourage the National Health Insurance Scheme."
Local Choice within an Informal Space	**Background, level of education and motivation of local actors influence the choices they make about primary health care**	**Community Physician** "level of education of LG Chairman also contributes to PHC effectiveness (most are just average)… the renumeration is attractive, therefore there is no interest of the community at heart."
Research Question: To what extent does information drive health care decisions?		
Health information as a monitoring tool	**Health information is subject to manipulation and divergent political agenda**	**PHC Doctor (Private Sector):** "Non-governmental parastatals records have accurate data reflecting health conditions but government information may be dubious."
Health information as health systems performance	**Diverse range of information quality, lack of feedback mechanism; performance indicators are primarily constructs**	**PHC Doctor (Public Sector):** "If you have people on the ground, there is usually no question about the reliability of data reported…" "The problem is that people don't do their job, they shirk their duties and make up figures…" "Some LG conduct research on the ground and feed it into policy and action…"

Weak State, Rogue Agent: Complementary Vices

The findings of the study suggest that where you have a weak principal, agents will operate predominantly through an informal decision space. The formal decision space therefore serves as a platform for breeding unaccountable local agents. However, in developing countries, it is not just the lack of an accountability structure (see Abouzahr *et al.* 2005) that necessarily leads to the poor delivery of primary health care and the failing health system. Rather, the motivation and capacity of local agents also have some influence in determining the quality of primary health care in a particular locality. In the absence of a competent State to enforce the boundaries of a formal decision space, self-seeking local government officials exploit the opportunity to indulge in unscrupulous activities with public finances at the expense of the local health system.

The access of poor people to health care facilities are not only curtailed but their right to influence issues regarding their health is also limited. For public health systems to be effective, people have to take an active part in shaping health care strategies (Macfarlane *et al.* 2000). This necessitates a rethinking for national health policy makers to institute a public health system that collaborates with local actors to reflect the diversity of local needs as indicated by the local communities (see Newell 1989).

Information is an Elusive Reality

Developing countries face a host of challenges at different stages and functions of the primary care information process (Godlee *et al.* 2004). At the technical level, although the process is fairly routinized, the reliability of the data collected rests on the competence and motivation of health workers. A lack of appreciation for data may be due to not understanding how this data actually fits into the bigger picture of health care delivery. However, without a visible feedback and data verification structure, this exercise would only be perceived as theoretical. As supported by this study, the managerial imperative which views information as a monitoring and control instrument (Berg 2001) has been widely criticised as narrowly conceived in the information systems field (Ciborra 2000, Kallinikos 2006) .

In conclusion, this study explores the significant contextual factors which have far-reaching implications for the implementation and use of health information systems for improving health care delivery in developing country context. As far as it is exploratory, the study has not been particularly concrete in investigating a grounded HIS project. The viewpoint of the researcher, which was substantiated through this study, is that most matters in developing countries (and especially in the domain of health care) do not warrant the centrality of technology because a rich understanding can often be obtained by studying the social and political foundations on which previous technological initiatives have been built.

REFERENCES

Aanestad, M., *et al.* (2005) "Strategies for Development and Integration of Health Information Systems: Coping with Historicity and Heterogeneity", *Information Systems Group Working Article: University of Oslo,* 5.

AbouZahr, C., & Boerma, T. (2005). Health Information Systems: The Foundations of Public Health. *Bulletin of the World Health Organization*, *83*(8), 578–583.

Adeyemo, A. (2005). Local Government and Health Care Delivery in Nigeria: A Case Study. *Journal of Human Ecology (Delhi, India)*, *18*(2), 149–160.

Alvarez, A. J. S. (2003). Towards an Interpretative Integrative Framework to Conceptualise Social Processes in Large Information Systems Implementations. *Information Technology for Development, 10*, 233–247. doi:10.1002/itdj.1590100403

Atkinson, S. (1995). Restructuring Health Care: Tracking the Decentralization Debate. *Progress in Human Geography, 19*(4), 486–503. doi:10.1177/030913259501900403

Atkinson, S., Fernandes, L., Caprara, S., & Gideon, J. (2005). Prevention and Promotion in Decentralized Rural Health Systems: A Comparative Study from Northeast Brazil. *Health Policy and Planning, 20*(2), 69–79. doi:10.1093/heapol/czi009

Atkinson, S., Medeiros, R., Oliveira, P., & Dias de Almeida, R. (2000). Going Down to the Local: Incorporating Social Organisation and Political Culture into Assessments of Decentralised Health Care. *Social Science & Medicine, 51*, 619–636. doi:10.1016/S0277-9536(00)00005-8

Berg, M. (2001). Implementing Information Systems in Health Care Organizations: Myths and Challenges. *International Journal of Medical Informatics, 64*, 143–146. doi:10.1016/S1386-5056(01)00200-3

Bergqvist, J., Dahlberg, P., & Ljungberg, F. (2006) *Scalability through Cultivation. Designing It Support for Co-Ordination Work* Last accessed: 6 February 2007 Last updated: Address: http://citeseer.ist.psu.edu/cache/articles/cs/23947/http:zSzzSzwww.dahlberg.sezSzpubzSzmaster.pdf/scalability-through-cultivation-designing.pdf.

Berman, P. (Ed.). (1995). *Health Sector Reform: Making Health Development Sustainable*. Boston: Harvard University Press.

Berman, P., & Bossert, T. (2000). *Appraising a Decade of Health Sector Reform in Developing Countries*. Washington, DC: Havard School of Public Health.

Bhasker, R. (1998). Philosophy and Scientific Realism. In Archer, M., Bhasker, R., Collier, A., Lawson, T., & Norrie, A. (Eds.), *Critical Realism: Essential Readings* (pp. 16–48). London: Routledge.

Blaauw, D., Gilson, L., Penn-Kekana, L., & Schneider, H. (2003). *"Organisational Relationships and the 'Software' of Health Sector Reform. Background Article Disease Control Priorities Project (Dcpp) Capacity Strengthening and Management Reform" Centre for Health Policy, Schoolff Public Health*. University of The Witwatersrand.

Bossert, T. (1979). Health Policies in Africa and Latin America: Adopting the Primary Care Approach. *Social Science & Medicine, 13*(C), 65.

Bossert, T. (1998). Analyzing the Decentralization of Health Systems in Developing Countries: Decision Space, Innovation and Performance. *Social Science & Medicine, 47*(10), 1513–1527. doi:10.1016/S0277-9536(98)00234-2

Bowker, G., & Star, S. (1999). *Sorting Things Out: Classification and Its Consequences*. Cambridge, MA: The MIT Press.

Braa, J. (2000) "Developing District-Based Health Care Information Systems: The South African Experience". in *Proceedings of IRIS 23. Laboratorium for Interaction Technology,* University of Trollhättan Uddevalla, Braa, J., *et al.* (2001) "A Study of the Actual and Potential Usage of Information and Communication Technology at District and Provincial Levels in Mozambique with a Focus on the Health Sector", *EJISDC,* 5 (2), pp. 1-29.

Braa, J., Monteiro, E., & Sahay, S. (2004). Networks of Action: Sustainable Health Information Systems across Developing Countries. *MIS Quarterly: Management Information Systems, 28*(3), 337–362.

Buse, K., & Watt, G. (1996). Aid Coordination for Health Sector Reform: A Conceptual Framework for Analysis and Assessment. *Health Policy (Amsterdam)*, *38*, 173–187. doi:10.1016/0168-8510(96)00855-X

Chatora, R., & Tumusime, P. (2004). Primary Health Care: A Review of Its Implementation in Sub-Saharan Africa. *Primary Health Care Research and Development*, *5*, 296–306. doi:10.1191/1463423604pc220oa

Chilundo, B., & Aanestad, M. (2003) "Vertical of Integrated Health Programmes? The Consequence for the Laboratory Information Systems in Mozambique". in *Electronic Proceedings of the IFIP TC8 & TC9. WG8.2 + 9.4 Working Conference on Information Systems Perspectives and Challenges in the Context of Globalization,* Athens, Greece, Chilundo, B. and M. Aanestad (2004) "Negotiating Multiple Rationalities in the Process of Integrating the Information Systems of Disease-Specific Health Programmes", *EJISDC,* 20 (2), pp. 1-28.

Ciborra, C. (Ed.). (2000). *From Control to Drift. The Dynamics of Corporate Information Infrastructures*. Oxford: Oxford University Press.

Ciborra, C. (2000). *From Control to Drift: The Dynamics of Corporate Information Infrastructure*. Oxford: Oxford University Press.

Ciborra, C. (2002). *The Labyrinths of Information: Challenging the Wisdom of Systems*. Oxford: Oxford University Press.

Collins, C., & Green, A. (1994). Decentralization and Primary Health Care: Some Negative Implications in Developing Countries. *International Journal of Health Services*, *24*(3), 459–475.

Cornia, G. A. (2001). Globalization and Health: Results and Options. *Bulletin of the World Health Organization*, *79*, 834–841.

Cornwall, A., Lucas, H., & Pasteur, K. (2000). Introduction: Accountability through Participation:Developing Workable Partnership Models in the Health Sector. *IDS Bulletin*, *31*(1), 1–13. doi:10.1111/j.1759-5436.2000.mp31001001.x

Cueto, M. (2004). The Origins of Primary Health Care and Selective Primary Health Care. *American Journal of Public Health*, *94*(11), 1864–1874. doi:10.2105/AJPH.94.11.1864

Deaton, A. (2003). Health, Inequality, and Economic Development. *Journal of Economic Literature*, *XLI*, 113–158. doi:10.1257/002205103321544710

Dobrow, M., Goel, V., & Upshur, R. (2004). Evidence-Based Health Policy: Context and Utilisation. *Social Science & Medicine*, *58*, 207–217. doi:10.1016/S0277-9536(03)00166-7

Eisenhardt, K. (1989). Building Theories from Case Study Research. *Academy of Management Review*, *14*(4), 532–550. doi:10.2307/258557

Filmer, D., Pritchett, L., & Hammer, J. (1998). *Health Policy in Poor Countries: Weak Links in the Chain?*Washington, D.C.: World Bank, Development Research Group, Poverty and Human Resources.

Gallup, J. L. and J. D. Sachs (2001) "The Economic Burden of Malaria", *The American Society of Tropical Medicine and Hygiene,* 64 (1,2), pp. 85-96.

Garrett, L. (2007) *The Challenge of Global Health* Foreign Affairs Last accessed: 1 March 2007 Last updated: Address: http://www.foreignaffairs.org/20070101faessay86103/laurie-garrett/the-challenge-of-global-health.html.

Geertz, C. (1973). *The Interpretation of Cultures*. New York: Basic Books.

Godlee, F. (2004). Can We Achieve Health Information for All by 2015. *Lancet*, *364*, 295–300. doi:10.1016/S0140-6736(04)16681-6

Goodman, N. (1978). *Ways of Worldmaking*. Indianapolis: Hackett.

Green, A. (1999). *An Introduction to Health Planning in Developing Countries* (2nd ed.). Oxford: Oxford University Press.

Griffith, J. A. G. (1966) Central Departments and Local Authorities. University of Toronto Press, Toronto, Ont.

Gupta, M., Gauri, V., & Khemani, S. (2003). *"Decentralized Delivery of Primary Health Services in Nigeria. Survey Evidence from the States of Lagos and Kogi" The world Bank*. Africa Region.

Gwatkin, D. (2000). Critical Reflection: Health Inequalities and the Health of the Poor. What Do We Know? What Can We Do? *Bulletin of the World Health Organization*, *78*(1), 3–18.

Hall, J. J., & Taylor, R. (2003). Health for All Beyond 2000: The Demise of the Alma-Ata Declaration and Primary Health Care in Developing Countries. *The Medical Journal of Australia*, *178*(1), 17–20.

Heeks, R. (2006). Health Information Systems: Failure, Success and Improvisation. *International Journal of Medical Informatics*, *75*, 125–137. doi:10.1016/j.ijmedinf.2005.07.024

Jamison, D., & Mosley, W. (1991). Disease Control Priorities in Developing Countries: Health Policy Responses to Epidemiological Change. *American Journal of Public Health*, *81*(1), 15–22. doi:10.2105/AJPH.81.1.15

Jeppsson, A., & Okuonzi, S. A. (2000). Vertical or Holistic Decentralization of the Health Sector? Experiences from Zambia and Uganda. *The International Journal of Health Planning and Management*, *15*(4), 273–289. doi:10.1002/hpm.597

Kallinikos, J. (2006). *The Consequences of Inffor-mation. Institutional Implications of Technological Change*. Cheltenham: Edward Elgar.

Kimaro, H., & Nhampossa, J. (2005). Analysing the Problem of Unsustainable Health Information Systems in Less-Developed Economies: Case Studies from Tanzania and Mozambique. *Information Technology for Development*, *11*(3), 273–298. doi:10.1002/itdj.20016

Klein, H., & Myers, M. (1999). A Set of Principles for Conducting and Evaluating Interpretive Field Studies. *Management Information Systems Quarterly*, *23*(1), 67–93. doi:10.2307/249410

Lee, K. (1998). Shaping the Future of Global Health Cooperation: Where Can We Go from Here? *Lancet*, *351*, 899–902. doi:10.1016/S0140-6736(97)11455-6

Littlejohns, P., Wyatt, J. C., & Garvican, L. (2003). Evaluating Computerised Health Information Systems: Hard Lessons Still to Be Learnt. *BMJ (Clinical Research Ed.)*, *326*, 860–863. doi:10.1136/bmj.326.7394.860

Loewenson, R. (1993). Structural Adjustment and Health Policy in Africa. *International Journal of Health Services*, *23*(4), 717–730.

Macfarlane, S., Racelis, M., & Muli-Musiime, F. (2000). Public Health in Developing Countries. *Lancet*, *356*, 841–846. doi:10.1016/S0140-6736(00)02664-7

Magnussen, L., Ehiri, J., & Jolly, P. (2004). Comprehensive Versus Selective Primary Health Care: Lessons for Global Health Policy. *Health Affairs*, *23*(3), 167–176. doi:10.1377/hlthaff.23.3.167

Masaiganah, M. S. (2004). Primary Health Care for the People: Health Policy in Tanzania. *Development*, *47*(2), 136–139. doi:10.1057/palgrave.development.1100041

McGrail, K., & Black, C. (2005). Access to Data in Health Information Systems. *Bulletin of the World Health Organization*, *83*(8), 563.

McMichael, C., Waters, E., & Volmick, J. (2005). Evidence-Based Public Health: What Does It Offer Developing Countries? *Journal of Public Health*, *27*(2), 215–221. doi:10.1093/pubmed/fdi024

McPake, B., & Banda, E. (1994). Contracting out of Health Services in Developing Countries. *Health Policy and Planning*, *9*(1), 25–30. doi:10.1093/heapol/9.1.25

Mengiste, S., & Nielsen, P. (2006) *Scaling Health Information Systems in Developing Countries: On the Essence of Being Installed Base Friendly* Last accessed: 6 February 2007 Last updated: Address: http://www.itu.dk/iris29/IRIS29/14-5.pdf.

Mills, A. (2004). The Performance of Different Models of Primary Care Provision in Southern Africa. *Social Science & Medicine*, *59*(5), 931–943. doi:10.1016/j.socscimed.2003.12.015

Murray, C., & Frenk, J. (2001). World Health Report 2000: A Step Towards Evidence-Based Health Policy. *Lancet*, *357*, 1698–1700. doi:10.1016/S0140-6736(00)04826-1

Myers, M. (1997). Qualitative Research in Information Systems. *MISQ Quarterly*, *21*(2), 241–242. doi:10.2307/249422

Myers, M. D., & Newman, M. (2007). The Qualitative Interview in Is Research: Examining the Craft. *Information and Organization*, *X*(x).

Newell, K. (1989). The Way Ahead for District Health Systems. *World Health Forum*, *10*(1), 80–87.

Niessen, L., Grijseels, E., & Rutten, F. (2000). The Evidenced-Based Approach in Health Policy and Health Care Delivery. *Social Science & Medicine*, *51*, 859–869. doi:10.1016/S0277-9536(00)00066-6

Okuonzi, S. A., & Macrae, J. (1995). Whose Policy Is It Anyway? International and National Influences on Health Policy Development in Uganda. *Health Policy and Planning*, *10*(2), 122–132. doi:10.1093/heapol/10.2.122

Paglin, M. (1974). Public Health and Development: A New Analytical Framework. *Economica, New Series*, *41*(164), 432–441. doi:10.2307/2553354

Peters, D., & Chao, S. (1998). The Sector-Wide Approach in Health: What Is It? Where Is It Going? *The International Journal of Health Planning and Management*, *13*, 177–190. doi:10.1002/(SICI)1099-1751(199804/06)13:2<177::AID-HPM504>3.0.CO;2-T

Pettigrew, A. (1997). What Is a Processual Analysis? *Scandinavian Journal of Management*, *13*(4), 337–348. doi:10.1016/S0956-5221(97)00020-1

Rhodes, R. A. W. (1986). *The National World of Local Government*. London: Allen and Unwin.

Sachs, J. (2004). Ending Africa's Poverty Trap. *Brookings Articles on Economic Activity*, *1*, 117–240. doi:10.1353/eca.2004.0018

Sahay, S., & Walsham, G. (2006). Scaling Health Information Systems in India: Challenges and Approaches. *Information Technology for Development*, *12*(3), 185–200. doi:10.1002/itdj.20041

Sayer, A. (2000). *Realism and Social Science*. London: Sage.

Scott, S. (2000) "Lived Methodology: A Situated Discussion of 'Truth and Method' in Interpretive Information Systems Research" *London School of Economics. Department of Information Systems Working Article Series 91*

Shaw, V. (2005). Health Information System Reform in South Africa: Developing an Essential Data Set. *Bulletin of the World Health Organization*, *83*(8), 632–636.

Smith, B. C. (1997). The Decentralization of Health Care in Developing Countries: Organisational Option. *Public Administration and Development*, *17*, 399–412. doi:10.1002/(SICI)1099-162X(199710)17:4<399::AID-PAD976>3.0.CO;2-P

Smith, M., & Madon, S. (2008). Integrated Health Information Systems in Tanzania: Experience and Challenges. *EJISDC*, *33*(1), 1–21.

Stansfield, S. (2005). Editorial - Structuring Information and Incentives to Improve Health. *Bulletin of the World Health Organization*, *83*(8), 562–563.

Starfield, B., Shi, L., & Macinko, J. (2005). Contribution of Primary Care to Health Systems and Health. *The Milbank Quarterly*, *3*, 457–502. doi:10.1111/j.1468-0009.2005.00409.x

Tarimo, E., & Fowkes, F. (1989). Strengthening the Backbone of Primary Health Care. *World Health Forum*, *10*(1), 74–79.

Valsiner, J. (2000). Data as Representations: Contextualizing Qualitative and Quantitative Research Strategies. *Social Sciences Information. Information Sur les Sciences Sociales*, *39*(1), 99–113. doi:10.1177/053901800039001006

Waitzkin, H. (2003). Report of the Who Commission on Macroeconomics and Health: A Summary and Critique. *Lancet*, *361*, 523–526. doi:10.1016/S0140-6736(03)12491-9

Walsham, G. (1995). Interpretive Case Studies in Is Research: Nature and Method. *EJISDC*, *4*(2), 74–81.

Walsham, G. (2006). Doing Interpretive Research. *EJISDC*, *15*, 320–330.

Walt, G., & Gilson, L. (1994). Reforming the Health Sector in Developing Countries: The Central Role of Policy Analysis. *Health Policy and Planning*, *9*(4), 353–370. doi:10.1093/heapol/9.4.353

WHO. (1978) "Declaration of Alma-Ata". in *International Conference on Primary Health Care,* Alma-Ata, USSR,6-12 September, WHO (2000) "The World Health Report 2000" *WHO* Geneva.

WHO. (2001). *Commission on Macroeconomics and Health. Macroeconomics and Health: Investing in Health for Economic Development.* Geneva: WHO.

World Bank. (1993). *The World Development Report 1993: Investing in Health.* New York: Oxford University Press.

Yin, R. K. (2003) *Case Study Research: Design and Methods,* (Third Edition) Sage. Third Edition, London.

Chapter 4
Wireless Technology and Clinical Influences in Healthcare Setting:
An Indian Case Study

Abdul Hafeez Baig
University of Southern Queensland, Australia

Raj Gururajan
University of Southern Queensland, Australia

ABSTRACT

This chapter argues that current techniques used in the domain of Information Systems is not adequate for establishing determinants of wireless technology in a clinical setting. Using data collected from India, this chapter conducted a first order regrssion modeling (factor analysis) and then a second order regression modeling (SEM) to establish the determinants of clinical influences as a result of using wireless technology in healthcare settings. As information systems professionals, the authors conducted a qualitative data collection to understand the domain prior to employing a quantitative technique, thus providing rigour as well as personal relevance. The outcomes of this study has clearly established that there are a number of influences such as the organisational factors in determining the technology acceptance and provides evidence that trivial factors such as perceived ease of use and perceived usefulness are no longer acceptable as the factors of technology acceptance.

INTRODUCTION

In the last few years, high expectations, technological developments, and effective and efficient services have been shown to be prerequisites for improvements in the healthcare domain (Rogoski, 2005; Versel, 2008). Latest trends in the healthcare sector include the design of more flexible and efficient service provider frameworks aimed at providing health services to all stakeholders.

DOI: 10.4018/978-1-60960-183-6.ch004

In order to implement such frameworks, wireless technology is increasingly being used in the healthcare sector. A decrease in the cost of wireless devices and improved awareness of the benefits by using related wireless applications are two of the contributing factors towards the increased use of wireless technology in this sector (R. Gururajan, Hafeez-Baig, & Gururjan, 2008; R. Gururajan, Quaddus, Fink, Vuori, & Soar, 2005). Even though the future of this technology and its usability is promising, its adoption is still in its infancy, which is attributed to the complex and critical nature of the healthcare environment. In the current competitive and complex business environment, technology developments have played a critical role in delivering high quality of care (Reinecke, 2004). However, there is limited knowledge and empirical research on the effectiveness and adoption of wireless technology in general, and in the Indian healthcare system in particular.

Recent research has established that investment in emerging Information Technology (IT), including Information Systems (IS), can lead to productivity gains only if they are accepted and effectively used by respective stakeholders. Consequently, acceptance and utilization of IT/IS in the healthcare environment have been central themes in the information systems literature. Therefore, the fundamental focus of this research is to investigate and examine the influence of internal and external determinants on the usefulness of wireless technology. Further, this research also assesses how its acceptance contributes to the adoption of wireless technology. We believe that this research is the first of its kind attempted in the Indian healthcare domain and it employs empirical evidence to explore the impact of wireless technology and its usefulness in the Indian healthcare system. The Indian healthcare domain is at the forefront in adopting the latest medical technologies and applications, as evidenced by media reports and, as such, it constitutes an excellent context for validating existing adoption theories and extending them.

The main contribution of this research includes the identification of a set of drivers and barriers to using wireless technology in a given Indian healthcare setting. In addition to this, for the first time, a set of clinical factors influencing the adoption of wireless technology has been identified and validated using a second order regression model.

LITERATURE REVIEW

The concept of wireless technology in healthcare is discussed in many studies (Dyer, 2003; Hu, Chau, & Liu Sheng, 2002; Sausser, 2003; Simpson, 2003; Siracuse, Pharm, & Sowell, 2008; Versel, 2008; Wisnicki, 2002; Wu & Wu, 2007; Zhang, 2007). For example, Wisnicki (2002) provides details of how broadband technology, an essential component of wireless technology, can be used in healthcare. While prior studies agree that wireless applications have the potential to address the endemic problems of healthcare, very limited information can be found about the determinants of such applications (Raj Gururajan, Clint Moloney, & Don Kerr, 2005; Raj Gururajan, Toleman, & Soar, 2004). In general, the majority of the works reviewed are descriptive about the benefits of wireless handheld devices in healthcare in general, and medicine in particular. There are only a small number of studies that provide evidence-based information concerning these devices in healthcare (Fischer et al. 2003; Sax et al. 2005)(Hafeez-Baig, 2007). Furthermore, five major studies in the area of healthcare (evaluated by (Spil & Schuring, 2006) testing the Technology Acceptance Model (TAM) produced findings which were inconsistent with the body of knowledge in non-healthcare settings. With 'Perceived Ease of Use' and 'Perceived Usefulness' as the major TAM attributes, these studies found that in the health environment, 'Perceived Usefulness' is an important attribute in technology adoption, while 'Perceived Ease of Use' was found to have no effect (Spil & Schuring, 2006). This is different to findings reported in non-health IS studies, where both attributes were found to be reliable technology adoption predictors. Therefore, further empirical investigation is required to explain the reasons why this variation exists in healthcare. In addition, there is a need to explore if further attributes exist which may influence the adoption of wireless applications in the healthcare environment.

TECHNOLOGY ADOPTION IN HEALTHCARE CONTEXT

In healthcare literature, the discussion on wireless technology falls into three periods. For example, studies prior to and including 2000 discussed the status of wireless technology and the possible role the technology can play in healthcare. Studies between 2000 and 2003 discussed how wireless technology can be deployed in healthcare and the potential benefits the technology can bring to healthcare. It should be noted that these studies were only 'discussion' type studies. Majority of these studies did not provide any empirical evidence as to the use or acceptance of wireless technology in healthcare domains. Studies from 2004 till current date have collected data to establish the usefulness of wireless technology in healthcare. These studies, to some extent have focussed on the PDAs as these devices have been found to be useful in nursing domain for clinical data management.

The studies between 2000 and 2003 discussed a number of potentials of wireless technology in clinical domains. For example, how broadband technology can be used in healthcare was discussed by (Wisnicki, 2002), ability to address prevailing healthcare staff crisis by adopting intelligent solutions using agent and wireless technology that can identify the need and match the need with available resources in a timely and efficient manner was outlined by (Davis, 2002), better compliance with the rigorous regulatory framework was highlighted by (Wisnicki, 2002), reduction in medication errors and hence the benefits that can be realised was discussed by (Turisco, 2000), provision for greater flexibility and mobility of healthcare workers in performing their work was portrayed by (Athey & Stern, 2002), effective management of the increasingly complex information challenges and improved access to those information from anywhere at anytime was discussed by (Stuart & Bawany, 2001). Our review clearly identified that all these studies were only implying the potential of wireless technology and did not provide any empirical evidence.

While prior studies agreed that wireless applications have the potential to address the endemic problems of healthcare, very limited information can be found about the determinants of such wireless applications in order to establish the adoption of technology in a given healthcare context (Raj Gururajan, et al., 2005; Raj Gururajan, et al., 2004). During the period of 2004 – 2006, studies emerged in the area of technology acceptance, specifically focussing on the acceptance of wireless technology in healthcare domains. These studies were empirical in nature and were testing the available models of technology acceptance or a variation in order to ascertain whether previous models hold good for a new technology in a specific domain. These studies were reported in a book titled 'E-Health Systems Diffusion and Use', published by Idea Group Publishing in 2006 (Spil & Schuring, 2006). These studies are summarised below:

Predicting Internet Use: Applying the Extended Technology Acceptance Model to the Healthcare Environment (Chismar & Wiley-Patton, 2006) – This study empirically established that only perceived usefulness is significant and ease of use was not significant.

The dynamics of IT adoption in a major change process in health delivery (Lapointe, Lamothe, & Fortin, 2006) – This study established that TAM as devised by (Davies, Bagozzi, & Warshaw, 1989) is not adequate for health systems because adoption/resistance factors may be group related as opposed to the fundamental basis of TAM which is individualistic, influence of intra and inter organisational factors, linkages to cultures, environmental factors as well as the complexity of the environment.

Introducing electronic patient records to hospitals: Innovation adoption paths (Suomi, 2006) – This study found that relative advantage, strong network externalities available, rich availability of information through different communication channels are key factors for innovation and adoption. It should be noted that these are not discussed in the TAM models.

User acceptance and diffusion of innovations summarised (Spil & Schuring, 2006) – This summary established that perceived usefulness is a predictor of technology acceptance in healthcare. Ease of use was not found to be significant.

Understanding physicians' use of online systems: an empirical assessment of an electronic disability evaluation system (Horan, Tule, & Hilton, 2006) – This study found that in order to diffuse technology in an organisation, it is important to ascertain physicians' behaviour, their workflow practices and their perceptions regarding the value of specific information systems.

In essence, the recent studies appear to be indicating that the current models of technology acceptance or its derivatives are not suitable to predict the adoption factors of wireless technology in healthcare environment. Strong support can also be derived from three specific studies that have tested TAM models in healthcare. The first study conducted by (Jayasuriya, 1998) established that ease of use was not significant in a clinical domain. The second study by (Chau & Hu, 2002) echoed similar sentiments. The third study by Hu et al. (Hu, Chau, & Tam, 1999) also found similar findings.

Further, recent studies conducted by (Howard, Gururajan, Hafeez-Baig, & Howard, 2006) also established that ease of use was not significant while determining factors of adoption in a clinical domain in regard to wireless technology. Further, (Ivers & Gururajan, 2006) also found that there are other factors beyond the TAM models influencing the acceptance of technology (Versel, 2008).

Interviews conducted with Queensland nursing staff members in Australia (R. Gururajan, C. Moloney, & D. Kerr, 2005) revealed that Clinical Influences of wireless technology is far more significant than ease of use factor as established in TAM. Another focus group discussion with the Western Australian senior health managers (R. Gururajan, M. Quaddus, et al., 2005) also indicated that aspects of Clinical Influences such as integration of clinical data may be a significant factor than the ease of use factor. (Howard, et al., 2006) also identified Clinical Influences is far more influencing than the ease of use factor while determining factors of adoption of wireless technology in the Indian healthcare domain.

However, the recent findings that the ease of use factor not showing strong significance in healthcare domain while determining wireless technology adoption warrants explanation as this is different to many other reported studies in the generic IS domain where both attributes (ease of use and perceived usefulness) were reported to be reliable predictors.

This variation requires further empirical investigation in order to explain the reason behind this variation specific to healthcare. Therefore, there is a need to identify attributes that assist in the adoption of wireless applications in healthcare environment. We argue that the initial validity of many technology acceptance models was predominantly established by testing the model with students as surrogates in a generic software application domain. This environment is very different to the healthcare environment, where the skills are at different levels. Further, the healthcare environment is complex, sensitive and time critical. These could be some of the reasons why TAM did not perform as expected in healthcare settings.

In addition, in the recent variant of technology acceptance, namely, UTAUT, (Venkatesh, Morris, Davis, & Davis, 2003) reviewed eight prominent models of user acceptance and managed to create a unified view. The unified model comprised of seven constructs. The first four – performance expectancy, effort expectancy, social influence and facilitating conditions – were theorised to be direct determinants. The last three – attitude towards technology, self efficacy and anxiety – were theorised to be indirect. All the seven constructs were found to be significant determinants of technology usage by Venkatesh et al ((Venkatesh, et al., 2003).

In terms of attitude, Venkatesh et al. (Venkatesh, et al., 2003) defined it as an individual's overall affective reaction to using a system. The model depicts four constructs relating to this determinant – attitude towards behaviour, intrinsic motivation, affect towards use and affect. (Spil & Schuring, 2006) verified that in three cases the relation between attitude and behavioural intention is significant. Therefore, this determinant cannot be indirect. If there is significance between attitude and behaviour intention, then there is a direct relationship.

Therefore, there appears to be a basis to identify factors that contribute to the adoption of technologies in healthcare settings. Given that wireless technologies have started making in-roads in healthcare, the overarching purpose of the research is to identify the factors that influence the adoption of wireless technology in the Indian healthcare system. The rationale of the purpose is justified by the fact that India is a leader in software technologies, especially medical applications. Further, India is emerging as 'health tourism', due to the advancement in medical technology and reduction in cost in offering high quality health services—as highlighted by various print media. However, our initial review of available literature indicated that this area is under-researched. Collectively, these aspects led to the following research question:

What are the determinants for the adoption of wireless technology by physicians in the Indian healthcare system?

The first stage of this study is focused on answering the research question qualitatively and the second stage on answering the research question quantitatively. Details as to how the research question was answered are provided in the research methodology section below.

METHODOLOGY

An examination of existing IS studies indicated that there is a necessity for a suitable research method. Most of the reviewed studies follow a quantitative approach which involves an instrument being administered onto a domain with perhaps a lesser understanding of the domain issues. For this study it was felt that if technology issues are to be studied with respect to a specific domain, then user involvement with the technology issues forms a major part in establishing the adoption (or inhibiting) factors. By necessity, this would occur prior to administering quantitative instruments (e.g. survey). This, in turn, requires an understanding of research philosophy, values of inquiry that would guide the study, and the choice of relevant research techniques required to conduct the investigation in order to answer the research questions.

Further, there appears to be limited information available in the Indian IS domain to guide the principles of this study. This study is relatively new and, hence, requires a rigorous justification as to the choice of research methods employed. We also believe that due to aspects associated with various regulatory issues impacting the Indian health system, unique factors of technology acceptance, as well as usefulness, may emerge. Our initial meetings with Indian physicians also suggested that there is a divide in terms of technology usage between private and public hospitals, where private hospitals are rich in technology use and public hospitals are not. On the other hand, in many traditional studies in IS, either quantitative or, to some lesser extent, qualitative methods are used—but not both. In recent years this has been cited as a weakness (see (Mingers, 2001) for a detailed argument on this). Taking this into account, this study investigates the suitability of both approaches in order to answer the research question.

We recognise that the foundation for any research will be grounded on the researcher's fundamental philosophical view of the world (Myers, 1997). The choice of tools, including research techniques, instruments, and methods such as qualitative and quantitative, are not inherently linked to a particular philosophical position, as these positions are generic in nature. It is the contextual framework within which they are applied that provides consistency to an inquiry. While the choice of tools and methods are not linked to the philosophical view, the articulation—which is commonly the process of explaining choices of research methods and its related choice of research instruments—helps determine the philosophical disposition. This is usually achieved by asking questions on the beliefs, perceptions, experiences, advantages and disadvantages in order to determine this disposition. This may even include a researcher's personal experience within that domain, or their expertise in explicating the information using any approach that may be suitable to that domain. This has prompted us to follow a qualitative approach as the first phase of the study. We argue that this approach facilitates direction to the second phase of the study where quantitative evidence can be collected to establish causality between the dependent and the independent variables.

The research question dictates the need for quantitative research methods, while the behavioural component of the same investigation dictates qualitative research methods. The rationale for this approach is based on the notion that behavioural components require a thorough understanding of how users apply wireless technology in a given setting in order to understand behavioural issues. To extract 'tacit' aspects, this is best accomplished by applying a qualitative approach. A quantitative instrument can then be developed to extract the quantitative aspects, such as the opinion scores.

Health professionals view the term 'wireless technology' in different ways, either as a product or a process. The combined domain of wireless technology and healthcare is relatively new in the Indian IS domain. While IS studies have discussed the impact of Information & Communication Technology (ICT) tools and associated behavioural intentions on healthcare users, limited information can be found as to how the combination of wireless technology and healthcare settings would influence users who are already conversant with novel and advanced medical technologies (Spil & Schuring, 2006). The workplace or organizational factors that influence such combinations are yet to be explored in detail. Such an exploration has close association with the choice of research method as these methods pave the way for proper inquiry into the factors that determine technology acceptance in a given setting. On this basis, the suitability of one research method over another has to be carefully weighed. Consequently, this study identified an exploratory approach to be suitable for the initial investigation. This approach is particularly favourable in confirming the direction of the study, variables chosen for the study, and in helping refine the literature. The exploratory study can also possibly eliminate some variables, while providing opportunities for including emerging variables.

QUALITATIVE DATA COLLECTION

As argued, for the first stage of this research the investigators used a qualitative approach to collect initial sets of themes for the adoption of wireless technology in the Indian healthcare system. For this purpose, 30 physicians operating in Indian healthcare were identified randomly. These physicians were interviewed by an independent member (external to the team) who identified the attributes for the adoption of wireless technology by physicians in the Indian healthcare system. This approach was deliberate to address criticisms of 'bias' in the interview process. Further, due to linguistic issues, we required a person with proficiency in both Indian language and English. The interview questions were derived from existing literature. The first stage of the data collection concentrated on Indian hospitals with some form of wireless technology already in use. The physicians were also chosen based on their wireless technology awareness or working experience. They were drawn from both private and government hospitals. The interviews were conducted over a 45-60 minute period and recorded using a digital recorder. Once they were recorded, the interviews were transcribed.

QUANTITATIVE DATA COLLECTION

This study developed a survey instrument from the interview data. The main reason for this digressed attitude was that previously tested instruments in the technology domain were not relevant to healthcare setting and were found to be inadequate in answering the research question. The data from the interviews were used to develop specific ranges of questions to gather a more detailed view from the wider population. This survey instrument was pilot tested to capture the information reflecting the perceptions and practice of those adopting the wireless technology in the Indian healthcare system. Particularly, it focussed on what internal and external environmental factors affect the adoption of wireless technology and the extent of this influence. The survey was then distributed to over 300 physicians randomly chosen from the telephone book and a total of 200 responses were received. The survey responses were then entered into a spreadsheet file. A Visual Basic interface was written to generate numerical codes for various elements of the survey for data analysis using SPSS. The coded spreadsheet file was then copied onto a SPSS file format.

DATA ANALYSIS

Qualitative data was analysed using the NVivo (version 7) application, which helped identify the initial themes from the interviews. Quantitative data were analysed using SPSS, which helped identify the factors and their correlation for the adoption of wireless technology in the Indian healthcare setting.

Qualitative Data Analysis

Qualitative data was manually coded to extract themes that had an impact on wireless technology acceptance as stated by the physicians. In total, 63 themes were extracted from the interviews. The initial themes include awareness, cost factors, advantages and disadvantages, medical errors, information sharing, current state of technology, usefulness and role of wireless technology, and technology awareness. On the basis of the interviews and the literature review, the themes were classified into drivers and inhibitors as shown in the following table. This list of drivers and inhibitors was expected to provide a direction for the development of the survey instrument for the collection of quantitative data to capture the wider community views and to generalize the outcome of the research. This grouping is presented in Table 1.

The content of the Table 1 is consistent with findings of previous studies conducted by Gururajan et al. (2004; 2005). This prompted conducting a quantitative study in order to establish causality among dependent and independent variables, as well as external validity and generalisability.

Table 1. The factors driving and inhibiting wireless technology adoption in healthcare

Drivers	Barriers
Save-time	Legal barriers
Improve-clinical-workflow	Administrative purpose
Efficiency-in-communication	Communication with physicians
Delivery-of-high-qual-info	Patient education
Better-quality-of-service	Communication with colleagues
Save-effort	Obtain lab results
Improve-clinical-performance	Note taking
More-contact-time-with-patients	Electronic medical records
Improved-delivery-of-information	Device usage barrier
Reduce-overall-cost	Benefit evaluation barrier
Positive-impact-on-patient-safety	Resource barrier
Reduce-inaccuracies	Electronic prescribing
Improve-public-image	
Reduce-medical-errors	
Easy-access-to-data	
Attract-more-practitioners	
Reduce-workload	

Quantitative Data Analyses

In order to ensure statistical reliability, suitable tests were run on the entire instrument, as well as selected group of variables. For example, the reliability test returned a Cronbach alpha value of 0.965 for the instrument indicating high reliability (Zikmund, 1994). We ran this test because the instrument was generated from the interview data and, hence, it was necessary to establish statistical reliability. In addition, reliability tests were also run for three factor groupings, namely, drivers, inhibitors of adoption and other technology factors. The reliability tests returned values of 0.941, 0.447 and 0.536, respectively, indicating that the data were suitable for factor analysis testing.

As a second step, survey data were analysed for factor analysis using SPSS. It is evident from Table 2 that two factor component matrix identified drivers and the barriers for the adoption of wireless technology in the Indian healthcare setting. This finding is consistent and aligned with the findings of the qualitative data collection stage (i.e. first stage) of this research.

The drivers identified through this research were further tested for factor groupings through data reduction technique provided by SPSS. The analysis resulted in Table 3.

The driving factors of adoption yielded three categories of factors, namely, 'organisational', 'management' and 'clinical'. The organisational components include wireless technology drivers that can generate specific benefits for organisations. The management components represent the benefits that healthcare managers can realise using wireless technology. The clinical components encompass clinical drivers of using wireless technology.

A similar factor model was generated for the inhibitors. The model resulted in Table 4.

Similar to the drivers, the inhibitors also resulted in three specific categories. The 'technology' category includes technology factors that inhibit wireless adoption in the Indian healthcare. The 'resource' category encompasses resource barriers that are currently being encountered in the healthcare setting. Finally the 'usage' category is comprised of inhibiting factors, which are associated with usage issues.

In addition to the two factor groups, namely drivers and inhibitors, we also identified a third. We named this 'Clinical Influences' and its components are shown in Table 5.

Table 2. Driving & inhibiting of wireless technology adoption in healthcare from data analysis of survey result

Drivers	Loading values	Barriers	Loading values
Improve-clinical-workflow	.798	Poor technology barrier	.605
Tech-support	.764	Time for training barrier	.572
Delivery-of-high-qual-info	.760	Tech expertise barrier	.554
Save-time	.757	Benefit evaluation barrier	.503
Better-quality-of-service	.749	Legal barriers	.465
Save-effort	.743	Solutions barrier	.444
Improved-delivery-of-information	.732	System migration barrier	.442
Efficiency-in-communication	.730	Technical support barrier	.436
More-contact-time-with-patients	.725	Lack of support barrier	.352
Improve-clinical-performance	.702	Device access barrier	.316
More-training	.699	Device comfort barrier	.248
Improve-public-image	.695	Funding barrier	-.225
Easy-access-to-data	.692	Security as barrier	.224
Positive-impact-on-patient-safety	.679	Device usage barrier	.208
Reduce-inaccuracies	.659		
Reduce-workload	.657		
Reduce-medical-errors	.650		
Reduce-overall-cost	.634		
Attract-more-practitioners	.600		
Org-culture	.464		

Table 3. The factors driving wireless technology adoption in healthcare from data analysis of survey result

Descriptions	Organizational	Management	Clinical
Save-effort	.716		
Reduce-overall-cost	.708		
Reduce-inaccuracies	.703		
Save-time	.667		
Easy-access-to-data	.659		
Attract-more-practitioners		.769	
Improve-public-image		.680	
Tech-support		.680	
Reduce-workload			.817
Improve-clinical-performance			.797

Table 4. The factors inhibiting wireless technology adoption in healthcare from data analysis of survey result

Descriptions	Technology	Resource	Usage
Poor technology barrier	.625		
Time for training barrier	.582		
Solutions barrier	.575		
Benefit evaluation barrier	.528		
Tech expertise barrier	.527		
System migration barrier	.511		
Funding barrier		-.749	
Resource barrier		-.690	
Technical support barrier			.542
Device usage barrier			.519

Table 5. The factors 'Clinical Influences' of wireless technology adoption in healthcare from data analysis of survey result

Descriptions	General Communication	Clinical Communication	Records Management
Obtain lab results	.837		
Administrative purpose	.770		
Electronic prescribing	.670		
Medical database referral	.632		
Patient education		.727	
Communication with colleagues		.707	
Communication with patients		.676	
Drug administration		.596	
Communication with physicians		.548	
Electronic Medical Records			.764
Generating exception list			.738
Note taking			.617
Disease state management			.563

This factor group yielded three components. The first component deals with the general communication aspects facilitated by wireless technology in healthcare settings. The second component refers to clinical communication using wireless technology. The third component is specific to records management. In summary, the data analyses yielded three specific categories of factors which can affect the adoption of wireless technologies in the healthcare setting. These comprise adoption drivers, inhibitors, and Clinical Influences.

HYPOTHESES FORMULATION AND TESTING

Based on the evidence collected, the three sets of factors, namely, drivers, barriers and Clinical Influences, contribute to the acceptance of wireless technology in healthcare. We hypothesise that the drivers positively impact on Clinical Influences', whereas the barriers have a negative impact on it. While the drivers and barriers include factors beyond the technology aspects, their respective influences are restricted to the clinical domain as this is where the usefulness of wireless technology can be experienced. Therefore, the following two hypotheses were generated for testing:

H1: Drivers of wireless technology positively impact on "Clinical Influences".
H2. Barriers to wireless technology negatively impact on "Clinical Influences".

A "Structural Equaction Modeling (SEM) model was developed in order to test the hypotheses. The rationale for using SEM includes: SEM is used for confirmatory factor analysis (CFA); the pattern of loadings of items on the latent constructs is explicit; SEM provides strong convergent and discriminant validity; p-value of t-value is significant (over 0.50 level) for constructs; and measurement items load highly on theoretically assigned factors and not highly on other factors.

SEM MODEL DEVELOPMENT

In order to develop the SEM model, an AMOS version 16 was used. A description of items used in building the SEM model can be found in Table 6. Initially, the individual drivers, barriers and "Clinical Influences" were tested for CFA (Confirmatory Factor Analysis) scores and these were found to be reliable. When the CFA was found to be satisfactory, a model was built with clinical influences as dependent variable on drivers and barriers. The final outcome is shown in Figure 1.

Figure 2 shows that the factor loading (the number on the path: for example, for the construct Drivers, has 0.16, 0.21, and .48). The drivers and clinical influneces load highly (over 0.8 for most of the items), indicating a high reliability. Further, all variables have a t-value of over 2.0 to indicate high convergent validity.

Upon construct validation, a simple SEM (consolidated) model was developed to test the hypotheses. The model consists of clinical influneces as the dependent variable, and drivers ("Organizational" (O), "Clinical" (C), and "Management" (M)) and barriers ("Usage" (U), "Technology" (T), and "Resources" (R)" (M) as independent variables. The model was run with AMOS Graph program and the screenshot shown in Figure 3 displays the values along the link from Drivers to Clinical Influences, and Barriers to Clinical Influences.

According to (Holmes-Smith, 2000) to analyse a model for the data fit, the following five measurements need to be analysed carefully:

1. Chi-square (X^2 acceptable fit: $p > 0.05$)
2. Normed Chi-square (X^2/df acceptable fit $1 < X^2/df < 2$)
3. Goodness-of-fit index (GFI- acceptable fit value, $0.95<GFI<1$, reasonable fit value would be $0.90<GFI<0.95$)
4. Tucker-Lewis Index (TLI- acceptable value; $TLI>0.95$; reasonable value of fit $0.9<TLI<0.95$ and lack of model parsimony would be $TLI>1$)
5. RootMean-Square Error of Approximation (RMSEA- acceptable fit value: $RMSEA<0.05$; reasonable level of: $0.05<RMSEA<0.08$)

Above criteria was used to analyse the data fit for each of the construct before computing the composite variables. Figures 4, 5 and 6 show the values of each variable separately for initial model and the improved acceptable model for each of the composite model.

Data reduction and technique for Compatibility Variable

Figures 4, 5, and 6 show the data fit for the improve model. This was achieved by appropriate after the analysis of the suggestions provided "Modification Indies" provided by SEM along with the analysis of the adequate theoretical support. Objective was to achieve the improved measure of data fit for the empirical data while keeping integrity of the theoretical support. Results shows that changes in the model has resulted all

Table 6. Description of items used in building the SEM model and their reliability

Variables	Initial	Descriptions	Reliability
Drivers	D1	Reduce-workload	**0.885**
	D2	Improve-public-image	
	D3	Improve-clinical-performance	
	D4	Attract-more-practitioners	
	D5	Save-time	
	D6	Save-effort	
	D7	Tech-support	
	D8	Reduce-overall-cost	
	D9	Easy-access-to-data	
Barriers	B1	Funding barrier	**0.539**
	B2	Resource barrier	
	B3	Solutions barrier	
	B4	System migration barrier	
	B5	Benefit evaluation barrier	
	B6	Time for training barrier	
	B7	Poor technology barrier	
	B8	Tech expertise barrier	
	B9	Technical support barrier	
	B10	Device usage barrier	
clinical influneces	CI 1	Electronic medical records	**0.850**
	CI 2	Medical database referral	
	CI 3	Electronic prescribing	
	CI 4	Obtain lab results	
	CI 5	Disease state management	
	CI 6	Adminstrative purpose	
	CI 7	Generating exception list	
	CI 8	Patient education	
	CI 9	Note taking	
	CI 10	Drug administration	
	CI 11	Communiation with physicians	
	CI 12	Communication with colleagues	

the five indicator showed that empirical data fitted the improve measurement model.

Once the data reduction techniques was used to individual variables and data was found to fit as per (Holmes-Smith, 2000) incies, we draw the initial SEM model with Barriers (B) and Drivers (D) as an independent variables and clinical influneces (CI) as dependent variable in the model.

As can been seen from Figure 5 above five of the popular measured provided by (Holmes-Smith, 2000) is provided under the diagram. First two values (Chi-square, and Normed Chi-square) were not at acceptable level, however values of other three (Goodness-of-fit index, Tucker-Lewis Index, and RootMean-Square Error of Approximation)

Figure 1. Initial model

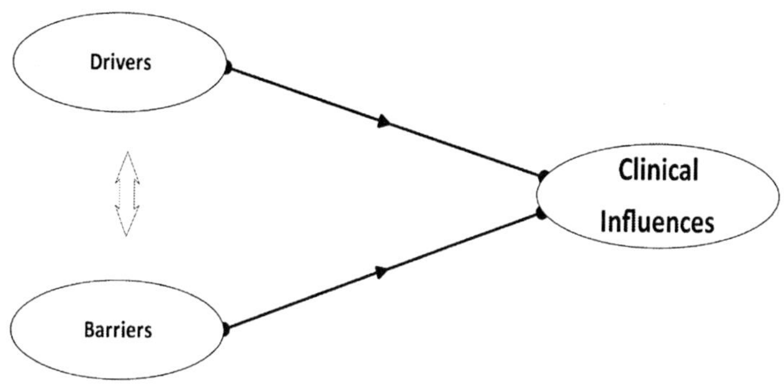

Figure 2. SEM Model: $X^2 = 41.6$, $df = 23$, $p = 0.010$, $X^2/df = 1.810$, GFI = 0.955, TLI = .932, RMSEA = 0.065 (Data fit the improved model)

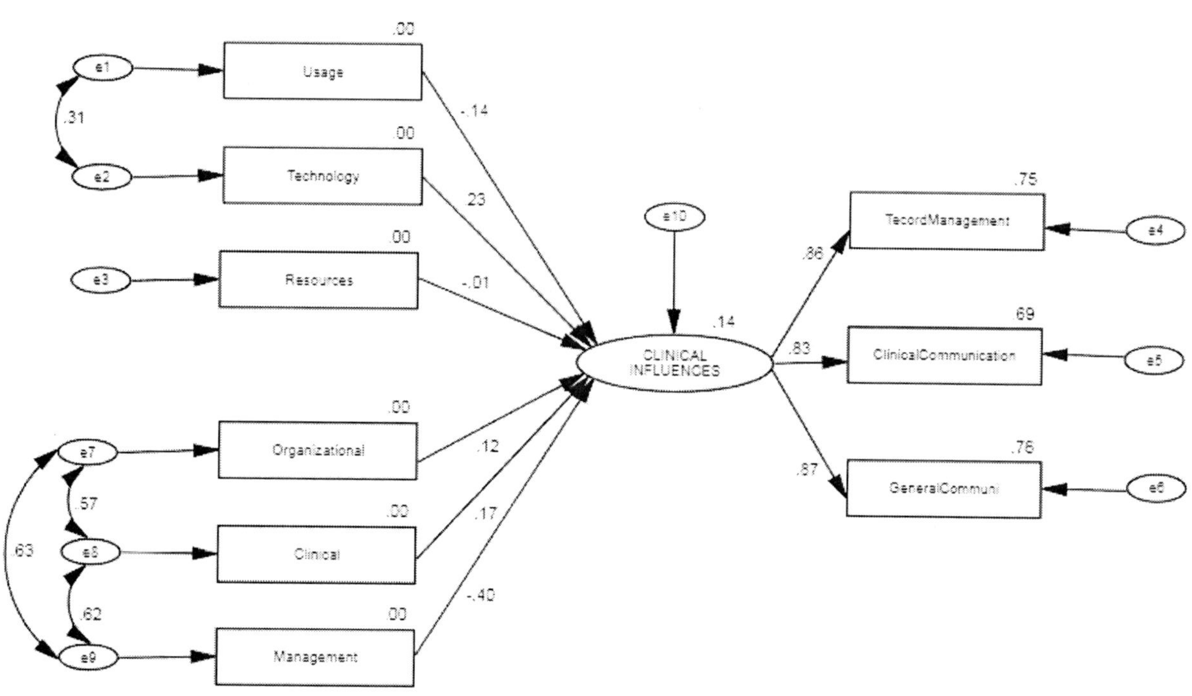

Figure 3. Drivers: $X^2 = 27.5$, $df = 14$, $p = 0.017$, $X^2/df = 1.964$, GFI = 0.961, TLI = .963, RMSEA = 0.070 (Data fit the improved model)

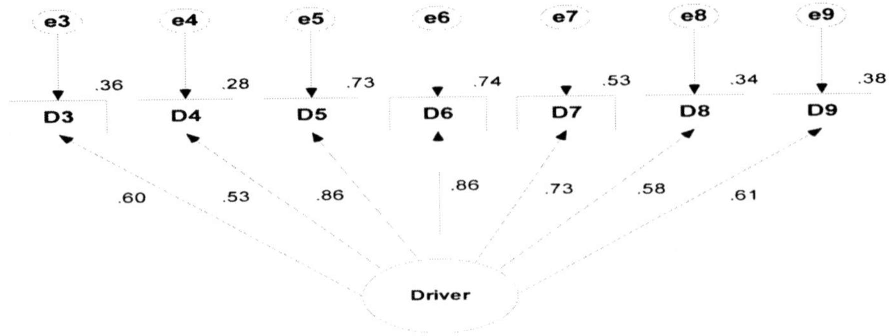

Figure 4. Drivers: $X^2 = 37.3$, $df = 25$, $p = 0.054$, $X^2/df = 1.492$, GFI = 0.959, TLI = .900, RMSEA = 0.050 (Data fit the improved model)

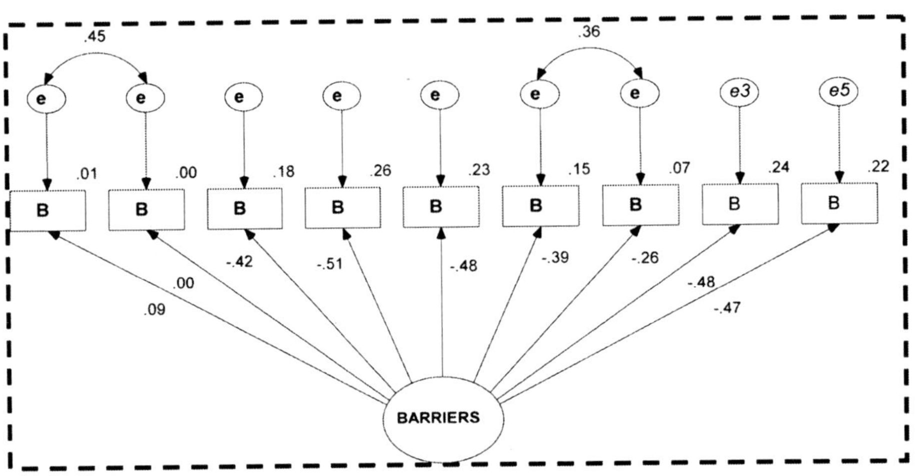

Figure 5. Clinical Influences: $X^2 = 30.8$, $df = 12$, $p = 0.054$, $X^2/df = 1.492$, GFI = 0.959, TLI = .900, RMSEA = 0.050 (Data fit the improved model)

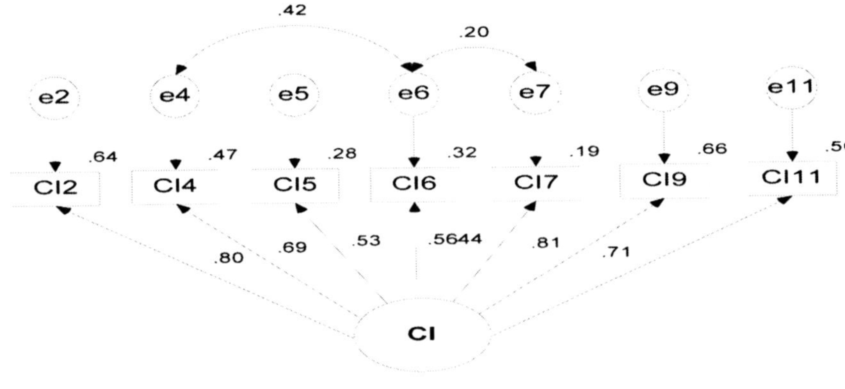

Figure 6. Clinical Influneces: $X^2 = 9.0$, $df = 7$, $p = 0.252$, $X^2/df = 1.28$, GFI = 0.986, TLI = .992, RMSEA = 0.038 (Data fit the improved model)

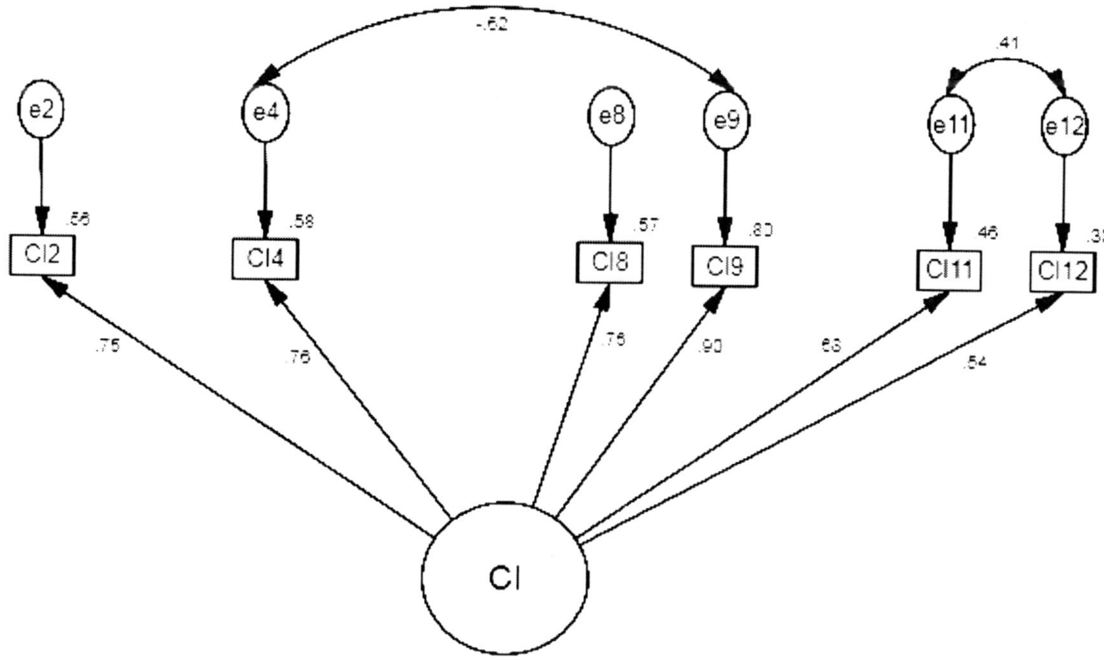

were not at acceptable level. It was concluded that the data did not adequately fit the model.

Figure 5 shows the data fit for the improve model. This was achieved by appropriate after the analysis of the suggestions provided "Modification Indies" provided by SEM along with the analysis of the adequate theoretical support. Objective was to achieve the improved measure of data fit for the empirical data while keeping integrity of the theoretical support. Results shows that changes in the model has resulted all the five indicator showed that empirical data fitted the improve measurement model.

Figure 2 provides the visual results of aggregating the items of the measurement model of stage two of the process, which provided the evidence for the data fit the model for the empirical data. As a result we produced a composite variable for "Drivers", "Barriers", and "Clinical Influences" in the complete model for the existing data in order to analyse the influence of drivers and barriers on the clinical influences. Data fit of the model and the indices measures are $X^2 = 41.6$, df = 23, $p = 0.010$, $X^2/df = 1.810$, GFI = 0.955, TLI = .932, and RMSEA = 0.065.

In Figure 2, the latent variable "Clinical Influences" (CI), set of possible predictors, "Usage" (U), "Technology" (T), "Resources" (R), "Organizational" (O), "Clinical" (C), and "Management" (M) are the observed variables. CI is itself indicated by three items, "Technological Management" (TM), "Clinical Communication" (CC), and "General Communication" (GC). As can be seen, the overall structural model fit was good. Criteria used to determined: $X^2 = 41.6$, with 23 df, $X^2/df = 1.810$, CFI = , AIC = , GFI = 0.955, TLI = .932, and RMSEA = 0.065,. Based on these results we proceeded to test the two hypothesis mentioned above (H1, and H2) previously proposed. These hypotheses stated that drivers have positive impact and barrier have negative impact on the clinical influneces. The result supported theses

Figure 7. SEM Initial Model: $X^2 = 548.0$, $df = 202$, $p = 0.000$, $X^2/df = 2.713$, GFI = 0.817, TLI = .755, RMSEA = 0.094 (Data did not fit the improved model)

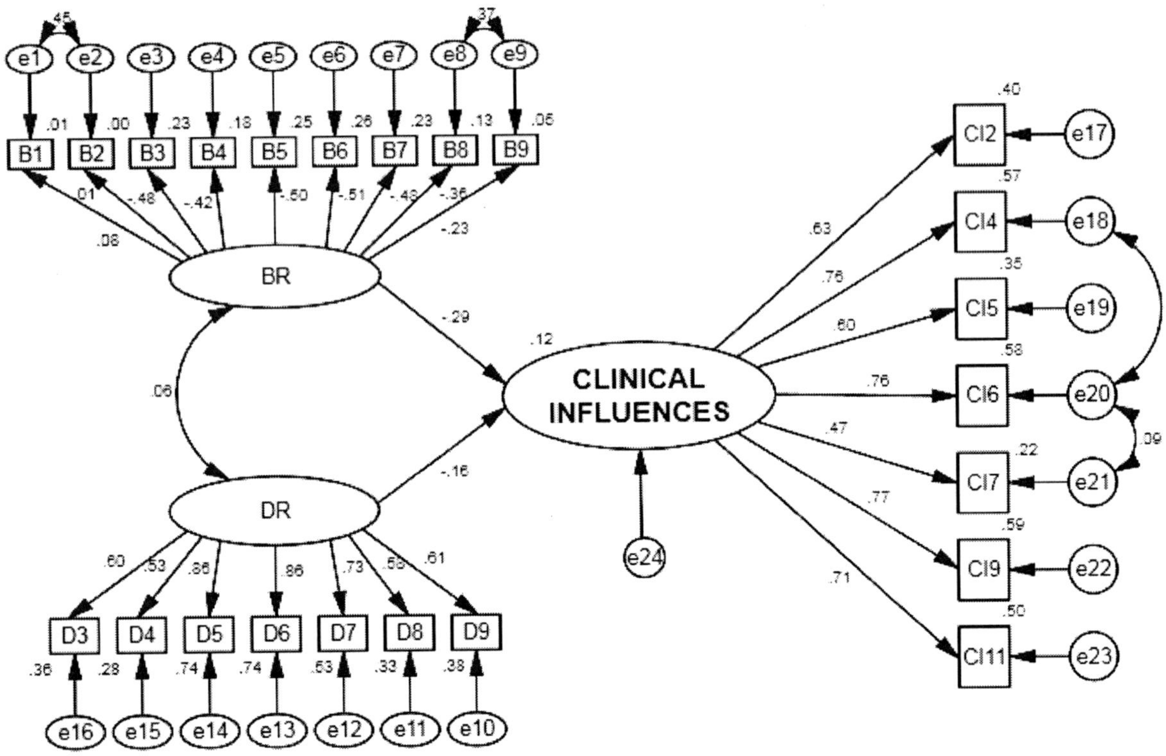

hypothesis, for example in the case of drivers, "Organizational, (t=1.56, $p > 0.01$)", "Clinical, (t=2.14, $p < 0.01$)", and "Management, (t=4.4, $p < 0.01$)" shows that clinical and management drivers are positively contributing to the Clinical Influences, where as the contribution of organizational is not significant. Whereas barrier have vary limited scope, "Usage, (t= -1.98, $p > 0.01$)", "Technology, (t=3.13, $p < 0.01$)", and "Resources, (t= -0.685, $p > 0.01$)". Drivers and barriers are the predictive of the Clinical Influences; results indicate that drivers have stronger influence on the Clinical Influences of the wireless technology than the barrier.

DISCUSSIONS

The Confirmatory Factor Analysis agrees with the outcomes derived from the interview qualitative data in that the set of drivers, barriers and clinical influences are indeed the determinants of wireless technology in the Indian healthcare. Within these three determinants, we are able to identify usage, technology and resources influencing the Clinical Influences. The predictor 'usage' is influenced by the usefulness of technology as identified in recent studies. This study also conforms to the notion that 'ease of use' is not a major influence on technology adoption in the Indian healthcare.

In terms of Clinical Influences, we are able to assert that record management, clinical communication and general communication to be the three major aspects. Our qualitative study had already

Figure 8. SEM Model: $X^2 = 78.9$, $df = 50$, $p = 0.006$, $X^2/df = 1.577$, GFI = 0.939, TLI = .910, RMSEA = 0.055 (Data fit the improved model)

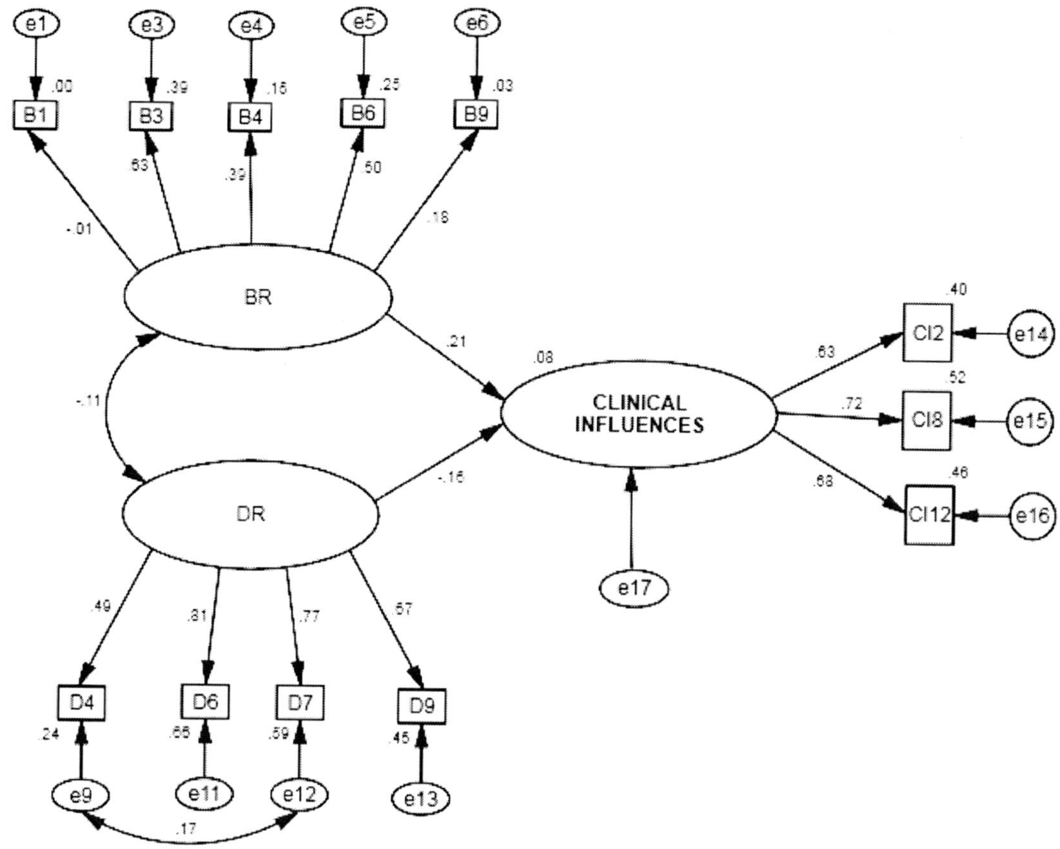

given us some indication to these predictors. Our interviews revealed that the greatest benefits of wireless technology in clinical settings would be records management because it is possible for clinicians to access patient data at the point of care. We also understood that it is possible to use smart phone type technology to send patient conditions to other clinicians in order to get advice. In terms of general communication, our interview transcripts indicate that it si now possible to provide patient education using the wireless technology.

Thus, wireless technology can be used to facilitate access to clinical information and communications between clinicians, maximise clinician time, increase patient safety, and accomplish the strategic and business goals of health organisations. Taken together, these factors have a direct impact on Clinical Influences and its effectiveness. However, achieving Clinical Influences with wireless handheld devices can be a challenge and has several implications.

Firstly, the highest security standards must be achieved. This includes direct end-to-end data encryption, authentication, authorisation, maintenance of audit logs and session management (Chen et al. 2004). While high security standards are essential, their implementation is likely to affect usability. For example, the download and encryption of patient information from the server where it is stored into a wireless handheld device may not be prompt. Sax et al. (2005) argue that clinicians may experience increasingly longer time lags when they carry out increasingly more complex procedures. This is likely to adversely affect Clinical Influences and, hence, decrease user acceptance.

Closely associated with security is also the issue of patient confidentiality, which is of significant importance and concern. Although wireless handheld devices have locking security features and password protection functions which activate during periods of inactivity, the frequent use of these functions during the clinicians' busy daily schedules may have an impact on Clinical Influences.

A crucial lesson learnt in this study was in the use of qualitative and quantitative components. We approached the healthcare professionals to seek their opinions on the benefits of using wireless technology. This stage was followed up with a survey instrument. We conducted a first order regression analysis to regress the 90 or so factors explored into a set of manageable factors. The lesson was quite valuable because as outsiders (coming from an Information Systems background), we were able to appreciate the complexities of healthcare information systems. Similarly, our open minded approach enabled healthcare professionals to appreciate IS related aspects. We also found out through our informal discussions that the study would have been a stereo-type study had we approached a quan-qual type mixed method because we would have been restricted by what was available in the literature to derive our quan part and this would have restricted our qual part.

To our own surprise, we found both IS and health literature to be limited in catching up with wireless technology related attitude and perception data. While the technology literature such as the IEEE provided us with the technical knowledge, human aspects have not yet been discussed in IS and healthcare literature. The results established through a second order regression are consistent with what we found for the Australian Healthcare (published elsewhere).

We measured only perceptions and attitudes in this study. While there is sufficient information available through interviews on the type of savings and benefits that can be attained by using wireless technology in healthcare, it is still not clear as to the exact quantification of these. Therefore, it would be useful to measure this by employing a wireless technology in a clinical setting and then collecting some evidence as to the savings and benefits.

In essence, the study has clearly identified a number of organisational factors and context factors influencing technology adoption in a clinical setting, rather than merely identifying trivial factors. The factors identified in this study are drawn from the experiences and oipinions of clinical professionals who are current with their profession and who are involved in critical yet timely decision making. Thus, teh factors identified in this study add value to administrators of healthcare settings.

REFERENCES

Athey, S., & Stern, S. (2002). The impact of information technology on emergency health care outcomes. *The Rand Journal of Economics*, *33*(3), 399–388. doi:10.2307/3087465

Chau, P. Y. K., & Hu, P. J.-H. (2002). Investigating healthcare professionals' decision to accept telemedicine technology: An empirical test of competing theories. *Information & Management*, *39*, 297–311. doi:10.1016/S0378-7206(01)00098-2

Chismar, W. R., & Wiley-Patton, S. (2006). Predicting Internet Use: Applying teh Extended Technology Acceptance Model to the Healthcare Environment. In Spil, T. A. M., & Schuring, R. W. (Eds.), *E-Health Systems Diffusion and USe: The Innovation, the USer and the USE IT Model*. Hershey, PA: Idea Group Publishing.

Davies, F. D., Bagozzi, R. P., & Warshaw, P. R. (1989). User acceptance of computer technology: A comparison of two theoretical models. *Communications of the ACM, 35*(8), 982–1003.

Davis, R. (2002). Pursue front end solutions to revenue problems. *Healthcare Financial Management, 56*(8), 30–36.

Dyer, O. (2003). Patients will be reminded of appointments by text messages. *British Medical Journal, 326*(402), 281. doi:10.1136/bmj.326.7402.1281-a

Gururajan, R., Hafeez-Baig, A., & Gururjan, V. (2008). *Clinical Factors And Technological Barriers As Determinants For The Intention To Use Wireless Handheld Technology In Healthcare Environment: An Indian Case Study.* Paper presented at the 16th European Conference on Information Systems, National University of Ireland, Galway.

Gururajan, R., Moloney, C., & Kerr, D. (2005). *Drivers for wireless handheld technology: views from Queensland nurses.*

Gururajan, R., Moloney, C., & Kerr, D. (2005). *Drivers for wireless handheld technology: views from Queensland nurses.* Paper presented at the Australian Business & Behavioural Sciences Association (ABBSA) Conference, Cairns, Australia.

Gururajan, R., Quaddus, M., Fink, D., Vuori, T., & Soar, J. (2005). *Drivers and Barriers to adoption of wireless handheld system in WA healthcare: Selected views.* Paper presented at the HIC 2005, Melbourne.

Gururajan, R., Toleman, M., & Soar, J. (2004, 25-27 July). *Necessity for a new technology acceptance model to predict adoption of wireless technology in healthcare.* Paper presented at the Let's Make a Difference with Health ICT, HIC Conference.

Hafeez-Baig, A. (2007). *Technology Management, Data management, Improved outcomes, Efficiency and Software limitation influencing the use of wireless technology for healthcare in Pakistan* Paper presented at the 6th IEEE/ACIS International Conference on Computer and Information Science (ICIS 2007) Melbourne.

Holmes-Smith, P. (2000). *Introduction to Structural Equation Modeling Using AMOS 4.0: Course Notes*. Melbourne, Australia: SREAMS.

Horan, T. A., Tule, B., & Hilton, B. N. (2006). Understanding physician use of online systems: An empirical assessment of an electronic disability evaluation system. In Spil, T. A. M., & Schuring, R. W. (Eds.), *E-Health Systems Diffusion and Use: The Innovation, the User and the USE IT Model*. Hershey, PA: Idea Group Publishing.

Howard, A., Gururajan, R., Hafeez-Baig, A., & Howard, S. (2006). *Clinical Usefulness of Wireless Technology in Healthcare: An Indian Study.* Paper presented at the The Australasian Conference on Information Systems, University of South Australia.

Hu, P. J., Chau, P. Y. K., & Liu Sheng, O. R. (2002). Adoption of telemedicine technology by health care organisations: An exploratory study. *Journal of Organizational Computing and Electronic Commerce, 12*(3), 197–222. doi:10.1207/S15327744JOCE1203_01

Hu, P. J., Chau, P. Y. K., & Tam, K. Y. (1999). Examining teh technologya cceptance model using physician acceptance of telemedicine technology. *Journal of Management Information Systems, 16*(2), 91–112.

Ivers, B., & Gururajan, R. (2006). *Management issues in telecommunications: videoconferencing & telehealth.* Paper presented at the International Conference on Recent Trends in Information Systems Proceedings, India.

Jayasuriya, R. (1998). Determinants of microcomputer technology use: Implications for education and training of health staff. *International Journal of Medical Informatics*, *50*, 187–194. doi:10.1016/S1386-5056(98)00067-7

Lapointe, L., Lamothe, L., & Fortin, J. (2006). The dynamics of IT adoption in a major change process in healthcare delivery. In Spil, T. A. M., & Schuring, R. W. (Eds.), *E-Health Systems Diffusion and Use: The Innovation, the User and the USE IT Model*. Hershey, PA: The Idea Group Publishing.

Mingers, J. (2001). Combining IS research methods: Towards a pluralist methodology. *Information Systems Research*, *12*(3), 240–259. doi:10.1287/isre.12.3.240.9709

Myers, M. D. (1997). Qualitative research in Information Systems. *Management Information Systems Quarterly*, *21*(2), 241–242. doi:10.2307/249422

Reinecke, I. (2004). *Managing Information in Health*. Melbourne National Health Information Summit.

Rogoski, R. (2005). Wireless by Design. *Health Management Technology*, (January): 1–7.

Sausser, G. D. (2003). Thin is in: web-based systems enhance security, clinical quality. *Healthcare Financial Management*, *57*(7), 86–88.

Simpson, R. L. (2003). The patient's point of view -- IT matters. *Nursing Administration Quarterly*, *27*(3), 254–256.

Siracuse, M. V., Pharm, D., & Sowell, J. G. (2008). Doctor of Pharmacy Students' Use of Personal Digital Assistant. *American Journal of Pharmaceutical Education*, *72*(1), 1–7.

Spil, T. A. M., & Schuring, R. W. (2006). *E-Health system Diffusion and Use*. Hershey, PA: Idea Group Publishing.

Stuart, D., & Bawany, K. (2001). *Wireless Services*. United Kingdom: Gartner.

Suomi, R. (2006). Introducing electronic patient records to hospitals: Innovation adoption paths. In Spil, T. A. M., & Schuring, R. W. (Eds.), *E-Health Systems Diffusion and Use: The Innovation, the User and the USE IT Model*. Hershey, PA: Idea Group Publishing.

Turisco, F. (2000). Mobile computing is next technology frontier for health providers. *Healthcare Financial Management*, *54*(11), 78–82.

Venkatesh, V., Morris, M. G., Davis, G. B., & Davis, F. (2003). User Acceptance of Information Technology: Toward A Unified View. *Management Information Systems Quarterly*, *27*(3), 425–478.

Versel, N. (2008). Use of Mobile and Wireless Technology Jumps in Hospitals. *Digital HealthCare*, from http://www.digitalhcp.com/DigitalHealthCare_Content.aspx?id=72018

Wisnicki, H. J. (2002). Wireless networking transforms healthcare: physician's practices better able to handle workflow, increase productivity (The human connection). *Ophthalmology Times*, *27*(21), 38–41.

Wu, K., & Wu, X. (2007). *A Wireless Mobile Monitoring System for Home Healthcare and Community Medical Services*. Paper presented at the Bioinformatics and Biomedical Engineering, 2007. ICBBE 2007. The 1st International Conference on.

Zhang, D. (2007). Web content adaptation for mobile handheld devices. *Communications of the ACM*, *50*(2), 75–79. doi:10.1145/1216016.1216024

Zikmund, W. (1994). *Business Research Methods* (International Ed. ed.). Orlando, FL: The Dryden Press.

Chapter 5
Factors Affecting the Adoption of ICT for Health Service Delivery in Namibia:
The Role of Functional Literacy and Policy Implications

Blessing M. Maumbe
Eastern Kentucky University, USA

Meke I. Shivute
Polytechnic of Namibia, Namibia

Vesper T. Owei
Cape Peninsula University of Technology, Republic of South Africa

ABSTRACT

The article examines ICT use in health service provision in Namibia. The patterns of ICT use for health services by patients, public and private health service providers are not yet fully understood. This study describes ICT applications in health service delivery to patients in the Khomas and Oshana regions of Namibia. The study interviewed 134 patients and 21 health service providers. Factor analysis on ICT use identified three main factor groupings namely, 'high technology', 'mobile technology' and 'traditional technology'. Multinomial regression results showed the major factors affecting multiple ICT awareness in the two regions as functional literacy, diverse sources of health information services, age and educational level of the patients. Logistic regression results on individual ICT use identified functional literacy, personal privacy, cost of ICT, age, education, and positive perceptions about ICT applications in improving health services as statistically significant factors influencing adoption by both rural and urban patients in Namibia.

DOI: 10.4018/978-1-60960-183-6.ch005

INTRODUCTION

The use of Information and Communication Technologies (ICT) in the provision of health services is growing rapidly throughout Sub-Saharan Africa and the developing world. As ICT are deployed in health service delivery (HSD), there is a need to understand how individuals are using the new devices to access health services. Namibia is one of the few African countries that have demonstrated leadership in ICT utilization (SIDA, 2002; Hesselmark & Miller, 2002:36), and HSD seems to provide growing opportunities for the application of these modern technologies.

For the effective use of ICT for health services to occur, both patients and health service providers (HSP) must be willing and able to use the new devices in health service provision. In addition, the use of ICT for HSD must be socially inclusive; that means both rural and urban-based patients must be exposed to the new ways of health service provision. Moreover, social inclusivity requires that both young and old, rich and poor, able-bodied and physically challenged, and individuals of various backgrounds must have equal access opportunities.

However, the emerging patterns of ICT use for health services by Namibian patients are not fully understood. Similarly, the use of ICT by public and private health service providers remains unknown, yet this may influence how they deliver services to their patients in the future. Given the gap that exists between the understanding of (i) the patterns of ICT use by patients and (ii) the degree or the extent to which ICT are being used for HSD by HSPs in Namibia. It is of paramount importance that knowledge is amplified of how this growing phenomenon is unfolding. Therefore, successful utilization of ICT for HSD requires that digital divide constraints, patient technology demand patterns, service provider access and utilization, and public policy among others are seriously addressed.

Failure to understand the key factors affecting ICT use for health services by patients may lead to gaps in enabling policies, ineffective policy formulation, or a total absence of policy. In turn, this may lead to a general lack of ICT awareness or it might affect the effective use of ICT in HSD in general. Without doubt, HSPs in both private and public health sector play a central role in the provision of ICT-based health services. In order to improve our understanding of the circumstances surrounding ICT use for health services, this particular article seeks to examine; (i) the factors affecting the use of both individual and multiple ICT by Namibian patients (ii) Highlight key constraints that inhibit patient's access to ICT for health services, and (iii) Recommend policy considerations for improving the uptake of ICT for HSD in Namibia. In order to address the above stated issues, this study analyzes the type of ICT being used in HSD to patients in the Khomas and Oshana regions of Namibia, an urban and rural setting respectively.

The rest of the article is structured as follows: In the next section, background information on transformations in HSD in Namibia is presented. Then secondly, the significance and limitations of the study will be described. Thirdly, institutional policies in support of ICT for HSD in Namibia will be examined focusing on government ICT policy and its implications for HSD and this is followed by a presentation on the theoretical framework of the study. Fourthly, the next Section presents the methodology used to collect and analyze data. And finally, the results and discussion of the findings will be presented and this will lead into the concluding remarks and recommendations for future research.

BACKGROUND: TRANSFORMATIONS IN HEALTH SERVICE DELIVERY (HSD) IN NAMIBIA

As in most developing countries, Namibia is at the threshold of expanding its ICT use in HSD to promote sustainable development and the knowledge society (Schware, 2003; Crede & Masell, 1998). In today's information society, health professionals need to maximize the potential benefits offered by ICT as a means to improve public access to health care and information (Wallace: 1997:88).

The Government of the Republic of Namibia (GRN) has developed a general ICT policy which was an outcome of several consultative workshops. This policy was aimed at shaping the use of ICT in the country, starting with the education sector. The policy provided the basis for the telecommunications policy and regulatory framework of 1999 (Namibia, 2002:19). In addition, there have been policy reforms in terms of ICT implementation in Namibia (Hesselmark & Miller, 2002:5). According to the Namibian National Information and Communication Infrastructure (2006), the country has been active in ICT policy formulation and in developing the necessary infrastructure for the information society. The country's telecommunications and Internet infrastructure is very advanced by African standards, (United Nations Economic Commission for Africa, 2006). It is important to observe that although a general ICT policy has been developed and implemented, there is still no official policy on ICT use for HSD.

A GRN's national development plan entitled "Namibia Vision 2030" aims to "improve the quality of life of the people of Namibia to the level of their counterparts in the developed world by 2030" (Namibia, 2004c: 7). The 2030 vision pertaining to ICT status in Namibia aims to advance ICT to achieve social and economic transformations in the country. As the cost of ICT continue to fall while the capabilities increase, ICT are bound to be applied throughout all the development sectors of the economy for the benefit of society (Namibia, 2004c: 79). One of the weaknesses of the "Namibia vision 2030" is that it does not describe the current state of ICT for HSD in Namibia, but it simply focuses on what is aimed to be achieved by the year 2030.

The Ministry of Health and Social Services (MOHSS) has adopted a decentralization policy to improve health service provision and management by devolving authority to the thirteen regional directorates of the MOHSS (Namibia, 2003:31). The thirteen regional directorates manage service delivery in all health districts. The provision of health services in Namibia is divided proportionally between the government (i.e., provides 70-80%), missions (i.e., provide 15-20%) and the private sector which provides 5 percent of the health services. Delanyo (2001:2) explains that the non-governmental HSPs in Namibia are mainly in the form of various religious missions, which are subsidized by the government and include hospitals, health centers and clinics, mainly in the rural areas of the northern part of the country. For example, the missions (i.e., Lutheran, Anglican, and Roman Catholic) are non-profit providers, and they are 100 percent subsidized by the MOHSS (Namibia, MOHSS, 2004b:5). The organization of health services in Namibia is depicted in Figure 1.

Given this background on health services provision, what is important to note is the fact that the state of health services is poised for a major improvement with the introduction of ICT in the Namibian health sector. ICT are used to support HSD to all the thirteen regions and thirty four districts. The main aims of using ICT tools such as personal computers is to analyze, document, and distribute the planning, implementation and evaluation of health information, and also to assist with resource allocation and direct changes in policies and strategies. Furthermore, the use of ICT aims to improve the delivery of quality health services and improve the effectiveness of strategies, monitor performance over time and identify

Figure 1. Organization of health service delivery in Namibia

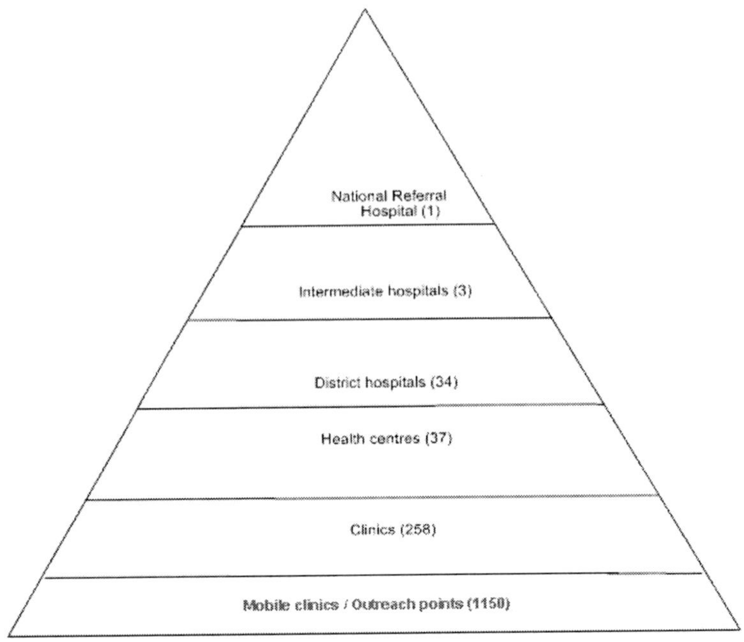

health facilities that need support and supervision (Haoses-Gorases, 2005).

According to Baldwin, Clarke, Eldabi and Jones (2002:312), ICT plays an increasingly crucial role in delivering healthcare nowadays. In Namibia, ICT applications to support HSD are growing, partly because the MOHSS has completely decentralized and computerized the health information system (HIS) to the regional and district level (Namibia, 2004a:26). The foregoing shows that ICT are being used to some extent to support HSD, even though there is need for improvement on the efficiency and effectiveness of the processes at the operational levels.

This study describes and analyzes factors that influence the adoption of ICT for HSD in Namibia with specific reference to the role of functional literacy and policy implications.

MOTIVATION, SIGNIFICANCE AND CONTRIBUTION OF STUDY

Given the growing importance of ICT use for socio-economic development in Africa, it is crucial to study the use of ICT in improving HSD in Namibia. It is crucial so that health services are diffused to communities in remote locations and those faced with health emergencies that require immediate diagnosis and intervention. There are signs of growing ICT related developments in the area of HSD in Namibia. HSD encompasses the provision of information for health care, prevention and treatment. By examining the literature and conducting a survey with both the patients and HSPs, recommendations can be made to policy makers on how to effectively deploy ICT in delivering health services in Namibia. The results of this study can be used to provide lessons for other African countries and draw some insights for policy and further research work.

LIMITATIONS OF THE STUDY

The limitations of this research are threefold; (i) it covers only two regions of Namibia, (ii) targets a specific age group of patients (i.e. those who were 15 years and older at the time of the study), and (iii) the fact that these results are drawn from a cross-sectional survey that are specific to the time of the study. We recognize the fact that ICT uptake is constantly evolving and the value of longitudinal studies should not be underestimated. It is also important to emphasize that this study does not address the use of ICT for the treatment, prevention or caring of patients with a specific disease ailment. Such more specialized studies will help provide valuable contribution to ICT applications in HSD.

LITERATURE REVIEW

Potential Impacts: ICT has the potential to radically change the way health services are delivered to patients and improve the quality of health services by providing easy access to health information. The potential use of ICT as a means to improve the quality of health services is widely acknowledged worldwide, and health institutions are striving to identify ways to deliver their services more efficiently and effectively. ICT can be utilized to minimize geographic isolation for the population in rural areas, and they can facilitate access, dissemination, utilization and exchange of information on combating debilitating diseases such as malaria, tuberculosis and HIV/AIDS (Yamuah, 2005:1). Chandrasekhar (2001:851) adds that ICT has the potential to be used as a mechanism to increase the transparency and efficiency of governance, which in turn would improve the availability and delivery of health services. ICT encourages easy dissemination of disease treatment and disease control and it also helps to reduce costs on patient transfers (Yamuah, 2001:2). Telemedicine is a good example of this, as it simply allows exchange of health information and delivery of health care across distances by using telecommunications (Rao, 2001:223).

Benefits: Numerous benefits in ICT use for health services abound. For instance, ICT use can facilitate the delivery of information in a reliable manner and enhance communication in the health sector. Technologies like the Internet and e-mail have the ability to send information in a fast, efficient and cheap fashion, which can provide remarkable improvements in access to information and care in the health sector (Pradhan, 2003:157). Historically, traditional technologies such as telephones have improved delivery of health services to patients, especially those in remote areas, and they continue to play a major role in this process. Mcwhirter (2003:341) suggested a wide range of ICT options and amongst them a bedside television that has been used as a source of health information for patients in hospitals in England. Radio has also been widely used as a means of communication especially in rural areas to better communicate health information to communities in remote areas. Kenny (2002: 141) reviewed the potential efficacy of radio and telephones and concluded that such ICT are powerful and sustainable tools that meet diverse information needs of the poor and that traditional technologies are less expensive than high technology such as Internet. In Uganda, FM radio transmission and modern graphics transmitted via the TV stations are one-way communication channels that are being utilized to deliver health service information to patients (Kasusse, 2005:148). Similarly, mobile computing or technology which includes laptops, palmtop computers, Personal Digital Assistants (PDAs) etc., are examples of portable ICT that are increasingly being used for health services (Hameed 2003:100) and are making health procedures more accurate and efficient thereby reducing the risk of human error (Chao, Jen, Hung, Li & Chi, 2006:1;Chau and Turner 2006: 307). PDAs have proven useful in African countries such Uganda

(Satellife Inc, Uganda Chartered Healthnet and Makerere University in 2003).

Challenges: While there are many benefits offered by using ICT in the health sector, there are a number of challenges which need to be tackled before the benefits are realized. Yamuah (2005:2) states that developing countries are facing a lot of challenges that hinder ICT use. The challenges in the health sector may be summarised as outdated modes of data collection, lack of electronic means to capture data, dependency on manual processes in hospitals for administrative, diagnosis and referral services in Africa and other developing countries, and low literacy rates among health providers that in turn affect ICT utilization, since literacy is critical for ICT use. The literacy problem is actually spreading from computers to new ICT, such as PDAs, 3G mobile phones, etc. Infrastructure constraints such as low distribution of reliable telecommunications and grid power in community health units, and lack of technical support have been identified as a hindrance in ICT use and the high establishment costs for ICT projects given limited budget for health services. The barriers in using ICT to enhance health services relate both to the specific use and access to certain ICT.

Computer use in HSD: Over the past decades, the use of computers in HSD has increased. Computers are being used particularly in large public hospitals and also in different applications such as Health Information Systems (HIS), computer-based psychological testing applications and individual patient monitoring in the intensive care units (Egan & Liu, 1995:357). Rao (2001:222) states that computers have become indispensable to the healthcare industry. The Internet has been widely used in health care industry and it has brought remarkable changes in the way services are delivered. It has been used especially in developed countries to supply health related information, such as diseases symptoms, research in the medical fields, etc. The Internet plays a vital role in the health sector and it has improved the process of delivering services to patients. According to Seror (2001:2), the Internet provides rapid access to medical information and expert consultation, and this will help in the process of delivering services in developing countries. Tele-health is one of the key ICT uses which include health services, education and research supported by the Internet, and it affects the way health services are provided (Seror, 2001:2).

INSTITUTIONAL POLICIES IN SUPPORT OF ICT FOR HEALTH SERVICE DELIVERY

Policies play a vital role in the use of ICT in any sector. According to Galloway and Mochrie (2005:41) policies have been developed for a number of ICT related issues. Galloway and Mochrie (2005:41) stated that policies may best intervene to support rural ICT development for economic sustainability or advantage. Policies should be developed with clear objectives and specific goals in mind, regarding expected achievements of the health institutions. In East Africa, ICT policies are being coordinated at the regional level with the aim to increase socio-economic development. The ICT policy framework in Eastern Africa is designed to foster sustainable development in various areas including the health sector (UN, 2003:2). In Asia, Quibria, Ahmed, Tschang and Reyes-Macasaquit (2003:819) state that policies to promote ICT involve key investments in education, infrastructure, creation of favorable institutions, fostering new institutional innovations and international cooperation. Schware (2003:3) argues that governments and health institutions should have policies and strategies on ICT implementation. Maumbe and Owei (2007:1) are of the opinion that in order to achieve long term success in e-service delivery and e-government policy development, it is critical to examine the socio-economic context and identify key constraints that inhibit the formulation and implementation of appropriate policies.

However, governments cannot merely set up their own policies but they must adhere to the international standards. Namibia (2002:33) has adopted a position that local government policy standards and related processes should be internationally benchmarked and must also facilitate interoperability within an international, voluntary and consensus-based environment for standards setting. The international standards bodies such as International Telecommunication Union guide Namibian policies and standard formulations. According to Maumbe and Owei (2007:1), the area of e-government and ICT policy development and implementation has received less attention in Africa, and South Africa is not an exception despite making great strides in e-government development.

At the time of the study, the Namibian MOHSS did not have an ICT policy developed specifically for the delivery of health services to patients. But there is a national ICT policy that the MOHSS adheres to. According to the interview with the directorate of policy and planning in the MOHSS the ministry adheres to policies set up by the public service management committees. However, it was established that the policy for HSD was in draft form at the time of the study and was still to be implemented. Even though, there is no ICT policy specifically for HSD in Namibia, there have been initiatives in other sectors such e-education. The ICT policy for education has been implemented with the aim of articulating the relevance, responsibility, and effectiveness of integrating ICT in education with a view to meeting the challenges of the 21st century (Tech/na, 2007:1). In this regard, Namibia is deemed to benefit from a similar focused ICT policy for HSD.

THEORETICAL FRAMEWORK FOR TECHNOLOGY ADOPTION IN HEALTH SERVICE DELIVERY

The use of ICT such as PDAs, PC, mobile devices etc. in the health sector has grown and both patients and health service providers need to be aware of these changes. According to Schaper & Pervan (2004), applications such as electronic patient records, telemedicine, clinical information systems will become common place in the health industry. However, the key question should be if such applications are implemented, will the stakeholders adopt or use the applications or ICT provided to them? Understanding the adoption factors and diffusion of ICT is paramount.

Damanpour (1991) study on adoption of health innovations reports that managerial attitudes towards change have positive influence on innovation adoption. Ma and Liu (2004) used the Technology Acceptance Model (TAM) to explain the usage of information technology. Johnson (2005) argues that TAM explains perceived ease of use and perceived usefulness predicts attitude toward use of technology. Further, the author adds that "attitude toward use predicts the behavioral intention to use". Davis (1989), defined perceived usefulness as the extent to which a person believes that using technology would enhance job performance and perceived ease of use refers to the extent to which a person believes that using the technology would be free of mental effort. According to Gagnon et, al, (2005) successful implementation of telehealth will ultimately depend on both human factors and organizational (and managerial or operational) factors.

A number of studies have used TAM as a basis for discovering the effect of external variables on the internal beliefs, attitudes, and intentions of users. A study by Lu, yu, Yiu and Yao (2003) developed a TAM for wireless Internet via mobile devices. Their study focuses on explanatory factors for use of wireless Internet and mobile devices. Lu, yu, Yiu and Yao (2006), conducted a comparison study whereby they compared various theories on technology adoption.

In contrast, the Theory of Planned Behavior (TPB) is believed to provide more specific information that can better guide development (Mathieson, 1991). TPB speculates that individual behavior is determined by behavioral intentions where behavioral intentions are a function of an individual's attitude toward the behavior, the subjective norms surrounding the performance of the behavior, and the individual's perception of the ease with which the behavior can be performed (behavioral control) (Ajzen, 1991). The TPB theory was later extended and integrated with TAM by Taylor and Todd (1995). The integrated model further incorporated additional factors that were not present in TAM.

The Unified Theory of Acceptance and use of Technology (UTAUT) explains end user intentions to apply an information system (IS) and subsequent usage behavior. According to Venkatesh et. al.,(2003), the theory consists of four key constructs namely, performance expectancy, effort expectancy, social influence, and facilitating conditions that are direct determinants of usage intention and behavior (dependent factors). Independent factors such gender, age, experience, and voluntariness of use are hypothesized to mediate the impact of the four key constructs on usage intention and behavior (Venkatesh et. al., 2003).

Not much research has been done to understand factors affecting multiple technology adoption in health service provision to patients. This particular study uses a different approach based on (i) the multiple nature of the ICT being adopted for health services. Secondly, the study setting is unique in that it compares the circumstances affecting ICT use for HSD among both rural and urban patients in a developing country context. The selection of variables affecting adoption draws upon common categories of independent variables that were used in previous studies namely, attitudinal, demographic, facilitative, managerial/operational, geographical, and performance related variables. A selection of previous studies and models used on technology adoption are summarized in Table 1.

Since this study focuses on the adoption of several ICT for HSD, it will employ multinomial and logistic regressions to determine significant factors that influence the aggregate use of these modern technologies and to draw policy implications. Those two models help us to understand factors affecting multiple as well as individual ICT adoption respectively. The empirical model uses key factors such as functional literacy, sources of health information services and demographic variables (e.g. age, gender, and level of education) to explain ICT use for HSD to patients. Table 2 summarizes the different categories of independent variables used in the empirical models. Based on the fore-going information; the next section will therefore describe the methodology used to collect and analyze data from respondents.

METHODOLOGY

The study examined ICT use in HSD in Namibia's rural and urban areas. The main focus of our study was on how patients and HSP use ICT in HSD. The study also examined patient views, constraints they face in using ICT to access health services, as well as government ICT policy and its implications for HSD.

Location of the Study

The study was conducted in the Khomas and Oshana regions of Namibia. The rationale for choosing these regions is that Khomas is representative of a typical urban area while Oshana region is situated in the northern part of the country which is primarily a rural setting. By conducting the survey in two different geographical areas, the researchers sought to make comparisons of any geographical and socio-economic differences and or similarities in ICT use for HSD.

Table 1. Selected technology adoption studies

Author	Model description	Data Collection (Sample Size)	Factors	Remarks
Davis (1989)	Technology acceptance model (TAM)	Cluster analysis used to determine the structure of the substrata.	-Near-term usefulness -Long-term usefulness -Ease of use -Behavioral intention to use	Developed the TAM to validate perceived usefulness & ease of technology use.
Lu, et.al., (2003)	Technology Acceptance Model (TAM) for wireless Internet via mobile devices	Empirical study used to examine the entire TAM for wireless Internet model.	Behavioral intention -Usage behavior -Performance expectation -Effort expectancy -Social influence -Facilitating conditions-age, gender, experience, willingness to use.	TAM for wireless Internet proposes a framework for understanding, explaining and predicting factors that influence individual acceptance of wireless Internet and mobile devices.
Chau and Hu (2001)	Comparison of TAM, Theory of Planned Behavior (TPB) and decomposed TPB models.	An empirical survey was used to get responses on telemedicine technology acceptance from more than 400 physicians in public tertiary hospitals in Hong Kong.	-Behavioral intention, attitude -Subjective norms -Perceived behavioral control -Perceived usefulness -Perceived ease of use compatibility	The model was limited to explaining technology acceptance by individual physicians.
(Venkatesh et. al., 2003).	Unified theory of acceptance and use of technology (AUT).	Longitudinal field studies conducted among individuals being introduced to a new technology in four different organizations.	-Individual differences, -Technology complexity, -Facilitating conditions -Social influences - Wireless trust environment - Near-term usefulness -Long-term usefulness -Nature of use-voluntary versus mandatory -Ease of use	The Unified Theory of Acceptance and Use of Technology (AUT) explains 70 percent of the variance in intention to use technology.
Gagnon et. al., (2005)	Contingency Analyses	Telephone interviews to 32 hospitals participating in Extended Telehealth Network of Quebec.	Identification of organizational factors affecting telehealth adoption.	Adoption affected by larger geographical, economic, and socio-political environment.

Khomas region is located in the central part of Namibia and it is 37,007 square km^2, and this is where the capital city Windhoek, is situated. The region consists of various health facilities that include a national referral hospital, an intermediate hospital, two health centers, seven clinics, three private hospitals, private clinics and thirty-three outreach points. The region has the highest population which stands at 264,616 compared to other regions in the country, and the population per hospital is 121,278 (Namibia, 2006). Access to ICT in the Khomas region is expected to be higher than Oshana, as the community tends to have better access to infrastructural resources. However, access to infrastructure cannot be taken to imply actual use, because it is possible that the community might have access to various ICT but may not necessarily utilize them. Nonetheless,

Table 2. Description of variables

Variable	Variable Description	Measurement/Scale
Dependent variable		
ICTAWARE	ICT awareness	[1] = Traditional technology, [2]= Mobile technology, [3]= High technology
Demographics/Patient Characteristics		
AGE	Age	Years
GENDER	Gender	[1]=Female, [0]=Male
EDUCATION	Level of education	Count/scale 1= Primary 2= Secondary 3=College 4 =University
RACE	Race	[1]=Black, [2[=Colored [3]=White
INCOME	Household income range	N$
LOCATION	Region	[1]=Khomas,[0]= Oshana
Operational/Management Variables		
INFOSCOUNT	Number of health information sources	Count variable
LITCOUNT	Number of ICT a patient can operate	Count variable
PRIVACY	Number of ICT contacts one is willing to share	Count variable
Perception variables		
STC	Skills and training capability	[1]= yes, [0] = no
STPERCEPT	Service convenience	[1]= yes, [0] = no
AFFORDP	Perception on affordability	[1]= yes, [0] = no
PEPINFRA	Perception on infrastructure	[1]= positive perception on infrastructure [0]= otherwise
PEPTRNW	Perception on training	[1]= positive perception on training [0]= otherwise

Source: Survey data, 2006

Khomas region tends to have better health facilities as it is more developed than the Oshana region.

On the other hand, Oshana region is the smallest region (5,290 km^2) with a population of 167,797, hence it is densely populated (Namibia, 2004a:1). The Oshana region forms the second largest population concentration in Namibia after Windhoek, but it lacks basic infrastructure and most of the services and facilities normally found in urban areas (Anon, 2007). The Oshana health directorate is divided into fifteen health facilities, one Intermediate Hospital (regional), four health centers and twelve clinics. The district also has twenty-eight outreach points. The Intermediate hospital is the ultimate referral point in the Oshana region and it is responsible for providing essential back up services and support for clinics and health centers in the region. Health centers are smaller than Intermediate hospitals and they are found in two types, namely, day care health centers and rural health centers (Namibia, 1998:16). The latter is common to Oshana region. The population per hospital in the Khomas region is 169,147 (Namibia, 2006).

Table 3. Number of questionnaires administered in the Khomas and Oshana health facilities

Type of health facility	Number of questionnaires administered with patients	Number of Health service providers interviewed
Khomas region	72	10
Oshana region	62	11
Total	134	21

Source: Survey data, 2006

DATA COLLECTION

Primary Data

Two separate surveys on patients and HSPs were conducted. The surveys were carried out in private and public health facilities in the Khomas and Oshana regions to explore ICT use by both patients and HSPs. The surveys were conducted during the period from July 2006 to August 2006. Given the privacy and confidentiality associated with health studies, permission to conduct the research study was first obtained from the Permanent Secretary of the MOHSS before data could be collected. Respondents were given the opportunity to not participate on the survey and were informed that their answers will be kept anonymous and their personal information will not be disclosed publicly. In addition, prior to the implementation of the actual survey, the structured questionnaires were pre-tested to improve the logical flow and rephrase vague questions that both patients and HSPs had some difficulty understanding. In that regard, pre-testing the questionnaires helped to evaluate the clarity of the instructions on the questionnaires and exclude sensitive health questions.

A total of 21 HSP were interviewed to determine factors that influence their use of ICT in delivering health services and specifically how ICT was being used to serve patients. The questionnaire for patients sought to establish kinds of ICT used when seeking health services, and obtain their views on ICT related services rendered by HSPs. The researcher made sure that all the patients who participated in the study were screened based on (i) if they had visited a health facility in the past three months and, (ii) if they were at least 15 years of age. Data was collected from a total of 134 patients in both the Khomas and Oshana regions. Table 3 shows the number of responses from questionnaires in different health facilities.

Secondary Data

Firstly, secondary data was sought *from various government publications such as white papers and public health policy documents. The research examined Namibia's ICT policy development and specifically its implications for the health sector. Secondly,* GRN officials from the P*olicy and Planning Directorate in the MOHSS were interviewed to further investigate* policies that engender ICT use in HSD. Secondary data obtained from the review of public policy documents and personal communications with government officials from the Policy and Planning Directorate provided useful insights on Namibia's readiness for ICT use in HSD.

Sampling Procedure

The first step involved the identification of the target population to be studied. The target population in terms of a geographical area studied was the HSPs and patients in health institutions in the Khomas and Oshana regions. The sampling procedure was therefore designed to produce a representative sample of patients from various public and private health facilities in the two regions. The selection procedure of the population sample was based on

Figure 2. Summary of steps in data analysis procedure Source: Survey data, 2006

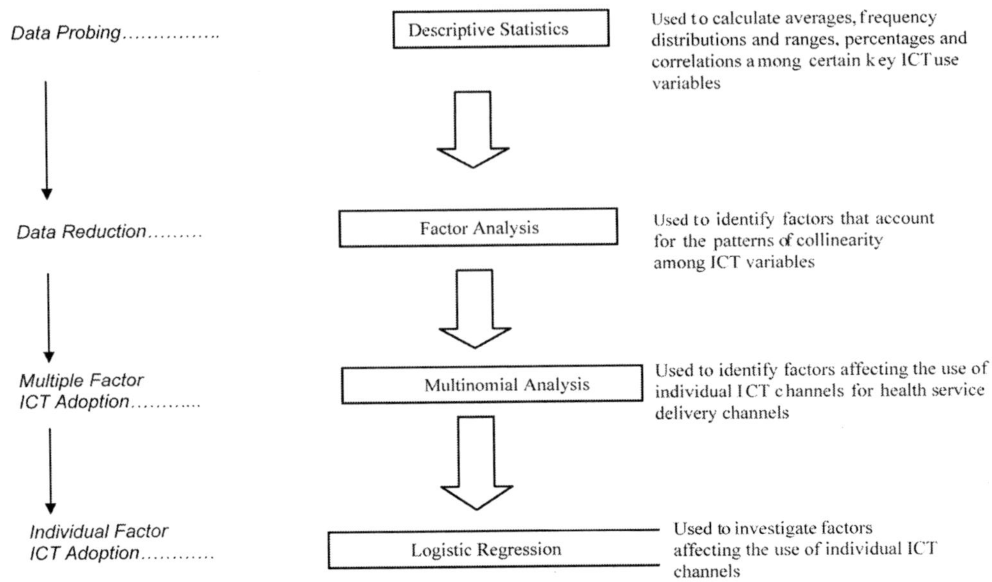

two sampling methods, namely multistage stratified sampling and purposive random sampling. Multi-stage stratified sampling sought to capture different regional health facilities and purposive random sampling sought to include only those patients who met a specific qualifying criteria as already highlighted above.

TECHNIQUES OF ANALYSIS

The analysis was conducted in a series involving four steps. The steps that were used in the analysis are (i) descriptive statistics, (ii) factor analysis, (iii) multi-nominal regression and (iv) binary logistic regression. A summary of the steps or techniques used for data analysis are depicted in Figure 2.

Descriptive Analysis

This was used to calculate averages, frequency distributions, ranges, percentages and correlations among certain key ICT use variables as well as between ICT use and patient demographics.

Factor Analysis

Factor analysis was conducted *on eight ICT based HSD channels used in the study areas namely, PC, email, Internet, fax, mobile, radio, telephone and television. The aim was to find out if they could load on a common component in the component matrix. Kaiser- Meyer-Olkin and Bartlett's test was conducted to test if the variables were suitable for factor analysis. Bartlett's test was found to be statistically significant for the combined data set*

Multinomial Analysis

Multinomial regression was used to identify factors affecting the use of multiple ICT channels for HSD. The ICT awareness variable was developed using results obtained from the factor analysis which generated three categories which were labeled, 'high technology', 'mobile technology' and 'traditional technology'. A chi-square test was conducted to identify important variables affecting ICT awareness.

Results from the chi-square test were then used to identify variables that were used in the multinomial model. Since there were multiple responses for ICT use, multinomial regression analysis was carried out to determine factors influencing the use of multiple ICT in HSD in Khomas and Oshana region. The dependent variable (ICTAWARE) was determined based on the patient's usage and ownership of ICT.

Logistic Regression Analysis

The data was analyzed further using a logistic regression model to investigate factors affecting the use of individual ICT channels. *Logistic regression analysis was conducted on pre-selected "high technology" and "mobile technology" channels to determine the specific factors driving individual ICT use.Booysen (2006: 46) explains that logistic regression analyzes the relationship between one dependent variable and a number of independent variables. The selected ICT based channels used as dependent variables in the two separate Logistic regression models were (i) PC and (ii) mobile phones respectively.*

RESULTS AND DISCUSSION

The analysis of the results from the Khomas and Oshana regions was carried out to identify patterns of ICT use for health services in the two regions.

Descriptive statistics were conducted on data obtained from patients. Initially, the data sets from the urban and rural health institutions were analyzed separately to describe the ICT use patterns by region. Exploratory factor analysis was conducted to identify factors that explain patterns of collinearity among the eight ICT-based communication channels. Results of factor analysis identified three main factor groupings namely, '*high technology*', '*mobile technology*' and '*traditional technology*'. These factors were then used in the multinomial regression analysis to investigate factors affecting awareness of multiple ICT use by the patients. *Logistic regressions were used to reinforce the results from the multinomial regression analysis by identifying specific factors that influence individual ICT use by patients.*

Results of Patient Demographics

Patient's demographic characteristics by region are presented in Table 4. Out of a total of 134 respondents from both Khomas and Oshana regions, 71 percent of the respondents were female. The largest group of patients (47%) was in the 21 to 30 years age group from both regions. The majority of patients (89%) were black and (60%) have at least completed secondary education and 15% had finished college. The majority (61%) of the patients surveyed reported a household income of less than N$5000.

Comparison of the Khomas and Oshana Regions

The study compared the patterns of ICT use in the two regions. These comparisons covered mainly ICT health information sources, ICT-based communication channels, and their use in HSD.

Figure 3 shows the distribution of sources of information used by patients in the two regions. The two main ICT channels that were being used by patients as their sources of health information are radio and television (TV). Patients in the Khomas region tend to have more access to TV which was expected due to the fact that Khomas is in an urban area. Similarly, Internet use as a source of health information is higher in the Khomas (13%) than in the Oshana region (8.2%).

However, community health services rendered by health workers are higher in the Oshana (55%) than Khomas region (39%). The majority of patients indicated that they depend on multiple sources of health information. In addition, patients from both regions indicated that they also obtain their health information from other sources such

Table 4. Namibian patient demographics by region, 2007

	Khomas region		Oshana region		*Both regions*	
Demographics	**Total** N=72	%	**Total** N=62	%	*Total N=134*	%
Gender						
Female	54	71	44	69	98	73
Male	18	24	18	28	36	27
Age Distribution						
Under 21	11	15	8	13	19	14
21-30	30	40	33	52	63	47
31-40	16	21	11	17	27	20
41-50	9	12	6	9	15	11
51-60	5	7	2	3	7	5
61 and older	0	0	2	3	2	1
Education						
Primary [grade 1- 7]	4	5	7	14	11	8
Secondary [grade 8- 12]	46	61	34	65	80	60
Tertiary College	10	13	10	19	20	15
University	9	12	1	2	10	7
Other	n/a	n/a	n/a	n/a	13	10
Race						
Black	59	82	61	98	120	90
White	3	4	0	0	3	2
Colored	10	14	1	2	11	8
Household Income						
Less than N$ 5,000	43	57	38	59	82	61
N$5001-10000	24	32	14	22	37	27
N$11000-15000	3	4	5	8	5	4
N$16000 and more	none	none	2	3	5	4
Not disclosed	n/a	n/a	n/a	n/a	5	4

Source: Survey data, 2006

as, newspaper, pamphlets from health facilities, health education offered by nurses at health facilities, local or national campaigns and also through telephone enquiries to a health facility.

From the foregoing results, it is evident that ICT use is comparatively higher in the Khomas than in the Oshana region. Khomas being an urban region where most relatively high income people live this could be partly the reasons why access to, and use of ICT is higher than in the Oshana region. Combined data analysis results (i.e. Figure 3) clearly show that radio (90%) was the leading source for health information followed by national TV (58%), community health workers (48%), Internet (13%) and mobile phone (12%). It is interesting to note that mobile phone usage for HSD is still evolving despite more than 90 percent penetration rate recorded during the survey demonstrating a high mobile phone usage in general.

Figure 3. Distribution of information sources used by patients in the Khomas and Oshana regions Source: Survey data, 2006

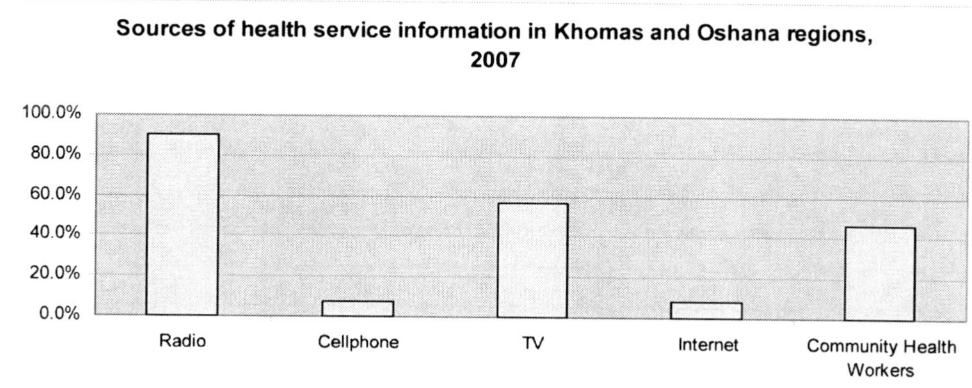

Table 5. Principal component analysis showing eigenvalues for components and percent of variation explained by each component, 2007

Component/ Variable	Initial Eigenvalues			Extraction Sums of Squared Loadings		
	Total	% of Variance	Cumulative %	Total	% of Variance	Cumulative %
1	2.602	32.524	32.524	2.602	32.524	32.524
2	1.737	21.713	54.236	1.737	21.713	54.236
3	1.012	12.649	66.886	1.012	12.649	66.886
4	.949	11.867	78.753			
5	.623	7.793	86.546			
6	.439	5.485	92.031			
7	.366	4.577	96.608			
8	.271	3.392	100.000			

Factor Analysis Results on ICT Use for Health Service Delivery

The study revealed that eight ICT-based channels were used for HSD by patients in Khomas and Oshana regions of Namibia. These ICT-based channels are namely, (i) personal computer, (ii) e-mail, (iii) Internet, (iv) mobile phone, (v) television, (vi) telephone, (vii) fax and (viii) radio. Exploratory factor analysis was conducted to identify common factor loadings that explain collinearity among the eight ICT variables. A correlation matrix was computed to test variables and confirm whether factor analysis was appropriate for the data. Bartlett's and Kaiser-Meyer-Olkin (KMO) tests were conducted to test for factorability of the data. The Bartlett's test result for sphericity was 276.720 and it was statistically significant at 1 percent level. The result of Kaiser-Meyer-Olkin (KMO) measure of sampling adequacy for this data was 0.677. Both tests indicated appropriateness of using factor analysis in this study.

It is considered that all factors that achieved eigenvalues greater than 0.5 were significant and conversely, those that were less than one were excluded. The number of components and the respective eigenvalues are shown in Table 5.

Table 6. Factor loadings on the component matrix for ICT use in the health service delivery system in Namibia, 2007

	Component		
	1	2	3
USEPC	.789	.098	.005
USEMAIL	.839	.009	.021
USEINT	.797	-.186	.023
USEMOB	.133	.908	-.002
USERADI	.051	.922	-.005
USETV	.163	-.040	.821
USETEL	.287	-.072	-.580
USEFAX	.716	-.106	-.009

Source: Survey data, 2006

Extraction Method: Principal Component Analysis

Source: Survey data, 2006 Principal component analysis (PCA) was the method used for factor analysis. This method aims to minimize the large number of variables to a small set of uncorrelated variables (Hair, Anderson, Tatham & Black: 1995). The PCA produced 8 components of which three were retained, and they had eigenvalues greater than or equal to one. The factor loading cut off point was 0.5. Table 6 shows the structure matrix and the loadings of the specific technologies on different components. The technologies that were grouped under component one are; personal computer, e-mail, Internet and fax. This group comprised of relatively modern technologies and was thus labeled '*high technology*'.

Table 6 shows that the technologies that loaded on component 2 were mobile phone and radio. One of the major characteristics for these technologies is the mobility aspect; and as a result this group was labeled '*mobile technology*'. Telephone and television loaded on component 3, and these technologies comprised traditional media channels and were therefore labeled '*traditional technology*'. According to Hopkinson and Pujari (1999: 282), factor loadings indicate the correlation between the variables and the factors such that variables with large loadings on the factors are grouped together. In this study, a factor loading of the value 0.50 and above is considered good and significant.

The study also examined ICT related constraints in delivering health services to patients. To uncover the constraints, an analysis of the factors that influence ICT use was conducted. However, since the study examined multiple ICT use in HSD, understanding factors affecting such use required a determination of awareness levels of the different technologies.

As already highlighted, the ICT awareness variable was determined using the results of the factor analysis. The awareness variable was based on the use of the three technology groups identified above. For instance, level one referred to the use of '*traditional technology*', level two '*mobile technology*' and level three '*high technology*' in that particular order. Therefore, the index for ICT awareness comprised four different levels namely; high technology, mobile technology, traditional technology, and no awareness. However, the results show that respondents fell into the first two categories. No respondent showed complete lack of ICT awareness on "traditional" technologies as stated above.

Table 7. Model fitting information for multinomial regression, 2007

Model	Model Fitting Criteria	Likelihood Ratio Tests		
	-2 Log Likelihood	Chi-Square	df	Sig.
Intercept Only	122.750			
Final	12.857	109.892	26	.000

Source: Survey data, 2006

Table 8. Chi-squared goodness-of-fit

Model	Model Fitting Criteria	Likelihood Ratio Tests		
	-2 Log Likelihood	Chi-Square	df	Sig.
Intercept Only	122.750			
Final	12.857	109.892	26	.000

Source: Survey data, 2006

All the variables except one have communality values above the cut off value of 0.5. This suggests that all the variables were adequately represented by the 3 components identified. A multinomial model regression was conducted to investigate factors affecting awareness of multiple ICT channel use for HSD.

Multinomial Logistic Regression Results

The independent variables that were included in the model are, demographics (e.g. age, gender, education etc), sources of health service information, functional literacy, attitude towards privacy and confidentiality, ICT use in HSD, and perception variables on ICT training appreciation and ICT infrastructure. Multinomial logistic regression predicts categorical outcomes with a potential of more than two categories (Statistical Package for the Social Sciences, 2007).

The model fit results of the multinomial regression are presented in Table 7. The model was found to be statistically significant at 1 percent level of significance. Salkind (2004:144) defines statistical significance as the degree of risk one is willing to take that one will reject a null hypothesis when it is actually true. He further explains that significance level is the "risk that is associated with not being 100 percent confident that what one has observed in an experiment is due to the treatment or what was being tested" (Salkind, 2004:144).

The results of chi-squared goodness of fit are reported in Table 8. The Pearson chi-square and a deviance (likelihood ratio) chi-square indicated a 1.000 significance level and this shows a good prediction of the ICT awareness (ICTAWARE) variable. The result (1.000) is not significant; therefore the model fits the data adequately. Lee, Kwon and Schumann (2005:429) explain that values that are greater than 0.05 in deviance statistics indicate a good fit with the data, and this makes the model acceptable. Garson (1998: 1) also states that the chi-square statistic test is desired to have an outcome of non-significance, as this indicates that the model has adequate fit for the data. The chi-square goodness of fit intends to find out how well a set of data "fits" an existing set (the observed data set), (Salkind, 2004: 266). Discrepancies between the model and data are also measured in the goodness of fit test. Li, Tan and Xie (2003:299) refers to the goodness of fit as the degree to which the structural equation model fits the sample data. The results of the Cox

Table 9. Multinomial logistic regression results for the Khomas and Oshana regions, 2007

Effect	Model Fitting Criteria	Likelihood Ratio Tests		
Variables	-2 Log Likelihood of Reduced Model	Chi-Square	df	Sig.
Intercept	12.857	.000	0	.
Age	34.162	21.305	5	.001 ***
Race	17.503	4.646	2	.098 *
Education [EDUC]	21.513	8.656	3	.034 **
Functional Literacy [LITCOUNT]	77.352	64.495	5	.000 ***
Sources of health information (INFSCOUN]	31.473	18.615	5	.002 ***
Privacy [INFCOUNT]	19.141	6.284	3	.099 *
Use of ICT for health services [ICTHEALT]	13.733	.876	1	.349 ns
Willingness to develop ICT skills [DEVICTSK]	15.876	3.019	1	.082 *
Perceptions on health services [PEPSERV]	19.273	6.415	1	.011 **

Source: Survey data, 2006
Notes:
***Significance at 1 percent level
** Significance at 5 percent level,
* Significance at 10 percent level
Ns = Not significant

and Snell and McFadden R-square were 0.603 and 0.880 respectively, and this indicates that the model is highly robust.

Table 9 present the significant variables from the multinomial regression results. The results show that there are three key variables that were statistically significant at 1 percent level, and these are functional literacy (LITCOUNT), age, and sources of health information services (INFOSCOUNT). This finding suggests that functional literacy, access to diverse information sources for health services and age particularly influence multiple uses of ICT channels. Education (EDUC) and a positive perception on health services (PEPSERV) were statistically significant at 5 percent level. Perceptions on health services entail views from patients on whether or not they perceived private and or public ICT services positively or negatively. These results clearly show that patient's ability to effectively utilize the ICT channel (i.e. functional literacy); access to diverse sources of health services information, better educational attainment and age are the most important factors that influenced multiple ICT channel use in HSD in Namibia, particularly in Khomas and Oshana regions. Logistic regression was conducted to further confirm key factors that affect the adoption of individual ICT channels. The results are presented in the next section.

Results of Binary Logistic Regression on Individual ICT Channel Use

According to Agresti (2002: 175), the logistic regression model compares the observed counts and fitted values by using either likelihood ratio (G^2) or Pearson X^2 statistic. The logistic regression analysis was conducted to ascertain factors that influence individual ICT channel use for health services. In order to identify key factors affecting individual ICT channel adoption, a likelihood ratio chi-square X^2 test of independence was initially conducted to establish associations between the

Table 10. Binary logistic regression results for personal computer use in the Khomas and Oshana regions, 2007

	PC			
Variable	B	S.E	Sig.	Exp (B)
Age	-.815	.368	.027**	.443
Education [EDUC]	.467	.241	.052*	1.595
Functional Literacy [LITCOUNT]	3.258	.753	.000***	26.004
Privacy for health information [IMPORTP]	2.965	1.291	.022**	19.386
ICT Improves health services [ICTIMPR]	-3.230	1.898	.089*	.040
Perception on infrastructure [PEPINFRA]	1.773	.945	.061*	5.887

Source: Survey data, 2006
Notes:
***Significance at 1 percent level
** Significance at 5 percent level,
* Significance at 10 percent level
Ns = Not significant

eight ICT based communication channels and the independent variables.

A backward-wald selection method was used to identify the most significant variables influencing ICT adoption leading to the selection of a final model. In this method, variables specified for the model are entered into the model together and they are removed from the model based on their significance of Wald statistic. The pre-selected ICT channels were personal computer and mobile phone. The aim was to select at least one ICT from the "high technology" and "mobile technology" groups and identify major factors affecting its use by Namibian patients.

PC Adoption Results

Table 10 presents the logistic regression results for PC which represents the "high technology" ICT group. Results for PC show seven significant variables namely, functional literacy, age, education, perception on importance of personal privacy in health information, perception that ICT improves health services and perception on infrastructure support. Functional literacy was highly statistically significant at 1 percent level and has a positive effect on the likelihood of PC use. Functional literacy represents the ability for one to operate various ICT communication channels. Results showed that unitary increase in functional literacy (LITCOUNT) increases the odds of using PC by 26 times. This variable had the greatest effect on PC adoption in both Oshana and Khomas regions of Namibia. This result is consistent with the findings of the Multinomial regression model. Perception on the importance of privacy of health information for patients (IMPORTP) was statistically significant at 5 percent level and it had a positive (19.386) effect on the likelihood of PC use. This implies that an increase in positive perception on the importance of privacy of health information increases the likelihood of PC use by 19 times. This means that patients that had a positive perception on the importance of privacy of their health information were more likely to adopt PC as they are confident that it secures their private health information. Age was also statistically significant at 5 percent level, but had a marginal positive effect on PC adoption. Education (EDUC), perception on ICT infrastructure and perception that ICT improves health services (ICTIMPR) had a positive effect

Table 11. Binary logistic regression results for mobile phone

	Mobile phone			
Variable	B	S.E	Sig.	Exp (B)
Functional Literacy [LITCOUNT]	2.747	.699	.000***	15.592
Privacy [INFCOUNT]	2.569	.899	.004***	13.048
Contact details willing to share [SHAREC]	-6.620	3.589	.058*	.001
Willingness to develop ICT skills [DEVICTSK]	21.125	11209.486	.998	1E+009
Perception on infrastructure [PEPINFRA]	3.212	1.595	.044**	24.835
Perception on ICT cost [ICTCOST]	-2.246	1.091	.040**	.106

Source: Survey data, 2006
Notes:
***Significance at 1 percent level
** Significance at 5 percent level,
* Significance at 10 percent level
Ns = Not significant

on the likelihood of PC use at 10 percent level of statistical significance.

Mobile Technology Adoption Results

Logistic regression results on mobile phone are shown in Table 11. Functional literacy (LITCOUNT) and privacy (INFCOUNT), meaning the number of ICT channels with personal contact details that the patient is willing to share were statistically significant at the 1 percent level of significance. It is important to note that functional literacy was highly significant in both the PC and mobile phone logistic regression results. This implies that functional literacy measured by the patient's ability to operate the modern ICT is critical for their adoption.

Furthermore, a unitary change in functional literacy increases the odds of using mobile phone by 15 times. The result of privacy (INFCOUNT) indicate that a unit increase in the number of ICT related contact details that a patient is willing to share increases the likelihood of mobile phone use by up to 13 times.

A positive perception on infrastructure and the cost of ICT were statistically significant at 5 percent level. A unit increase on the perceptions on infrastructure increases the likelihood of mobile phone usage by approximately 25 times. In addition, a positive perception on the cost of purchasing a mobile phone had a positive effect on the likelihood of mobile phone usage, although the magnitude was marginal. Furthermore, the willingness to share personal contact details specifically with HSP was statistically significant at 10 percent level. This means that individuals who are predisposed to sharing their ICT contact details with HSP are more likely to use mobile phone, although the effect is marginal in this case as well.

Policy Implications of Findings

In finding answers to the research questions posed, literature was reviewed to get a better understanding of the status of ICT in Namibia and other developing countries. From the literature it has been established that:

1. There was no ICT policy specifically for HSD in Namibia at the time of study, but it was only in draft form. However, a general national ICT policy for the Republic of Namibia and a general Information Technology for the public service are in existence and these

were further used to comprehend current ICT policies.

2. The ICT policy for education has been implemented with the aim of articulating the relevance, responsibility, and effectiveness of integrating ICT in education with a view to meeting the challenges of the 21st century (Tech/na, 2007:1). A similar policy is needed in the health sector to promote the adoption of ICT for HSD. Key considerations should be given to enhance the use of ICT in the HSD in Namibia. These will be presented in the next section.

CONCLUSION

This study investigated the use of ICT for HSD in Namibia. The results showed that there was widespread ICT use for health services by Namibian patients. The study identified eight different ICT-based channels that were being used in one way or the other for health services. These were television, radio, telephone, mobile phones, personal computers, Internet, email and fax.

Television and radio stood out as the leading sources of ICT-channels for HSD, although there was clear evidence of widespread use of mobile phones and also personal computers to an extent. Results for multinomial regression and binary logistic regressions showed that the key factors affecting ICT use for HSD were functional literacy, sources of health services information, age, level of education, and a positive predisposition towards ICT use for health services among others. From a public policy standpoint, the study suggests the need for the Government of the Republic of Namibia to actively pursue the opportunities presented by ICT such as personal computer and mobile phones to complement traditional ICT-based HSD channels such as radio and television.

It is also recommended that a comprehensive ICT-based HSD policy be drafted to guide strategies and procedures for HSD in the Namibian health sector. Results of the study demonstrate the presence of a relatively high potential to use ICT to transform HSD in Namibia.

Furthermore, the results of this study can be used to provide insights into ICT use in HSD in other African countries. Future studies should probe ICT use in private or public health care focusing on a specific patient group or functional area, e.g. HIV and AIDS, maternity, emergency services etc. Alternatively, a similar study could assess the willingness to use modern technologies such as mobile phones, as there are likely future platforms for HSD; and some risks and benefits associated with such applications.

REFERENCES

Agresti, A. (2002). *Categorical Data Analysis* (2nd ed.). Canada: John Wiley & Sons. doi:10.1002/0471249688

Ajzen, I. (1991). The theory of planned behavior. *Organizational Behavior and Human Decision Processes, 50*(2), 179–211. doi:10.1016/0749-5978(91)90020-T

Anon. (2007). Khomas region. Wikipedia. http://en.wikipedia.org/wiki/Khomas [date accessed: 28 May 2007].

Baldwin, L. P., Clarke, M., Eldabi, T., & Jones, R. W. (2002). Telemedicine and its role in improving communication in healthcare. [October.]. *Logistics Information Management, 15*(4), 309–319. doi:10.1108/09576050210436147

Booysen, C. (2006). *The application of discriminant analysis and logistical regression as methods of compilation in the research function in youth rugby*. Pretoria: University of Pretoria.

Chandrasekhar, C. P., & Ghosh, J. (2001). Information and communication technologies and health in low income countries: the potential and the constraints. *Bulletin of the World Health Organization, 79*(9), 850–855.

Chao, C.C., Jen, W.Y., Hung, M.C., Li, Y.C. & Y.P. Chi. (2006). An innovative mobile approach for patient safety services: The case of a Taiwan health care provider.

Chau, P. Y. K., & Hu, P. J. H. (2001). Information technology acceptance by individual professional: a model comparison approach. *Decision Sciences*, *32*(4), 699–719. doi:10.1111/j.1540-5915.2001.tb00978.x

Chau, S., & Turner, P. (2006). Utilization of mobile handheld devices for care management at an Australian aged care facility. [Winter.]. *Electronic Commerce Research and Applications*, *5*(4), 305–312. doi:10.1016/j.elerap.2006.04.005

Crede, A., & Masell, R. (1998). *Knowledge societies...in a nutshell: Information technology for sustainable Development*. Canada: IDRC Books.

Davis, F. D. (1989). Perceived usefulness, perceived ease of use, and user acceptance of information technology. *Management Information Systems Quarterly*, *13*(3), 319–340. doi:10.2307/249008

Delanyo, D. (2001). Namibia country briefing paper. Department for international Development Health systems resource centre for the UK DFID. http://www.dfidhealthrc.org/shared/publications/Country_health/Namibia.pdf [date accessed: 10 March 2006].

Egan, G. F., & Liu, Z. (1995). Computers and networks in medical and Healthcare systems. [May.]. *Computers in Biology and Medicine*, *25*(3), 355–365. doi:10.1016/0010-4825(95)00016-W

Equity Network for Southern Africa (EQUINET). (2005). Equity in health Care in Namibia Towards needs-based allocation formula. MOHSS World Health Organization. EQUINET policy paper number 26, Windhoek, Namibia. http://www.healthnet.org.na [date accessed: 12 May 2006].

Gagnon, M., Lamothe, L., Fortin, J., Cloutier, A., Godin, G., Gagne, C., & Reinharz, D. (2005). Teleadoption in hospitals: an organizational perspective. *Journal of Health Organization and Management*, *19*(1), 32–56. doi:10.1108/14777260510592121

Galloway, L., & Mochrie, R. (2005). The use of ICT in rural firms: a policy-oriented literature review. *Info*, *7*(3), 33–46. doi:10.1108/14636690510596784

Garson, G. D. (1998). Statnotes: Logistic regression. Raleigh, North Carolina: Carolina State University. http://www2.chass.ncsu.edu/garson/pa765/logistic.htm) [date accessed: 2 April 2006].

Geldenhuys, E., Herbst, D., & Dixon, B. J. Schnetler, J. (ed) & Stoker, D., J. (1989). Survey methods and practice. Revised Ed. Pretoria: Opinion Survey Centre. HSRC.

Greenfield, T. (Ed.). (2002). *Research methods for postgraduates* (2nd ed.). London: Arnold.

Groves, R. M., Fowler, F. J., Couper, M. P., Lepkowski, J. M., Singer, E., & Tourangeau, R. (Eds.). (2004). *Survey Methodology*. New Jersey: John Wiley & Sons.

Hair, J. F., Anderson, R. E., Tatham, R. L., & Black, W. C. (1995). *Multivariate Data Analysis with Readings* (4th ed.). London: Prentice-Hall.

Hameed, K. (2003). The application of mobile computing and technology to health care services. [May.]. *Telematics and Informatics*, *20*(2), 99–106. doi:10.1016/S0736-5853(02)00018-7

Haoses-Gorases, L. (2005). Utilization of Health Information System (HIS) in Namibia: Challenges and opportunities faced by the health care delivery system. Paper presented at the international workshop on Strategies for Permanent Access to Scientific Information in Southern Africa: Focus on Health and Environmental Information for Sustainable Development, Pretoria, 5-7. September 2005.

Hesselmark, O., & Miller, J. (2002). A country ICT survey for Namibia. http://www.cyberzoo.co.za/download/milless/newdocs/Namrep%20 v5.pdf [Date accessed: 10 March 2006].

Hopkinson, G. C., & Pujari, D. (1999). A factor analytic study in hedonic consumption. [April.]. *European Journal of Marketing*, *33*(3/4), 273–290. doi:10.1108/03090569910253053

Johnson, A. M. (2005). The technology acceptance model and the decision to invest in Information security. Southern Association of Information systems conference. Savannah, Georgia, USA, 25-26, 2005.

Kenny, C. (2002). Information and communication technologies for direct poverty alleviation: costs and benefits. *Development Policy*, *20*(2), 141–157. doi:10.1111/1467-7679.00162

Laurence, G. G., & Paul, R. Y. (eds). (2000). Reading and Understanding more multivariate statistics. American Psychological Association.

Lee, E., Kwon, J., & Schumann, D. W. (2005). Segmenting the non-adopter category in the diffusion of Internet banking. *International Journal of Bank Marketing*, *23*(5), 414–437. doi:10.1108/02652320510612483

Lu, J., Yu, C., Liu, C., & Yao, J. E. (2003). Technology acceptance model for wireless Internet. *Electronic Networking Applications and Policy*, *1*(3), 206–222. doi:10.1108/10662240310478222

Ma, Q., & Liu, L. (2004). The technology acceptance model: a meta-analysis of empirical finings. *Journal of Organizational and End User Computing*, *16*(1), 59–74.

Mathieson, K. (1991). Predicting user intention: comparing the technology acceptance model with the theory of planned behavior. *Information Systems Research*, *2*(3), 173–191. doi:10.1287/isre.2.3.173

Maumbe, B. M., & Owei, V. (2007). e-Government policy development in South Africa: distributional issues and implementation hurdles. *Proceedings of the 2007 conference of the IST Africa*, Maputo, 9-11 May 2007: Ireland, IIMC International Information Management Corporation Ltd.

Mcwhirter, G. (2003). The potential for using hospital bedside TV services in England to provide patients with access to information. [December.]. *Aslib Proceedings*, *55*(5/6), 339–345. doi:10.1108/00012530310498914

Munukka.K. (2005). Bridging the digital divide? Development of information society in Namibia-Conceptions of the local actors. University of Tempere.

Namibia, M. O. H. S. S. (2004b). The technical efficiency of District Hospitals in Namibia. Windhoek: Directorate: Policy, Planning and Human Resources Development. Mcwhirter, G. (2003). The potential for using hospital bedside TV services in England to provide patients with access to information. [December]. *Aslib Proceedings*, *55*(5/6), 339–345.

Namibia. (2004)c. Namibia Vision 2030: Policy Framework for Long-Term National Development. Windhoek: National Planning Commission Secretariat.

Namibia. Ministry of Foreign Affairs, Information and Broadcasting. (2002a). Information and communication technology policy for the Republic of Namibia. http://www.uneca.org/aisi/nici/Documents/ICT%20Policy%20Document%20 Ver%208.2.pdf [date accessed: 8 March 2006].

Namibia. Ministry of Health and Social Services. (2005). Follow-up to the declaration of commitment on HIV/AIDS (UNGASS): Namibia Country Report. Windhoek: Directorate: Special Programmes (HIV/AIDS, TB & Malaria).

Namibia. Ministry of Health and Social Services.2006.Health Facilities. http://www.healthnet.com.na [date accessed: 20 April 2006].

Namibia. MOHSS. (2003). Namibia National Health Accounts November 2003.Windhoek: Directorate: Policy, Planning and Human Resources Development.

Namibia. MOHSS. (2004a). Annual Report of Oshana region: 2003-2004.Windhoek: Ministry of Health and Social Services.

Namibia.MOHSS.(1998).The referral system. Performance audit report of the Auditor General. Windhoek.

Pradhan, M. R. (2003). ICTs application for better health in Nepal. [April-June.]. *Kathmandu University Medical Journal*, *2*(6), 157–163.

Quibria, M. G., Ahmed, S. N., Tschang, T., & Reyes-Macasaquit, M. (2003). Digital divide: determinants and policies with special reference to Asia. [October.]. *Journal of Asian Economics*, *13*(3), 285–309.

Quibria, M. G., Tschang, T., & Reyes-Macasaquit, M. (2002). New information and communication technologies and poverty. *Journal of the Asia Pacific Economy*, *7*, 11–825. doi:10.1080/1354786022000007852

Rao, S. S. (2001). Integrated health care and telemedicine. [June.]. *Work Study*, *50*(6), 222–229. doi:10.1108/EUM0000000006034

Salkind, N. J. (2004). Statistics for people who (think they) hate statistics. 2nd ed. London: Sage.

Schaper, L., & Pervan, G. (2004). A model for information and communication technology acceptance and utilization by occupational therapists. http://s-cah-vishnu.infotech.monash.edu.au/dss2004/proceedings/pdf/72_Schaper_Pervan.pdf, [date accessed: 5 June, 2008].

Schware, R. (2003). Information and communications technology (ICT) agencies: functions, structures, and best operational practices. [June.]. *Information*, *5*(3), 3–7.

Schware, R. (2003). Information and communications technology (ICT) agencies: functions, structures, and best operational practices. [June.]. *Information*, *5*(3), 3–7.

Seror, A. (2001). The Internet, Global Healthcare Management Systems, and Sustainable Development: Future Scenarios. [August.]. *The Electronic Journal on Information Systems in Developing Countries*, *5*(1), 1–18.

Statistical Package for the Social Sciences (SPSS). (2007). *SPSS regression models*. http:/www.spss.com/regression [date accessed: 9 April 2007].

Statistical Package for the Social Sciences (SPSS). (2007). *SPSS regression models*. http:/www.spss.com/regression [date accessed: 9 April 2007].

Stevens, J. P. (2002). *Applied multivariate statistics for the social sciences* (4th ed.). London: Lawrence Erlbaum Associates.

Taylor, S. and Todd,P.A.(1995). Understanding information technology usage: a test of competing models, information systems Research, 6(2): 144:174.

Tech/na. (2007). ICT Integration for Equity and Excellence in Education. http://www.tech.na/download/ICTPolicy2005_15March2005.pdf [date accessed: 30th May, 2007].

(2007)... *Technovation*. doi:.doi:10.1016/j.technovation.2006.12.008

United Nations Economic Commission for Africa (UNECA). (2006). National Information and Communication Infrastructure (NICI) Policies and Plans (e-strategies), Namibia. http://www.uneca.org/aisi/nici/Namibia/namibia.htm [date accessed: 1 November 2006].

Venkatesh, V., Morris, M. G., Davis, G. B., & Davis, F. D. (2003). User acceptance of information technology: Toward a unified view. *Management Information Systems Quarterly*, *27*(3), 425–478.

Wallace, S. (1997). Health information in the new millennium and beyond: the role of computers and the Internet. [May.]. *Health Education*, *97*(3), 88–95. doi:10.1108/09654289710162488

Yamuah, L. K. (2005). ICT in the African health sector: towards healthy nations with ICT Wealth. i4d magazine: May 2005. http//:www.i4donline.net/may05/africanhealth.asp (date accessed: 20 June 2006).

This work was previously published in International Journal of Healthcare Delivery Reform Initiatives, edited by Matthew W. Guah, pp. 63-87, copyright 2009 by IGI Publishing (an imprint of IGI Global).

Chapter 6
Information Completeness:
A Qualitative Analysis of Indoor Air Quality (IAQ)

Gary Hackbarth
Northern Kentucky University, USA

John McQuade
J.P. Morgan, USA

ABSTRACT

Medical information is readily online to patients, family's doctors and others in search of enhanced or supplementary information arising from healthcare concerns. To a large extent, this information varies greatly in terms of information quality and depending on the healthcare information source, is often incomplete. This study used an indirect qualitative analysis of the information completeness of 31 Indoor Air Quality (IAQ) checklists using CATPAC and found that these sources differed in both the depth and breathe of information provided. We suggest that users of healthcare information may be underserved and that healthcare information providers might act in a more collaborative way to better balance the presentation of their information in terms of depth and breathe of presented content.

INTRODUCTION

Healthcare providers, patients, family, and friends are increasingly seeking medical information to discover, research, and evaluate the credibility of healthcare information found on the web, informational pamphlets, books, magazines, and advice from healthcare professionals (Kang, Yoo, & Ko, 2006). The easy availability of healthcare information online has led to concerns over the quality of health information rather than the way in which users interact with health information systems (Williams, Nichols, Huntington, & McLean, 2002). Poor quality or incomplete information may

DOI: 10.4018/978-1-60960-183-6.ch006

lead to discomfort, a wrong diagnosis, confusion, or perhaps death in extreme cases (Ammenwerth & Shaw, 2005; Smith, Wilson, & Henry, 2005). Users of healthcare information often evaluate the attributes of information quality in terms of the timeliness, accuracy, and completeness contained in the message (Cline & Haynes, 2001; Shankaranarayanan & Yu, 2006) but often see a high degree of information variability (Lindars & Spickett, 2000). While critical thinking skills are important in evaluating the timeliness and accuracy of medical type information, we often neglect to consider the completeness of information (Hsu, Li, & Zhi, 2004) because users often are not provided fundamental information that enables informed decision making (Hoffman-Goetz & Clarke, 2000).

Information completeness is about the depth and breadth of information provided to healthcare consumers about a particular topic. However, unlike accuracy and timeliness where users can receive cues (dates, references, etc.), users who are not experts lack the experience to gauge the completeness and credibility of the information they are receiving as it is tainted by the perspective of the information provider (Cline & Haynes, 2001). Prior medical studies note the importance of breadth and depth of information but they provide little insight into how a user might determine whether or not the information is complete (Williams, et al., 2002). Qualitative research is a useful methodology in developing new insights where a theory driven approach might overlook other factors. Thus, this study uses a qualitative approach to evaluate definitive information (collected facts and data about a particular subject, i.e. Indoor Air Quality) in order to determine the extent to which an informational set is complete and can be evaluated by a healthcare consumer.

Following the introduction, this article discusses medical information quality, information quality, completeness, and a qualitative methodology to study information completeness. The article concludes with a discussion of results, study limitations, implications for future research, and culminates with conclusions.

MEDICAL INFORMATION QUALITY

Healthcare consumers seek medical information to take better care of themselves and participate in a more informed way when they interact with a healthcare professional (Quintana, Feightner, Wathen, Sangster, & Marshall, 2001). In one study focusing on children requiring cardiac surgery for congenital heart disease, 58% used the Internet related to their child's diagnosis and 74% used the Internet for educational purposes before their child's diagnosis of congenital heart disease (Ikemba, et al., 2002). Traditionally, healthcare consumers read brochures, books, magazines or asked professionals to gain additional knowledge. Today, online medical information is readily available with many biomedical journals offering free Internet access as soon as articles are published or at least within the last two years of publication (Hundie, 2002). Weiler (2000) reported that two thirds of online users from the United States who searched for healthcare information reported success 90% of the time yet, there were few measures present to ensure accuracy (Weiler & Pealer, 2000). Unfortunately, information delivery channels may reflect inaccurate, incomplete and dated information that reaches users who have no way to evaluate the quality of the information they are receiving (Goldsborough, 2001).

Inaccurate and incomplete information can be costly. In one cited case, parents found a website with information from a purported tertiary care pediatric medical center based in the United States regarding advice "not" to hydrate a child who suffered from diarrhea (Crocco, Villasis-Keever, & Jadad, 2002). The parents faithfully followed this advice even as their child became progressively more ill. Ultimately the child required admittance to the tertiary care Pediatric Gastroenterology service at McMaster University Medical Center where the child was started on Pedialyte and solid foods. The child soon recovered. The parents were obviously upset and concerned they had received the wrong information. In fact they had received inaccurate and incomplete information. Upon review, it was obvious they had not misrepresented the information found on the website, rather, the information they followed did not conform to standards of care found in any available clinical practice guidelines (Crocco, et al., 2002). This example is perhaps extreme but points out the potential variability of the medical information available to healthcare consumers and the importance of cross checking and evaluating multiple sources of information.

A study of 75 postmenopausal osteoporosis websites concluded that few websites provided comprehensive medical information or complete information and that the content and quality of these websites were highly varied and biased (Perez-Lopez & Perez-Roncero, 2006). A similar study evaluating the quality of information found on the Internet related to rheumatoid arthritis found that the Internet was a poor source of information, quality information was hard to find, was time consuming and recommended that standards were needed to regulate who and what was published on the Internet (Culver & Chadwick, 2005). Further, some healthcare studies of the Internet recommend the Internet not be used as a single source of patient information unless they are professionally endorsed. In a study of Osteosarcoma, less than 10% of relevant websites were of high informational value (Liu & Liu, 2006). Similar studies in this vane found wide variations in the quality of information concerning Cervical Cancer, Multiple Sclerosis, Colorectal Cancer, Dental Education, Prostrate Cancer, Osteoporosis, Retinopathy, Menopause, cosmetic surgery, cancer risk and brain trauma informational sources (Atreja, et al., 2005; Black & Penson, 2006; Chestnutt & Reynolds, 2003; Cheung, Morze, Jones, & Venkatesh, 2006; Ekman, Hall, & Litton, 2005; John, 2006; Ko, Brown, Frost, & Woosley, 2006; Lewiecki, Rudolph, Kiebzak, Chavez, & Thorpe, 2006; Lopez, 2004; Martins & Morse, 2005; Selman, Prakash, & Khan, 2006; Smarritto, Mitrofanoff, Haddad, & Pavy, 2003).

INFORMATION COMPLETENESS

Information Quality (IQ) is a value or quality determination of the content of information contained in a collection of data. It is a subjective judgment by users and importantly, such determinations can vary among users and by uses of that information. It has been suggested that three of the most important and commonly addressed information quality dimensions are accuracy, timeliness, and completeness (D. Ballou & Pazer, 1985; Fox, Levitin, & Redman, 1994; Klein, 2001; Wang & Strong, 1996). Timeliness and accuracy have been addressed in depth many times (D. Ballou & Pazer, 2003; Donald Ballou, Wang, Pazer, & Tayi, 1998; D. P. Ballou & Pazer, 1995; Mullen, Fontaine, & Muller, 2002) however, information completeness has been addressed to a lesser extent in the literature (D. Ballou & Pazer, 2003; Morey, 1982; Xu & Koronios, 2004/2005).

The Encarta English dictionary (North America) defines "complete" as having every necessary part or everything that is wanted. Kahn (2002) defined completeness of an information product as the extent to which data elements are not missing in a data set and are of sufficient breadth and depth for the task at hand (Kahn, Strong, & Wang, 2002). Ballou and Pazer (2003) examined the concept of completeness theorizing that completeness be thought of as two independent concepts; structural completeness and content completeness. Structural completeness is like filling out a form where we make sure all the elements are there, that is, the form is completely filled out. Content completeness requires the user to have all the necessary information to make a successful decision. As a search for information takes place, from the user's perspective, there must be a acceptable balance between the accuracy and completeness, or precision, of the information being received, so that the evaluation of the information search task is viewed as being successful (Bharati, 2002/2003). Precise rather than fully complete information is required because users do not want to be overwhelmed with information that clouds the few vital facts needed to make an accurate decision. In this sense, information completeness must be a balance between depths and breathe of available information in a particular context.

In our view, it is difficult for decision-makers to determine the validity or completeness of content that could have been conveyed without knowing the details of the processes and the origin of the data used for creating the content that is being evaluated. To some extent, we can review multiple informational sources to clarify or test information however; we believe that most decision-makers have neither the expertise nor the time to seek out additional information to determine what content may or may not have been conveyed from a single informational source. Although many quality assessment instruments are available, few can be used by health care consumers and in fact, few disclose their quality criteria (Bernstam, Shelton, Walji, & Meric-Bernstam, 2005).

Previous studies evaluating information completeness and quality used trained judges, medical experts, or pre-determined content criteria gleamed from selected content sources. A study of questionable websites on nonexistent nutritional supplements found that 50% of respondents were unable to identify the websites with the most trustworthy features (Ivanitskaya, O'Bole, & Casey, 2006). In another study of quality rating instruments, few were found to be of practical use by the intended audience (Bernstam, et al., 2005). More importantly, in another study of health information, of a total 172 websites studied, 85% contained accurate information but 65% of this information was incomplete and only 24% made reference to reliable sources (Sproule, Tansey, Burns, & Fenelon, 2003). When healthcare websites have attempted to develop scoring systems to evaluate quality, they have done poorly (Christopher, Hardwick, & McKenzie, 2003; Gagliardi & Jadad, 2002). What would be useful is a technique for uninformed users to be able to assess content for completeness (missing content) themselves but also determine some sense of relative importance of specific content.

QUALITATIVE METHODOLOGY

This study used CATPAC to conduct a content analysis of 31 Indoor Air Quality (IAQ) Checklists. Inductive content analysis is based in grounded theory and has been used to understand e-mail discussion groups, listservs, and other archived textual information (Glasser & Strauss, 1967; Lincoln & Cuba, 1985; Pennington, Wilkinson, & Vance, 2004). Informatic methods are essential for good quality control, especially for frequently changing information (Mitchell, Fomous, & Fun, 2006). In fact, qualitative methods may overcome the limitations of expert users who seem unable to conduct advanced searches and evaluate complex information even if they think their research skills are good or excellent.

Having chosen qualitative methods to evaluate potential data sets, we chose checklists as an indirect source of information to evaluate. We felt we could capture the majority of available checklists in print about a particular topic and keep content at a manageable level. Further, checklists represent a unique evaluation of content by experts in a specialized healthcare area. Experts creating checklists refine the content of an area and then ask questions of the user as to whether or not particular symptoms, situations, factors, events, etc. have occurred. Content has already been filtered by experts with the type and number of questions in a checklist being an indirect measure of depth and breadth of a topic area. Checklists are a precise way for experts to eliminate extraneous information, focus on a particular context, seek out the most accurate information, and capture what they think are a set of complete facts needed to make an evaluation. Given, that some checklists are designed for the non-expert, or those at least familiar with a particular healthcare problem, we have an opportunity to evaluate a data set that is both structurally and content complete.

Several Environmental Protection Agency (EPA), state government, and independent scientific studies have consistently identified indoor air pollution as an important environmental health problem (United States Environmental Protection Agency, 1997). For our purposes, we felt that many people sought information regarding the etiology, diagnosis, management and treatment of respiratory diseases related to Indoor Air Quality (IAQ). IAQ is an important issue for most Americans who spend up to 90% of their time indoors. IAQ refers to the quality of air inside buildings inclusive of pollutants and thermal conditions (heat and humidity) that affect the health, comfort, and performance of occupants. An important manifestation of information sharing in this environment is the IAQ checklist. IAQ stakeholders promulgate checklists as a way to identify IAQ problems in order to develop remedies to IAQ deficiencies. In the context of IAQ, our research hypothesis suggests a lack of completeness of information related to IAQ informational products and users seeking IAQ information.

Evaluation of these 31 checklists, summarized in Appendix A, required the copying of all checklists into a single text file for use in CATPAC, a self-organizing artificial neural network computer program used for analyzing text (http://www.galileoco.com). CATPAC reads and understands text by learning the inter-relationship among words and phrases in the text. There is no pre-coding of text nor is it necessary for the analyst to predetermine any categories in advance (Doerfel & Barnett, 1999). It allows categories to emerge from the data by allowing IAQ checklists to develop into meaningful conceptual groupings. The most fundamental output of the program is a matrix containing the mean response computed for every pair of concepts. CATPAC assigns a neuron to each major word in the text and then runs a scanning window. Neurons representing each word are paired with other neurons creating word-by-word paired comparisons resulting in a Dendogram (cluster analysis) which shows the pattern of relationships between key words and further identifies clusters of key symbols (concepts).

An alternative presentation of the data is a multidimensional scaling technique (perceptual mapping) that reveals the positions key concepts occupy in space. Mathematically, this is a process of converting a matrix (similar to covariance or correlation matrix) of distances to Cartesian coordinates. The stronger the relationship between symbols, the closer they are positioned in multidimensional space. The program can also provide descriptive and inferential statistics, including standard deviations, standard errors, indices of skewedness and kurtosis, sample size, minimum and maximum values, and other global statistics. These statistics provided no meaningful insight into data from past studies and thus, for this study as well, we can be satisfied with a straight forward analysis presenting frequency tables, dendograms, and perceptual maps useful in prioritizing IAQ issues (Colfer, Woelfel, Wadley, & Harwell, 2001). While the program is not particularly difficult to use, some thought, preparation, and book keeping skills are needed to make sense of the data. Table 1 summaries the process needed to create, correct, and organize a CATPAC text file.

RESULTS

Our initial analysis resulted in the creation of two text files; one related to IAQ for buildings (17 Checklists), including schools, and a second for homes (14 Checklists). Each of the checklists clearly showed two very different set of circumstances regarding air quality issues and will be

Table 1. Checklist analysis methodology

Step 1	Gather data collected from articles, books, pamphlets and internet sources.
Step 2	Consolidate data into a text file for analysis by CATPAC software (http://www.galileo.com). Develop initial analysis including word frequency, key word grouping, and relationships. This process allowed us to determine we needed two text files, one for buildings and one for residential dwellings.
Step 3	As shown in Appendix B, words are changed in the raw data when a plural form of the word or an abbreviation of a word could skew the analysis. For example "fan" and "fans", "CO2" and "carbon dioxide" or "air conditioner" which we changed to "airconditioners". In a situation like "air conditioners", we combined two words into one word to maintain the meaning of the two words together, and keeping the word "air" from being grouped with the individual word "air", which would have a different meaning for the checklist.
Step 4	Create an exclude file that eliminates unnecessary and redundant words. Excluded words are shown in Appendix C. Words are systematically eliminated one at a time until a text file remains that can be interpreted clearly. Most excluded words are direct or indirect articles, such as 'a', 'an' and 'the', as well as conjunctions, 'and' and or, or other common words unrelated to IAQ research. We also excluded vague or meaningless words within the context of the checklists. For example, problems may seem like a topic of IAQ but it turned out to be too vague. Another example is the word heating, which, when investigated within the raw data text file, was actually ambiguous, covering more than one topic or being not important to the context of the word grouping. Excluding words is an interactive process requiring words to be excluded in differing orders to assure a consistent result. Both researchers agreed on excluded words after conducting separate analyses.

Table 2. Building checklist key word frequency

Key Word	Frequency	Percentage
SMOKING	56	3.1
FILTERS	58	3.2
CHEMICAL	59	3.3
PAINT	63	3.5
HUMIDITY	63	3.5
CARBON DIOXIDE	65	3.6
TEMPERATURE	67	3.7
PRESSURE	67	3.7
CARPET	68	3.8
DRAIN	71	3.9
DUST	74	4.1
HEALTH	78	4.3
SMOKE	86	4.7
MOLD	88	4.9
LEAKS	92	5.1
MOISTURE	110	6.1
POLLUTANT	111	6.1
ODORS	114	6.3
WATER	179	9.9
FANS	242	13.4

discussed later. The length and complexity of individual checklists varied greatly in that building checklists contained a high of 668 and a low of 26 questions, while home checklists had a high of 84 and a low of 8 questions. The same exclude file was used for both text files.

Building Checklists

Table 2 is the Building IAQ Checklist frequency word list in ascending order for the 20 most used words. Frequency is the total number of times a word was used followed by its percentage compared to the total number of words. One may infer that those who created building checklists considered issues related to "fans" the most important and "smoking" of lesser importance based on word use frequency.

Figure 1 shows a Dendogram of inter-relationships between words grouped into named categories. An important part of the data analysis is the grouping of key words into concepts. Both authors agreed independently to the naming of these grouped words into concepts. The naming of these concepts is not done by CATPAC, but as a qualitative assessment of the data and knowledge of IAQ checklists. Respiratory Health Issues, Water, and Heating, Ventilation, and Air-conditioning (HVAC) Equipment represent common themes across the various building checklists. The column heights in Figure 1 represent relative intensity of the relationships between key words while the horizontal axis represents the relative strength of the relationship. The Respiratory Health group includes Carbon Dioxide, Smoke, chemical fumes, and paint fumes. These substances may be dispersed throughout a building atmosphere in small quantities or in some cases with considerable discomfort. Technical controls are often inadequate for early detection with the first sign of recognition often the human nose or eye. Positive pressure is also present in this grouping which is a function of the efficiency of the HVAC system and is required to keep pollutants from entering a building.

Water related issues grouped together in Figure 1 are the most commonly mentioned words in Table 2 and form the substantive portion of most building IAQ checklists. Water, humidity, moisture, drains and leaks create an environment behind walls, under floorboards or above ceilings ripe for mold growth. Odors often emanate from damp dark places. Fans are necessary to remove or circulate moisture in the air, help dry moist areas, remove odors, or filter particulates through air filters.

Figure 2 shows the building checklist multidimensional perceptual map with groupings

Figure 1. Building checklist dendogram

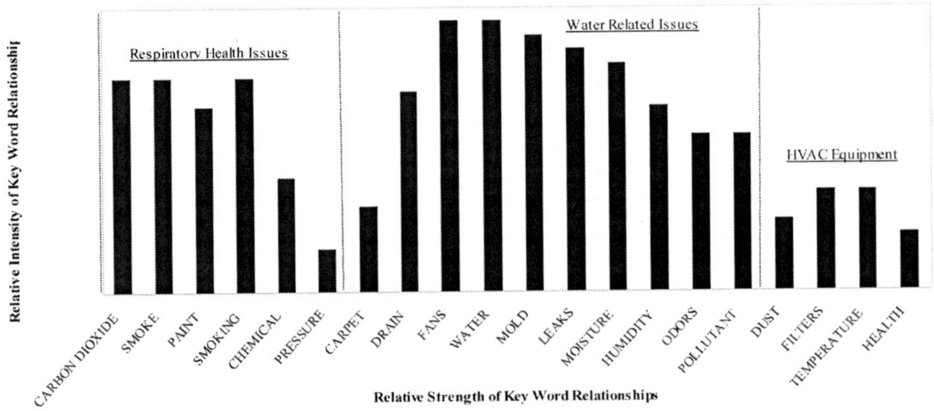

Figure 2. Building checklist multidimensional perceptual map with groupings

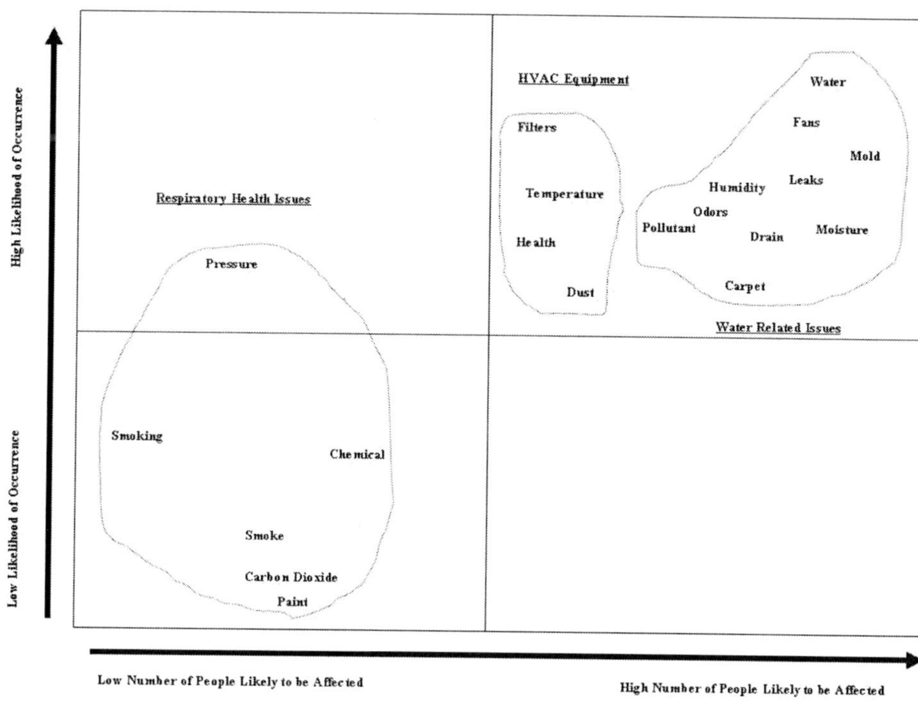

useful in prioritizing IAQ issues. The ordinate represents the likelihood of a particular IAQ issue occurring from low to high while the while the abscissa relates to the impact of a particular IAQ problem from low to high. Also associated with the ordinate are higher manageability costs and with the abscissa the cost of correcting IAQ problems. While severity may be relative, factors like smoke and paint fumes occur infrequently and can be managed easily through Standard Operating Procedures (SoPs) and other administrative procedures. Short exposure to smoke and fumes may not have long lasting health effects in most cases. Water issues are harder to control, thus they are more unmanageable and may result in more frequent, longer exposures to molds resulting in more intense health issues.

Home Checklists

Table 3 is the ascending IAQ Checklist frequency word list for homes. "Mold" and "Lead" are the two most frequently appearing words in home IAQ checklists while "Disease", "Pets", and "Allergies" are less frequently used. The word "Gas" is in reference to gas appliances. The Dendogram shown in Figure 3 groups these key words into seven separate but related concepts. These groupings are Water related issues I, Water related issues II, Respiratory Health, Allergens, Pets, Radon, and Lead paint issues.

Water issues in buildings cause similar problems in homes. Water I reflects water drainage from home air-conditions where drip pans may overflow causing damage or condensation. Water II reflects water intrusion from other sources like leaking roofs. Mold is associated with Water II,

Table 3. Home checklist key word frequency

Key Word	Frequency	Percentage
DISEASE	20	2.0
PETS	22	2.2
ALLERGIES	24	2.4
FILTER	26	2.6
AIR CONDITIONERS	27	2.7
SYMPTOMS	32	3.2
RADON	34	3.4
ASTHMA	35	3.5
PAINT	36	3.6
DAMP	41	4.1
SMOKE	42	4.2
MOISTURE	44	4.4
CARPET	46	4.6
GAS	53	5.2
DUST	64	6.3
CARBON MONOXIDE	70	6.9
HEALTH	81	8.0
WATER	89	8.8
LEAD	110	10.9
MOLD	114	11.3

perhaps because Water I moisture is easier to discover and correct.

The Respiratory Health group seems to focus on the effect of contaminants which are potential precursors of respiratory problems. For instance, Smoke and carbon monoxide may cause systems of asthma or related diseases. The Pet group is very specific and focuses on pets as a source of allergies, through saliva, urine, and dander. Lead Paint and Radon gas are also very specific home issues with known medical consequences. The Allergens group similarly represents the importance of clean carpets, exposure to formaldehyde from older carpets, and the way dust becomes trapped within carpets. Air filters exist to reduce these airborne particulates.

Figure 4 shows the home checklist multidimensional perceptual map with groupings. The ordinate represents the likelihood of a particular IAQ issue occurring from low to high while the while the abscissa relates to the number of people likely to be affected by a particular IAQ problem from low to high. Clearly, there is a greater dispersion of IAQ issues in homes compared to buildings. Similar to buildings, water issues are harder to manage and reflect the worry over mold induced illnesses. Closely aligned with allergens are pet IAQ issues. Of interest, radon is not an issue in buildings nor is lead paint. The key word disease seems to act as a linking word or concept between allergens and respiratory issues.

Figure 3. Home checklist dendogram

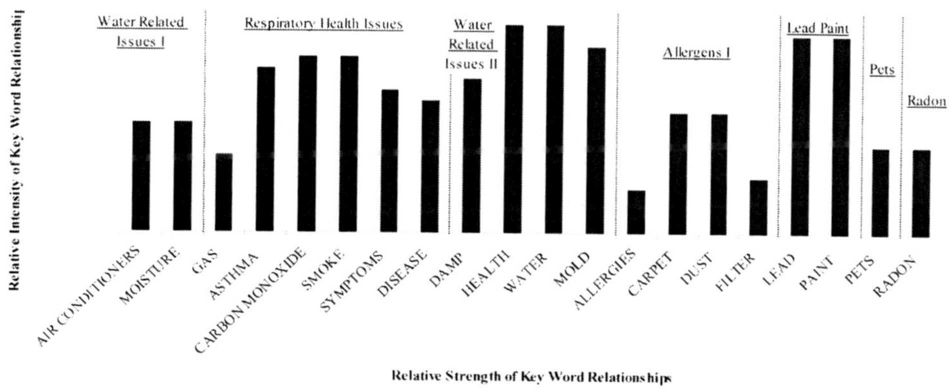

Figure 4. Home checklist multidimensional perceptual map with groupings

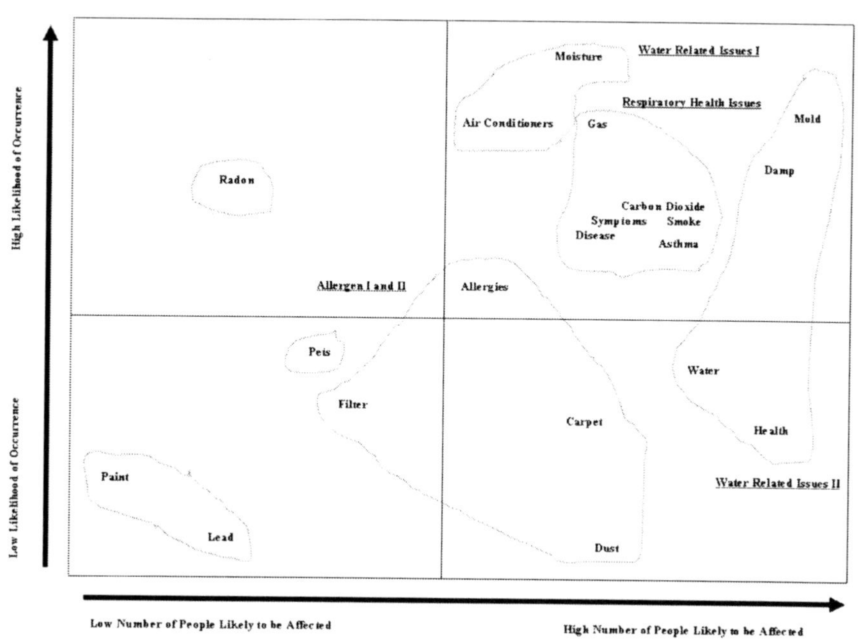

Our initial analysis suggested two contexts for evaluation, buildings and homes. To better understand these differences, we recombined checklist text files while using the same exclude file to overlap the depth and breathe of the completeness of information presented in the checklists. Figure 5 compares key word frequencies between Building and Home checklists. Stripped black indicates home checklist keywords and black, building IAQ checklists. The overlap areas focus on water, moisture, damp, and the associated growth of mold. There is concern about filters, smoke, and paint with a similar focus on the impact of carpeting. Carpeting may cause fumes, collect dust, and must be cleaned regularly to maintain clean air.

Of equal interest is where the two types of checklists differ. Building checklists are concerned about smoking, pressure, temperature, drains,

Figure 5. IAQ checklist key word comparisons

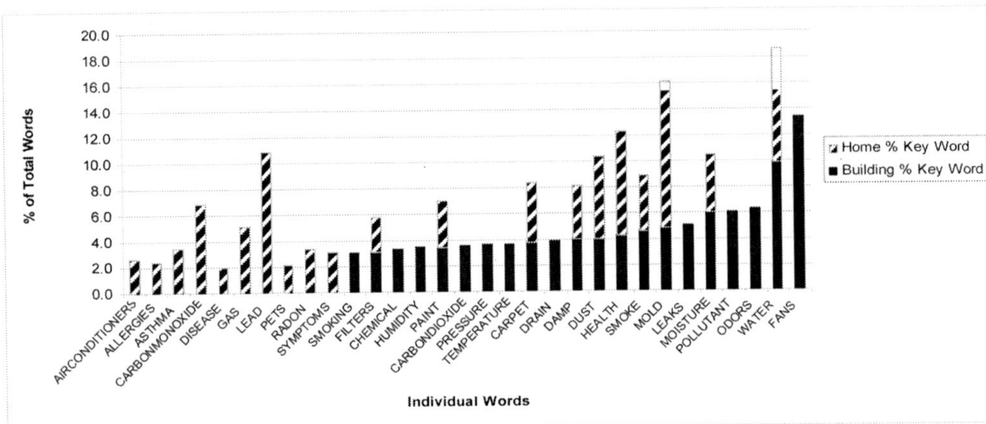

leaks, pollutants and odors, probably related to HVAC systems. Existing laws restrict smoking in public places, which does not intrude into residential homes, but it would seem that home checklists should include such a question as an obvious contributor to poor IAQ. Another interesting observation is building checklists concern themselves with drains while home checklists do not even though homes with basements typically have drains that run off the furnace/AC unit and many homes have sump pumps.

Similarly, building checklists do not address asthma, allergies, symptoms and disease. We know the "Sick Building" syndrome exits yet building checklists are not proactive in seeking evidence of its existence (Agency, 1991). Older buildings may have window air conditioners, which present the same water and mold issues as homes. Further, lead paint, radon, pets, and gas are important home checklist issues but are not concerns for building checklists.

To gather a deeper appreciation of the differences between building and home IAQ checklists we plotted concepts developed from the individual dendograms (Figures 2 and 4) and key words (Tables 2 and 3) by individual checklist found in Appendix A. This allowed us to create tables that reflect the extent to which keywords and concepts exist within individual checklists. Such tables reflect the extent to which keywords and concepts are shared between individual checklists as evaluated by the authors. We placed an "X" at each intersection in Tables 4 and 6 when the key word existed within the checklist. An "X" was placed at each intersection in Tables 5 and 7 when more than half of the number of key words within a checklist concept existed. While arbitrary, this methodology gave us a practical sense of the coverage (depth and breathe) of key IAQ issues found in individual checklists.

When one compares Tables 4 and 6, one readily notes that home checklists are more similar than building checklists. Differences between Tables 5 and 7 suggest greater concept sharing between home checklists than building checklists. This may reflect greater differences in building checklists than home checklists even though building checklist appeared to be more homogenous with only three major concepts.

Table 4, the Building Checklist Keyword and Concept Comparisons table, readily shows that not all key words represent every concept suggesting that individual concepts do not reflect best practice even within a single checklist. The higher-level view of Building Checklist Concept comparisons shown in Table 5 is even more revealing. A large number of building checklists (9 of 17) fail to represent even a single concept. The percentages

Table 4. Building checklist keyword and concept comparisons

Building Checklists	Respiratory Health Issues						Water Related Issues										HVAC Equipment			
	CARBON DIOXIDE	SMOKE	PAINT	SMOKING	CHEMICAL	PRESSURE	CARPET	DRAIN	FANS	WATER	MOLD	LEAKS	MOISTURE	HUMIDITY	ODORS	POLLUTANT	DUST	FILTERS	TEMPERATURE	HEALTH
EPA: Indoor Air Pollution		X	X	X			X			X				X			X			X
Handbook of Indoor Air Quality Management	X			X						X		X		X		X	X		X	
Indoor Environmental Quality		X													X		X		X	X
IAQ Case Studies Reference Guide								X	X	X		X	X	X			X	X		
Indoor Air Quality Issues						X		X	X	X				X	X				X	
Indoor Air Quality & HVAC Workbook	X	X		X	X	X	X	X	X	X	X			X	X		X	X	X	
Air Quality Sciences		X		X											X					X
EPA: HVAC checklist						X		X	X	X		X						X		
EPA: IAQ Management checklist				X		X												X		X
EPA: School Air Quality checklist		X	X	X	X	X	X	X	X	X	X	X	X	X	X	X	X	X	X	X
EPA: Mold Remediation						X	X	X		X	X	X	X	X					X	

continued on following page

Table 4. continued

Centers for Disease Control: schools	X		X	X			X			X		X		X			X	X		
California Indoor Air Quality Program Schools (EPA)		X	X	X	X	X	X	X	X	X	X	X	X	X	X	X	X	X	X	X
IOMA's Safety Director's Report				X	X					X		X			X	X		X		X
EPA: Building Air Quality Action Plan		X		X	X	X		X					X		X	X		X		
CDC: IAQ Management checklist				X		X												X		X
EPA: Water Damage Cleanup							X		X	X	X		X	X						
PERCENT OF TOTAL	18	41	24	65	29	53	41	47	41	71	29	47	35	59	47	29	47	59	41	47

found at the bottom of table 5 reflect the coverage across checklists, suggesting stakeholders using a single Building IAQ checklist may not be receiving a complete (depth and breathe) picture of IAQ issues.

Tables 6 and 7 tell an equally revealing story for home checklists. Not all concepts are represented within individual checklists. However, only 1 of 14 checklists fails to represent a single concept suggesting a broader consensus of what should be in an IAQ home checklist, which is further reflected in the percentages found at the bottom of Table 7. Home checklists also show a higher percentage across all concepts of IAQ information when compared to the building checklists with the exception of water related issues. While we must be careful not to read more into these tables, it is clear that home and building checklists differ, and that key concepts are not consistently represented across IAQ stakeholders.

DISCUSSION

This study sought to discover the extent to which healthcare information from IAQ checklists were incomplete and suggest a qualitative methodology to aid a novice user in evaluating depth and breathe of content. We found variability of depth and breathe of content across checklists with identifiable key words and associated groupings. A novice user using CATPAC could follow the study methodology and arrive at a similar understanding of IAQ checklists. It is the identification of key words and grouped concepts from the dendograms and spatial mappings that would give a novice healthcare information investigator a starting position to understand the problem(s) they are facing. Further, they have a way to evaluate the completeness of the information they are receiving. Thus they have a tool not so much as to

Table 5. Building checklist and concept comparison

Building Checklists	Concepts		
	Respiratory Health Issues	**Water Related Issues**	**HVAC Equipment**
	1	**2**	**3**
EPA: Indoor Air Pollution			
Handbook of Indoor Air Quality Management			
Indoor Environmental Quality			X
IAQ Case Studies Reference Guide		X	
Indoor Air Quality Issues			
Indoor Air Quality & HVAC Workbook	X	X	X
Air Quality Sciences			
EPA: HVAC checklist			
EPA: IAQ Management checklist			
EPA: School Air Quality checklist	X	X	X
EPA: Mold Remediation		X	
Centers for Disease Control: schools			
California Indoor Air Quality Program – Schools (EPA)	X	X	X
IOMA's Safety Director's Report			
EPA: Building Air Quality Action Plan	X		
CDC: IAQ Management checklist			
EPA: Water Damage Cleanup		X	
PERCENT OF TOTAL	23.5%	35.3%	23.5%

answer questions but to discover what questions they need to ask.

We found that Home and Building checklists differed. Some checklists were more complete and reflect greater emphasis on the identification of health related factors. We can see this in the conceptual breakout of lead, radon and the cause of allergies. Clearly, water related issues are a high priority in terms of management attention and health concerns. Mold is especially of concern in both home and building checklists reflecting its ranking as the number one IAQ issue. For homeowners, mold is a health issue, whereas for building managers, it may be more of a legal or liability issue.

In general, Respiratory Health Issues reflect concern over what building and home occupants breathe in. Regular HVAC maintenance seems to be an important consideration for both homes and buildings. Smoke and Carbon Monoxide are related words. This makes sense intuitively, as Carbon Monoxide is a result of many people breathing a limited air supply and is potentially deadly as a result of a fire or malfunctioning furnace. A reduction of particulates by using air filters or removing problematic carpets, pets, or other sources of respiratory discomfort is of corresponding interest.

Allergy groups are rated as mid- level importance in the home perceptual map. They are more of a concern in homes than buildings, where you will be more likely to encounter pets as well as thicker pile carpets. Radon is present in the home checklist with a fairly high manageability cost.

Table 6. Home checklist keyword and concept comparisons

Home Checklists	Water Related Issues I		Respiratory Health Issues						Water Related Issues II				Allergens I				Lead Paint		All er gens II	Radon
	AIR CONDITIONERS	MOISTURE	GAS	ASTHMA	CARBON MONOXIDE	SMOKE	SYMPTOMS	DISEASE	DAMP	HEALTH	WATER	MOLD	ALLERGIES	CARPET	DUST	FILTER	LEAD	PAINT	PETS	RADON
American Lung Assoc		X	X		X	X			X		X	X		X	X	X	X	X		X
BSIconnection.com	X			X							X	X	X	X		X			X	
Cook Heating & AC						X	X						X	X					X	X
AirCareOnline											X	X				X			X	
American Academy of Allergy, Asthma & Immunology			X	X	X		X	X		X	X	X		X	X		X	X	X	
Shafer s Heating and Air	X	X	X	X		X					X		X		X				X	X
American Lung Assoc Maine	X	X	X	X		X					X		X		X				X	X
University of WI Healthy Home	X	X	X	X		X	X		X	X	X	X	X		X	X			X	X
University of WI IAQ checklist	X	X	X	X	X	X			X	X	X	X	X	X	X	X			X	X
Consumer Federation of America		X	X	X		X	X	X		X	X	X		X		X	X	X		X
U.S. Consumer Product Safety Commission						X	X			X										
HUD			X	X	X	X		X	X	X		X	X	X	X		X	X	X	X
ALA: Top Ten Tips for a Healthy Home	X	X	X		X	X				X	X	X		X	X					X
Building Sciences Corp: Mold Remediation in Occupied Homes	X	X							X	X	X	X			X			X		
Percent Total	50	57	64	57	36	71	36	21	36	57	77	71	50	57	64	43	29	36	64	64

Table 7. Home checklist concept comparisons

Home Checklists	**Concepts**						
	Water Related Issues I	**Respiratory Health Issues**	**Water Related Issues II**	**Allergens I**	**Lead Paint**	**Allergens II**	**Radon**
American Lung Assoc			X	X	X		X
BSIconnection.com				X		X	
Cook Heating & AC						X	X
AirCareOnline						X	
American Academy of Allergy, Asthma & Immunology		X	X		X	X	
Shafer s Heating and Air	X					X	X
American Lung Assoc Maine	X					X	X
University of WI Healthy Home	X		X	X		X	X
University of WI IAQ checklist	X	X	X	X		X	X
Consumer Federation of America		X	X		X		X
U.S. Consumer Product Safety Commission							
HUD		X	X	X	X	X	X
ALA: Top Ten Tips for a Healthy Home	X		X				X
Building Sciences Corp: Mold Remediation in Occupied Homes	X		X				
	42.8%	28.6%	57.1%	35.7%	28.6%	64.3%.	64.3%

However, it does not show up in checklists with regular consistency to bring it into the high issue severity category. This may be because radon is a regional issue. A Lead paint group is present in the home perceptual map, located near the origin. This group's relative importance is rather low, as houses built since the mid 1970s have not used lead paint. Therefore, the issue has become less important over the years, except when renovating older homes.

It was interesting that building checklists focused on identifying and tracking down various causes of IAQ pollution before they occurred, perhaps because of liability issues. Home checklists, often devised by healthcare providers, focused on individuals and the identification of the causes of IAQ after a illness or problem manifested itself. Building checklists pay a closer level of detail to the overall HVAC system and subcomponents. Building maintenance and periodic monitoring of the HVAC system is necessary to ensure its efficiency and reliability. Moisture and respiratory health were common themes in both building and home checklists. Water in conjunction with temperature is the cause of mold, mildew and fungi. The cleanliness of carpets and reduction of dust are major objectives of both building and home maintainers.

The authors much like any other healthcare information seekers, would not understand all the in and outs of IAQ prior to doing the analysis. We learned and evaluated information as we went along. We did not start out as IAQ experts nor are we now. This is an important point. The purpose of this research and the methodology used was to see if a healthcare information seeker could look at a group checklists from various sources and develop a framework that would provide a grouping of concepts and ideas that would lead to better questions for the experts and some sense of the depth and breathe of IAQ or similar healthcare issues. Previous studies found that experts evaluated information as being incomplete, but the difference in this study is that non-experts can follow a similar methodology, placing themselves in a better position to seek and understand information from expert sources.

LIMITATIONS AND FUTURE DIRECTIONS

This research is limited in that we do not have all the IAQ checklists. An expanded list might provide additional insights and additional concepts. Other researchers might create a different exclude list altering the concepts and key words we report in this exploratory study. The way we chose to determine concepts and their comparison within individual checklists might be altered by other techniques or the addition of more checklists in the analysis. Additionally, an extension to the study could ask subject matter experts to compare and contrast qualitative results with their own expertise.

The lack of consistency across building and home checklists and within individual checklists suggests the need for more e-collaboration between stakeholders with requisite sharing of processes and IAQ knowledge. E-collaborative technologies encourage online interactions and support a move to self sustaining interactive environments (Andrews, 2002). Greater collaboration could result in checklists that are more complete. Today, stand alone software packages to track IAQ problems and resolutions for building managers, such as Solutions Software Corp's IAQ Manager (http://www.env-sol.com/Solutions/IAQ.html) exist but are not well known. These products, like so many checklists that we have analyzed, keep track of isolated IAQ developments for users who buy the product but do not have the ability to share with others and spread the knowledge.

Communities of Interest may represent an interesting way to resolve completeness issues. Such groups may have diverse interests but by being able to share these diverse views under a single umbrella, violable information would be more complete (Mullen, et al., 2002). It is also clear that there must be more effort to improve communication and information exchange between health consumers, professional, official organizations (Childs, 2004). Qualitative tools make it possible to develop informational sources that will allow health consumers to discriminate between high and low quality online information treatment. Another example application called DISCERN, changed consumer attitudes toward health information to being more critical or systematic (Charnock & Sheppard, 2004). DISCERN (http://www.discern.org.uk) provides users a brief questionnaire to assess the quality of written information on treatment choices for health problems.

Another area of further exploration in IAQ is country differences and cultural differences. Many cultures keep windows open and refrain from or do not have air conditioners because of fuel costs. Different cultures maintain and build buildings differently. Clearly, there would be an impact on the completeness and perhaps interpretation of information that is gathered impacting a user's evaluation of medical information.

CONCLUSION

This study is about a qualitative process to better filter information from the perspective of a non-expert analyzing healthcare information when they have little or no understanding of the topic of interest at the start of the process. We found that information completeness varied between Home and Building checklists and between checklists. Clearly healthcare consumers seeking checklists to improve their IAQ accept tremendous variability of information in terms of the depth and breathe of IAQ information. We believe our approach in this study is generalizable to other healthcare issues and provides a non-expert a contextual view of the data we analyzed. CATPAC provided a list of key words, dendograms, and perceptual maps that helped organize text into explainable concepts.

As a qualitative tool, CATPAC can give the non-expert some sense of the depth and breathe of available information given a large enough data set. Rather than rely on medical professionals or medical information providers to provide content and evaluate context, the non-expert can do their own assessment to determine what information is missing (incomplete) and to be able to ask more insightful questions.

To some extent, stakeholders tailor information for their particular purposes and their outlook may be tempered to the detriment of healthcare consumers who do not have the time or expertise to evaluate multiple informational sources. Checklists may exist for different purposes or are customized for specific deficiencies while overlooking factors too expensive to correct or factors not normally considered. Our approach represented an independent assessment of information completeness that may serve to enlighten and assist information seekers in developing nameable concepts they can use to frame the information they are receiving and perceive what they are not receiving.

Qualitative assessment of information quality and completeness do not guarantee the correctness of information a user of healthcare information is receiving but it might increase the level of confidence they have in their healthcare provider. Healthcare providers might seek to provide more complete information with users being more informed and able to more fully understand their situation. We also believe healthcare stakeholders would benefit from e-collaboration with other providers by sharing best practices, operating procedures and shortcuts in a central repository of knowledge. Ultimately, we would like users of healthcare information to evaluate the depth, breathe, and context of information they are receiving for themselves and not rely solely on others for their information value judgments.

REFERENCES

Agency, U. S. A. a. R. E. P. (1991). Indoor Air Facts No. 4 (revised) Sick Building Syndrome. [Government publication].

Ammenwerth, E., & Shaw, N. T. (2005). Bad Health informatics can kill--is evaluation the answer? *Methods of Information in Medicine*, *44*(3), 215–231.

Andrews, D. C. (2002). Audience-specific online community design. *Communications of the ACM*, *45*(4), 64–68. doi:10.1145/505248.505275

Atreja, A., Mehta, N., Miller, D., Moore, S., Nichols, K., Miller, H., et al. (2005). One size does not fit all: using qualitative methods to inform the development of an Internet portal for multiple sclerosis patients. Paper presented at the AMIA Annual Symposium, Cleveland, OH.

Ballou, D., & Pazer, H. (1985). Modeling data and process quality in multi-input multi-output information systems. *Management Science*, *31*(2), 150–162. doi:10.1287/mnsc.31.2.150

Ballou, D., & Pazer, H. (2003). Modeling completeness versus consistency tradeoffs in information decision contexts. *IEEE Transactions on Knowledge and Data Engineering*, *15*(1), 240–243. doi:10.1109/TKDE.2003.1161595

Ballou, D., Wang, R., Pazer, H., & Tayi, G. K. (1998). Modeling Information Manufacturing Systems to Determine Information Product Quality. *Management Science*, *44*(4), 462–484. doi:10.1287/mnsc.44.4.462

Ballou, D. P., & Pazer, H. L. (1995). Designing information systems to optimize the accuracy-timeliness tradeoff. Information Systems Research: ISR: A Journal of the Institute of Management Sciences, 6(1), 51-72.

Bernstam, E. V., Shelton, S. M., Walji, M., & Meric-Bernstam, F. (2005). Instruments to assess the quality of Health Information on the World Wide Web: What can our Patients Actually Use? *International Journal of Medical Informatics*, *74*, 13–19. doi:10.1016/j.ijmedinf.2004.10.001

Bharati, P. (2002/2003). People and information matter: Task support satisfaction from the other side. *Journal of Computer Information Systems*, *43*(2), 93–102.

Black, P. C., & Penson, D. F. (2006). Prostrate Cancer on the Internet--information or misinformation? *The Journal of Urology*, *175*(5), 1836–1842. doi:10.1016/S0022-5347(05)00996-1

Charnock, D., & Sheppard, S. (2004). Learning to DISCERN online: applying an appraisal tool to health websites in a workshop setting. *Health Education Research*, *19*(4), 440–446. doi:10.1093/her/cyg046

Chestnutt, I. G., & Reynolds, K. (2003). Perceptions of how the Internet has impacted Dentistry. *British Dental Journal*, *11*(2), 161–165.

Cheung, B. K., Morze, C. J., Jones, M. A., & Venkatesh, B. (2006). Information on the Internet about head injury pertaining to intensive care: less quantity and more quality is needed. *Critical Care and Resuscitation*, *8*(2), 100–106.

Childs, S. (2004). Developing Health Website Quality Assessment Guidelines for the Voluntary Sector: Outcomes from the Judge Report. *Health Information and Libraries Journal*, *21*(2), 14–26. doi:10.1111/j.1740-3324.2004.00520.x

Christopher, J., Hardwick, R., & McKenzie, F. M. (2003). Information contained in miscarriage-related websites and the predictive value of website scoring systems. *European Journal of Obstetrics and Gynecology*, *106*, 60–63. doi:10.1016/S0301-2115(02)00357-3

Cline, R. J., & Haynes, K. M. (2001). Consumer Health Information Seeking on the Internet: The State of the Art. *Health Education Research*, *16*, 671–692. doi:10.1093/her/16.6.671

Colfer, C. J. P., Woelfel, J., Wadley, R. L., & Harwell, E. (2001). Assessing people's perceptions of forests: Research in West Kalimantan, Indonesia. In Colfer, C. J. P., & Byron, Y. (Eds.), *People Managing Forests: The Links between Human Well-Being and Sustainability* (pp. 135–154). Washington, D.C.: Resources for the Future.

Crocco, A. G., Villasis-Keever, M., & Jadad, A. R. (2002). Two Wrongs Don't Make a Right: Harm Aggravated by Inaccurate Information on the Internet. *Pediatrics*, *109*(3), 522–523. doi:10.1542/peds.109.3.522

Culver, M., & Chadwick, A. (2005). Internet Information on Rheumatoid Arthritis: An Evaluation. *Musculoskeletal Care*, *3*(1), 33–43. doi:10.1002/msc.24

Doerfel, M. L., & Barnett, G. A. (1999). A Semantic Network Analysis of the International Communication Association. *Human Communication Research*, *25*(4), 589–603. doi:10.1111/j.1468-2958.1999.tb00463.x

Ekman, A., Hall, P., & Litton, J.-E. (2005). Can we Trust Cancer Information on the Internet? - A Comparison of interactive cancer Risk Sites. *Cancer Causes & Control*, *16*(6), 765–772. doi:10.1007/s10552-005-1722-3

Fox, C., Levitin, A., & Redman, T. C. (1994). The notion of data and its quality dimensions. *Information Processing & Management*, *30*(1), 9–19. doi:10.1016/0306-4573(94)90020-5

Gagliardi, A., & Jadad, A. R. (2002). Examination of instruments used to rate quality of health information on the Internet: chronicle of a voyage with an unclear destination. *BMJ (Clinical Research Ed.)*, *9*, 569–576. doi:10.1136/bmj.324.7337.569

Glasser, B. G., & Strauss, A. L. (1967). *The discovery of grounded theory*. New York: Aldine.

Goldsborough, R. (2001). Mastering Computers: Can the Internet be trusted? *Tech Directions*, *61*(4), 13–14.

Hoffman-Goetz, L., & Clarke, J. N. (2000). Quality of Breast cancer sites on the World Wide Web. *Canadian Journal of Public Health*, *91*(4), 281–284.

Hsu, L. L., Li, H., & Zhi, Z. (2004). Establishing evaluation indicators in health and medical websites. *Hu Li Za Zhi*, *51*(3), 47–52.

Hundie, K. (2002). free medical journals Website: an exemplary service. *Campus-Wide Information Systems*, *19*(3), 113–116.

Ikemba, C. M., Kozinetz, C. A., Feltes, T. F., Fraser, C. D., McKenzie, D., & Shah, N. (2002). Internet Use in Families with Children requiring Cardiac Surgery for Congenital Heart Disease. *Pediatrics*, *109*(3), 419–422. doi:10.1542/peds.109.3.419

Ivanitskaya, L., O'Bole, I., & Casey, A. M. (2006). Health Information Literacy and Compentencies of Information Age Students: Results from Interactive Online Research readiness Self-Assessment (RRSA). *Journal of Medical Internet Research*, *8*(2), 1–15. doi:10.2196/jmir.8.2.e6

John, A. K. (2006). A Critical Appraisal of Internet Resources on Colorectal Cancer. *Colorectal Disease*, *8*(3), 217–223. doi:10.1111/j.1463-1318.2005.00882.x

Kahn, B. K., Strong, D. M., & Wang, R. Y. (2002). Information quality benchmarks: product and service performance. *Communications of the ACM*, *45*(4), 184–193. doi:10.1145/505248.506007

Kang, S. W., Yoo, J. S., & Ko, I. S. (2006). Development of a-health information website: evaluation categories with items for diabetes mellitus. *Studies in Health Technology and Informatics*, *122*, 777.

Klein, B. D. (2001). User perceptions of data quality: Internet and traditional text sources. *Journal of Computer Information Systems*, *41*(4), 9–15.

Ko, Y., Brown, M., Frost, R., & Woosley, R. L. (2006). Brief Report: Development of a Prescription Mediation Information Webliography for Consumers. *Journal of General Internal Medicine*, *21*(12), 1313–1316. doi:10.1111/j.1525-1497.2006.00620.x

Lewiecki, E. M., Rudolph, L. A., Kiebzak, G. M., Chavez, J. R., & Thorpe, B. M. (2006). Assessment of Osteoporosis Quality. *Osteoporosis International*, *17*(5), 741–752. doi:10.1007/s00198-005-0042-5

Lincoln, Y. S., & Cuba, E. G. (1985). *Naturalistic Inquiry*. Newbury Park: Sage.

Lindars, E. S., & Spickett, J. T. (2000). The content and efficacy of environmental public health journal homepages. *Asia-Pacific Journal of Public Health*, *12*(1), 32–36.

Liu, Y., & Liu, M. (2006). Osteosarcoma: Evaluation Information on the Internet. Telemedicine and e-Health, 12(5), 542-545.

Lopez, F. R. P. (2004). An Evaluation of the contents and Quality of Menopause Information on the World Wide Web. *The European Menopause Journal*, *49*, 276–282.

Martins, E. N., & Morse, L. S. (2005). Evaluation of Internet Websites about Retinopathy of Prematurity Patient Education. *Journal of Ophthalmology*, *89*, 565–568.

Mitchell, J. A., Fomous, C., & Fun, J. (2006). Challenges and Strategies of the Genetics Home Reference. *Journal of the Medical Library Association*, *94*(3), 336–342.

Morey, R. C. (1982). Estimating and improving the quality of information in the MIS. *Communications of the ACM*, *25*(5), 337–342. doi:10.1145/358506.358520

Mullen, D. R., Fontaine, M. A., & Muller, M. J. (2002). Understanding the Benefit and Costs of Communities of Practice. *Communications of the ACM*, *45*(4), 64–68.

Pennington, T., Wilkinson, c., & Vance, J. (2004). Physical Educators Online: What is on the Minds of Teachers in the Trenches? *Physical Educator*, *61*(1), 45–56.

Perez-Lopez, F. R., & Perez-Roncero, G. R. (2006). Assessing the content and quality of information on the treatment of postmenpausal osteoporosis on the World Wide Web. *Gynecological Endocrinology*, *22*(12), 669–675. doi:10.1080/09513590601012603

Quintana, Y., Feightner, J. W., Wathen, C. N., Sangster, L. M., & Marshall, J. N. (2001). Preventive health information on the Internet. Qualitative study of consumers' perspectives. *Canadian Family Physician Medecin de Famille Canadien*, *47*(9), 1759–1765.

Selman, T. J., Prakash, T., & Khan, K. S. (2006). Quality of Health Information for Cervical Cancer Treatment on the Internet. *BMC Women's Health*, *6*, 9. doi:10.1186/1472-6874-6-9

Shankaranarayanan, G., & Yu, C. (2006). Supporting data quality management in decision-making. *Decision Support Systems*, *42*(1), 302. doi:10.1016/j.dss.2004.12.006

Smarritto, S., Mitrofanoff, M., Haddad, T., & Pavy, B. (2003). Do we need a chart of quality for websites related to cosmetic surgery? *Annales de Chirurgie Plastique et Esthetique*, *48*(4), 222–227.

Smith, D. E., Wilson, A. J., & Henry, D. A. (2005). Monitoring the Quality of Medical News Reporting: Early Experiences with Media Doctor. Medicine and the Media--Research (MJA), 183(4), 190-193.

Sproule, J. A., Tansey, C., Burns, B., & Fenelon, G. (2003). The Web: friend or foe of the hand surgeon. *Hand Surgery*, *8*(2), 181–185. doi:10.1142/S0218810403001716

United States Environmental Protection Agency. O. o. A. a. R. O., Indoor Environments Division (6604J) (1997). An Office Building Occupant's Guide to Indoor Air Quality. [Web page]. (EPA-402-K-97-003).

Wang, R. Y., & Strong, D. M. (1996). Beyond accuracy: What data quality means to data consumers. *Journal of Management Information Systems: JMIS*, *12*(4), 5–33.

Weiler, R. M., & Pealer, L. N. (2000). The Site Legend: twelve components of a new strategy for providing website documentation. *The Journal of School Health*, *70*(4), 148–152. doi:10.1111/j.1746-1561.2000.tb06461.x

Williams, P., Nichols, D., Huntington, P., & McLean, F. (2002). Surfing for health: user evaluation of a health information website. *Health Information and Libraries Journal*, *19*(1), 98–108. doi:10.1046/j.1471-1842.2002.00374_2.x

Xu, H., & Koronios, A. (2004/2005). Understanding Information Quality in E-Business. *Journal of Computer Information Systems*, *45*(2), 73–82.

APPENDIX A. CHECKLIST SOURCES

Table 8.

Name	Reference/ Date	Type	Questions
EPA: Indoor Air Pollution	pamphlet, 1995	Building	63
Handbook of Indoor Air Quality Management	Moffat, 1997	Building	103
Indoor Environmental Quality	Godish, 2001	Building	57
IAQ Case Studies Reference Guide	Benda, 1999	Building	26
Indoor Air Quality Issues	Hansen, 1999	Building	50
Indoor Air Quality & HVAC Workbook	Burton, 1995	Building	724
Air Quality Sciences	Web site, N/A	Building	13
American Lung Assoc	Web site, N/A	Home	81
EPA: HVAC checklist	Web site, N/A	Building	218
EPA: IAQ Management checklist	Web site, N/A	Building	42
EPA: School Air Quality checklist	Web site, N/A	Building	668
EPA: Mold Remediation	Web site, N/A	Building	30
BSIconnection.com	Web site, N/A	Home	57
Cook Heating & AC	Web site, 2002	Home	8
AirCareOnline	Web site, 2004	Home	11
American Academy of Allergy, Asthma & Immunology	Web site, N/A	Home	84
Centers for Disease Control: schools	Web site, N/A	Building	34
Shafer's Heating and Air	Web site, N/A	Home	28
American Lung Assoc Maine	Web site, N/A	Home	28
California Indoor Air Quality Program – Schools (EPA):	Web site, N/A	Building	668
University of WI Healthy Home	Web site, N/A	Home	15
University of WI IAQ checklist	Web site, N/A	Home	56
Consumer Federation of America	Web site, N/A	Home	45
U.S. Consumer Product Safety Commission:	Web site, N/A	Home	15
HUD	Web site, N/A	Home	24
IOMA's Safety Director's Report	Periodical, 2004	Building	30
EPA: Building Air Quality Action Plan	Web Site, N/A	Building	100
CDC: IAQ Management checklist	Web Site, N/A	Building	42
EPA: Water Damage Cleanup	Web site, 2004	Building	12
ALA: Top Ten Tips for a Healthy Home	Web site, 2000	Home	10
Building Sciences Corp: Mold Remediation in Occupied Homes	Web site, 2002	Home	75

APPENDIX B. WORD CHANGES

Table 9.

Original Word	Changed To	Original Word	Changed To
area	areas	area	areas
systems	system	problems	problem
co	carbon monoxide	fan	fans
carpets	carpet	pollutants	pollutant
air conditioner	airconditioners	carpets	carpet
air conditioners	airconditioners	CO2	carbon dioxide

APPENDIX C: EXCLUDED WORDS

Building and Home Checklists

Table 10.

N	yes	complaints	HAD	MID	THOUGH	OF
d	will	flowing	WITH	OWN	WOULD	ON
e	supply	damper	ALSO	VERY	COULD	ONE
g	classroom	dirt	FROM	EVERY	SHOULD	OR
air	flooring	hvac	WERE	EACH	ABOUT	OUT
quality	outdoor	surfaces	WHILE	SOME	BECAUSE	S
number	cleaning	windows	THEN	MUCH	BECAME	SAME
iaq	materials	USE	NOW	ONLY	OFF	SEE
checklist	clean	MAKE	HERE	GAVE	EXCLUDE	SINCE
information	return	WHO	THERE	BEING	A	SO
indoor	problem	WHAT	CAME	WHICH	AN	STILL
help	date	WHERE	INTO	HIS	ANOTHER	SUCH
properly	equipment	WHEN	DURING	HERS	AS	TAKE
appropriate	occupants	HOW	THEY'D	BEEN	AT	THAN
i	regularly	WHY	AFTER	USING	BACK	THOSE
need	handling	IT'S	MRS	HER'S	BE	THROUGH
used	staff	ITS	MISS	WENT	BEFORE	TO
confirm	maintenance	THE	MISTER	MADE	BESIDES	TOO
completed	exposure	BUT	THEY	UNTIL	BETWEEN	UP
local	intakes	ANY	MAY	SAID	BY	WAY
school	operating	CAN	SHALL	SAY	COME	WE
building	under	THIS	DID	TRIED	DO	WELL

Table 10. continued

N	yes	complaints	HAD	MID	THOUGH	OF
activities	products	THAT	DIDN'T	TRY	EVEN	YOU
check	floor	AND	ISN'T	EITHER	HE	Page
areas	storage	HAVE	SHE	OTHER	HI	Q
room	students	FOR	HER	MORE	HIMSELF	Procedures
control	potential	ARE	HIM	LESS	IF	Management
system	near	HAS	YET	ALL	IN	
unit	time	THEM	GET	ONTO	IS	
supplies	inspection	THESE	KEPT	DONE	IT	
location	containers	OUR	GIVE	SAW	JUST	
airflow	food	YOUR	THUS	DOES	LIKE	
sources	good	YOURS	VERILY	NOT	MANY	
work	occupied	OURS	GOES	BOTH	MOST	
exhaust	source	THEIRS	GONE	NEITHER	MUST	
rooms	traps	THEIR	ECT	NOR	MY	
ventilation	provide	WAS	GOT	ALTHOUGH	NO	

This work was previously published in International Journal of Healthcare Delivery Reform Initiatives, edited by Matthew W. Guah, pp. 1-24, copyright 2009 by IGI Publishing (an imprint of IGI Global).

Chapter 7
Preparing Healthcare Organizations for New IT Systems Adoption: A Readiness Framework

Robert Breas
National IT Institute for Healthcare (NICTIZ), The Netherlands

Matthew Waritay Guah
Claflin University, USA

ABSTRACT

Information systems exist for hospitals but even the most advanced systems concentrate on relatively simple coordination, resource allocation and documentation aspects of healthcare operations. At the same time the need to improve health care performance by means of more sophisticated IT systems is widely felt. In practice, however, the adoption of new IT is usually a difficult and a very slow process. To analyse the underlying reasons, we identified a set of key bottlenecks in the IT adoption process by interviewing large groups of healthcare actors. We conclude that health care organizations should be better prepared in order to facilitate easier IT systems' adoption. To do so, a readiness framework is considered to be helpful, the contours of which are sketched in this article. It is also discussed how, based on clarified clinical pathways, workflow management can assist in framing optimization of resource utilisation, clinical decision-making, staff training and quality improvement in healthcare delivery.

INTRODUCTION

Recent drive to automate hospital information has focused on the formal implementation of electronic health records. These systems are largely relational databases that focus on transaction-based intra-enterprise applications. Yet only a limited number become fully functional, scalable, distributed systems with interoperability. Based on these

DOI: 10.4018/978-1-60960-183-6.ch007

observations, it is widely felt that more sophisticated information systems are needed to support health care performance based on the concept of clinical pathway optimisation. The adoption however of such integrated distributed information systems takes place at a very slow rate (Aarts 2005; Stoop 2005). Underlying reasons given in popular literature relate to the misunderstanding of healthcare business processes.

Healthcare processes are very complex and dynamic due to the involvement of clinical and administrative tasks, large data volumes, large numbers of patients and personnel with different tasks requiring specific knowledge. Healthcare is a business where many changes occur (i.e. (new) treatments, drugs, equipment, protocols, and legislation). These changes have their influence on the instantiated processes that need adjustment (Anyanwu et al; 2003).

Observation of the dynamic character of healthcare system and the implementation of IS at Erasmus MC (medical centre) led towards the following research question.

Which internal factors of IS implementation affect healthcare organizations' readiness for new systems?

The following sub-questions assisted in finding answers to the central research question.

- What are the consequences of IS implementation in health care?
- What is the impact of IS implementation on organization?
- What initial choices need to be made before an IS implementation decision in a healthcare organization?

The article is structured as follows. The next section describes the potential workflow management (WfM) and how WfM affects healthcare IS. That will be followed by a brief description of actor network theory (ANT) before a sketch on key bottlenecks related to the introduction of new IT as found in the scientific literature and selected by using criteria taken from change management. The design and results of the empirical research will integrate the content into a coherent view that is used to sketch a readiness framework for new IT adoption in complex healthcare environment. Finally, we discuss the high potential of WfM to provide optimised healthcare, provided that the healthcare organisation at stake has been sufficiently prepared for adopting of WfM systems. We finalize this article by presenting our conclusions.

What is Workflow Management?

In the last couple of years notion was growing about whether data processing in complex organizations should not only be based on integrated data management, but also on integrated process management. Organization processes usually define the order and time of data creation and alteration. Workflow management (WfM), also referred to as structured process management, is an important ingredient for data processing and data management in many cases. Automated support is needed to effectively and efficiently execute process management in complex environments and situations. WfM, from a general perspective, can be seen as administrative logistics. Like physical logistics where the right goods are delivered at the right place and time, WfM takes care of delivering the right information at the right time and by the right person (Grefen, 2001).

Workflow is an abstraction of a business process. Normally a workflow comprises a number of logical steps, known as tasks. These tasks consist of dependencies among tasks, routing rules and participants. A task can require human involvement, or it might be executed automatically by IS applications (Cardoso et Al, 2004). Some well established definitions of WfM in literature are given below.

The ultimate goal of workflow management is to make sure that the right persons execute the proper activities at the right time (Orlikowski, 2000). Although it is possible to do workflow management without using a workflow management system, most people associate WfM with WfM systems.

Cardoso (2002) defines WfM as a workflow model, which is customized to accommodate specific business process structures. Workflows are designed based on business processes. These processes already exist in an organization and need to be improved or managed better. Once the design phase of the model is completed, instances are created to carry the actual steps described in a given workflow. During their execution, the workflow instances can access legacy systems, databases, applications and can interact with users. Workflow systems are flow-independent; they control a data flow among tasks is graphically described during the workflow design phase. This makes applications independent from the underlying workflow system.

Workflow management is a technology supporting the reengineering of business and information processes (Georgakapoulos, 1995). WfM involves:

a. Defining workflows, e.g., describing those aspects of a process that are relevant to controlling and coordinating the execution of its tasks. It will require the skills of individuals or information systems to perform each task.
b. Providing for fast (re)design and (re)implementation of processes such as business needs and information systems change. To effectively support WfM, organizations must evolve their existing computing environments to a new distributed environment that:
   - Is component-oriented, i.e. it supports integration and interoperability among loosely coupled components corresponding to Heterogeneous, Autonomous and Distributed (HAD) legacy, current and new systems;
   - Supports workflow applications corresponding to business or information process implementations accessing multiple HAD systems;
   - Ensures the correctness and reliability of applications in the presence of concurrency and failures;
   - Supports the evolution, replacement, and addition of workflow applications and component systems as processes are reengineered.

The remaining of this section aggregates the above definitions for a more comprehensive one that suits the article's optimal objectives. The above definitions share three factors of importance to our interest in healthcare IS implementation: people, processes, and IS. The other definitions weren't complete on those factors, and lacked at least one of them. Our agreed definition of WfM is the customisation of workflow to accommodate specific business process structures. The goal is to have the right persons execute proper activities at the right time. Workflows are designed based on existing business processes in an organization that need to be improved or managed better. Therefore they support the reengineering of business and information processes. They define aspects of processes that are relevant and necessary for controlling and coordinating the execution of functional tasks. This will require the skills and input of individuals and the usage of Information Systems to perform each task. During the execution of tasks, workflow instances support integration and interoperability among loosely coupled components corresponding to Heterogeneous, Autonomous and Distributed (HAD) legacy and new systems. WfM must also be able to access legacy systems, databases, applications and set-up an interaction with users. It also must ensure the correctness a reliability of applications in the presence of concurrency and failures. Used applications are independent from the underlying workflow system.

The addition of all these factors may not be able to explain why adoption of new IT is so difficult (Guah, 2000). The difficulty is not due to problems related with software or hardware or to limitations of technologies in use. Systems fail because they are built on the wrong assumptions, incorporate problematic models of medical work or implementation is not seen as an organisational change (Berg et al. 2003).

Reflecting these observations, we recognize that organizations might not be well prepared for adopting new IT solutions. This case study on lack of readiness for IS implementation in healthcare organization contains interviews with a set of relevant healthcare actors in Erasmus MC, the largest medical centre in The Netherlands. The main goals of the case study were:

a. to show what we have found as the key bottlenecks in the IT adoption process,
b. based on these key bottlenecks found (and those presented in literature) to sketch the contours of a readiness framework to present in this article, and
c. to illuminate why and how, after having finished the preparation phase, workflow management has great potential to improve quality in complex healthcare delivery (Breas, 2007).

This research shows conflict between the tendency to build internal but somewhat restrictive systems and the need to plan for future interoperability, multi-functionality and scalability by the hospital management to avoid a too limited operational success and acceptance.

Actor Network Theory

Actor-Network Theory (ANT) is a well-known theory from within the field of science and technology studies that has developed conceptual constructs to deal with the processes through which technologies are developed and influence societies. Though ANT has a relatively short history, it is a multi-disciplinary field and unlike the field of information systems, it allows a deeper devotion to theoretical and explanatory studies, without assuming an intellectual responsibility for guiding professional practice (Latour, 1999).

The authors have selected ANT as a framework for analysis due to a number of reasons:

- It is well established with an important hinterland of work explaining, critiquing, developing and applying the theory; including application to information systems in the healthcare sector (Heathfield, Pitty, & Hanka, 1998);
- It has been comparatively stable, with later presentations building on the original theory, probably because the theory is "owned" by a particular group of followers (Latour, 1986);
- It overcomes some important limitations of the "IT as an enabler" perspective of general management science literature that are based on technological determinism and can thus be presented as a complementary approach to information system research.

ANT Concepts

The "actor-network" concept was developed by Michel Callon, Bruno Latour and John Law during the course of the 1980s as a recognition that actors build networks combining technical and social elements and that the elements of these networks, including those entrepreneurs who have engineered the network, are, at the same time, both constituted and shaped within those networks (Law, 1999).

The unique position of technologies in ANT recognizes that IT does not evolve under the impetus of scientific logic unlike common suggestions by technological determinism. IT does not possess an inherent momentum that allows it to do what Latour (1986) describes as passing through a neutral social medium. Bijker and Law (1992) similarly concludes that "technologies mirror societies" considering they are continuously shaped and reshaped by the interplay of a range of heterogeneous forces within the networks. Therefore IT is as much an actor in the networks as are the human parties.

Papers on ANT often develop their arguments in an empirical context (Latour, 1999; Law, 1999) with tales that tend to be heroic. They narrate how actors, within a specified period, manage to constitute themselves and their networks; thus treating the world as a set of related bits and pieces with no social order. There are only endless attempts at ordering through the formation and stabilization of networks (Latour, 1999). By telling stories and tracing histories rather than taking snapshots, ANT proves itself as "a pragmatic, recursive sociology of process with an interest in the uncertain processes that generate power and size" (Law, 1999). By clarifying power relationships in organizational settings, ANT helps us understand how actors are defined, associated and obliged to remain faithful to their alliances.

Bottlenecks

At this moment healthcare organisations are focussing more on the existing processes. Klischewski and Wetzel (2001) proclaim a couple of sticking points that exist in the healthcare environment concerning processes.

- The first sticking point they discuss is the lack of overall responsibility for either the process or it's planning. The process mostly relies on the ability and commitment of individual providers to flexibly shape the service according to their special insights about the patient's case (Klischewski and Wetzel, 2001). A lack of fixed responsibilities seems to be the crux of this problem;
- Secondly, there is a problem relating to the exchange of patient information. Clear rules are needed for documentation of patient records and the exchange of patient information;
- The third point concerns the monitoring of the process status. The healthcare providers involved have little oversight about the complete process, its current status or further development. Healthcare providers often lack information about deviations from tacitly assumed ways to proceed, or are unable to obtain this knowledge (Klischewski and Wetzel, 2001).

What often is forgotten, while implementing an IS related product, is that such an implementation will fundamentally affect the structure and processes in a health care organization. This is a core reason for failure of the implementation (Berg et al. 2003).

What is needed is a mutual transformation of the organization and the (level of) technology. Work tasks and information flows will be affected or changed. This will also affect relationships between (groups of) health care professionals. Discussions about data access among health care professionals will be inevitable and can lead to political and social issues (Berg et al. 2003).

An IS implementation should not be run as only a technical project. Organizational structures, routines and roles should be managed as well. This means that adequate user involvement is extremely important by development and by implementation of IS that must be accepted by the different users. A good fit between work processes, and involved characteristics like roles, and IS is evident. System specifications and implementation plans should be discussed among the different users and IS department. Interdependencies between work tasks should be made clear and less abstract for the users and IT-department during such discussion (Berg et al. 2003).

These identified sticking points by Klischewski and Wetzel result in a set of requirements regarding the software support for inter-organizational services in healthcare, or in other words Workflow Management. They claim four main requirements for the design process:

- **Flexibility support:** The support of the process has to provide flexibility and dynamic selection and configuration of services as the process moves on. The steps in the process also need to be transparent to the parties involved;
- **Interoperability:** Patient information between different physicians and other healthcare providers must be exchangeable and shareable. Therefore software components must be compatible with each other for digital information exchange;
- **Customer Orientation:** Service delivery has to consider the possibly changing customer concern and the subtleties in customer satisfaction. This goes beyond efficiency criteria of underlying processes and has to do with understanding the customer concern and with service customization, e.g. the availability of services;
- **Agreement Process:** The parties involved have to formulate the entire service process, e.g. the kind of service delivery, IS support (Klischewski and Wetzel, 2002).

These requirements are directly related to financial aspects, which also have an important role in healthcare. For this article the financial aspects were considered out of scope.

EMPIRICAL RESEARCH

Three methods of data collection were adopted. First, the researchers assembled a range of academic, government and industry studies on the healthcare sector in The Netherlands. This material proved invaluable for understanding some of the societal, economic, political, cultural and technical differences in today's healthcare delivery and that of the past decades. Second, we attended various meetings, workshops and exhibitions on Duthcare healthcare systems. Some of these events were focused on general topics (i.e. IT in healthcare, patient services, hospital management and professional best practice), with others more focused upon specific activities. These events generated many useful research contacts

We engaged in primary data collection, conducting around 25 open-ended and semi-structured interviews during the nine months period, with a range of actors (i.e. health service professionals and administrators, clinicians, IT researchers, and Erasmus MC IT deparmental staff).

Data Collection

Data was collected using questionnaire in the Obstetrics department and the outpatient clinic. Goal of the case study was to determine the level of efficiency and make measurements for pinpointing where more efficiency could be achieved. Two important aspects of the case study were the process analysis and the time measurement research, were every worker (from secretary till physician) had to register time spent on their tasks. This data was used to find out what and where the primary bottlenecks for IS and healthcare were. Figure 1 demonstrates the bottlenecks observed in the decision structure:

- Decisions are made by people who don't have a clear overview of the work floor;
- Lack of involvement of different actors with different functions during decisions;
- The IS department's primary task is to respond to the requested demand;
- Responsibilities about project tasks are ambiguous.

Figure 1. Business and IT roles, adapted for the Erasmus MC (Adapted Maes, 1999)

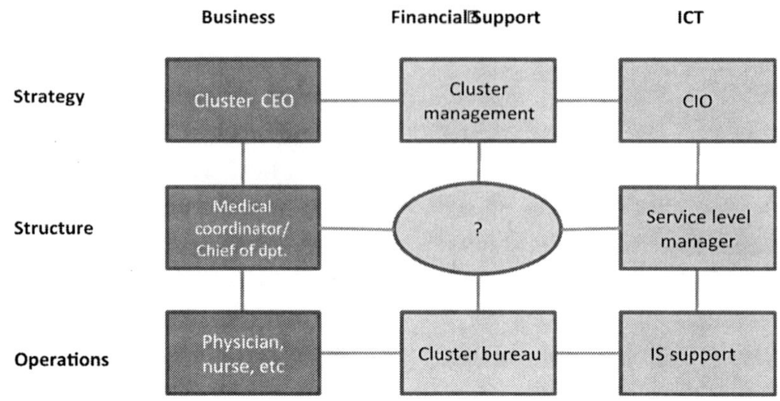

Lack of Alignment between Existing Processes and IS

Many IS implementations, which were reviewed in this case, weren't based on the workflow of the specific unit. This means that as a result, systems did not have a high compatibility with processes. Other than that, functionalities within implemented systems weren't used to the full capacity. Without a good alignment with processes, IS implementations were not optimal effective and efficient as they could be. A better alignment can result in better patient quality and a reduction in costs.

Involvement of Relevant Actors at Decision Moments

At this moment the medical staffs are the only ones making decisions about which systems to use and what the necessary specifications are needed. The staffs cooperate with the IS department and have information meetings in which decisions are made only from their perspective. Input from other actors, such as physician assistants and nurses, are not taken into consideration. This group are the end users of the specific system because the staff physicians are less involved in the primary care process. Lacking the input of that group is eventually a loss for the workability of the system/ application.

Due to staff lack of full knowledge on the level of operational management, their decisions carry a risk of an IS implementation resulting in incomplete fit with the unit. To recapitulate, the people who have to work with the system are very important. They are responsible for the unit to function well. Involvement of more actors is needed to make sure that IS implementations can have a good fit within the unit.

Existence of Inefficient Administration

Across Erasmus MC, most units have high numbers of information systems. E.g. the Obstetric unit uses twenty-three mini-systems just for registering different kinds of patient information. The people who work at the Obstetric unit perceive this high number of used systems as normal. Due the vastness of systems, a lack of communication between them exists. As a result a lot of patient information has to be inputted more than once, which means redundancy. Another danger of redundancy is clarity about where the most recent patient information is registered and whether this information is retrieved. In our opinion this has a negative effect on the quality of patient care. Further research on this topic is necessary.

Decision Structure

As stated earlier this chapter, many decisions are made by the medical staff. The disadvantage they have is the lack a good oversight of the primary process. Their knowledge is better suited on the tactical and strategic levels of the unit. In combination with the lack of a balanced involvement of actors during the decisions made during development this results in non-optimal decisions about IS. A clear structure for making decisions is necessary. The decision structure must consist of three layers, the strategic, tactical and operational layer. The different actors with their different area of knowledge are categorized in such a way that decisions are optimal knowledge supported.

These four bottlenecks contribute to a low adoption of IS within the hospital with a coherent view in Figure 1.

The horizontal lines, between business and IS, represent common language and understanding. Semantics are of great importance among lines of communication. There is a need for a common discussion between people on the business side and people on the IS side. The horizontal lines represent transfer operational resources and experiences towards sustainable strategic assets (Maes, 1999).

Within the model, all different roles must be fullfilled and anchored. This is needed for a good communication flow between people which have the same semantics. The emphasis must also lay on communication (Gartner 2005). For the case of the Erasmus MC, the important central role as process managers is not fullfilled. Also the roles of physician, nurse etcetera on the operational business side and the service level manager aren't anchored that well. As a result alignment of business and IS is very hard, perhaps impossible, to achieve.

Contours of Readiness Framework

Adjusting the decision structure is necessary to gain efficiency. In the new categorization decisions are made by the actors who have the best knowledge within their layer. The relation of the IS department must be of a more cooperative character instead of a customer/principal relation. The IS department can also act as mediator between the management layer of the unit and with their own project group this way. The result must be a general oversight on the project by the IS department and not just on a split up of the project into the layers. For this to work, the most important change must be made by the people. They are the enabler for change.

Nevertheless, IT is increasingly becoming an important actor based on its changing roles in the delivery of healthcare. As IT becomes "enabler" of necessary organizational change with the Dutch healthcare sector the effect of IT projects will depend on the individual circumstances (Westert and Verkleij, 2006). The mainstream literature has avoided hypotheses of causality between IT innovation and particular organisational or societal effects in critical industries like healthcare (Guah, 2009).

Beside that decisions must be made at the right place: other than the requirements that are described above, Grefen (2001) defines an additional set of criteria for WfM. His criteria set out what kind of data is needed to develop and create a WfM. Grefen (2001) defined the following criteria:

- **Process Specification:** The process specification contains a detailed description of the workflow process. By saving this specification in a database, elements within the specification become accessible;
- **Organization Specification:** The specification of the organization contains the description in which the workflows have to be executed. In this organization model,

descriptions of actors, functions, groups etc. are developed;

- **Information Specification:** The structures of information, which are manipulated by workflows according to the information model of the WfM, are described in this point;
- **Situations in Current Cases:** The situation on "current" cases contains relevant situation and context information for the execution of every case;
- **Historical Information:** Historical information is the information of cases of which the implementation is completed. This information is merely used within the function of an archive. This information can also be aggregated.

These criteria should be used as a guidance principle when developing and arranging WfM.

POTENTIAL FOR WFM IN HEALTHCARE

Uncertainties Faced by Current Decision Structure

The medical staff that may lack a good oversight of the primary process makes many decisions. Their knowledge is better suited on the tactical and strategic levels of the unit. In combination with the lack of a balanced involvement of actors during the decisions made during development this results in non-optimal decisions about IS. A clear structure for making decisions is necessary. The decision structure must consist of three layers, the strategic, tactical and operational layer. The different actors with their different area of knowledge are categorized in such a way that decisions are optimal knowledge supported.

The observed bottlenecks of the decision structure are:

- Decisions are made by people who don't have a clear overview of the work floor;
- Lack of involvement of different actors with different functions during decisions;
- The IS department's primary task is to respond to the requested demand;
- Responsibilities about project tasks are ambiguous.

Adjusting the decision structure is necessary to gain efficiency. In the new categorization the actors who have the best knowledge within their layer make decisions. The relation of the IS department must be of a more cooperative character instead of a customer/principal relation. The IS department can also act as mediator between the management layer of the unit and with their own project groups this way. The result must be a general oversight on the project by the IS department and not just on a split up of the project into the layers. For this to work, the most important change must be made by the people. They are the enablers for change.

The Current Decision Structure Must be Adjusted on the Following Points:

- Decisions must be made at the right place: This automatically means that the right persons make the decisions. The knowledge of the medical staff is mostly on the tactical and strategic level. Their knowledge on the operational level is much less. Their interest also differs from the other actors. The primary task of the medical staff is about research and education. These are the factors they will be judged upon at the end of the year. The physician assistants are the ones that are mostly responsible for giving care to the patient. The incentives of the medical staff differ much from the incentives nurses or physician assistants have. Decisions are influenced by the role and incentives of the decision maker. A clear structure for the levels of decisions is therefore necessary.

- IS knowledge is necessary: at this moment the IS department finds themselves solely responsible for the executions of the demand by the customer within the hospital. The relations between the IS department and organizational units, was observed as a principal/customer relation. This relation must be transferred to more of a team relation. This can be reached if one or more representatives from the IS department, depending on the situation, should be present at the different management layers.

What could be another solution is the mediator or middleman. This middleman should give advice on the business level of the unit. The middleman can be seen as an information manager. This function requires that mediation between the different management layers takes place and that the functionalities of the system are specialized.

The result of this structure must be that the quality of consultation and the focus is improved. The advantage is that the execution lines are shorter and results can be achieved sooner. As a result of this, the people will experience more involvement of the IS department. This experience can influence the creation for a good basis for the IS implementation. The shared responsibility for the succeeding of the project will enhance each other. Without reorganizing the decision structure, readiness for the implementation of an IS will be low.

Resolution of Implementation Problem

Healthcare work is a social process. It involves simultaneously dealing with sick individuals, each of which have their own problems and needs, and is connected with other physicians and organizational units. Because of the nature of healthcare work, standard organizational solutions never wholly fit the individual needs of a patient. Healthcare workers are therefore constantly compromising between the problem and solution to give the best care to the patient (Berg et al. 2003). Standardisation of healthcare pathways could provide a possible solution for giving better suited healthcare for the patient and centralizing the patient within the process.

A clinical pathway is the care process that a patient goes through during sickness. It starts with a health complaint and ends after the patient is treated for the health complaint. A clinical pathway displays all the care activities of the treatment that a patient has to follow. Care activities are organized around the patient. This must reduce inter-doctor variation, minimize delays in a treatment and decrease resource use (Lin et al, 2000). A clinical pathway coordinates the treatment procedure and also defines the quality of care that is provided at each activity (Smagghe et al, 2005). The main goal of a clinical pathway is to improve the quality of care while costs are decreased.

The advantage of a clinical pathway overview is the possibility to plan care activities in advance. Most appointments in healthcare are dependent of previous care activities or appointments and of available capacity at other locations within the organization, e.g. an x-ray is needed before the first consult with a physician. The description of the steps within the process helps to make the pathway mutual dependency insightful and offers a better planning. Criteria for quality can also be fixed within the clinical pathway (Bal and Bont, 2005).

When talking about planning up-following care activities in a clinical pathway, it is interesting to take a closer look at Order Management. The goal of clinical pathways is to organize the care activities around the patient. It provides the corresponding ideal sequence and timing of physician and staff actions to achieve the predefined goals with optimal efficiency (Pearson et al 1995). Reasons to use clinical pathways are thus mostly about improving the quality of care and/or reducing costs of a certain product of service. Strongly

Figure 2. Shows the order management process

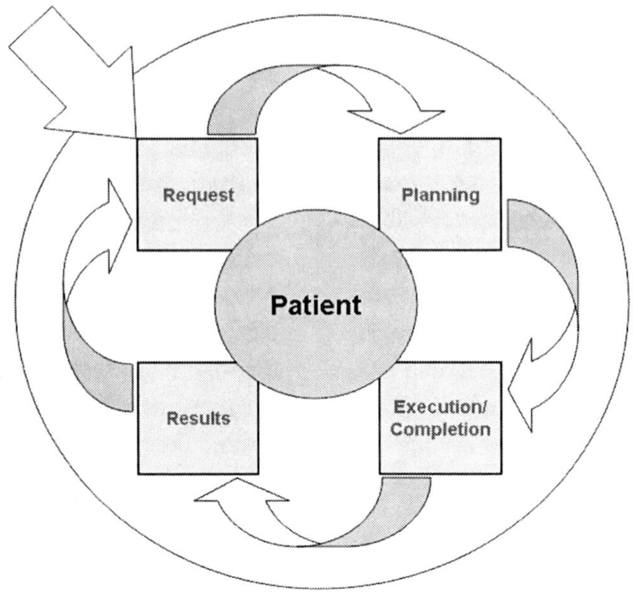

related is the timely execution of the treatment within the clinical pathway.

Implementation of clinical pathways can be difficult for the following reasons:

- A great deal of time, skill and effort is needed to find and analyse the highest quality evidence available. This quality is essential when making clinical pathways;
- Medical knowledge is changing on a continuous basis. Therefore clinical pathways should also be improved continuously, to be certain that the highest quality is obtained;
- A clinical pathway cannot have all the answers on individual cases;
- Implementation of clinical pathways can face organizational and/or cultural challenges. For example the resistance from physicians against standardisation of medical work (Smagghe et al, 2005).

Order Management (OM) is not about replacing paper forms for electronic versions. OM is about the facilitation of health care workers for initiating and protection of the total sum of health care activities that incorporate the treatment of the patient. OM is the electronic guarding of the healthcare pathway.

The goal of OM is:

- Providing quality on a consistent level;
- Supporting working on a basis of protocols, standardisation;
- Input control and decision support;
- The realisation of time reduction;
- during the application and execution of applications;
- Monitoring the progress of the clinical path.

Examples where OM would prosper are on the area of: medication, radiology, the operating theatre, laboratory, nursing activities, and transport requests. These aspects should always be taken in account when setting up an OM system (Reingoud, 2006).

Functionalities of OM are:

- Monitoring of individual activities in the clinical pathway;
- Giving oversight of individual activities within the clinical pathway;
- Giving oversight in time, for planning purposes;
- Identifying status change and deviations of the predefined norms;
- On clinical paths based access for (lab) results and reports;
- Order application;
- Order planning;
- Order execution;
- General oversight;
- Placing and interfacing the information in the Electronic Patient Record (Reingoud 2006).

For a patient to be treated effectively in a clinical pathway, integration of processes is a key aspect for success. This change can only be achieved when changes in the organisational structures are met. This process includes registering a planned activity (electronically) and the activity being requested, planning of the activity's execution, returning the status of the activity, giving feedback on the activity. Across all of these steps, having the data available electronically can provide opportunities for monitoring of the process.

Order execution comprehends the, administrative, status of the patient in the pathway. Within OM, there is a process of continuous feedback. With this feedback and general oversight of the physician, continuous improvement of the process of the patient is possible. As a result the patient gets the most optimal treatment and unnecessary researches will not be done.

When a patient has an appointment with the physician the physician sends out a request, e.g. a blood test. This request is planned in time with needed resources such as personnel. When the execution of the request takes place the physician who gave the order gets a notification. The next step is that results are returned to the physician and choices about further care activities can be taken.

CONCLUSION

The article has argued why the WfM is important by sketching key issues related to the research problem. The authors have also identified the bottlenecks as suggested in the scientific literature. These bottlenecks are often due to the difficulty in involving physicians during IS implementation, especially if they do not perceive a need to change clinical working practices. Notwithstanding, Erasmus MC has been heralded in The Netherlands as a teaching hospital with technology that would make medical care more cost effective and increase patient safety. Occasionally, there exists perception that making the delivery of care more time and resource efficient is not a clinical necessity. This article has shown that such perception of IS in the healthcare sector is a result of a rather poor understanding of the long-term benefits of improving patient care by changing medical work practices.

The research also showed a rich picture of WfM that includes practical issue of use and implementation and policy issues related to organization strategy and changing healthcare practices in The Netherlands. While the authors acknowledge the complexity of integrating those issues into a comprehensive approach, this article suggest there could be times when less restrictions apply to who can enter orders for the purpose of increasing patient care quality. That's because focussing on subatomic tasks to increase patient safety could occasionally result in decrease in patient safety in the overall process of care. Finally, IS implementation process interacts with an overall healthcare systems that includes healthcare workers at various levels of the healthcare delivery process or patient pathway. The healthcare organization is therefore at the central of any work in this critical sector. Attention must therefore be given to situations when clashes might occur between the rationality of IS that is expressed in technical and functional specifications and the actual use of such system by a healthcare worker. The decision whether to use the system, how to use the system and when to use the systems then becomes more important than just the cost and benefit of implementing a new healthcare information system.

RERFERENCES

Aarts, J. E. C. M. (2005). Understanding implementation: a sociotechnical appraisal of the introduction of computerized physician order entry systems in Dutch and American hospitals. Unpublished doctorial thesis Erasmus.

Anyanwu K., A. Sheth, J. Cardoso, J. Miller, K. Kochut (2003). Healthcare Enterprise Process Development and Integration. Journal of Research and Practice in Information Technology, Vol. 35, No. 2. May 2003.

Bal, R., & de Bont, A. 2005 Taakherschikking en ICT in de Zorg. In: Kennis in Netwerken: Jaarboek ICT en samenleving 2005. J. de Haan & C. van 't Hof 2006. Amsterdam: Uitgeverij Boom. 2005 (113-126).

Berg, M., Aarts, J., & van der Lei, J. (2003). ICT in Healthcare: Sociotechnical approaches. *Methods of Information in Medicine*, *42*, 297–301.

Bijker, W. E., & Law, J. (Eds.). (1992). *Shaping Technology/Building Society: Studies in Sociotechnical Change*. Cambridge, MA: MIT Press.

Breas, R. A. (2007). Workflow Management, "the" challenge for health care. An unpublished Masters thesis, Erasmus University Rotterdam.

Cardoso, J. (2002). *Workflow Quality of Service and Semantic Workflow Composition*. Athens, GA: Department of Computer Science, University of Georgia.

Cardoso, J., Bostrom, R. P., & Sheth, A. (2004). Workflow management systems vs. ERP systems: Differences, Commonalities, and Applications. [Kluwer Academic Publishers]. *Information Technology Management*, *5*, 319–338. doi:10.1023/B:ITEM.0000031584.14039.99

Ciborra, C., & And Hanseth, O. (1998). From tool to Gestell, agendas for managing the informtaion infrastructure. *Information Technology & People*, *11*(4), 305–327. doi:10.1108/09593849810246129

Doolan, D.F., & Bates, D.W., James, and B.C. (2003). The use of computers for clinical care: a case series of advanced U.S. sites. *Journal of the American Medical Informatics Association*, *10*(1), 94–107. doi:10.1197/jamia.M1127

Freed, D. H. (2004). Hospitalists: evolution, evidence, and eventualities. *Health Care Management (Philadelphia, Pa.)*, *23*(3), 238–256.

Georgakolpoulos, D., & Hornick, M. (1995). An overview of Workflow Management: From process modelling to workflow automation infrastructure. *Distributed and Parallel Databases*, *3*, 119–153. doi:10.1007/BF01277643

Gerrard, M. (2005). "Business/IT Alignment a Critical Factor When Determining IT's Role", Gartner Report. (http://www.gartner.com)

Grefen, P.W.P.J. (2001). Workflow Management: Geautomatiseerde ondersteuning voor integrale procesbesturing. Alphen aan den Rijn: Samsom.

Guah, W. M. (2009). *Managing very large IT projects in businesses and organizations* (pp. 99–115). PA: IGI Global.

Heathfield, H., Pitty, D., & Hanka, R. (1998). Evaluating Information Technology in Healthcare: Barriers and challenges. *British Medical Journal*, *316*, 1959–1961.

Klischewski, R., & Wetzel, I. (2001). *Serviceflow Management for Health Provider Networks* (pp. 313–319). Hamburg: Jahrestagung.

Klischewski, R., & Wetzel, I. (2002). *Service flow Beyond Workflow?*Concepts and Architectures for Supporting Inter-Organizational Service Processes.

Latour, B. (1986) The Powers of Association in Law, J. (ed), Power, Action and Belief: A New Sociology of Knowledge? Routledge & Kegan Paul, London, UK

Latour, B. (1999) On Recalling ANT in Law, J. and Hassard, J. (eds) Actor Network Theory and After, Blackwell Publishers, Oxford

Latour, B. (2005). *Reassembling the Social: An Introduction to Actor-Network-Theory*. Oxford: Oxford University Press.

Lin, F., Chou, S., Pan, S., & Chen, Y. 2000. Mining Time Dependency Patterns in Clinical Pathways. Proceedings of the 33rd Hawaii International Conference on System Sciences - 2000

Maes, R. (1999). *Reconsidering Information Management Through a generic Framework*. University of Amsterdam.

Orlikowski, W. J. (2000). Using technology and constituting structures: a practice lens for studying technology in organizations. *Organization Science*, *11*(4), 404–428. doi:10.1287/orsc.11.4.404.14600

Pearson, S. D., Goulart-Fisher, D., & Lee, T. H. (1995). Critical Pathways as a strategy for improving care: Problems and Potential. *Annals of Internal Medicine*, *123*(Issue 12), 941–948.

Reingoud, A. (2006). *EMC Order Management Adviesrapport. Version 1.1, July 2006*. Erasmus MC Rotterdam.

Smagghe, D., Segers, M., Spy-Anderson, P. J., Benamou, N., & Eddabbeh, N. 2005. Model of Good Practice Tools for Risk Reduction and Clinical Governance. In: The Journal on Information Technology in Healthcare 2005 (3) 114: 117-124.
Stoop, A.P. (2005). Evaluating ICT applications in health care. Studies from a Sociotechnical Perspective.Universal Press, Veenendaal

This work was previously published in International Journal of Healthcare Delivery Reform Initiatives, edited by Matthew W. Guah, pp. 25-38, copyright 2009 by IGI Publishing (an imprint of IGI Global).

Chapter 8
Physician Characteristics and EMR Attitudes

David Meinert
Missouri State University, USA

Dane K. Peterson
Missouri State University, USA

ABSTRACT

Despite the numerous purported benefits of Electronic Medical Records (EMR), the medical profession has been extremely reluctant to embrace the technology. One of the barriers believed to be responsible for the slow adoption of EMR technology is resistance by many physicians who are not convinced of the advantages of using EMR systems. This study examined potential characteristics of physicians that might help identify those individuals that are most likely to pose a threat to the successful implementation of an EMR system in a multi-specialty clinic. The results demonstrated that older physicians and physicians with only minimal computer skills are more likely to have negative attitudes regarding EMR technology. Medical specialists were most likely to have positive attitudes with respects to the use of EMR systems, while primary care physicians were most likely to have doubts regarding the purported benefits of EMR technology.

PHYSICIAN CHARACTERISTICS AND EMR ATTITUDES

An Electronic Medical Record (**EMR**) is a computerized system that contains a patient's long-term legal health record generated by encounters at one particular medical practice. Thus an EMR electronically stores such items as x-rays, prescriptions, physician's notes, structured data, diagnostic images, wave forms, scanned images of paper documents, and other types of medical documentation. EMR technology offers a number

DOI: 10.4018/978-1-60960-183-6.ch008

of potential benefits, including improved quality of patient care, more efficient healthcare workflows, and reduced costs (Thompson, Osheroff, Classen, & Sittig, 2007). Improvement in the quality of patient care can be credited to several attributes of an EMR system including superior documentation, flexible data organization, integrated systems, and assisted clinical decision making (Shekelle, Morton, & Keeler, 2006).

Because of the many potential benefits associated with EMR technology, a number of experts believe the market for EMR systems will grow rapidly over the next decade. A recent study projected a13.5 percent growth rate for EMR technology in the U.S. over the next four years (Pizzi, 2007). This study estimated that the 2005 EMR market of $1 billion will grow to more than $4 billion by the year 2015. The prospects for market growth in the EMR industry are further enhanced by evidence suggesting that the U.S. represents only a small proportion of the market potential for EMR technology. Enormous growth is also anticipated on the global level, making EMR software an exceptional opportunity not only for the current market players, but also for new entrants into the market.

Despite the numerous benefits associated with EMR systems, there is extensive documentation indicating that the healthcare industry in the United States has been extremely reluctant to embrace the technology (Fonkych & Taylor, 2005). As a whole, the healthcare industry is almost 20 years behind the rest of the nation's industries in the adoption of information technology (Ilie, Courtney, & Slyke, 2007). The financial service industry for example spends nearly $200 billion a year on information technology, while the healthcare industry spends only about one-tenth of that amount ("From clipboards to keyboards," 2007). Estimates of the number of hospitals in the U.S. that have adopted the technology range from about 30 to 56 percent depending largely on how EMR systems are defined (Fonkych & Taylor, 2005). The slow growth rate has prompted possible intervention by the U.S. government to facilitate the implementation of EMR systems. In 2004, the U.S. federal government announced a framework to accelerate the adoption of health information technology, with the goal of having electronically stored medical records for most Americans within the next decade (Health IT Strategic Framework, 2004).

The slow adoption pace for EMR systems has been attributed to a number of barriers, such as privacy concerns and interoperability. In hospital settings, one of the key obstacles to successful EMR implementation is resistance among physicians. Physicians may be reluctant to accept EMR technology for a number of reasons, including the perception that the use of an EMR system requires extensive training and interferes with the quality of physician-patient interaction. Many physicians are skeptical about claims that EMR systems reduce errors, increase productivity and the overall assertion that the benefits of EMR technology outweigh the costs (Handy, Whiddett, & Hunter, 2001). While the validity of these issues have been addressed in a number of previous studies, it is important to note that physician acceptance of EMR technology is dependent on the physicians' perceptions and not necessarily the actual value of EMR technology.

Since physicians must use EMR systems in their day to day work, physician acceptance is crucial to widespread adoption of EMR technology (Mazzoleni et al., 1996). Many unsuccessful attempts to implement EMR technology have been attributed to the physicians' dissatisfaction with the EMR system (Van Der Meijden, Tange, Troost, & Hasman, 2003; Wager, Lee, & White, 2002). This is exemplified by several highly publicized EMR implementation fiascos, including the Cedars Sinai Medical Center in Los Angeles, in which physicians revolted and forced the administration to scrap a $34 million computer system (Connolly, 2005).

On the other hand, instances in which physicians approached the adoption of EMR technology with a positive attitude were often associated with successful implementations (Darr, Harrison, Shakked, & Shalom, 2003). Thus, a better understanding of the factors that are associated with physicians' attitudes toward the adoption of EMR systems is a key to achieving the substantial benefits associated with EMR technology (Reardon & Davidson, 2007). Therefore, this study examined the perceptions of physicians associated with a multi-purpose clinic to identify potential barriers to the acceptance of EMR technology. Such information may be useful in developing EMR training programs to enhance the prospects for successful EMR implementation.

PHYSICIANS' PERCEPTIONS REGARDING EMR TECHNOLOGY

One concern for many physicians is the amount of training time required to become proficient users of EMR technology. Although most EMR vendors claim extensive training is not required, adequate training appears to be crucial for the successful implementation of EMR systems (Miller & Sim, 2004). The exact amount of training required to become a proficient user of EMR technology is difficult to ascertain, since the necessary training time appears to be dependent on a number of factors (Bergeron, 2006; Ovretveit, Scott, Rundall, Shortell, & Brommels, 2007; Vanmeerbeek, 2004). For instance, it appears the specific type of EMR system being implemented, the training method employed, and the general computer proficiency of the physicians influence the required amount of training time (Aaronson, Murphy-Cullen, Chop & Frey, 2001; Kirshner, Solomon, & Chin, 2004). Thus, it appears that in some instances, the empirical evidence supports the concerns of many physicians that extensive training time may be necessary. Consequently, the present study examined physicians' views regarding the willingness of their colleagues to expend the time necessary to become proficient EMR users.

Quality of care, particularly the significance of physician-patient interaction, has been a primary concern among many physicians (Russell & Spooner, 2004). At issue is whether incorporating computers in the examination room detracts from the quality of communication between the physician and the patient (Aaronson et al., 2001). The results from empirical investigations appear to be mixed. For instance, one study reported that gazing at the computer monitor was inversely related to physician engagement in psychosocial questioning, emotional responsiveness to the patient, and overall psychosocial exchange during patient visits (Margalit, Roter, Dunevant, Larson, & Reis, 2006). In addition, keyboarding activity (physician order entry) has been reported to adversely influence the medical dialogue between physicians and patients. On the other hand, other investigations have not observed any negative consequences associated with the use of computers in the examination room (McGrath, Arar, & Pugh, 2007). In fact, some evidence suggests equipping examination rooms with computers may a positive effect on physician-patient interactions (Hsu, Huang, Fung, Robertson, & Jimison, 2005).

The conflicting results regarding use of EMR systems and physician-patient interaction may be the result of differences in the level of EMR experience among the physicians. That is, use of computers in the exam room may be less likely to interfere with physician-patient interaction as physician become more experienced with EMR systems (Rouf, Whittle, Lu, & Schwartz, 2007). This conclusion is based on objective methods of investigating physician-patient interaction, such as eye contact with the patient. However, the successful implementation of EMR systems may be more influenced by physicians' attitudes than such factors as amount of eye contact. Thus, the present investigation examined physicians' perceptions regarding the influence of EMR systems on quality of patient care.

One of the many claims made by vendors is that the use of EMR systems can result in a reduction of medical errors. Certainly, medical errors in hospital settings are both prevalent and costly (Crane & Crane, 2006), and there is some empirical evidence that the use of EMR technology can reduce medical errors. For instance, one study reported that use of EMR technology reduced documentation errors by over five percent (Gearing et al.2006). However, a review of the literature suggested that using EMR technology does not always result in a reduction of errors (Sidorov, 2006). One comprehensive investigation examined 17 measures regarding the quality of care in ambulatory settings. The results credited EMR technology with improvement for two outcome measures, but EMR technology resulted in a worse outcome for one measure, and no differences on the remaining 14 measures (Linder, Bates, Middleton, & Stafford, 2007). Thus, there would appear to be some valid reasons why physicians may not perceive EMR technology as a useful means for reducing medical errors. The present investigation provides a current examination of how physicians' view the effectiveness of EMR technology to reduce medical errors.

Increased productivity, or the number of patients seen per day, is another benefit often touted by EMR vendors (Joos, Chen, Jirjis, & Johnson, 2006). Although increased productivity is widely claimed as one of the benefits of EMR technology, there is only a modest amount of evidence to support the proposition and much of the evidence is anecdotal (Gonzales & Puri, 2008; Thakkar & Davis, 2006). Thus it is quite reasonable to expect physicians to be skeptical about the claimed benefits associated with increased productivity (Handy, Whiddett, & Hunter, 2001). Given the conflicting evidence, it would seem beneficial in this study to examine the current perceptions of physicians regarding the usefulness of EMR technology for increasing physician productivity.

A number of studies have attempted to assess the overall cost/benefits of EMR technology (Gearing et al., 2006). Developing an effective and valid assessment procedure has proven to be a difficult task (Thompson et al. 2007). However, the majority of the evidence suggests that the benefits of EMR technology outweigh the considerable costs of the technology (Hillestad et al., 2005; Simon & Simon, 2006). Even in instances in which physicians were initially skeptical about cost/benefits of EMR technology, the objective evidence indicated a substantial return on investment (Mullen, & Donnelly, 2006). To ascertain how the empirical evidence has influenced physicians' perceptions of EMR technology, this study examined physicians' views on the cost/benefits of EMR systems.

Finally, this study asked physicians if they believe their colleagues were aware of the benefits of EMR technology, whether the clinic should adopt EMR technology, and if EMR technology is adopted, will it be necessary for administration to mandate the use of the system in order to achieve successful implementation.

Attitudes and Physician Characteristics

Most theories on the diffusion of information technology suggest that the attitudes and perceptions of users is a key to successful implementation (Bagozzi, Davis & Warshaw, 1992). Thus, a number of studies have examined potential relationships between characteristics of physicians and attitudes regarding EMR technology with the hope of identifying the physicians most likely to resist EMR implementation. The goal is to determine which physicians represent the greatest obstacle to successful EMR implementation and thus, the physicians who would benefit the most from EMR training programs. Some of the primary factors investigated include the physician's age, computer sophistication, and medical specialty.

With respect to age, most studies have found that younger physicians are more likely to use EMR technology (Burt, Hing, & Woodwell, 2005; Terry, 2005). However, while younger physicians may be more likely to use EMR technology, some studies have reported that younger physicians are also more likely to have negative attitudes regarding the EMR system they are currently using (Darr et al., 2003; Terry, 2005).

Several researchers have suggested that a lack of computer sophistication among physicians may impede the implementation of EMR technology (Anderson, Asher, & Wilson, 2007; Rabinovitch, 2007: McGowan, Passiment, & Hoffman, 2007). Although there appears to be a substantial need for improvement in the computer skills among some physicians, studies examining the relationship between computing skills and EMR acceptance has produced contradictory results. Some studies have found a positive association between level of computer sophistication among physicians and use of EMR technology, while other studies did not observe a significant relationship between these variables (Joos et al. 2006).

Studies examining EMR adoption by medical specialty have also failed to produce consistent results. While some studies have found primary care physicians are most likely to use EMR technology (Terry, 2005), other studies have reported medical specialist are more likely to adopt to EMR systems (Audet et al., 2004; Burt et al., 2005; Corey & Grossman, 2007).

Study Objectives

To date, most studies examining EMR adoptions have reported general findings in terms of system "availability" or "usage." Unfortunately, such studies provide minimal understanding of what drives physician acceptance or resistance of EMR systems. While global measures such as "availability" and "usage" provide information regarding the rate of adoption of EMR systems they fall short of providing detailed insight into variables relevant to their successful widespread implementation.

The objective of the present investigation was to examine the attitudes of physicians at one large multi-specialty hospital regarding EMR technology. In addition, the study examined how perceptions regarding EMR technology were related to age, computer sophistication, and medical specialty of the physicians. Identifying which physicians are likely to have positive attitudes regarding EMR technology could assist hospital administrators and technology managers identify potential "innovators". Innovators, or early adopters, can play an important role as "opinion leaders" in the diffusion of information technology (Andrews, Pearce, Sydney, Ireson, & Love, 2004). Similarly, identifying physicians that are most likely to be resistant to EMR technology may provide administrators with information on who may benefit the most from technology training. Studies have shown that proper training improves attitudes toward EMR technology, even among physicians who were initially resisted the adoption of EMR systems (Kirshner, Salomon, & Chin, 2004).

METHODOLOGY

Sample

To examine physicians' attitudes regarding EMR systems, a mail survey of 358 physicians affiliated with a large, multi-specialty clinic in the Midwest was conducted. The clinic is a physician-led, professionally managed group practice in an integrated health-care system. Although some of the physicians had prior experience using EMR technology in other settings, the survey was conducted before the clinic had implemented an EMR system.

Targeting physicians at one multi-specialty clinic made it possible to obtain a high response rate to the questionnaire, avoiding a common problem encountered by many similar studies. In addition, the clinic was only in the preparation stage for adopting EMR technology. Thus most of the physicians had only read about EMR technology, but had little experience with specific EMR

Table 1. Percent of physicians agreeing with each item

Concerns	Percent Agreeing
1. Physicians will devote the time necessary to be trained using an EMR	68.3
2. An EMR will improve the quality of patient care	76.6
3. An EMR will reduce the number of errors	82.6
4. An EMR will increase a physician's productivity	60.2
5. The benefits of an EMR system will outweigh the costs	72.0
6. The clinic's physicians are familiar with EMR functions and benefits	43.8
7. The clinic should implement an EMR system	79.6
8. EMR usage will have to be mandated	71.5

systems. Hence, their opinions were not likely to be overly influenced by use of one specific EMR system.

Questionnaires were mailed to physician homes, with follow-up mailings to non-respondent's homes (3 weeks later) and offices (5 weeks later). Preaddressed, postage-paid return envelopes were provided. A total of 266, or 74 percent, of the questionnaire were returned. Five of the questionnaires (1.4%) were excluded because at least half of the items were not completed. Thus, useable data was obtained from 261 (73%) respondents. The high response rate and percentage of usable questionnaires was a result of reminders by administrators and physician-executives to participate in the research. These reminders were conveyed via email, weekly newsletters and staff meetings.

Questionnaire

The questionnaire asked respondents to rate their degree of agreement regarding eight items on a forced Likert scale (no neutral point) ranging from 1 - strongly agree to 6 - strongly disagree. The eight items are listed in Table 1. These items were derived through an examination of the literature, discussions with administrators at the multi-specialty clinic and physicians in other clinics. The questionnaire also contained items to assess the physician's age, computer sophistication, and medical specialty. As in previous studies (Audit et al., 2004; Burt et al., 2005), physician age was classified as under 35, 35 to 44, 45 to 54, and over 54. Based on the same reasoning, medical specialty was classified as Primary Care, Surgical, and Medical Specialist. It was determined that computer sophistication was best assessed by a single item that asked respondents to rate their "Knowledge/experience working with Windows based applications (e.g., Word, PowerpPoint, Excel)" on a scale from 1 – "Proficient" to 4 – "Non-existent". Due to the small number of respondents indicating non-existent computer skills (n = 22), the last two categories were combined (i.e., minimal and non-existent computer skills).

RESULTS

The percent of physicians agreeing with each statement (respondents checking 1, 2, or 3 on the Likert scale) is displayed in Table 1. The physicians generally agreed that EMR technology would be beneficial. That is, nearly 80 percent of the physicians agreed that the clinic should implement an EMR system and 72 percent agreed the benefits will outweigh the costs. However, the physicians were somewhat pessimistic regarding the acceptance of EMR technology by their colleagues. Only 43.8 percent of the physicians believe that their colleagues are familiar with the benefits of EMR technology and 79.6 percent believe the clinic will need to mandate the use of EMR systems in order to achieve widespread use of the technology.

Only 55 of the 261 respondents were females. Statistical tests indicated no gender differences on any of the eight dependent measures. Thus, all subsequent analyses were based on all 261 respondents without including gender as a separate factor. A separate ANOVA was performed on each of the eight dependent measures. Of the three independent variables, a chi-square test indicated that only physician age and computer proficiency were significantly related. That is, younger physicians were more likely to rate themselves as proficient computer users and less likely to have minimal or non-existent computer skills (chi-square = 20.36, p = .002). Chi-square tests on the relationship between physician age and medical specialty and between computer proficiency and medical specialty were not significant.

The ANOVA results for physician's age are summarized in Table 2. The analysis indicated the difference between the age groups was significant for all items except mandated use of EMR systems and familiarity with EMR benefits. For each item in which significant age differences were observed, younger physicians had a more positive attitude regarding EMR technology.

The results for physician's computer knowledge are summarized in Table 3. As expected, physicians who were more proficient with computers were more likely to agree with the items. The difference between the groups was significant on all eight items.

Table 4 summarizes the results for physician specialty. The differences between physician specialties were significant for four of the items, namely quality of patient care, reduced errors, physician productivity, and familiarity with EMR benefits. Although the results were significant on only four of the eight items, the pattern of results were the same for all questions. That is, medical specialists were most likely to agree with the statements indicating a more positive attitude with respect to EMR technology. Primary care physicians were least likely to agree with the items.

Table 2. Attitudes and physicians' age

	Under 35	35 to 44	45 to 54	Over 54	F
Sample Size	23	97	91	44	
1. Physicians will devote necessary time to training	3.31	2.81	3.17	3.41	2.70*
2. EMRs improves quality of patient care	1.95	2.49	2.79	3.20	4.27**
3. EMRs reduce errors	1.82	2.27	2.54	2.86	3.76*
4. EMRs increase physicians' productivity	2.19	2.99	3.53	3.59	6.35**
5. EMR benefits outweigh costs	2.24	2.46	2.84	3.39	4.82**
6. Clinic should implement EMR systems	2.04	2.29	2.49	3.21	4.18**
7. EMR usage will have to be Mandated	2.86	2.57	2.80	3.07	1.10
8. Familiar with EMR functionsand benefits	3.62	3.72	3.71	3.98	0.61

* P < .05, ** p < .01

Table 3. Attitudes and physicians' computer proficiency

	Proficient	Adequate	Minimal/Non-existent	F
Sample Size	68	112	72	
1. Physicians will devote necessary time to training	2.74	2.93	3.63	11.62**
2. EMRs improves the quality of patient care	2.18	2.34	3.67	26.99**
3. EMRs reduce errors	1.94	2.21	3.20	20.90**
4. EMRs increase physicians' productivity	2.64	2.95	4.17	24.51**
5. EMR benefits outweigh costs	2.18	2.45	3.69	24.69**
6. Familiar with EMR functions and benefits	3.23	3.68	4.29	14.84**
7. Clinic should implement an EMR system	1.84	2.15	3.59	32.33**
8. EMR usage will have to be mandated	2.38	2.66	3.31	7.27**

* P < .05, ** p < .01

Table 4. Attitudes and physicians' specialty

	Primary Care	Surgical Specialist	Medical Specialist	F
Sample Size	106	35	107	
1. Physicians will devote necessary time to training	3.15	3.11	2.99	0.50
2. EMRs improves the quality of patient care	3.03	2.60	2.32	6.52**
3. EMRs reduce errors	2.72	2.29	2.16	5.10**
4. EMRs increase physicians' productivity	3.48	3.18	2.96	3.21*
5. EMR benefits outweigh costs	2.87	2.85	2.54	1.38
6. Familiar with EMR functions and benefits	4.00	4.00	3.39	8.28**
7. Clinic should implement an EMR system	2.72	2.47	2.25	2.40
8. EMR systems will have to be mandated	2.71	2.83	2.80	0.13

* P < .05, ** p < .01

CONCLUSION

One of the strengths of the present study was the high response rate (74%) which overcomes a limitation in some previous studies in which the results might be biased because the physicians completing the surveys may be those with the most interest in EMR technology. With the high response rate in this study, the results should be highly representative of the views of physicians working in multi-specialty clinics.

In general, the results suggest that physicians agree that EMR technology can be beneficial. The majority believed EMR technology can improve the quality of patient care, reduce errors, increase physician productivity, and believe the benefits of EMR technology outweigh the costs of implementing an EMR system. Consequently, nearly 80 percent of the physicians agreed that the clinic should implement an EMR system. However, only 43.8 of the physicians agreed that their colleagues were familiar with EMR functions/benefits and only 68.3 physicians believed their colleagues would be willing to devote the time necessary to be trained in using EMR technology. Thus, it is not be surprising that 71.5 percent of the physicians believe that in order to achieve successful implementation of an EMR system, the clinic will need to mandate the use of the technology.

The results overwhelmingly demonstrate that younger physicians have a more positive attitudes regarding EMR technology. Younger physicians were more likely to agree that EMR technology improves patient care, reduces errors, increases productivity, and that the benefits outweigh the costs. They are also more likely to agree the clinic should implement EMR technology. Similar results were found for computer proficiency. That is, physicians who rated themselves as proficient computer users had more positive attitudes regarding EMR technology than those with minimal or non-existent computer skills. As observed in many previous studies outside the medical profession, age and computer proficiency were highly related (Marquie, Jourdan-Boddaert, & Huet, 2002). Thus it is difficult to independently assess the importance of physician age and computer proficiency on physician attitudes.

The results of the present study also show that medical specialists are more likely to have a positive attitudes regarding EMR technology than surgeons, and surgeons are more likely to have a positive attitude with respect to EMR technology than primary care specialists. Thus the results are consistent with most previous investigation examining medical specialty (Audet et al., 2004; Burt et al., 2005; Corey & Grossman, 2007), but contradicts the of one recent investigation (Terry, 2005). The conflicting results of the latter study may be attributed to the classification categories used for medical specialty. Studies such as the current investigation that have classified physicians as primary care, surgeons, or medical specialist have generally produced consistent results.

LIMITATIONS AND CONCLUSION

There are limitations to all research and it is important to note those that may affect the implications of the present study. An obvious limitation is that all physicians were affiliated with the same multispecialty clinic. While this approach provided several advantages such as a high response rate and more control over physician experience with specific EMR systems, it limits the generalizations that can be made from the study. Clearly, replications with different subject population would add significantly to the literature. A second issue pertains to the classification of medical specialties. While the division into three medical specialties was based on procedures used in several previous studies, there are other classification schemes that have could be used (e.g., see Corey and Grossman, 2007). It may be useful in future studies to examine potential differences in perceived importance of EMR functions using alternative methods of classifying medical specialty. A third concern pertains to controlling for the degree of previous EMR experience. Thorough information on physicians' previous experience with EMR technology and the types of information physicians used to form their perceptions regarding EMR technology would be helpful to understanding differences in perceived usefulness of EMR technology. Future investigation may examine how perceptions change depending on specific sources of information available to physicians and their personal experiences with specific EMR systems.

In conclusion, the results indicate that resistance to EMR implementation may be most likely to occur among older, less computer proficient physicians, particularly among primary care physicians. The fact that younger physicians are more computer proficient may suggest medical schools are taking the advice of researchers who have been advocating a curriculum that devotes more time to teaching computer skills (McGowan et al., 2007). Thus, it may be expected that resistance to implementing EMR technology may diminish over time as younger physicians with greater computer skills enter the profession.

REFERENCES

Aaronson, J. W., Murphy-Cullen, C. L., Chop, W. M., & Frey, R. D. (2001). Electronic medical records: the family practice resident perspective. *Family Medicine*, *33*(2), 128–132.

Anderson, D. M., Asher, L. M., & Wilson, E. A. (2007). Physician computer skills: A prerequisite to the future in healthcare services. *The Journal of the Kentucky Medical Association*, *105*(2), 67–71.

Andrews, J. E., Pearce, K. A., Sydney, C., Ireson, C., & Love, M. (2004). Current state of information technology use in a US primary care practice-based research network. *Informatics in Primary Care*, *12*(1), 11–18.

Audet, A., Doty, M., Peugh, J., Shamasdin, J., Zapert, K., & Schoenbaum, S. (2004). Information technologies: When will they make it into physicians' black bags? *Medscape General Medicine*, *6*(4), 843–853.

Bagozzi, R. P., Davis, F. D., & Warshaw, P. R. (1992). Development and test of a theory of technological learning and usage. *Human Relations*, *45*(7), 659–686. doi:10.1177/001872679204500702

Bergeron, B. P. (2006). I have an EMR system – now what? *The Journal of Medical Practice Management*, *22*(3), 131–132.

Burt, C. W., Hing, E., & Woodwell, D. (2005). Electronic medical record use by office-based physicians: National Center for Health Statistics. Retrieved February 4, 2008 from http://www.cdc.gov/nchs/products/pubs/pubd/hestats/electronic/electronic.htm

Connolly, C. (2005, March, 21). Cedars-Sinai Doctors Cling to Pen and Paper. The Washington Post, p. A01. Retrieved February 4, 2008 from http://www.washingtonpost.com/wp-dyn/articles/A52384-2005Mar20.html

Corey, C., & Grossman, J. M. (2007). Clinical information technology adoption varies across physician specialties. Center for Studying Health System Change. Data Bulletin, Number 34. Retrieved February 4, 2008 from http://www.hschange.com/CONTENT/945/

Crane, J., & Crane, F. G. (2006). Preventing medication errors in hospitals through a systems approach and technological innovation: A prescription for 2010. *Hospital Topics*, *84*(4), 3–8. doi:10.3200/HTPS.84.4.3-8

Darr, A., Harrison, M. I., Shakked, L., & Shalom, N. (2003). Physicians' and nurses' reaction to electronic medical records. *Journal of Health Organization and Management*, *17*(5), 349–359. doi:10.1108/14777260310505129

Fonkych, K., & Taylor, R. (2005). The state and pattern of health information technology adoption. The Rand Corporation Monograph. Retrieved February 4, 2008 from http://www.rand.org/pubs/monographs/MG409/

From clipboards to keyboard (2007, May 19). The Economist, pp. 68-69.

Gearing, P., Olney, C. M., Davis, K., Lozano, D., Smith, L. B., & Friedman, B. (2006). Enhancing patient safety through electronic medical record documentation of vital signs. *Journal of Healthcare Information Management*, *20*(4), 40–45.

Gonzalez, C. M., & Puri, L. (2008). Productivity and cost implications of implementing electronic medical records into an ambulatory surgical subspecialty clinic. *Urology*, *71*(2), 173–177. doi:10.1016/j.urology.2007.09.024

Handy, J., Whiddett, R., & Hunter, I. (2001). A technology acceptance model for inter-organizational electronic medical records systems. *AJIS*, *9*(1), 39–50.

Health IT Strategic Framework. (2004), Office for the National Coordinator for Health Information Technology. United States Department of Health and Human Services. Retrieved February 4, 2008 from http://www.hhs.gov/healthit/preface.html

Hillestad, R., Bigelow, J., Bower, A., Girosi, F., Meili, R., Scoville, R., & Taylor, R. (2005). Can electronic medical record systems transform health care? Potential health benefits, savings, and costs. *Health Affairs*, *24*(5), 1103–1117. doi:10.1377/hlthaff.24.5.1103

Hsu, J., Huang, J., Fung, V., Robertson, N., & Jimison, H. (2005). Health information technology and physician-patient interactions: Impact of computers on communication during outpatient visits. *Journal of the American Medical Informatics Association*, *12*, 474–480. doi:10.1197/jamia.M1741

Ilie, V., Courtney, J. F., & Slyke, C. V. (2007). Paper versus electronic: Challenges associated with physicians' usage of electronic medical records. Proceedings of the 40th Hawaii International Conference on Systems Science.

Joos, D., Chen, Q., Jirjis, J., & Johnson, K. B. (2006). An electronic medical record in primary care: Impact on satisfaction, work efficiency, and clinical processes. AMIA Symposium Proceedings, 394-398.

Kirshner, M., Salomon, H., & Chin, H. (2004). An evaluation of one-on-one advanced proficiency training in clinicians' use of computer information systems. *International Journal of Medical Informatics*, *73*(4), 341–348.

Linder, J. A., Bates, D. W., Middleton, B., & Stafford, R. S. (2007). Electronic health records use and the quality of ambulatory care in the United States. *Archives of Internal Medicine*, *167*(13), 1400–1405. doi:10.1001/archinte.167.13.1400

Margalit, R. S., Roter, D., Dunevant, M. A., Larson, S., & Reis, S. (2006). Electronic medical record use and physician-patient communication: An observational study of Israeli primary are encounters. *Patient Education and Counseling*, *61*(1), 134–141. doi:10.1016/j.pec.2005.03.004

Marquie, J. C., Jourdan-Boddaert, L., & Huet, N. (2002). Do older adults underestimate their actual computer knowledge? *Behaviour & Information Technology*, *21*(4), 273–280. doi:10.1080/0144929021000020998

Mazzoleni, M. C., Baiardi, P., Giorgi, I., Franchi, G., & Cortesi, M. (1996). Assessing users' satisfaction through perception of usefulness and ease of use in the daily interaction with a hospital information system. Proceeding of the AMIA Annual Fall Symposium.

McGowan, J. J., Passiment, M., & Hoffman, H. M. (2007). Educating medical students as competent users of health information technologies: The MSOP data. *Medinfo*, *12*, 1414–1418.

McGrath, J. M., Arar, N. H., & Pugh, J. A. (2007). The influence of electronic medical record usage on nonverbal communication in the medical interview. *Health Informatics Journal*, *13*(2), 105–118. doi:10.1177/1460458207076466

Miller, R. H., & Sim, I. (2004). Physicians' use of electronic medical records: Barriers and solutions. *Health Affairs*, *23*(2), 116–126. doi:10.1377/hlthaff.23.2.116

Mullen, R., & Donnelly, J. T. (2006). Keeping it real--building an ROI model for an ambulatory EMR initiative that the physician practices espouse. *Journal of Healthcare Information Management*, *20*(1), 42–52.

Ovretveit, J., Scott, T., Rundall, T. G., Shortell, S. M., & Brommels, M. (2007). Improving quality through effective implementation of information technology in healthcare. *International Journal for Quality in Health Care*, *19*(5), 259–266. doi:10.1093/intqhc/mzm031

Pizzi, R. (2007). U.S. EHR market to approach $5 billion by 2015, Healthcare IT News, Retrieved February 4, 2008 from. www.healthcareitnews.com/story.cms?id=6332 - 31k

Rabinovitch, I. (2007, July). Speedy EMR implementations. Technology for Doctors.

Reardon, J. L., & Davidson, E. (2007). How do doctors perceive the organizing vision for electronic medical records? Preliminary findings from a study of EMR adoption in independent physician practices, Proceedings of the 40th Hawaii International Conference on Systems Science.

Rouf, E., Whittle, J., Lu, N., & Schwartz, M. D. (2007). Computers in the exam room: Differences in physician-patient interaction may be due to physician experience. *Journal of General Internal Medicine*, *22*(1), 43–48. doi:10.1007/s11606-007-0112-9

Russell, S. C., & Spooner, S. A. (2004). Barriers to EMR adoption in internal medicine and pediatric outpatient practices. *Tennessee Medicine*, *97*(10), 457–460.

Shekelle, P. G., Morton, S. C., & Keeler, E. B. (2006). Costs and benefits of health information technology. *Evidence Report/technology Assessment*, *132*, 1–71.

Sidorov, J. (2006). It ain't necessarily so: The electronic health record and the unlikely prospect of reducing health care costs. *Health Affairs*, *25*(6), 1745. doi:10.1377/hlthaff.25.6.1745-a

Simon, S. J., & Simon, S. J. (2006). An examination of the financial feasibility of Electronic Medical Records (EMRs): A case study of tangible and intangible benefits. *International Journal of Electronic Healthcare*, *2*(2), 185–200.

Terry, K. (2005, January 21). Exclusive survey: Doctors and EHRs, Medical Economics, Retrieved 2/4/08 from http://www.memag.com/memag/article/articleDetail.jsp?id=143144

Thakkar, M. & Davis, D. C. (2006). Risks, barriers, and benefits of EHR systems: a comparative study based on size of hospital. Perspectives in Health Information Management, August 14, 3-5.

Thompson, D. I., Osheroff, J., Classen, D., & Sittig, D. F. (2007). A review of methods to estimate the benefits of electronic medical records in hospitals and the need for a national benefits database. *Journal of Healthcare Information Management*, *21*(1), 62–68.

Van Der Meijden, M. J., Tange, H. J., Troost, J., & Hasman, A. (2003). Determinants of success of inpatient clinical information systems: A literature review. *Journal of the American Medical Informatics Association*, *10*(3), 235–243. doi:10.1197/jamia.M1094

Vanmeerbeek, M. (2004). Exploitation of electronic medical records data in primary health care. Resistance and solutions. Study in eight Wallon health care centres. *Studies in Health Technology and Informatics*, *110*, 42–48.

Wager, K., Lee, F. W., & White, A. W. (2002). *Life After a Disastrous Electronic Medical Record Implementation: One Clinic's Experience*. Hershey, PA: Idea Group Publishing.

This work was previously published in International Journal of Healthcare Delivery Reform Initiatives, edited by Matthew W. Guah, pp. 39-51, copyright 2009 by IGI Publishing (an imprint of IGI Global).

Chapter 9
Mobile Solutions for Managing Health Care

Esko Alasaarela
University of Oulu, Finland

Ravi Nemana
360Fresh, Inc., USA

Steven DeMello
University of California - Berkeley, USA

Nick S. Oliver
Imperial College, UK

Masako Miyazaki
University of Alberta, Canada

ABSTRACT

Wirhe project is an international collaborative study that focused on the future of healthcare needs, technology requirements and solutions for effective use of wireless platform for health care delivery. In this chapter, the authors present results of a Wirhe survey of 85 experts and individual interviews with 35 experts. The authors asked their opinions on the current status of adopting wireless equipment in health care, unmet needs in serving hospital in-patients and outpatients, and their views on the incorporation of wireless platform for future health care delivery and personal health management. Key findings are that 1) both remarkable quality improvements and process enhancements can be expected from thoroughly utilizing the wireless technologies and mobile solutions, 2) integration of personal health monitoring and professional health management is a key issue to be addressed and 3) health promotion and illness prevention will grow by utilizing mobile solutions. As a result of this study, they propose a framework that can be used in developing wireless health care solutions for managing diseases and related health problems. It can also be used to structure and stratify the needs by importance and utility, to anticipate which technologies and solutions are needed next, and to estimate how large the market size may be for industries.

DOI: 10.4018/978-1-60960-183-6.ch009

INTRODUCTION

Healthcare is a large industry that spends globally USD 6 trillion per year (in 2008). The US alone spent USD 2.3 trillion on health care in 2007, and spending was growing at a rate of 8 percent annually (Kalorama, 2007). According to the U.S. Department of Health and Human Services, healthcare spending in the U.S.A. will remain between 17 and 18 percent of the GDP until 2015 (http://www.cms.gov/NationalHealthExpend-Data/downloads/proj2009.pdf).

An aging population, rising costs of care, changes in environment such as global warming and industrial pollution, management of chronic disease, and enablement of self-care, among other challenges, challenge human health and health care systems in many countries, both developed and undeveloped. Mobile, wireless solutions offer an intriguing approach and value proposition to gather and provide information, maintain continuity of care, improve care coordination, and allow for advanced health services to be delivered, such as telemedicine. In addition, many leading information technology companies like IBM, Intel, Microsoft, Google, HP and Cisco have begun to focus on health care technology solutions that are converging / emerging toward an interoperable ecosystem that leverages wireless connectivity and mobility.

Online health record systems offer people the opportunity to input their health data including diagnostic and care history into forms, which they can share with their peers and all health professionals through the Internet. Kalorama's market study (2007) also shows rapid growth in IT; in particular, wireless technologies are seen to have big potential. They are expected to: improve patient care; reduce costs; streamline processes; help with regulatory compliance; and provide many other benefits. IT solutions may be directed at all phases of healthcare from prevention, through diagnostics into acute care, long-term disease care and rehabilitation in any setting. Healthcare professionals need real-time access to data at the point of care for improving their decision making and enhancing processes. Remote patient monitoring, e-prescription, asset management and tracking are also potential application areas of wireless technologies in health care.

The total market for wireless technologies in U.S. health care in 2005 was USD 1.8 billion, expected to grow 33 percent annually until 2010, reaching a total market size of USD 7.3 billion (Kalorama, 2007).

Microsoft Health Vault (http://www.healthvault.com/) is the first trial for a major generic commercial Personal Health Record (PHR). The dominance of Microsoft in personal computing makes this trial especially interesting. One big challenge is the connectivity throughout the health ecosystem and how users can browse their personal information in a wide range of health and wellness IT applications. Google emphasizes the continuity even more in their Health Data API service (http://code.google.com/apis/health/). They promote the use of a Continuity of Care Record (CCR) endorsed by the American Academy of Family Physicians and ASTM international as a standard of exchanging care information (http://www.astm.org/Standards/E2369.htm). The health record system has to communicate both with people and machines, and simultaneously maintain the high privacy and security of people's health data.

An IBM research team (Adams et al., 2006) summarizes the challenges of the world's health care this way: "Change must be made; the choices left to the stakeholders of today's health care systems are when and how. If they wait too long to act or do not act decisively enough, their systems could 'hit the wall' – in other words, be unable to continue on the current path – and then, require immediate and major forced restructuring."

Among IBM's recommendations are that: health care providers enhance management of chronic diseases and prevention of illness; consumers take personal responsibility for their health and maximize the value they get from the health care system; societies make better decisions regarding lifestyle expectations; and governments provide the leadership and political will power needed for innovative, sustainable solutions. Three methods to improve health care systems are proposed: 1) transforming value, 2) transforming consumer responsibility and 3) transforming care delivery.

The same IBM research team also describes the major changes needed in typical successful U.S. health plans in 2015; one of them is that business processes should be greatly improved and enhanced with IT-related capabilities (Adams et al., 2007).

Intel's research team (Intel Health, 2007) proposes rethinking the disease management process, emphasizing development of IT solutions for chronic diseases. Patients with chronic conditions account for 83% of US health care spending; 81% of inpatient stays; 91% of prescriptions; 76% of physician visits; and 98% of home health care visits (Anderson, 2004). New technical solutions could strengthen patients' long-term engagement in their care. Healthcare providers could have accurate, relevant and timely information from their patients. Patients could have intuitive, enjoyable and educational communication channels open to their care team and their families. In addition to periodic mailings and phone calls, communication could occur by e-mail, videoconferences, SMS messages and other mobile services. Touch screen and other user-friendly technologies should serve people with little or no IT experience.

A UK report on wireless based disease management (Wireless Healthcare, 2007) argues that wireless technologies play a key role within disease monitoring and modeling applications for AIDS, diabetes and influenza which are, especially in developed countries, diseases that significantly impact health care providers and pharmaceutical companies.

The California Healthcare Foundation (CHCF) (Adler, 2007) categorizes wireless applications of health care in two ways: 1) Monitoring applications for cardiac, diabetic etc. functions which can use portable, wearable or implantable sensors and work automatically and 2) Patient communication and supporting applications which can provide patients with information and feedback directly, and encourage them to take an active role in managing their health.

Many applications have been developed, for example, for cardiac monitoring (http://medicalconnectivity.com/), glucose monitoring (http://healthpia.us/, GlucoPhone, developed by HealthPia, South Korea), multiple vital signs monitoring (portable and wearable), and even implantable monitoring integrated in pacemakers (http://www.biotronik.de/, Cylos DR-T, developed by Biotronik, Germany). There are also applications for appointment reminders, health education and promotion, public health alerts, compliance monitoring and other treatment support and engagement. BeWell's Asthma Assistant (http://www.bewellmobile.com/) is an example.

CHFC defines issues of adoption of wireless technology. The health industry issues are uncertainty in reimbursement; unproven benefits; incompatibility of the health system for wireless applications; and privacy and security issues. The technical issues are potential information overload; lack of standards; market issues; incomplete coverage; network fragmentation; and the mismatch between the vivid cell phone market and the slow health care market.

The Continua Health Alliance (http://www.continuaalliance.org/) promotes a promising cooperative strategy to achieve continuity in care from the developer point of view (Carroll et al., 2007). There are more than 200 member companies who develop architecture, create use cases and define standards for better integrated health care services (CHA, 2009). The three target areas are: 1) disease management - managing a chronic disease outside of a clinical setting, 2) aging independently - using technology and services to live in one's own home longer, and 3) health and fitness - expanding personal health and wellness to where people live and play.

Alberta Health Service's Capital Health (Rowe, 2008) is a good example of applying continuum of care with evidence based practice. The challenge is to cover even the most complex patients in the vast rural areas of Canada with 2700 beds in 13 hospitals and 29 000 staff members including 2400 physicians serving 1.7 million people. The operation serves 10 000 home care clients monthly and 635 000 calls for health advice. Annually they have 956 000 patient days in hospitals, 1.3 million ambulatory visits, 436 000 emergency visits, 93 000 surgical procedures, 13 900 births. The Canada Health Act outlines the rules that provinces and territories must follow to receive federal funding for health care; these are 1) public administration; 2) comprehensiveness; 3) universality; 4) portability; and 5) accessibility. In these conditions it is inevitable to focus on a technology supported continuum of care. (http://www2.parl.gc.ca/content/lop/researchpublications/944-e.htm)

On the hospital side there are many indications that wireless technologies can support improved outcomes. Solovy (2007) lists ten lessons for hospitals and health systems to improve their outcome and quality including: 1) improve patient flow, 2) improve workflow, 3) improve whole processes, 4) measure results and 5) manage medication to drive quality to the bedside, 6) use smart alerts to improve care, 7) provide ubiquitous access to digital images, 8) do not forget the operating room, 9) plan for the worst and 10) remember that infrastructure is the key to the future.

There is much research and development work proceeding worldwide to save health care from financial crisis, including process reengineering, new service solutions development and new technology development. Wireless technologies offer interesting potential, but also face many challenges.

Present Status of Wireless in Health Care

This analysis is based on an international survey and interviews which were carried out during the first half of 2008 in America, Asia and Europe as a part of the Wirhe project, where an international strategy and roadmap plan for cooperative development of wireless technologies and solutions for health care was planned (Alasaarela, 2008).

The Wirhe strategy and roadmap plan was seen as important for several reasons: to increase understanding of the changes needed in the health care industry worldwide and how wireless and mobile solutions can be applied to enhance and improve it; to draw a roadmap with essential milestones; to plan a set of activities and efforts needed to reach the goals; to raise awareness of big challenges; and to define gaps in the process where wireless technologies can provide the solution. The Wirhe strategy and roadmap was funded and published by Tekes (a public technology and innovation fund in Finland) in October 2008 (Alasaarela, 2008).

University of Oulu was chosen as the responsible operator for the Wirhe project. To get a wide scope of understanding for the Wirhe project we collaborated first with the University of California Berkeley in Berkeley, CA, and the Health Technology Center (HealthTech) in San Francisco, CA. Imperial College in London joined the project team to develop the idea of our wireless framework, especially for wireless management of diabetes (Alasaarela & Oliver, 2009). The University of Alberta, Canada, joined to work on defining wireless solutions in rehabilitation[1].

In the first part of the Wirhe project we collected information and expert opinions about drivers and challenges in developing and adopting wireless solutions in health care (Alasaarela, Nemana & DeMello, 2009). This study was carried out during HIMSS conference 2008, in Orlando, Florida, by interviewing 70 participants who are experts on hospital information management. The main findings show that on average the most attractive and credible application is wireless alarming and calling for help. The second and third are mobile access to patient health records and vital signs monitoring. The results also showed that process change challenges are remarkably more difficult than technical challenges. The process change from the doctors' point of view is particularly severe. Among technical challenges usability of the mobile user interface is seen as the most difficult. Also according to this study, security of patient data is no longer among the most severe challenges.

In the second part of the Wirhe project we interviewed 85 experts from 15 countries through an Internet survey. A ZEF analysis method (http://zefsolutions.com/en/) was used to collect opinions and comments and to produce a report of bases, needs, vision, challenges, risks etc. with 699 comments, ideas and proposals of experts. We also interviewed 35 experts face-to-face (15 of them were participants of the ZEF survey) to deepen the scope. We also compared perspectives on wireless healthcare in Finland and in the United States (Alasaarela, DeMello & Nemana, 2009).

In addition, we collected a Wireless in Healthcare database including 160 products or solutions, 193 concurrent scientific and technical articles, 149 news articles during 2007-2008 and 41 conferences and exhibitions during 2008-2009.

The results were also analyzed and published in our Wirhe Framework paper (Alasaarela, Nemana, DeMello, Oliver & Miyazaki, 2009).

The ZEF Survey and Interviews

ZEF analysis is a two-dimensional graphical survey tool capable of z-score processing and is available on the Internet (http://zefsolutions.com/en). Examples of ZEF-charts can be seen in Figures 1-4. The respondents get an equivalent graphical survey form and work by pointing their evaluations on the answering field whose coordinates have been defined and indicated on the field axes.

The reports are calculated in the ZEF server as ZEF charts indicating the average points and deviation ellipses around them. The position of the numbers 1 to 10 on the charts in Figure 1, for example, reports averages and the height and width of the ellipses around the numbers are proportional to the deviation in the respective direction.

An absolute or z-scored method can be used in report processing. In the absolute process the original answers are used when processing the averages and deviations. In the z-scored process a normalization (z-scoring) method is used twice: first on each chart for each respondent's answers and second after averaging to the whole data chart by chart. The ZEF method gives full resolution to each respondent and also more accurate results than absolute processed charts. However, the normalized process can be used effectively only when finding comparative differences: better / worse, more / less attractive etc.

The ZEF survey content was planned by a small expert group[2] starting from the contents of our previous wireless strategy projects (Alasaarela, 2009). The question groups with the used dimensions (horizontal / vertical) are: A) Background questions (choice questions only); B) Bases and premises (Agreement level / Importance); C) Needs for development for inpatient use (Need 2012-14 / Need 2008-09); D) Needs for development for outpatient use (Need 2012-14 / Need 2008-09); E) Components of vision for 2014 (Attractiveness / Credibility); F) Threats and risks (Seriousness / Probability); G) Technical challenges (Degree of difficulty); H) Process development challenges (Degree of difficulty); I) Your message to the strategy team (Free text). In each question group there is at least one text box for writing free text comments and ideas.

The experts were invited via email and motivated by a raffle of a Nokia smart phone. They answered by clicking a link in their invitation mail to open their graphical ZEF survey form. Altogether 85 (46%) experts of 187 invited responded to our

Figure 1. Bases and premises according to 83 experts' answers to the 10 claims. Numbered spots are on their average points and the ellipses around are proportional to their standard deviations. Four small charts describe opinions of the same experts divided into groups that they represent. The ZEF method is a registered trademark of ZEF Solutions (http://zefsolutions.com/en)

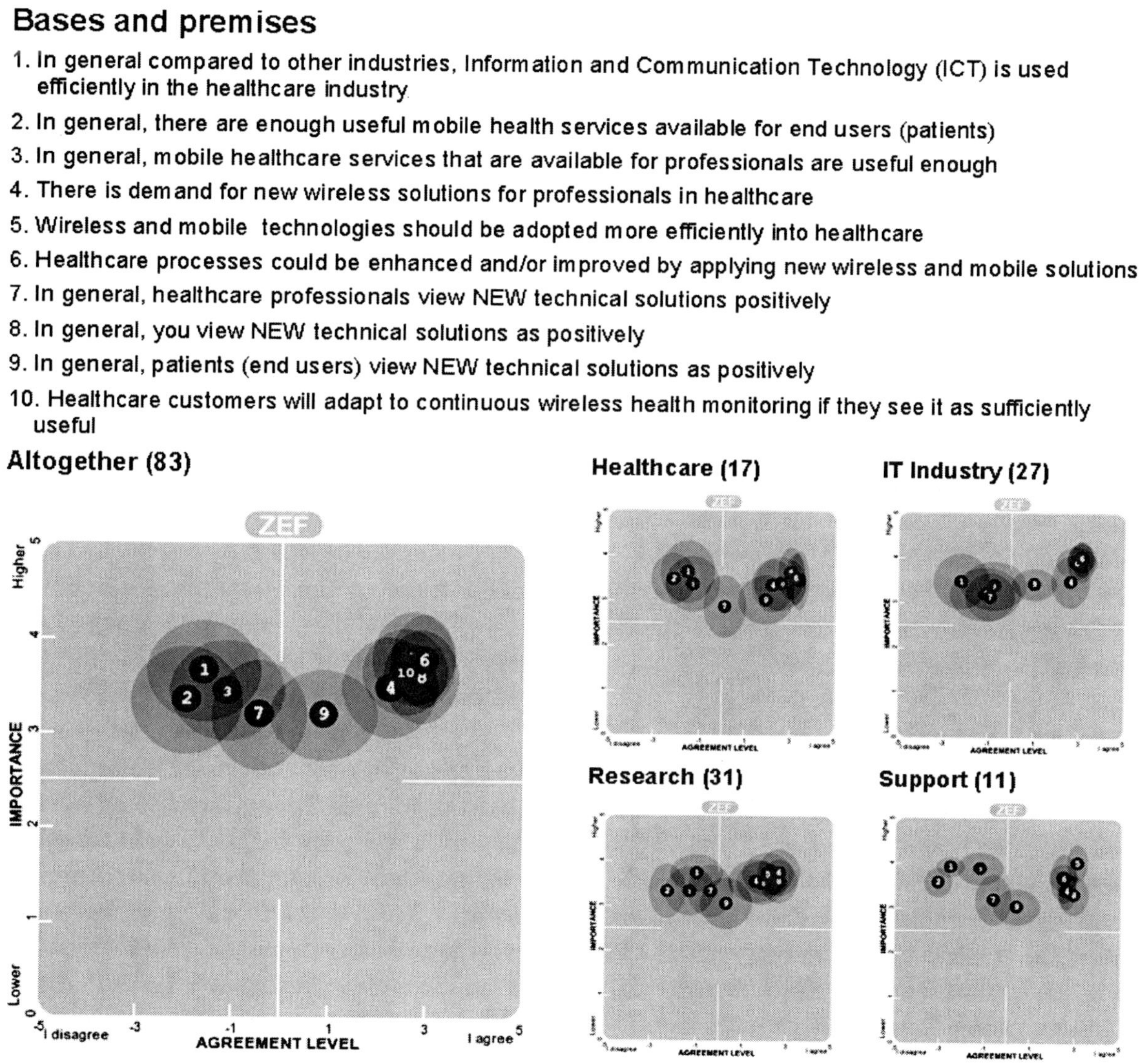

ZEF survey. A total of 39 ZEF survey respondents represented USA; 20 Finland; 7 South Korea; 6 UK; and 13 other countries (including Canada, Spain, Belgium, Sweden, Norway, Estonia, Hungary, Japan, the Netherlands, Germany and Switzerland). The respondents represented all-important expert groups: 1) health care services (19), 2) IT industry (27), 3) research (32) and 4) supporting (11).

The number of respondents varies in the reported question groups since the ZEF system gave access to each respondent according to their expert areas that they had selected in the background questions.

Background Questions

In the background questions of the Wirhe study the experts were asked to define their primary responsibilities in their jobs. They were allowed to select one or more responsibilities. 31.8% selected "Management/coordination," 47.1% "Technical research & development," 16.5% "Technology planning, acquiring and/or maintenance," 10.6% "Marketing / sales," 12.9% "Medical diagnosis and care," 2.4% "Nursing / nursing science" and 22.4% "Something else".

Experts were also asked to rate their familiarity with IT technology. The agreement percentages were: 97.6% in "I use mobile phone daily," 89.4% "I use wireless network (WLAN, WiFi) when needed," 76.5% "I use Bluetooth links when needed," 51.8% "I use 3G services when needed," 69.5% "I use GPS navigation when needed," 63.5% "I know ZigBee technology," 51.8% "I know UWB technology," 45.9% "I use PDA device daily and 21.2% "I use wireless network to browse patient records".

Bases and Premises

In general the experts believe that "ICT is not used efficiently in the health care industry" and "there are not enough useful mobile solutions available for end users" (numbers 1 and 2 in Figure 1). In addition the "mobile health care services available for professionals are not useful enough" (3). All groups, people from health care services, IT industry, research and supporting agree on these negative statements. An example comment: *"I have not seen an integrated total solution. There are lots of solutions tackling various different problems taking baby steps."*

The same people agree that "there is demand for wireless solutions" (4) for professionals, "wireless and mobile solutions should be adopted more efficiently" (5) into health care, and they would "enhance and/or improve health care processes" (6). In addition the same experts believe that "customers would adapt even continuous wireless health monitoring" (10) if they saw it as sufficiently useful. It is interesting to note that the error bars for the responses to the bases and premises section of the ZEF questionnaire are the smallest of all the sections. This indicates that there is significant overall agreement on general principles between experts in wireless health care, regardless of background. The spread of responses and the size of the error bars increase for more specific sections of the ZEF survey, though it should be noted that the number of experts polled differs between sections.

Some of the experts are concerned about the health care processes themselves, which would require major changes. They would not like to grant technology too big a role. The majority of comments were positive, like this one: *"Mobile solutions supported by privacy and security checks will be accepted as they will contribute to better, safer and more efficient care."*

Needs of Wireless for in-Hospital Use

The experts believe that in the short term the highest need is for "alarm buttons and systems" (number 11 in Figure 2). The highest needs both in the short and long term are "need for wireless networks" (1) themselves and "need for wireless access to an electronic patient record system" (4), "to an electronic prescription system" (5) and "to medical information" (6). In the long term "wireless sensor belts and wristbands" (10) are also needed.

The experts coming from health care services also stated a "need for wireless terminals" (2), and research experts estimate that the need with the greatest evolution over the forthcoming 5 years will be for "implantable sensors and care actuators" (9).

Patients would love to have services and information access through mobile and wireless devices.

Figure 2. Short and long term needs of wireless for in-hospital use according to 48 experts. The charts have been calculated by using a normalizing (z-scoring) method

Needs of wireless for in-hospital use

1. Need for wireless networks
2. Need for wireless terminals
3. Need for RFID-tags
4. Need for wireless access to an electronic patient record system
5. Need for wireless access to an electronic prescription system
6. Need for wireless access to medical information
7. Need for wireless access to inventory information
8. Need for wireless access to pharmaceutical information
9. Need for implantable sensors and care actuators
10. Need for wireless sensor belts and wristbands
11. Need for alarm buttons and systems
12. Need for location and tracking of patients
13. Need for location and tracking of instruments and devices
14. Need for developing wireless VoIP phone network

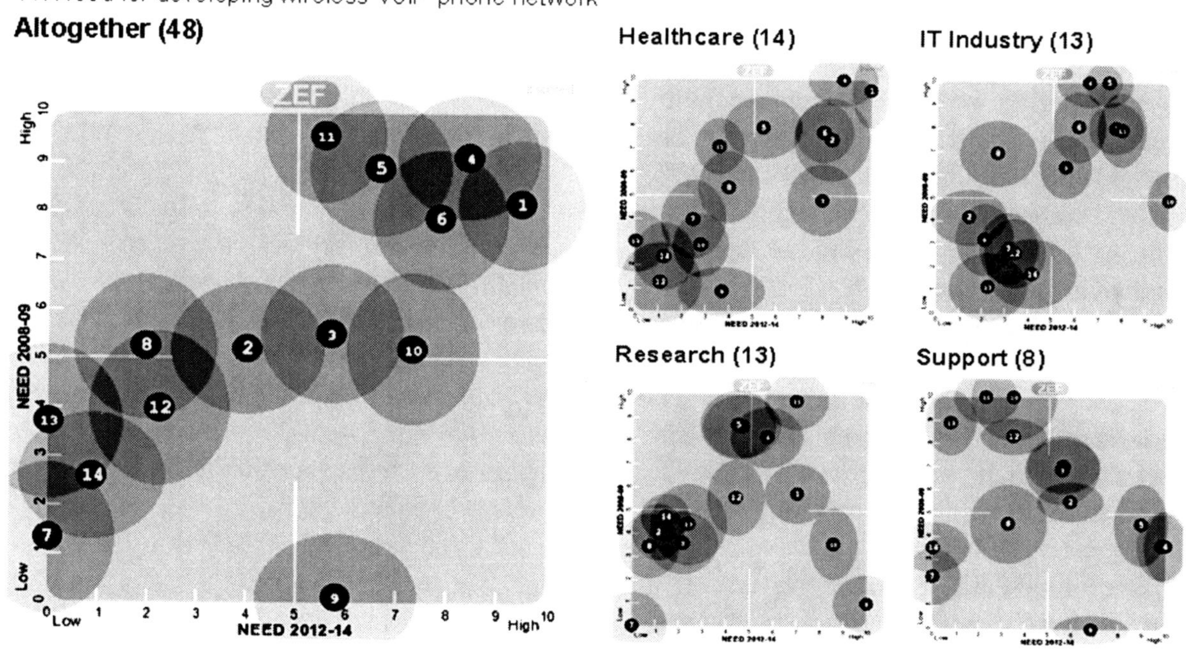

Needs of Wireless for Outpatient Use

One candidate is clearly higher than any other in our list of outpatient wireless needs, both short and long range: "home health care applications for special diseases" (1). The second is "sensor belts and/or wristband devices for remote monitoring" (2), especially, in the short term. Only experts from health care services raise "ubiquitous health services" (6) and "rural area home health care applications" (5) as more important long range. IT industry experts do not see ubiquitous health services as important as the three other mentioned above.

On the other hand these experts do not see any special "need for sensor floors, sensor walls or other ambient sensing systems" (3) which are usually seen as important in ubiquitous technology.

The text comments of the experts support the results above: *"Near future: remote monitoring and tele-assistance. Far future: sensor implants, implants improving body functions (for example vision, pain relief), artificial limbs connected to neural system."*

FUTURE OF WIRELESS IN HEALTHCARE

Vision and Goals for Future Development

In defining future vision and goals we used ZEF analysis to rate the attractiveness and credibility of questions or matters listed on a ZEF table. The thoroughly planned list of the asked choices for cores and components of vision can be seen in Figure 4. In the survey form each of them was described in greater detail.

In addition we asked the experts to write their comments and ideas about vision like: "Which objectives would be the most important to take into account?" and "Try to formulate your vision for wireless solutions in health care. What are the key issues? What are the key technologies? What are the expected benefits?"

The result of the ZEF analysis can be seen in Figure 4. After numerous discussions with experts the results were as follows. "Enhancing health care patient processes" (5) is the most credible and attractive component of the vision. The second is "mobile health care as a core of the vision" (2). The next two are "wireless monitoring at homes and in worksites" (8) and "ubiquitous computing in health care industry" (9). Two more: "integration as a core of the vision" (3) and "wireless health monitoring in hospitals" (7) are highly credible and attractive, especially, according to experts from health care services and research.

Although most of the original average points (calculated without z-scoring) are situated in the upper right corner (representing attractive and credible elements), numbers 1, 4 and 6 are clearly lower both in attractiveness and credibility than the other. Thus the wireless hospital and wireless location and tracking cannot be core elements on average in the future according to these experts.

The "international cooperation" (4) is an interesting detail in this study. It is the least attractive and least credible component of vision. Why? Perhaps the health care systems are so national by their inherent character that the experts can foresee such severe national challenges that they cannot credit any possibility of international cooperation. This analysis reveals that we have an especially hard challenge to obtain international cooperation.

The two text questions generated 92 answers which strengthen and detail the interpretation. Here are two samples:

An informed and empowered consumer is more compliant. Wireless technology facilitates monitoring at home and work. Key issues relate to privacy, security and reimbursement. The RFID, cell phones and ubiquitous technologies will continue to develop. This will produce significant cost savings to society as a result of better outcomes and fewer medical errors.

Key issues: The application of wireless technologies in health care lags behind other areas. It is important to come up with a platform that can be easily integrated with the existing devices. An open platform will allow researchers to test and implement their technologies. Key technologies: PDA or smart phones enabled with wireless technology. Developing robust sensing technology. Software to provide patients and clinicians with feedback. Expected benefits: Tremendous reduc-

Figure 3. Short and long term needs of wireless for outpatient use according to 44 experts. The charts have been calculated by using a normalizing (z-scoring) method

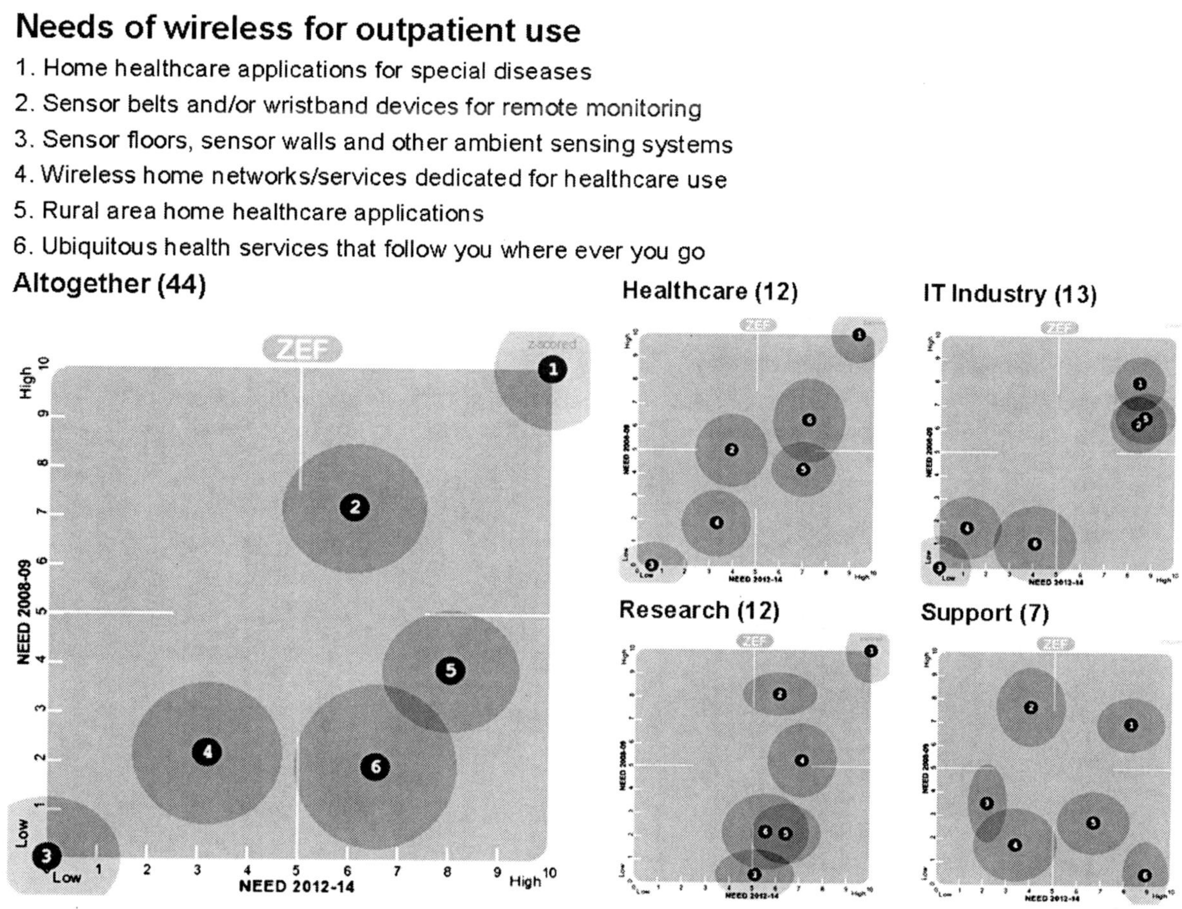

tion in health care costs. Increase in efficiency of clinicians. Convenience to patients.

Defined Vision 2014

According to the above studies and tens of face-to-face interviews of experts the vision 2014 was formulated as (Alasaarela, 2008):

Towards 2014 health care will become more mobilized and integrated – close to ubiquitous. The patient processes will be enhanced and supported by wireless monitoring and care services at homes and worksites as well as in hospitals. Wireless technologies and mobile solutions will be applied systematically to different disease groups according to a unified framework based on international development and standardization work.

The first part of the vision comes directly from the study results above. The second part –systematic application of wireless to different diseases - comes from discussions with experts. An estimation of prevalence and annual costs of some diseases in the USA can be seen in Table 1.

Major diseases compounded by aging and obesity problems form one of the biggest health care costs in the USA and even globally. Our hypothesis is that by utilizing wireless solutions

Figure 4. The main summary of the ZEF analysis of the vision components calculated by using z-scoring to get relative results

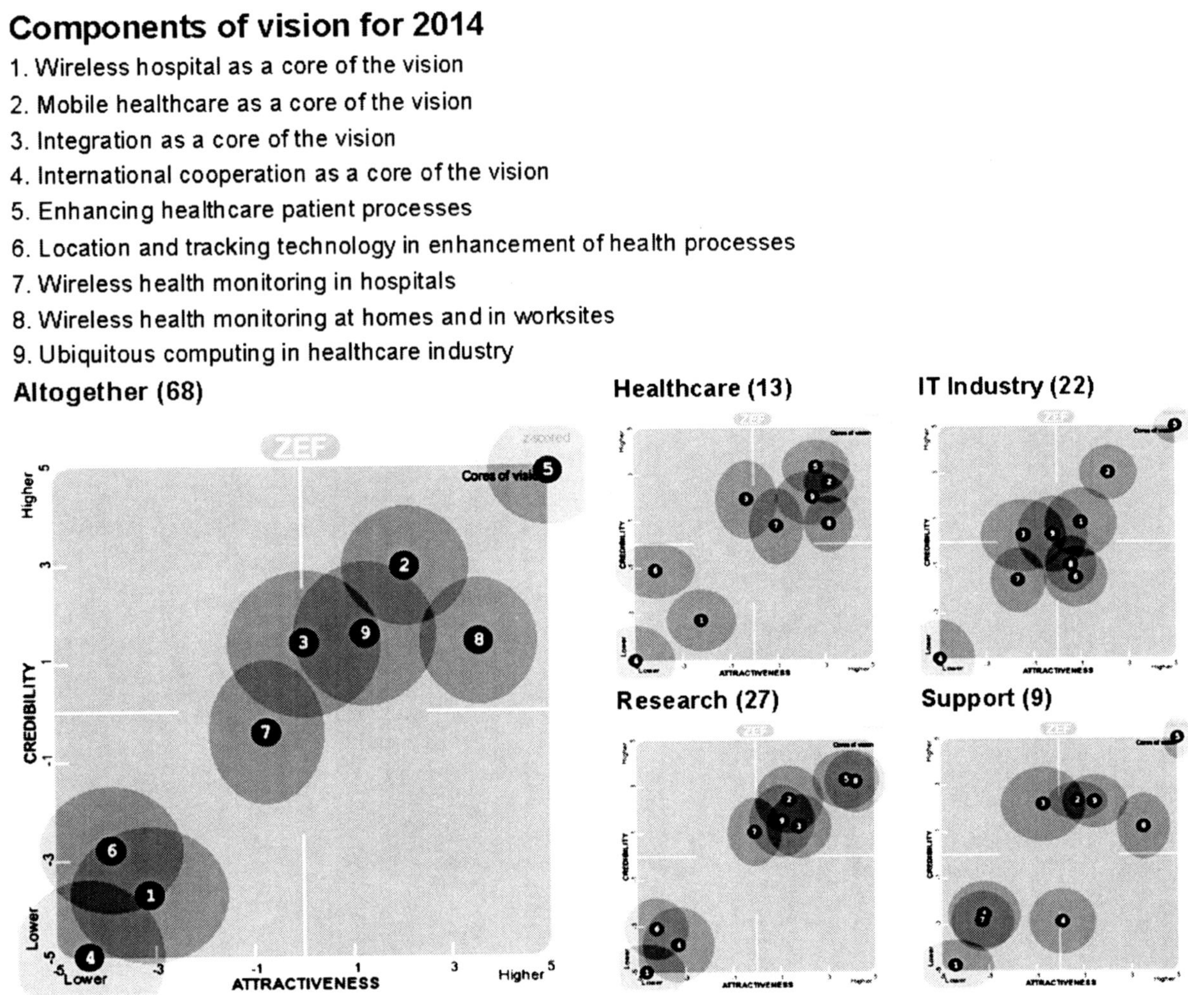

we can manage these costs more effectively. The main aim of this study is to offer a framework that will reveal the exact points in the health service continuum where mobile solutions will bring the most significant outcomes and improve the quality of care. The unified framework can be used to manage planning of wireless solutions for each health problem systematically.

Integration of Personal and Institutional Health Care

The future of wireless in health care can be viewed in four ways: 1) From the health professionals' point of view, how can health care processes be enhanced and improved by adopting wireless and mobile solutions? 2) From the patients' and citizens' point of view, how can disease and health management be enhanced, improved and better adapted to their daily lives? 3) From the providers' and governments' point of view, how can the whole

Table 1. The most expensive diseases in America (Herper, 2005)

Disease	*Annual costs*	**Patients in USA**
Heart conditions	$68 billion	20 million
Trauma	$58 billion	36 million
Mental Illness	$48 billion	31 million
Cancer	$48 billion	11 million
Respiratory Ailments	$45 billion	50 million
Hypertension	$33 billion	37 million
Arthritis and Joint Disorders	$32 billion	23 million
Diabetes	$28 billion	14 million
Back problems	$23 billion	18 million
Total	$383 billion	

health care industry be improved and made more efficient by promoting new wireless and mobile solutions? 4) From the engineers' technology point of view, how can modern wireless and mobile communication technologies be applied to solve problems in the health care industry?

In order to optimize the management of health care we need to combine the professionals' process-based thinking, the citizens' wellbeing, patients' disease-based thinking and the government and institutional return on investment (ROI) based thinking. This means integration of health care in a novel and fundamental way. Technologies are only tools to realize the solutions needed.

A health care process can be considered to be a chain of successive activities which health care professionals perform for the patient in a hospital or in the community. Broadly speaking, activities of the patient's own before coming to health services and after returning back home can also be considered to belong to this health care process. Therefore, wireless supported health care processes involve most of the same activities, which the patients receive in their wireless supported disease management programs.

The disease management concept is an entity, which comprises methods, systems, services, devices and products for diagnosing, caring for and monitoring a patient with a specific disease during the course of that disease. Mostly the term of disease management is attached to chronic illnesses, but now we broaden it to acute illness episodes as well. Perhaps, it would be better to speak of "health management concepts" or "healing support concepts".

Development of wireless supported disease management concepts requires a great deal of medical and nursing knowledge - much more than developing the devices and systems which are needed in only one phase of a health care process. This arises from a more holistic way of considering health processes.

By combining the three viewing angles we can formulate concepts to manage diseases with a wireless-supported continuum of care from preventive health management to care and rehabilitation services. This would lead to efficient, high quality care, financial savings and improved clinical outcomes which would not be possible without wireless and mobile solutions.

THE WIRHE FRAMEWORK FOR WIRELESS MANAGEMENT OF DISEASES

Each disease and health problem needs a specific diagnostic, care and monitoring concept, compris-

Figure 5. The Wirhe framework shows how the patient-driven disease management (left) and the professionals-driven health care processes (right) are integrated to form a unified service chain with many different paths for customers. Each text block refers to needs and solutions, both available and lacking. For example, supported care at home for a heart condition (arrhythmia) needs heart monitoring and requires a wireless ECG sensor with a means to transmit an alert and ECG sample to a professional health service unit as soon as abnormalities emerge in the data

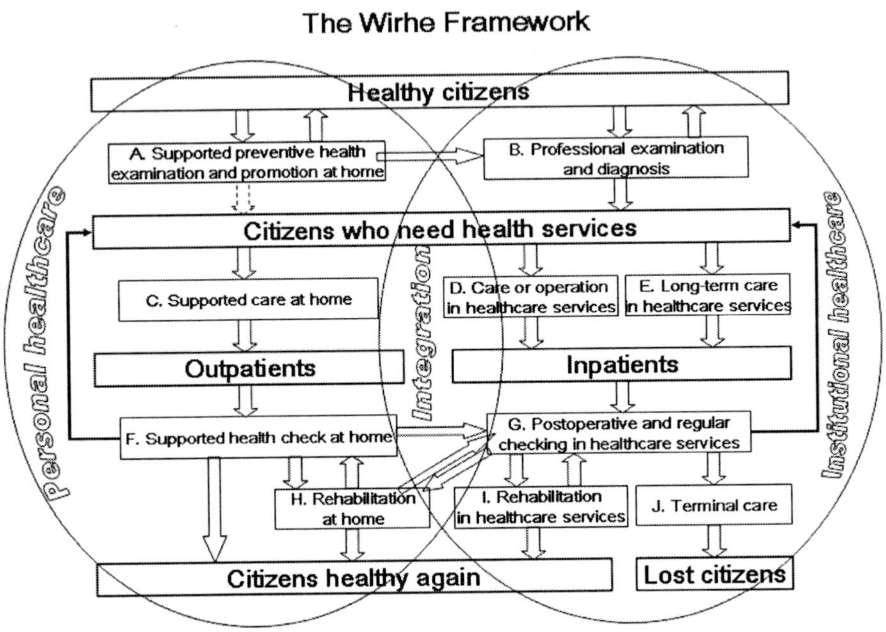

ing all-important phases starting from the first indicators of pathology and ending with no symptoms or indicators, demonstrating health. Disease prevention is also needed for specific risk groups (people with genetic or environmental risks).

Wireless support offers not only opportunities to manage diseases in a novel way, but also the opportunity to tailor the disease management concept individually for each patient, taking into account unique needs, wishes and lifestyles. The overall goal is that all patients continue their normal daily life despite their disease status and that wireless health care provides no additional burden to the patient.

Public, private and self-care can be seen as building blocks. They can be re-engineered to form a systematic framework (Figure 5) for developing the wireless supported health care. The existing wireless and mobile solutions can now be placed on the Wirhe framework.

Wireless support may be very different for different diseases. It might also be tailored to meet individual patient's needs, particularly if the patient has two or more chronic diseases.

Important blocks in the Wirhe Framework are:

A. Supported preventive health examination and promotion at home
B. Professional examination and diagnosis
C. Supported care at home
D. Care or operation in health care services
E. Long-term care in health care services
F. Supported health check at home
G. Postoperative health check and regular (continuous or sampled) health monitoring in health care services

H. Rehabilitation at home
I. Rehabilitation in health care services
J. Terminal care

Wireless networks and access points are needed in hospitals, clinics, and health centers as well as at home. Therefore, they are needed in most of the blocks. Cisco (http://www.cisco.com/) and Philips (http://www.philips.com) are well known global providers of wireless networks solutions with access points, controllers, etc.

Aruba Wireless Networks (http://www.arubanetworks.com/) provides user-centric wireless networks to integrate adaptive wireless LANs, identity-based security, and application continuity services for health care campuses, clinics, physician and home-offices.

Flo Healthcare (http://www.flohealth care.com/) markets mobile clinical workstations, wireless access points and accessories specifically for the health care industry. Wireless connection to information helps clinicians stay better connected with their patients.

Cardinal Health (http://www.cardinal.com/) markets their Alaris solution including system manager and gateway units, a safety net module and a connectivity program for facilitating data flow between key technologies. Their customers are located on five continents and include hospitals, medical centers, retail and mail order pharmacies, clinics, physicians, pharmacists and other health care providers.

Nortel Networks (http://www.nortel.com/) provides affordable, scalable IP voice and wireless mobility solutions and other IP based clinical applications including asset tracking and management systems.

Motorola Remote Patient Monitoring Solutions (http://www.motorola.com/) combine WLAN enabled mobile computers, voice over WLAN, leading clinical IT and medical device applications to help improve the speed and quality of medical treatment.

Next we describe briefly each block and give examples of the kind of needs and wireless solutions there might be in each block. Some of the blocks are not needed in all of the diseases. For example, diabetes is a life-long disease. Therefore, rehabilitation is seldom needed for diabetes itself; it is more often needed due to its co-morbidities. In addition, diabetes itself is not fatal, although it may lead to fatal complications (Alasaarela & Oliver, 2009).

A. Supported Preventive Health Examination and Promotion at Home

Preventive care and health promotion are some of the most important needs in the future. Many changes in human life-style, working environment, eating habits, environmental pollution etc. set new challenges to our health. We need new solutions to measure and monitor our health to diagnose evolving health problems as early as possible. We also need solutions to collect the right information at the right time about the right problem. In the future genetic information will become increasingly important, describing susceptibilities to prevalent diseases.

In fact, if we are able to assess our genetic risks, follow daily what we eat and drink, monitor the gamut of our physical and mental exercise and measure regularly our bio signals, we will have a clearer risk assessment of what diseases and other health problems we should be concerned about. Is it possible to develop wireless solutions to offer these services? What are the most important means to start from?

There are already many technologies and platforms available for these needs. Heart rate monitors are well known; for example Polar Electro's products (http://www.polar.fi), who have also developed analysis software for fitness and weight monitoring. Firstbeat Technologies (http://www.firstbeat.fi) has developed an HRV (Heart rate variability) analyzing method and software which utilizes heart rate data to find latent diseases.

Cell phone networks working on the 3G level are effective platforms for preventive health solutions. Many mobile services for managing fitness, weigh, nutrition and lifestyle are under development. Wireless devices for monitoring vital signs and specific physiological parameters can also be used by healthy people, especially if they belong to a high-risk group. The monitoring could also be linked to health providers and call centers.

B. Professional Examination and Diagnosis

The professional examination happens mostly within health services (in health centers, hospitals or clinics). Therefore, some of the wireless technologies which are available for care are available also for examination.

As an example, LifeWatch Corp. (http://www.lifewatchinc.com/) offer wireless blood pressure meters, oxygen saturation monitors, weigh scales, PDA monitors with Bluetooth connection and services for integrated monitoring and analysis.

Medixine Ltd. (http://www.medixine.com/) offers an integrated monitor system via a Bluetooth connection for measuring devices such as blood pressure meters, scales and glucometers. The data are forwarded to the Medixine server either via a mobile phone or a Bluetooth hub.

C. Supported Care at Home

Home health care is a rapidly proliferating market. At Medica 2009 (http://www.medica.de/) visitors could see many comprehensive solutions for managing chronic patients at home. Wireless technology is important both for patient's freedom to move at home and for continuous connection and support from care providers.

Among the most utilized products in the home health care market are the Honeywell HomMed solutions. HomMed is one of the leaders in telehealth and remote patient monitoring solutions (http://www.hommed.com/) and over half a million patients are served by HomMed solutions. They are dedicated to improving the quality of patients' lives and reducing the cost of health care by providing integrated solutions for home care. The products of HomMed are the Centry and Genesis telehealth monitors with a wide variety of peripherals, medication reminders and a central station. The solutions can be used to collect heart rate, blood pressure, oxygen saturation and other vital signs data and to process and display it for diagnostic and care development use.

Philips Electronics (http://www.healthcare.philips.com/us_en/) offers among other products a TeleStation hub for the transmission of vital signs data collected from the wireless measurement devices at a patient's home. It is also a medium for interactive communication between care providers and patients at home. They also offer Intellivue Telemetry Systems for SpO2, ECG and improved tachycardia assessment, which uses so-called smart-hopping technology to maintain seamless connections between the central station and telemetry devices. Their Classic Pendant Personal help button gives patients at home access to fast assistance by a simple alert touch. Philips offers also many wireless products for hospital and other institutional use.

MedApps is an emerging company (http://www.medapps.net) which offers portable devices and a web-based monitoring application to deliver an end-to-end mobile, wireless, health monitoring system. Their whitepaper lists benefits of mobile healthcare solutions as: 1) Reduce the need for in-office visits, 2) Enable fewer physicians to provide care to a larger number of patients, 3) Reduce hospitalizations and re-hospitalizations, and 4) Eliminate unnecessary transport (MedApps, 2010).

University of Alberta (a team lead by Dr. Masako Miyazaki) has developed a comprehensive home care solution, WWPM for chronic elderly patients (Miyazaki, 2008). The system was tested by a third party research team for a healthy population and clients' population in Capital Health.

The system was spun off from the University of Alberta and is now available through Kanata Health Solutions Ltd. (www.kanatahealth.ca)

BeWell Mobile (http://www.bewellmobile.com/) is offered to advance engagement of conditions such as asthma and diabetes patients in three ways: via Web Portal, eDiaries by cell phones and Reminders by SMS.

ExmoCare (http://www.exmocare.com/) develops, produces and markets wireless health care, wellness and biosensor products. Its operations are focused around its line of wireless biosensor wristwatches and recurring monthly service plans for remote chronic care, weight management and eventually diabetes care.

BodyTel Scientific (http://www.bodytel.com/) specializes in telemedical monitoring and management systems for chronic diseases, particularly diabetes.

Visual Telecommunications Network (http://www.vitelnet.com/) offers ViTel Net solutions for home health monitoring, referral, consultation and emergency telemedicine.

Confidant (http://www.confidantinc.com/) has developed mobile phone solutions helping people suffering from chronic diseases manage their health easily while maintaining an active lifestyle.

D. Care or Operation in Health Care Services

Wireless networks are already in daily use in most of the hospitals in the western countries. For example, when physicians and nurses go on their rounds they have their laptops or tablet PCs to maintain access to patient record and medical information systems. In addition, there are many technologies available to apply WLAN, Bluetooth, RFID or other wireless connections.

Alien Technology (http://www.alientechnology.com/) provides RFID tags, RFID readers and related services.

InnerWireless (http://www.innerwireless.com/healthcare.shtml) is a provider of comprehensive in-building wireless distribution systems, as well as wireless tracking and location solutions.

Medanets Oy (http://www.medanets.com/en/index.php) offers a solution where the measurement data are transferred into the information system via a wireless network, either automatically or with one entry. The information is immediately available to all system users.

Allscripts (http://www.allscripts.com/) offers mobile TouchChart solutions for physicians to quickly prescribe, check for drug interactions, access medical histories and review drug reference information. Providers can connect directly to the pharmacy via electronic fax and electronically exchange prescription data.

CardioNet (http://www.cardionet.com/) offers a solution for arrhythmia patients. They wear three chest leads with a small sensor that detects heart rhythm and wirelessly transmits to the monitor. LifeWatch Corp. (http://www.lifewatchinc.com/) has a similar arrhythmia solution LifeStar, with a single lead ECG.

Audio Riders' (http://www.audioriders.fi/) Carerider collects information from wireless sensors placed in beds and nursing chairs, which is then integrated with the intelligent job control of the service.

CRF Inc (http://www.crfhealth.com/) is the leading global provider of eDiaries and wireless data collection solutions for the biopharmaceutical industry.

Emfit (http://www.emfit.com/) is specialized in developing and manufacturing networked, IP-based nurse call systems with assistive non-body-contact vitals and movements monitoring, fall and wander alarms, and epileptic seizure alarms.

Medictes (http://www.medictes.fi/) is focused on health care data systems by offering communication tools, applications and solutions. Their MobiiliSanelu allows clinicians to dictate ubiquitously by a web application or cell phone. The saved dictations are available for listening and unpacking in real-time.

A wireless, battery-free, fetal vital signs sensor which monitors baby's vital signs day and night has been developed in the National Children's Hospital. RF System Laboratory is in charge of product development. They have also been working with NASA to support astronauts during space flight (http://www.rfnokko.com/nokkop2.html)

E. Long-Term Care in Health Care Services

The applications of long-term care differ from basic hospital care. Their aim is to help patients to live with minimal intrusion while being monitored frequently enough to detect changes in health status. Many long-term patients have several chronic conditions and wear monitoring devices for years, increasing technology costs. However, in present care models, these patients use the vast majority of health care resources. Therefore, the expected savings of implementing wireless solutions are higher.

Televital (http://www.televital.com/) offers VitalWare VMS integrated Electronic Patient Medical Record and real-time telemedicine software modules with auto-recognition and configuration architecture that enables plug-and-play for a wide variety of medical devices from different manufacturers.

Sensitron (http://www.sensitron.net/) has developed careTrends solution, which is an enterprise software and wireless vital signs collection and dissemination system, to improve patient quality of care and decrease health care costs.

IST International Security Technology (http://www.istsec.fi/en.php) offers automatic personal security systems monitoring and analyzing users′ activity levels. Their Vivago wristtop monitor consists of sensors and algorithms that allow body signals to be monitored and analyzed automatically and continuously.

Medtronic (http://www.medtronic.com/) is a manufacturer of medical technology solutions for people with chronic disease. Each year, 6 million patients utilize Medtronic's technology, used to treat conditions such as diabetes, heart disease, neurological disorders, and vascular illnesses. Their Minimed Paradigm system integrates an insulin pump with real-time continuous glucose monitoring and sends blood sugar test results wirelessly to an insulin pump – making integration of glucose and insulin data easier.

Toumaz Technology (http://www.toumaz.com/) is a specialist in ultra low power sensing technology. Their Sensium is a sensor interface and transceiver platform for a wide range of applications in health care, not only for chronic diseases but also for lifestyle management. The device includes a reconfigurable sensor interface, digital block with 8051 processor and an RF transceiver block.

F. Supported Health Check at Home

Patients may acquire some home devices and services to monitor their important health parameters, blood pressure, blood glucose, weight, temperature etc. An example of a chronic disease with a need for regular self-checking is diabetes. Most diabetics should measure their blood glucose several times per day using portable glucometers. Some of these glucometers have wireless capability to transmit data to personal computers for later review.

ProWellness (http://www.prowellness.com/fi/) has developed a mobile system for diabetics to monitor their health at home. Similar solutions are available from Medapps etc.

G. Postoperative and Continuous Checking in Health Care Services

Many patient monitors are available with wireless connections. When intensive monitoring is not needed it is better to have a light minimally invasive or non-invasive patient monitor and move the patient into an area where costs are lower. Light patient monitors are available from many companies.

For example, Welch Allyn (http://www.welchallyn.com/) offers Spot Vital Signs Lxi monitors which use a barcode scanner, and a wireless radio to capture and transfer patient vital signs quickly thus bringing wireless vital signs transmission capability from the bedside.

H. Rehabilitation at Home

There are wide range of technologies that have been used to provide remote delivery of rehabilitation by Occupational Therapists, Physical Therapists, Speech Pathologist and Audiologists. The most widely used modalities, as of 2010, are Skype, webcams, videophones, iPhone, PDA and websites containing health information. There are telecommunication infrastructure challenges depending on where you reside. If your clients are living in a remote community in Canada with broadband nodes, your access to high speed Internet would provide TV type broadcasting for patients with chronic illness and provide health education just in time. The majority of rehabilitation services can be augmented if therapists and clients can access necessary equipment. For example, Occupational Therapists at the Glenrose Hospital, Edmonton incorporates the Wii fit (NINTENDO) game for head injury patients' balance, cognitive and endurance building. Providing readily commercially available wireless games enhances patients' recoveries. The Rutgers University's Tele-Rehabilitation Institute engineers have worked with clinicians at the Indiana University School of Medicine to deploy systems in participants' homes for up to 10 months. A description of the modified system (combined a Sony PlayStation 3 console and a commercial gaming glove with custom-developed software and games to provide exercise routines aimed at improving hand speed and range of finger motion) is in IEEE Transactions on Information Technology in Biomedicine. (http://www.sciencedaily.com/releases/2010/03/100317144642.htm)

Many aspects of rehabilitation practice can be enhanced with objective measurement tools such as 3D motion analysis for Occupational Therapy and Physical Therapy, instead of goniometry and manual muscle testing which are susceptible to error in measurements.

Two important areas of telerehabilitation research are (1) demonstrating equivalence of assessment and therapy to in-person assessment and therapy, and (2) building new data collection systems to digitize information that a therapist can use in practice. The study reported by Barlow, Liu, Sekulic (2009) which compared outcomes of wheelchair seating and positioning interventions provided via telerehabilitation (n=10) and face-to-face (n=20; 10 in each of two comparison groups, one urban and one rural. Clients who received their seating assessment via telerehabilitation were as satisfied with the outcomes of the recommended interventions, and their goals were as likely to be met as clients who were assessed face-to-face. They were assessed sooner than a group of out-of-region clients who traveled to a specialized seating service. Naturally, the technology could not substitute for travel required by vendors in order to provide the required seating components.

Groundbreaking research in telehaptics (the sense of touch) and virtual reality may broaden the scope of telerehabilitation practice, in the future. (http://en.wikipedia.org/wiki/Telerehabilitation)

I. Rehabilitation in Health Care Services

It is obvious that health care and being healthy do not have any clear boundaries. It is a continuum of care throughout our life inside and outside of institutions. One way to look at this is the level of care you need or level of productivity you have accomplished. You may need a small device to help you to get back to work or need a wheelchair to get around. Institutional rehabilitation service can be augmented by having a secure wireless LAN so that health care providers can access clients' data at the point of care. There is a serious need to evaluate all the wireless products which are used in an institution so that industries can provide the equipment clients' needs without interfering with other wireless medical devices.

J. Terminal Care

In terminal care there are only few wireless solutions available. If the patient is immobile, wires are not disruptive and the advantages of wireless data are reduced. However, terminal care should be planned for future utilization of wireless technologies due to potential improvements in cost efficiency.

Hoana Medical (http://www.hoana.com/) markets a special bed solution (LifeBed™ System) which could work in terminal care. Patient vigilance system provides a solution for continuous observation of patient conditions. Unlike conventional monitoring systems no physical contact or connections are needed. Wireless solutions for palliation of symptoms in the dying patient might include pain monitoring, consciousness monitoring and analgesic or hypnotic drug delivery.

PATHS OF PATIENTS IN THE WIRHE FRAMEWORK

In Figure 6 we can see an example of a path followed by a patient in the Wirhe framework. The individual with no symptoms of diabetes uses only preventive services. However, if the process of home monitoring and preventive care reveals signs of diabetes he/she goes on to professional examination. If diabetes is not diagnosed he/she returns back to use only preventive services. If the diagnosis is made, he/she progresses through the framework to care in a clinic. After a satisfactory review in the hospital he/she returns home to use supported care services with supported health monitoring at home. This loop continues until there is a need to go to a professional health check, at which stage he/she can access inpatient or outpatient hospital care and his/her care will describe an alternative loop in the Framework until resolution.

If the patient can use the same mobile user interface to access the service systems at home, in the workplace and in health care organizations, he/she will not need to carry different devices with him/her. Suitable devices are smart phones, PDA devices and mini-PCs. One interface system means a big advantage to the patient user. The same would be useful to health professionals as well, although not so remarkable as for patients. In many cases the professionals benefits more from a big screen interface when they work in or close to their office and a mobile device when they go into the field.

Integration can be built on electronic health record (EHR) systems. Mobility means wireless access to patients' health records when and where needed and automatic (sometimes manual but mobile) wireless collection of health information from patients. If all products and services (mobile or fixed) are built around the EHR system, the integration comes through the operating system of the EHR. Therefore, it would be ideal if all EHR systems were to use the same architecture and interface policies (such as HL7 – Health Level Seven). Standardization is a key factor in both national and international integration.

The Continua Health Alliance (CHA) is developing health standards, protocols and practices. Integration between health institutions and systems is a severe problem not only in diabetes but widely in global health systems. Healthcare IT systems have been developed mostly by companies who compete against each other to maintain their customers. Alliances like CHA help companies to cooperate rather than compete.

DISCUSSION AND CONCLUSION

Wireless technology is a cost-efficient way to respond to the challenges for public health care systems posed by inevitable structural changes.

Figure 6. A typical path of diabetes patients when they proceed in health care services from healthy citizens to outpatient loop (Alasaarela & Oliver, 2009)

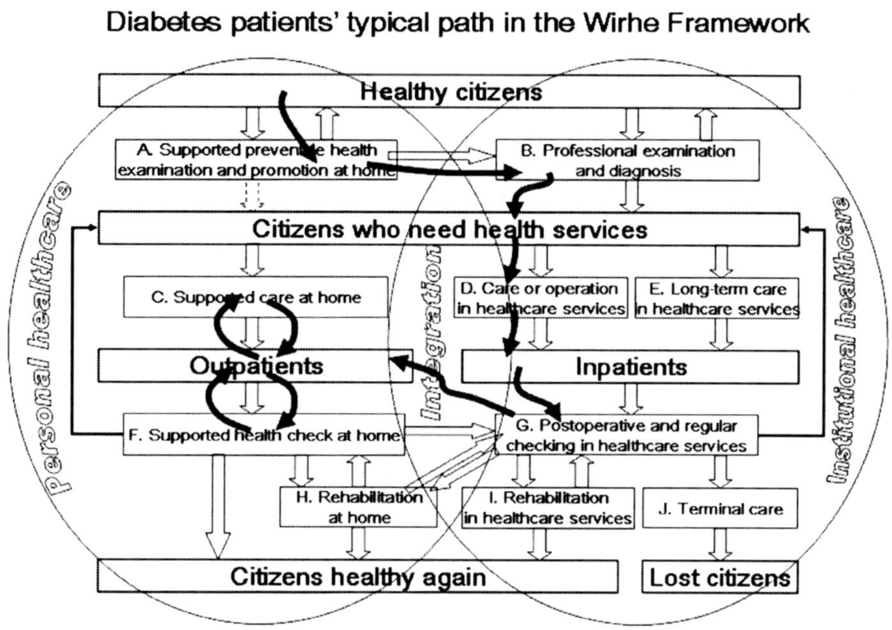

Due to demographic changes, the amount of patients will increase in upcoming years, while the relative amount of health care professionals is going to decrease. Despite these financial challenges, high quality treatment and organizational integrity must be maintained. An inevitable structural change is happening already.

The public health care systems are challenged to operate according to business requirements. The business baselines in developing health care systems are cost efficiency, patient-orientation, high quality at all operational levels and accessibility of services.

All these baselines can be improved by bringing real-time functions into health care systems accessed by wireless technologies. As human resources are decreased, a leading strategy is to develop technological solutions and preventive health care. Wireless technology is a relatively small, but strategically vitally important part of required IT solutions.

In the Wirhe Framework the viewpoints of health care professionals, citizens and government have been integrated to form a mutual fight against diseases and health problems. Now the wireless technologies and mobile solutions can be applied, in practice, according to the Wirhe framework. This allows a cost-efficient use of existing technologies; therefore, the focus can be shifted towards the development of unavailable products and services and unmet needs.

Wireless technologies can play a critical role in maintaining the independence of our elderly population, through support of safety monitoring (both within the home as well as tracking via GPS); assessment of gait (to predict the likelihood of falls); monitoring and transmission of vital signs and specific biological parameters (such as glucose levels); and the capability of triggering emergency alerts.

Alzheimer's patients would benefit from a wireless "safety net" that constantly tracks their location, assesses their level of cognitive awareness and capacity, and notifies family members and caregivers of behaviors or events.

Wireless support of food intake monitoring, tracking of dietary patterns, timely education and alerts, and even data support for meal services (using body chemistry and eating history to determine and order prepared meals) are all valuable applications to support those with obesity problems.

Even a small productivity increase in service processes will pay wireless technology investments back rapidly. For example, in diabetes alone, a USD 3 billion savings could be achieved if only 10% of patients adopt wireless treatment process, according to the Wirhe framework, resulting in a 20% resource savings. The very reasonable payback time for investments is only 2 years (Alasaarela & Oliver, 2009).

Real-time, wireless health care will benefit patients in numerous ways. Also the motivation and efficiency of health care professionals will improve markedly, as they can focus on care giving instead of bureaucracy. The main benefit will be faster, better and more efficient treatment processes, which will be of higher quality. Accordingly, waiting lists for treatment will shorten. In the future, wireless technology will improve productivity in health monitoring, outpatient activities and hospital activities.

In fact, wireless technology can be an important enabler of the structural change of public health care worldwide.

ACKNOWLEDGMENT

The authors would like to thank Riku Mäkelä, Tekes, Finland, for his great contribution in planning and practical implementation of the Wirhe project. In addition, they send their warmest thanks to the 105 experts, who gave their valuable contributions by participating in interviews and queries.

REFERENCES

Adams, J., Archbold, B., Mounib, E. L., & New, D. (2007). *Healthcare 2015 and U.S. health plans. New roles, new competencies. IBM Institute for Business Value*. IBM Corporation.

Adams, J., Mounib, E., Pai, A., Stuart, N., Thomas, R., & Tomaszewicz, P. (2006). [Win-win or lose-lose? *A portrait and a path to successful transformation*. IBM Institute for Business Value, IBM Corporation.]. *Health Care*, 2015.

Adler, R. (2007). *Health Care Unplugged: The Evolving Role of Wireless Technology*. Oakland, CA: California HealthCare Foundation.

Alasaarela, E. (2008). *Wirhe – Wireless Solutions in Healthcare. International strategy and roadmap towards 2014*. Helsinki: Tekes.

Alasaarela, E. (2009). Finnish Perspectives of Wireless in Healthcare. *International Journal of Electronic Healthcare*, *5*, 177–192. doi:10.1504/IJEH.2009.029224

Alasaarela, E., DeMello, S., & Nemana, R. (2009). Comparative National Perspectives on the Future of Wireless in Health Care: Finland and the United States. *Journal of Management and Marketing in Healthcare*, *2*(4), 1–18.

Alasaarela, E., Nemana, R., & DeMello, R. (2009, February), Drivers and challenges of wireless solutions in future healthcare. *International Conference on eHealth, Telemedicine, and Social Medicine, eTelemed'09*. Cancun, Mexico 1-7.2.2009. Available in IEEEXplore.

Alasaarela, E., Nemana, R., DeMello, S., Oliver, N. S., & Miyazaki, M. (2009, April-June). Wireless for Managing Healthcare – the Wirhe Framework. *International Journal of Healthcare Delivery Reform Initiatives*, *1*(2), 52–73.

Alasaarela, E., & Oliver, N. S. (2009). Wireless solutions for managing diabetes. *International Journal of Technology and Health Care*, *17*, 353–367.

Anderson, G. (2004). Chronic Conditions: Making the Case for Ongoing Care. *Partnership for Solutions*, Sept. 2004. Available at http://www.partnershipforsolutions.org/DMS/files/chronicbook2004.pdf, last accessed on 13 August 2010.

Barlow, I., Liu, L., & Sekulic, A. (2009). Wheelchair Seating Assessment and Intervention: A Comparison Between Telerehabilitation and Face-to-Face Service. International. *Journal of Telerehabilitation*, *1*(1).

Carroll, R., Cnossen, R., Schnell, M., & Simons, D. (2007). Continua: An Interoperable Personal Healthcare Ecosystem. *IEEE Pervasive Computing / IEEE Computer Society [and] IEEE Communications Society*, *6*(4). doi:10.1109/MPRV.2007.72

CHA. (2009). The Next Generation of Personal Telehealth is Here. Continua Overview Presentation. *Continua Health Alliance*. Available at http://www.continuaalliance.org/about-the-alliance.html, last accessed on 13 August 2010.

Herper, M. (2005). *The most expensive diseases*. Forbes. Available at http://www.forbes.com/2005/04/14/cx_mh_0414healthcosts.html, last accessed on 13 August 2010.

Intel Health. (2007). Reconceiving Disease Management: A Technology Perspective. *Whitepaper of Intel Health*. Available at http://www.intel.com/pressroom/kits/healthcare/DiseaseMgmt_whitepaper.pdf, last accessed on 13 August 2010.

Kalorama (2007). *Wireless Opportunities in Healthcare*. Rockville, MD:Kalorama Information.

MedApps. (2010). *m-Health's Enabling Role in Healthcare Reform*. Whitepaper of MedApps Inc. Available at http://www.medapps.net/RefDocs/MedAppsRole_HealthReform_041010.pdf, last accessed on 13 August, 2010.

Miyazaki, M., Rowe, M., Ohyanagi, T., Liu, L., Clark, C., Cook, A., & Duguay, R. (2008, April). Bidirectional wireless physiological monitoring of homecare clients. Presented in13th *Annual International Meeting of the American Telemedicine Association*.Seattle, Washington.

Rowe, M. (2008). *V-P Capital Health*. Alberta, Canada: Alberta Health Services.

Solovy, A. (2007). *Ten Lessons from the Top 100*. Healthcare's Most Wired, H&HN Hospitals and Health Networks.

Wireless Healthcare. (2007). *Wireless Based Disease Management*. *Wireless Healthcare*. Royston, UK: Steinkrug Publications.

ENDNOTES

1. Dr. Masako Miyazaki is the principal investigator of the "E-Health Edmonton Program-Development and Integration of Wireless Wearable Physiological Monitors" at the University of Alberta, Canada.
2. Participating persons: Steven DeMello and Ateret Haselkorn from Health Technology Center, Ravi Nemana from UC Berkeley, Riku Mäkelä, Kalevi Virta and Anne Turula from Tekes and Esko Alasaarela from the University of Oulu.

Chapter 10
Multi-Dimensional Criteria for the Evaluation of E-Health Services

Alalwany Hamid
Brunel University, UK

Alshawi Sarmad
Brunel University, UK

ABSTRACT

E-health is an emerging field in the intersection of information systems, healthcare and business, referring mainly to healthcare services delivered and enhanced through the use of information and communication technologies (ICT). An important area of research is the evaluation of e-health services. A holistic e-health evaluation framework should address the aspects that are hampering healthcare services from embracing the full potential of ICT towards successful e-health initiatives. In order to build a holistic evaluation framework for e-health services, this article suggests framework characteristics for the appropriate evaluation for e-health services. The article argues that e-health services evaluation framework should be criteria based. The criteria have to be multi-dimensional that grounded in, or derived from, one or more specific perspectives or theories. The proposed evaluation criteria in this article can serve as part of an e-health evaluation framework, improve our understanding of the role of information systems in health care, and develop our ability to deliver high quality services.

BACKGROUND

E-health is a very broad term encompassing various activities in an evolving field. This is reflected in the broad and various definitions of the term.

DOI: 10.4018/978-1-60960-183-6.ch010

An example of these definitions is the one that has been adopted by the World Health Organization. According to the Organisation, E-health can be defined as 'being the leveraging of the information and communication technology (ICT) to connect provider and patients and governments; to educate and inform healthcare professionals, managers and consumers; to stimulate innovation in care delivery and health system management; and, to improve our healthcare system' (Hans Oh et al., 2005).

The variety of e-health applications is considerable, ranging from a self-help guide about treating common health problems at home to a virtual clinic which allows diagnostic consultations between patients and practitioners at separate sites. In light of the dynamic and evolving meaning of e-health concept and the wide range of applications that the term e-health has covered, the questions are what the term e-health means and what is the e-health application that should be considered. In this paper although we employ e-health as a broad term, the scope will be limited to the service delivery aspect by electronic means of information, advice, and consultation.

E-health, which are basically enabled and driven by the use of information and communication technologies in healthcare, have the potential to change the healthcare industry worldwide in terms of their infrastructures, and the costs and quality of services (Wickramasinghe & Misra, 2004; Wickramasinghe & Goldberg, 2004). Despite the potential that e-health may bring to the healthcare sector, the sector is the slowest in moving to the form of e-health among other government services. Skinner (2003) argues that the slow progress is related to the fact that healthcare does not have the standards in place that other sectors do. Holliday and Tam (2004) have a broader explanation; they see that slow progress is more related to institutional, cultural and financial factors.

An important area of research is that of the evaluation of e-health services. It could contribute to important knowledge that can be used to support the value of existing e-health projects, and to increase the quality and efficiency of future e-health initiatives. Despite its importance, the evaluation of e-health services as many researchers agree, is both an under developed and under managed area in theory and practice (Brender, 2006; Friedman & Wyatt, 2000).

This study forms a part of a research that aims to develop, and assess a holistic evaluation framework for e-health services. Towards this aim, the objectives of this paper are; addressing the challenges in developing such a framework, suggesting framework characteristics for the appropriate evaluation for e-health services, and proposing a multi dimensional criteria for e-health evaluation. The proposed multi-dimensional criteria can serve as part of e-health evaluation framework, and also to provide useful and necessary tools to allow the development of successful e-health initiatives by assisting the healthcare organisation to identify and thus address areas that require further attention. The selection process of the proposed criteria will take into account the challenges faced at the intersection of the three areas, healthcare services, information systems, and evaluation methodologies.

THE RESEARCH APPROACH

According to Lowery & Evans (2004) and Myers & Avison (2002) that selecting an appropriate research approach is about setting a research strategy considering the underlying characteristics or assumptions about what constitutes valid research. Such strategy should guide the researcher through the research process by embodying a particular style and employing different research methods.

The process of selecting and deploying appropriate research approach for this study, is an important and critical issue, and should only be decided on after considering a number of factors including;

- The research question and its context (how to identify the key factors for the evaluation of e-health services?)
- The multi-dimensional aspects of e-health, as it has different roots and complex relationships associated with using information communications technologies, man-

agement as well as health regulations, and governments policies.
- The large number of stakeholders involve in e-health evaluation, each with their own particular needs, values and objectives.

As this study forms a part of a research project which will progress through a number of phases, the research will be based on a sequential multi-method approach (Creswell, 2003). Adopting the sequential multi-method approach paves the way to the use of the appropriate method for each research phase and creates the opportunity for multiple analyses about the same collected data.

This study represents one phase of the research project, and will be based partially on two lines of studies relating to the behaviour of users of new products or services. These studies are: diffusion of innovations (Rogers, 1995) and technology acceptance (Davis, 1989). The aim of using both studies is to build theoretical framework that aids in the selection process of the multi dimensional criteria. Broad examining and critical analysis of the existing evaluations initiatives specifically those who were based on e-health services case studies was also used to overcome the limitation of the theoretical framework.

In the next phase of the research project the authors will carry out an empirical validation and examination of the proposed evaluation criteria, the validation will be performed through case study methodology (Yin, 2003). This process is very important; it will address potential improvements, and verify the adaptability of the proposed criteria to various e-health contexts.

E-HEALTH EVALUATION CHALLENGES

The research in the area of e-health evaluation is a complicated and difficult subject (Brender, 2006; Friedman & Wyatt, 2000). The complexity and difficulty lies in the challenges encountered at the intersection of three research fields, each well-known for its complexity; healthcare services, information systems, and evaluation methodologies.

Healthcare services are characterized by having many stakeholders which are working in different disciplines and pursuing different goals (Alvarez, 2003; Connell & Young, 2007; Ray, 2007). Healthcare services are also dictated by complex regulations, especially those that apply to directly manage patients' information. The medical knowledge itself and methods of healthcare delivery are changing rapidly and require a high degree of formalized working practices (Friedman & Wyatt, 2000). The regulations of healthcare services particularly in developed countries is complex in its diversity and wide ranging in its scope, ruling the relation with patients, health professionals, the public, taxpayers, employers, educators, regulators, and many others across the country. The medical knowledge is an enormous and dynamic field, Mcconaghy (2006) states that the medical knowledge doubles approximately every five years. Moreover the main aspects of this knowledge require an interactive environment to be transferred or practiced.

Information systems and its evaluation as many researcher (Serafeimidis & Smithson, 2000; Jones & Hughes, 2001) assent is another complicated and difficult research field. Symons and Walsham (1988) argue that the complexity is due to the multiple perspectives involved, and the difficulties of quantifying benefits. Willcocks (1992) has a similar view but he also believes that the complexity of information systems evaluation is changing and becoming more and more complex nowadays. This is because the nature of information systems investments is changing both in terms of technological capability and the benefits they can deliver, as well as in terms of diffusion in most aspects of society. The evaluation of information systems in public sector has proved to be even more complex as an accurate evaluation requires conducting the evaluation process in more challenging context. To overcome the complexity and difficulty of information systems evaluation in public sector, it is necessary to address and consider a number of evaluation challenges in the development of the required evaluation framework. The first of these challenges is the investigation of various perspectives (Jansen, 2005), which may not only require addressing and meeting the general needs of a target group such as citizens, but also requires including the specific needs of the specific target groups of citizens that are using a particular service. The second challenge in evaluating information systems in public sector is in identifying and quantifying benefits. Beynon-Davies, (2005) states that it is difficult to determine the precise benefits associated with information systems in public sector. An explanation to this lies in the different goals and objective of the information systems investments in public sectors, the benefits gained by these initiatives will be different as well, and the assessment of these benefits also vary according to the different perspectives of the stakeholders for the value of these benefits. The third challenge in evaluating information systems in public sector is the fact that in order for the evaluation to be proper, it should consider the social and technical context of use. This is a result of the opinion that information systems research is as much a social science as an information systems science (Mingers & Stowell, 1997).

The establishment of an evaluation methodology is the last complex and difficult research field. The field is suffering from the limited experience of using methods, the unfamiliarity with evaluation techniques and the difficulty in interpreting results (Ballantine et al., 1999; Farbey et al., 1999; Powell, 1999). The limited experience of using methods in e-health evaluation is related to a certain extent to the gap between the theory and practice. Eng (2002) argues that this gap is a result of the tension between e-health research efforts in academic institutions and commercial organizations. He believes that the academic sector succeeds in developing scientifically rigorous evaluation methodologies, but these methodologies are not designed to answer real-world concerns. On the other hand, when commercial organizations conduct evaluations of e-health applications, they usually adopt methodologies with limited applicability to other situations. In adopting such methodologies, they maintain obtaining quick and practical answers because of market pressures.

Table 1 summarizes the challenges encountered at the intersection of healthcare services, information systems, and evaluation methodologies.

DEVELOPING AN EVALUATION FRAMEWORK FOR E-HEALTH SERVICES

The evaluation in the area of e-health services as many researchers argue, is dominated by economic and organizational aspects, has no standard framework for evaluating the effects and outputs of implementation and use, and the area in general is both under developed and under managed in theory and practice (Brender, 2006; Eng, 2001; Friedman & Wyatt 2000; Rahimi & Vimarlund, 2007). Nevertheless, there is a wide range of information system evaluation frameworks, some of them were proposed and used in a healthcare context.

Existing evaluation frameworks that have been proposed or used in e-health context are suffering from many limitations. These limitations include, that they are either designed to focus particularly on the supply side of the healthcare services (organizational perspective) or they are designed to target a specific user or a specific application of an e-health initiative. Moreover, the healthcare dimension is either ignored or not fully considered in the design and the implementation of these evaluation frameworks.

Though the development of a comprehensive evaluation framework for e-health services is be-

Table 1. The challenges encountered at the intersection of healthcare services, information systems, and evaluation methodologies

The Research Field	The challenges Encountered	References
Healthcare Services	Healthcare services are characterized by having many stakeholders which are working in different disciplines and pursuing different goals. Healthcare services are dictated by complex regulations. The medical knowledge is an enormous and dynamic field. The main aspects of medical knowledge require an interactive environment to be transferred or practiced.	Alvarez (2003) Connell and Young (2007) Ray (2007) Friedman and Wyatt (2000) Mcconaghy (2006)
Information Systems	The multiple perspectives involved. The difficulties of quantifying benefits. The nature of information systems investments is changing both in terms of technological capability and the benefits they can deliver, as well as in terms of diffusion in most aspects of society. Consider the social and technical context of use.	Walsham (1993) Beynon-Davies (2005) Jansen (2005) Willcocks (1992) Mingers, and Stowell (1997)
Evaluation Methodologies	The limited experience of using methods. The unfamiliarity with evaluation techniques. The difficulty in interpreting results.	Ballantine et al. (1999) Eng (2002) Farbey et al. (1999) Powell (1999)

yond the remit of this study, it is vital to examine the current evaluation frameworks in order to choose the appropriate evaluation approach and select the suitable framework that can accommodate the proposed criteria. We have selected for our analysis a number of evaluation approaches that we believe are more suitable for the evaluation in the healthcare context.

One of these approaches is focused mainly on the evaluation criteria, which can be called criteria-based evaluation approach. What is typical for this approach is that the information systems interface and the interaction between users and the systems work as a basis for the evaluation together with a set of predefined criteria. The chosen criteria rule the evaluation process and its results (Cronholm & Goldkuhl, 2003). In the same direction and based on what drives the evaluation, Cronholm and Goldkuhl (2003) identified another two approaches named goal-based and goal-free evaluations. The goal-based evaluations use goals from the organisational context to assess the information system. Goal-free evaluation is based on gathering data about a broad range of actual effects of the system and evaluating the importance of these effects in meeting demonstrated needs (Patton, 1990). Among the three previous approaches, the criteria based one is the most appropriate for e-health services evaluations. The appropriateness stems from the fact that e-health applications are principally complex in nature, hence they require an approach that can be derived from a multitude of perspectives and theories such as TAM or DOI.

Another group of evaluation approaches were introduced to address one or more of the perspectives of the system stakeholders. Freeman (1984) was among the first, who introduced the stakeholders' concept. Since then, several researchers have adopted the stakeholders approach in their research of information systems evaluation. However, there is only limited literature that recognizes healthcare stakeholders and their changing role in the evaluation of e-health services.

Moreover, even in the limited literature available on healthcare stakeholders, the description and identification of these stakeholders seems to be generally ignored (Mantzana & Themistocleous, 2006).

One of the popular and general approaches in categorizing e-health stakeholders is dividing them between supply side stakeholders (organizational perspective) and demand side stakeholders (users' perspective). According to Löfstedt (2007) most research in the area of e-government, and also in the development of e-services in public sector is dominated by supply side factors and there where none or a few efforts that focused on the demand side. Gustafson and Wyatt, 2004, acknowledged the dominant of supply side factors in the field of e-health as well. They stated that despite the fact that users are the most important stakeholder in the e-health evaluation, assessing e-health from users' perspective and addressing the key factors that influence the users' acceptance to the new adopted technologies is still lacking behind.

For practical reasons this study will focus on the demand side stakeholders. We believe that the acceptance and satisfaction of e-health services are dependent primarily on users' motivation to adopt and utilize these services, user utilization being important for the success of e-health services.

The stakeholder's evaluation approach is part of the school which suggested five levels of evaluation approaches for healthcare information systems, which are macro, sector, firm, application, and stakeholder. This suggests that different criteria would inevitably apply to each of these approaches (Connell & Young, 2007).

There is also another group of evaluation studies which is defined by the basis on which the evaluation is performed. In this direction Grover et al. (1996) categorize three approaches: Comparative, normative and improvement. In the comparative approach, the evaluation is based on comparing a particular system with other similar systems. The normative approach compares the system against a theoretical ideal system or, in essence, against best practice. The improvement approach is intended to assess how much the system has improved over time. In this study we intend to use only the comparative and normative approaches because the main aim is toward proposing evaluation criteria for proposed implementations rather than historical ones.

Furthermore, another group of evaluation studies classified evaluations based on when the assessment is performed (Brender, 2006; Cronholm & Goldkuhl, 2003; Grover et al., 1996). According to these studies the evaluation can be carried out during the analysis and planning phase, or during the development and the adaptation phases, or after the development has completed and the system is in use. An example of this kind of evaluation is process evaluation approach which is intended to evaluate the efficient use of resources, and is normally performed during the analysis and planning phase. There is also the response evaluation approach which assesses the users reaction to the system, and is usually performed during the final stage of implementation, or while the system is in use. The equity implementation model presented by Lauer et al. (2000) is an example of the response evaluation approach. The model was based on the equity theory (Adams, 1965), a well-established theory in the social sciences and was adopted in e-health assessments to examine and understand user reaction to the implementation of a system. Lauer et al. (2000) stated that the focus of this approach is on the effect of the changes that such a system brings about on the system users.

The last example in this group is the impact evaluation approach, which is intended to assess the overall social and technical impact of the system on users and organisations, and is normally performed while the system is in use. According to Grover et al. (1996), because the impact evaluation is the most comprehensive, it is the most difficult approach to undertake. The impact evaluation approach can be quite beneficial in evaluating e-health services because it would comprehensively recognize users and organisations needs, by measuring the acceptability as well as the risks and benefits of e-health services (Gustafson & Wyatt, 2004). In this study, the focus will be on the criteria that influence the user's reaction to the e-health services and the social, economical and technical effects of these services.

To conclude, we suggest that the appropriate evaluation framework for e-health services which can accommodate the proposed evaluation criteria would have the following characteristics:

- The framework has to be sufficiently generic to be applicable to a wide range of applications but also sufficiently detailed to provide effective guidance.
- The framework has to support the evaluator in making precise and effective choices at various stages of the evaluation process.
- The framework is criteria-based. The criteria can be grounded in, and derived from, one or more specific perspectives or theories.
- The framework only considers one stakeholder or a group of stallholders with a common perspective in an evaluation process. For example, as in the case of this study, the framework may consider the demand side perspective and specifically the criteria that influence the user's reaction to e-health services, and the impact of these services on the users.
- The framework combines both comparative and normative approaches toward proposing evaluation criteria for e-health services.

USERS' BEHAVIOUR TOWARDS NEW PRODUCTS OR SERVICES

There are many studies on the behaviour of consumers of new products and services, these studies were adopted in research to predict user's acceptance of innovations including e-health services. Towards aiding the selection process of the multi-dimensional evaluation criteria, this study will make use of two lines of these studies

The first one is Diffusion of Innovations Theory (DOI). DOI is one of the popular theories which were introduced by Rogers (1995) to explain how a new idea or innovation propagates in a social system. The theory is based on 50 years of research, and was adopted by many researchers in different research fields including the e-government research. For example, the theory was used by Carter and Belanger (2004) to assess the citizen adoption of e-government initiatives. Since being introduced, the diffusion of innovations theory was adopted in different ways in many studies including the use of the important part of the theory and the well-known S-shaped curve of adoption and the categorization of adopters.

In applying diffusion theory to e-health services evaluation, the most relevant points to recognize are the innovation perceived attributes identified by Rogers' study and their applicability to e-health services: Rogers (1995) describes the characteristics of an innovation in terms of its perceived attributes, and these attributes are responsible in controlling the rates of diffusion of the innovation. Rogers (1995) identified three primary perceived attributes, which are relative advantage, compatibility, and complexity. He added two other innovation attributes, which are trialability and observability.

From the five factors of DOI theory, we will only include in this study the primary ones, which are relative advantage, compatibility, and complexity. We believe that the other two, trialability and observability, are not pertinent for e-health services. Rogers (1995) considers trialability and observability as less important than the other three. Tornatzky and Klein (1982) have the same view, and they conclude that relative advantage, compatibility, and complexity are the most relevant factors to adoption research.

The second line of studies relating to the behaviour of users to new products or services is Technology Acceptance Model (TAM) (Davis, 1989). TAM is widely used to study user acceptance of technology. It was designed to examine the mediating role of perceived ease of use and perceived usefulness in their relation between systems characteristics as external variables and the probability of system use as an indicator of system success. However, as noted by several researchers (Hufnagel & Conca, 1994; Melone, 1990; Paul et al., 2003), TAM suffers from the absence of significant factors, including considering both human and social change processes and their affects on the adoption and utilization of new information systems. Paul et al. (2003) added that although technology acceptance model is useful, using TAM specifically in empirical research may give inconsistent results.

The technological acceptance model was used in the evaluation of e-services in the public sector by many research studies (Al-adawi et al., 2005;Carter & Belanger, 2004). The model was also applied to healthcare by Lapointe et al. (2002). In applying technology acceptance model to e-health services evaluation in this study, we will consider the mediating role of both perceived ease of use and perceived usefulness.

PROPOSED MULTI-DIMENSIONAL CRITERIA

E-government services evaluation and e-health services evaluation in particular are unable to reveal the full value of e-government projects without considering the perspectives of all the e-government services stakeholders and the e-government value measures presented by evaluation criteria consisted of all the key issues perceived by each of the stakeholders.

As mentioned earlier healthcare services are known to be a complex domain. This is related to the fact that healthcare is a safety critical area, dictated by a complex regulations. These regulations should be carefully considered in the selection process of the evaluation criteria, and in the description of the criteria used for a specific e-health service.

Hence, the proposed criteria are derived from two sources. The first source is two lines of studies relating to the behaviour of users of new products or services. The second source is a broad examination of the existing evaluations initiatives specifically those who were based on e-health services case studies. The first source represented by DOI and TAM which are popular and widely used theories, but still have their own merits and limitations. One of the main limitations of both theories is that they are not conclusive models and they suffer from the absence of significant factors. To adapt both theories for e-health context and overcome their limitations, critical analysis of e-health services case studies were used.

Considering the technical dimension, the economic dimension, and the social dimension in selecting and grouping the proposed evaluation criteria for this study, the criteria will be grouped in three sets of criteria, which are usability, direct costs and benefits, and trust. This classification should serve the deployment of the evaluation framework.

The Usability Criteria

The first set of evaluation criteria is the usability criteria. Usability in the proposed criteria may represent perceived ease of use and perceived usefulness as depicted by Davis (1989) technology acceptance model (TAM), or complexity as defined by Rogers (1995) diffusion of innovation.

Davis (1989) defines perceived usefulness as "the degree to which a person believes that using a particular system would enhance his or her job performance". He also defines perceived ease of use as "the degree to which a person believes that using a particular system would be free of effort". Rogers (1995) defines complexity as the "degree to which an innovation is perceived as difficult to understand and use"

We believe that perceived ease of use is predicted to influence perceived usefulness, since the easier a system is to use, the more useful it can be. We also believe that complexity and perceived ease of use are measures for the same issue. Therefore we are considering the three issues belonging to the same set and they will be represented by the usability criteria.

Usability has different interpretations and meanings depending on the context of use. Bevan and Macleod (1993) define usability as the quality of interaction within a particular context. Another description of usability which considers user's perspective is proposed by Nielson (1993), according to him, usability relates to how well users can use the functionality of a system or service in terms of what it can do. Researchers have provided broad dimensions and introduced long lists of aspects by which the usability can be assessed. These include accessibility (Steinfeld & Danford, 1999), functionality (Melander-Wikman et al., 2005; Nielson, 1993; Steinfeld & Danford, 1999), compatibility (Bevan et al., 2007; Chau & Hu 2001), user' satisfaction, easy to learn and use (Melander-Wikman et al., 2005; Nielson, 1993), and user interface (Melander-Wikman et al., 2005).

Accessibility is an important subset of usability. According to Terry, Ma, and Zaphiris (2003), accessibility means an effective and efficient user interface which is inclusive of more people in more situations and can achieve user satisfaction. Those people are different in their accessibily requirments and needs. A high percentage of them particularly those who suffer from disabilities or cronic illness are more likely in need than others for accessible and effective e-health services. Mont (2007) reported that an estimated 20 percent of American and Australian populations and 12.2 percent of British population have disabilities. Another research by Lenhart et al. (2003), shows a high percentage of about 38 percent of Americans with disabilities are using the Internet. The same research also shows that users with disabilities are more likely than the general population to use e-health services and have access to these services only from home.

Accessibility requirements for e-health services should generally accommodate all people, but particularly remove or reduce all the barriers that can hamper disabled people from fully benefiting from e-health services. One of the efforts for determining accessibility is the guidelines developed by the "Web Accessibility Initiative", a working group of the World Wide Web Consortium (Caldwell et al., 2007)

Despite the importance of accessibly in the evaluation of e-services in public sector and e-health services in particular, studies show that governments either ignored or did not pay enough attention to the accessibility importance. According to the Global e-government Survey conducted by World Market Research Centre and Brown University (2001), only 2% of government websites worldwide have some form of disability access and only 7% of the e-government websites were accessible. Another study by West (2000) show that only 15 percent of American government websites offer some form of disability access, such as TTY (Text Telephone) or TDD (Telephone Device for the Deaf) or are approved by disability organizations. The study also revealed that only 4 percent of American government websites offer foreign language translation features on their websites. Another example for ignoring accessibly in healthcare services is a cross-sectional study by Zeng and Parmento (2004). The study was aiming to evaluate the accessibility of consumer health information of 108 Web sites, and reported that no Web site met all the accessibly criteria in their assessing framework.

Compatibility is another important criterion to be included in the usability criteria. According to Rogers (1995), compatibility is measured by the degree to which an innovation is perceived as being consistent with the existing values, past experiences, and needs of potential users. Chau and Hu (2001) argued that compatibility is positively affecting user's attitude toward accepting new technologies in healthcare environments. They based their argument on the assumption that users would be more likely to consider technology useful if they perceived it to be compatible with their existing practices. In addition, users would consider technology easy to use if they did not need to change their practices significantly in an environment that can not cope with radical change.

Functionality is a broad criterion of the usability criteria which supposes to cover the user's requirements from a system to perform specific tasks in a specific situation; this includes accuracy, validity, robustly, speed and availability (Melander-Wikman et al., 2005).

User satisfaction is generally regarded as one of the most important measures of system or service success and should be included in the proposed usability criteria. The user satisfaction criterion can be measured by various dimensions including utility, reliability, efficiency, customization and flexibility (Horan et al., 2006).

Table 2 summarizes the proposed usability criteria, list of measuring aspects by which the criteria can be assessed and suggestions for measuring descriptions. The aim of proposing the measuring descriptions is to provide general guide for assessing these aspects. The applicability of the descriptions for specific context is out of the scope of this study.

The Direct Costs and Benefits Criteria

The second set contains the direct costs and benefits criteria. The criteria in this set are primarily based on Rogers's relative advantage. According to Rogers (1995), relative advantage is "the degree to which an innovation is seen as being superior to its predecessor". It is essentially a cost–benefit analysis of how useful a given innovation when compared with what is already available. Relative advantage represents mostly the economic return involved in the adoption of an innovation, but could also include the immediacy of reward, social prestige, or savings in time and effort (Rogers, 1995). The direct costs and benefits criteria have traditionally dominated the traditional information system evaluation process, and they were criticized by many authors (Farbey et al., 1995; Serafeimidis & Smithson, 2000) for their limited relevance to the role of information systems. This limitation is in their definition of stakeholders, targeting only direct tangible costs and benefits and being only based on accounting and financial instruments. On the other hand, many authors (Eng, 2002; Glasgow, 2007; Gustafson & Wyatt, 2004; Smaglik et al., 1998) argue that direct costs and benefits are important and should be considered in evaluating e-health services. Despite the above mentioned opinions regarding the limitations of using the economic issues in the evaluation; we tend to support the opinion of including them as part of the evaluation criteria because healthcare services have a high economic impact on governments and users comparing to any other services (Bower, 2005; Friedman & Wyatt, 2000; Gustafson et al., 2001).

One of the efforts in assessing the direct financial cost and benefits of e-health is the e-health impact project which was commissioned by the European Commission (DG Information Society and Media) (Stroetmann et al., 2006). The main aim of the project was to evaluate the economic and productivity impact of e-health services. The research project developed a generic economic assessment and evaluation framework for e-health applications, and was mainly focused on citizens' perspective in assessing ten e-health application cases. The ten cases were selected from across the European Union for their proven, sustainable e-health application. The result of the assessment, which was carried over a period of 15 years, indicates a positive, sustainable economic impact of these e-health services.

Table 3 summarizes the proposed direct costs and benefits criteria and suggestions for measuring descriptions for e-health services evaluation. Adopting the proposed evaluation criteria and their descriptions for a specific e-health service should take into account the relevancy of each of the evaluation criterion to the prevailing situation. This mainly depends on the maturity of the e-health initiative, and could lead to partial use of the evaluation criteria.

Table 2. The usability criteria and suggestions for measuring descriptions

Evaluation Criteria	Measuring Aspects	Suggestions for Measuring Descriptions
Easy to learn and use	Easy to learn	Measured by the time needed to learn to work with a service.
	Easy to use	Assessed by the simplicity of the service and how easy it is to understand and comprehend its functions
Accessibility	Content Accessibility	Measured by the degree of compliance with the Web Content Accessibility Guidelines
	User interface	Judged by the available options of user interfaces (e.g. Graphical interface, Multi-screen interface, Attentive User Interface).
	Disability access & translation	Is the system offering some form of disability access and foreign language translation features?
Compatibility	Compatibility	Assessed by how quickly and easily the e-service can fit into the whole health-care system.
Functionality	Accuracy	Measured by the degree to which information provided by the service is free of errors.
	Validity	Measured by the clarity and regularity of information updating.
	Robustly	Judged by the technical functionality of the service.
	Speed	Judged by the system response time; web page load time; download time.
	Availability	Assessed by the availability of the service 24hrs/7days per week and the existing of alternative choices.
User satisfaction	Utility	Assessed by the completeness and usefulness of the service content (Loiacono et al., 2002)
	Reliability	Judged by the appropriately of the service functions in terms of the technology as well as the accuracy of the content (Zeithaml et al. 2000).
	Efficiency	Judged by the time spent to complete the information task, quality of the information found, appropriateness of information found, and satisfaction with the outcome (Wang et al., 2005).
	Customization	Measured by the degree of service tailrarity to meet the needs of individual user (Burgess, 2004).
	Flexibility	Assessed by whether a system or a service provides choice of ways to state a need and delivers dynamic information (Zeithaml et al. 2000).

The Trust Criteria

The third set of the proposed evaluation criteria is the trust criteria. Trust has been acknowledged as a crucial property of information systems that provide e-services in a variety of contexts, because failing to address the trust aspects correctly may have a profound impact on the e-services (Fruhling & Lee, 2004; Presti et al., 2006). The aspects of trust must be tackled properly during the development and use of e-services. Trust can be defined as "the willingness of a party to be vulnerable to the actions of another party based on the expectation that the other will perform a particular action important to the trustor, irrespective of the ability to monitor or control that other party" (Mayer et al., 1995). Trust in e-health services is associated with data security and privacy of personal health data (Rodrigues, 2003). Given the sensitive nature of healthcare information, trust requires maintaining security in handling of patients' information, protecting their privacy, and assuring them that their personal information will be treated confidentially. Without this assurance, it will be difficult to promote the use of e-health services.

Table 3. The direct costs and benefits criteria and suggestions for measuring descriptions

Evaluation Criteria	Measuring Aspects	Suggestions for Measuring Descriptions
Costs	Money Saving	How much money the citizens are saving by using the e-health service.
	Time Saving	How much time the citizens are saving by using the e-health service.
Benefits	Effort Saving	Measured by the degree of convenience in using a particular e-health service.
	Quality	Assessed by the added value to the Citizens information and knowledge about their conditions, diagnoses, treatment options and healthcare facilities, as well as the appropriate timing of the service
	Access	Judged by access level comparing to the same quality of services through alternative channel.

Enhancing trust involves enhancing security measures. This requires a large variety of measures and principles. Slaymaker et al. (2004) identified several aspects for security to be considered in any e-health project. These aspects include: user authentication, encrypted data movement, data integrity, security breach detection, physical security, audit trails, client and server authentication, and availability.

Trust in e-health services is also associated with the privacy of personal health data. According to Davis et al. (1999) "Privacy is the state of being free from intrusion, and in the context of health care, it concerns the responsibility of a care provider to protect a patient from any disclosure (i.e., discovery by others), even unintentional, of personal health data by providing security to the patient and the patient's records".

Moor (1997), stated that the main consideration in developing policies for protecting privacy is to make sure that the right people, and only the right people, have access to relevant information at the right time. Moor (1997) also proposed a controlled and restricted access technique for managing privacy. The technique is based on setting up zones of privacy and provides the opportunity for different people to be authorized for different levels of access to different kind of information at different times.

In practice, studies show that governments and health organizations have different levels of consideration for trust, security and privacy in their initiatives. An example is the study of Jarvinen (2005) which concludes that governments and health organizations have low levels of consideration for privacy. The study which covers 39 American health organizations reveals numerous examples of practices that make the customer vulnerable can be found in the analysed healthcare privacy policies. These practices include the absence of an adequate privacy notice, not give the users reasonable control over their information and the use of technical and confusing language in the privacy policies that make it difficult for the user to fully understand them. Another study by West (2000) also confirms similar finding. The study shows that there is very low consideration to the security and privacy in the American e-government websites. The study reveals that only 7 percent of American government websites have a privacy policy, and another 5 percent show some form of security policy. On the other hand, there are positive examples for the consideration of security and privacy such as the privacy provisions in Canada or quality seals for e-government services which was introduced in Austria (Aichholzer, 2003).

Table 4 summarizes the proposed trust criteria and suggestions for measuring the aspects of the criteria. Although the table provides clear and useful set of criteria, the criteria are general and it may be necessary to modify them to suite

Table 4. The trust criteria and suggestions for measuring descriptions

Evaluation Criteria	Measuring Aspects	Suggestions for Measuring Descriptions
Security	User authentication	Measured by how strong the user authentication is and if its key capabilities are sufficient for e-Health services
	Encrypted data movement	Assessed by the suitability of the technology used to protect the transfer of data.
	Data integrity	Determined by if the information is complete, whole, valid and digitally signed when required
	Security breach detection	Judged by the ability of the system to monitor and look for suspicious activity on the network.
	Physical security	Assessed by how secure is the area that holding the database equipments and if it is located in an area with limited and controlled access.
	Audit trails	Judged by the ability of the system to record the modification of data, to keep the most up to date version of data and to retrieve old versions of data.
Privacy	Responsibility	Measured by the degree of protection supplied by the healthcare organization for patient information from any disclosure.
	Access Control	Assessed by the degree of control on different level of access to different kind of information at different time.
	Confidentiality	Measured by the degree of compliance with the UK Data Protection Act (1998)

specific e-health initiative. The aim of proposing the measuring descriptions is to provide general guide for assessing the criteria aspects. The applicability of the description for specific context is out of the scope of this study.

CONCLUSION

This paper argues that the first requisite towards developing a holistic evaluation framework for e-health services is to deal effectively with the complexities, and overcoming the barriers through a multi stage strategy. The e-health services evaluation complexities are correlated mainly to the multi-disciplinary nature of the field and the challenges at the intersection of three areas, each well-known for its complexity, healthcare services, information systems, and evaluation methodologies. The paper starts with a summarization for these challenges.

Working towards building a holistic evaluation framework through a multi stage strategy, the paper suggests framework characteristics for the appropriate evaluation for e-health services. The paper argues that e-health services evaluation framework should be criteria based, while the criteria have to be multi-dimensional that grounded in, and derived from, one or more specific perspectives or theories, and cannot be entirely framed within the bounds of a single theory or perspective. Understanding the multi-disciplinary nature of e-health services evaluation and the challenges that it faces is the first requisite towards dealing effectively with the complexities, and overcoming the barriers of e-health services evaluation.

The paper provides a set of clear and useful e-health evaluation criteria that can be used as part of e-health evaluation framework, and to address areas that require further attention in the development of future e-health initiatives.

The proposed criteria were mainly derived from two sources. The first source was two lines of studies relating to the behaviour of users of new products or services. The second source was a broad examining of the existing evaluations initiatives, specifically those who were based on e-health services case studies. Hence, general evaluation criteria were proposed that cover the technical, economic and social dimensions. The proposed evaluation criteria can also be adapted to a specific e-health service by analysing the criteria that apply in that situation.

The limitation of this paper lies in the absence of empirical validation and examination of the proposed evaluation criteria that has not yet been applied in the fieldwork. Hence, the proposed factors require an empirical validation which will be performed by the authors in the next stage of this research using multiple case study strategy and will form the basis for further research.

ACKNOWLEDGMENT

A previous version of this work appeared in the *Handbook of Research on Advances in Health Informatics and Electronic Healthcare Applications: Global Adoption and Impact of Information Communication Technologies;* edited by: Dr. Khalil Khoumabti, Dr. Yogesh Dwivedi, Dr. Aradhana Srivastava and Dr. Banita Lal

REFERENCES

Adams, J. S. (1965). Inequity in social exchange. In Berkowitz, L. (Ed.), *Advances in experimental social psychology*. New York: Academic Press.

Aichholzer, G. (2003). Scenarios of e-Government in 2010 and implications for strategy design. *Electronic Journal of E-government*. Available at http://www.ejeg.com

Al-adawi, Z., Yousafzai, S., & Pallister, J. (2005). Conceptual Model of Citizen Adoption of E-government. *The Second International Conference on Innovations in Information Technology (IIT'05).*

Alvarez, R.C. (2003). The promise of e-health: a Canadian perspective. *e-Health International, 1*(1), 4.

Ballantine, J. A., Galliers, R. D., & Stray, S. J. (1999). Information Systems Technology Evaluation Practices: Evidence from UK Organizations. In Willcocks, L. P., & Lester, S. (Eds.), *Beyond the IT Productivity Paradox* (pp. 123–149). Chichester, England: John Wiley & Sons.

Bevan, N., & Macleod, M. (1993). Usability assessment and measurement. In Kelly, M. (Ed.), *The management and measurement of software quality*. Ashgate Technical/Gower Press.

Bevan, N., Petrie, H., & Claridge, N. (2007). Strategies for Providing Guidance on Usability and Accessibility. In *Proceedings HCI International 2007*. Springer.

Beynon-Davies, P. (2005). Constructing Electronic Government: the case of the UK Inland Revenue. *International Journal of Information Management, 25*(1), 3–20. doi:10.1016/j.ijinfomgt.2004.08.002

Bower, A. (2005). *The diffusion and value of healthcare information technology.* Published by the RAND Corporation, Library of Congress Cataloging-in-Publication Data

Brender, J. (2006). *Handbook of Evaluation Methods for Health Informatics*. Elsevier Academic Press Publications.

Burgess, L. (2004, October 13-15). A Conceptual Framework for Understanding and Measuring Perceived Service Quality in Net-based Customer Support Systems. *CollECTeR LatAm Conference*, Santiago, Chile.

Caldwell, B., Cooper, M., Reid, L., & Vanderheiden, G. (2007, December). *Web Content Accessibility Guidelines 2.0.*

Carter, L., & Belanger, F. (2004). Citizen Adoption of Electronic Government Initiatives. In *Proceedings of 37th Annual Hawaii International Conference on System Sciences*, Big Island, Hawaii.

Chau, P., & Hu, P. (2001). Information Technology Acceptance by Individual Professionals: A Model Comparison Approach. *Decision Sciences*, *32*(4). doi:10.1111/j.1540-5915.2001.tb00978.x

Connell, N., & Young, T. (2007, June). Evaluating healthcare information systems through an "enterprise" perspective. *Information & Management*, *44*(4), 433–440. doi:10.1016/j.im.2007.04.002

Creswell, J. W. (2003). *Research Design. Qualitative, Quantitative, and Mixed Methods Approaches*. Thousand Oaks, CA, USA: Sage.

Cronholm, S., & Goldkuhl, G. (2003, September 25-26). Six Generic Types of Information Systems Evaluation. *The 10th European Conference on Information Technology Evaluation (ECITE-2003)*, Madrid.

Davis, F. (1989). Perceived Usefulness, Perceived Ease of Use and User Acceptance of Information Technology. *Management Information Systems Quarterly*, *13*(3), 319–340. doi:10.2307/249008

Davis, L., Domm, J., Konikoff, M., & Miller, R. (1999, Jan–Feb). Attitudes of First-year Medical Students toward the Confidentiality of Computerized Patient Records. *Journal of the American Medical Informatics Association*, *6*(1).

Eng, T. R. (2001). *The e-health landscape: A terrain map of emerging information and communication technologies in health and health care*. Princeton, NJ: The Robert Wood Johnson Foundation.

Eng, T. R. (2002). E-health research and evaluation: challenges and opportunities. *Journal of Health Communication*, *7*(4), 267–272. doi:10.1080/10810730290001747

Farbey, B., Land, F., & Targett, D. (1995). A Taxonomy of information systems applications: the benefits evaluation Ladder. *European Journal of Information Systems*, *4*, 41–50. doi:10.1057/ejis.1995.5

Farbey, B., Land, F., & Targett, D. (1999). Evaluating Investments in IT: Findings and a Framework. In Willcocks, L. P., & Lester, S. (Eds.), *Beyond the IT Productivity Paradox* (pp. 183–215). Chichester, England, UK: John Wiley & Sons.

Freeman, R. E. (1984). *Strategic Management: A stakeholder Approach*. Cambridge: Ballinger Publishing Co.

Friedman, C., & Wyatt, J. (2000). *Evaluation methods in medical informatics*. New York: Springer-Verlag.

Fruhling, A., & Lee, S. (2004, September). Designing Trustworthy e-Health Services for Rural Consumers. *MedInfo. American Medical Informatics Association Proceedings*.

Glasgow, R. E. (2007). E-health evaluation and dissemination research. *American Journal of Preventive Medicine*, *32*(5Suppl), S119–S126. doi:10.1016/j.amepre.2007.01.023

Grover, V., Jeong, S. R., & Segars, A. H. (1996). Information Systems Effectiveness: The Construct Space and Patterns of Applications. *Information & Management*, *31*(4). doi:10.1016/S0378-7206(96)01079-8

Gustafson, D., Hawkins, R., Pingree, S., McTavish, F., Arora, N., & Salner, J. (2001). Effect of computer support on younger women with breast cancer. *Journal of General Internal Medicine*, *16*, 435–445. doi:10.1046/j.1525-1497.2001.016007435.x

Gustafson, D., & Wyatt, J. (2004). Evaluation of e-health systems and services. *British Medical Journal*, *328*, 1150. .doi:10.1136/bmj.328.7449.1150

Hans, O., Rizo, C., Enkin, M., & Jadad, A. (2005, February 24). What is e-health? *A Systematic Review of Published Definitions. Journal of Medical Internet Research*. doi:.doi:10.2196/jmir.7.1.e1

Holliday, I., & Tam, W. (2004). E-health in the East Asian tigers. *International Journal of Medical Informatics*, *73*(11-12), 759–769. doi:10.1016/j.ijmedinf.2004.08.001

Horan, T., Abhichandani, T., & Rayalu, R. (2006). Assessing User Satisfaction of E-Government Services: Development and Testing of Quality-in-Use Satisfaction with Advanced Traveler Information Systems (ATIS). *Proceedings of the 39th Hawaii International Conference on System Sciences.*

Hufnagel, E. M., & Conca, C. (1994). Use Response Data: The Potential for Errors and Biases. *Information Systems Research*, *5*, 48–73. doi:10.1287/isre.5.1.48

Jarvinen, O. (2005). *Privacy Management of E-health, Content Analysis of 39 US Health Providers' Privacy Policies*. Publication of Turku School of Economics and Business Administration. *Series*, *A-3*, 2005.

Jones, S., & Hughes, J. (2001). Understanding IS Evaluation as a Complex Social Process: A Case Study of a United Kingdom Local Authority. *European Journal of Information Systems*, *10*(1).

Lapointe, L., Lamothe, L., & Fortin, J. P. (2002). The dynamics of IT adoption in a major change process in healthcare delivery. *Proceedings of the 35th HICSS conference,* Big Island, Hawaii.

Lauer, T., Joshi, K., & Browdy, T. (2000, Jan–Feb). Use of the Equity Implementation Model to Review Clinical System Implementation Efforts. *Journal of the American Medical Informatics Association*, *7*(1),

Lenhart, A., Horrigan, J., Rainie, L., Allen, K., Boyce, A., & Madden, M. (2003). *The ever-shifting Internet population. A new look at Internet access and the digital divide.* Washington, DC: Pew Internet & American Life Project.

Löfstedt, U. (2007). E-Government Services in Local Governments – A study of Development in Swedish Municipalities. *Journal of Organisational Transformation and Social Change*, *4*(2), 157–167. doi:10.1386/jots.4.2.157_1

Loiacono, E. T., Watson, R. T., & Goodhue, D. L. (2002). Webqual: A Web Site Quality Instrument. In *Proceedings of the AMA Winter Marketing Educators' Conference*, Austin, TX, USA.

Lowery, D., & Evans, K. G. (2004). The iron cage of methodology. *Administration & Society*, *36*(3), 306–327. doi:10.1177/0095399704265298

Mantzana, V., & Themistocleous, M. (2006). A Method for the Identification of Actors Involved in the Adoption of Innovations in Healthcare Organizations. In *Proceedings of the 39th Hawaii International Conference on System Sciences.*

Mayer, R. C., Davis, J. H., & Schoorman, F. D. (1995). An integrative model of organizational trust. *Academy of Management Review*, *20*(3), 709–734. doi:10.2307/258792

Mcconaghy, J. (2006). Evolving Medical Knowledge: Moving Toward Efficiently Answering Questions and Keeping Current. [Elsevier Inc.]. *Primary Care: Clinics in Office Practice*, *33*(4), 831–837. doi:10.1016/j.pop.2006.10.002

Melander-Wikman, A., Jansson, M., & Gard, G. (2005). The MobiHealth Usability Evaluation Questionnaire. *E-health International Journal.*

Melone, N. P. (1990). A Theoretical Assessment of the User Satisfaction Construct in Information Systems Research. *Management Science*, *36*, 76–91. doi:10.1287/mnsc.36.1.76

Mingers, J., & Stowell, F. (1997). *Information Systems: An Emerging Discipline? Information Systems Series* (pp. 239–266). London: McGraw-Hill.

Mont, D. (2007). *Measuring Disability Prevalence* (SP Discussion Paper NO. 0706). Available at: http://siteresources.worldbank.org/DISABILITY/Resources/Data/MontPrevalence.pdf.

Moor, J. H. (1997). Towards a Theory of Privacy in the Information Age. *Computers & Society*, *27*(3), 27–32. doi:10.1145/270858.270866

Myers, M. D., & Avison, D. (2002). *Qualitative Research in Information Systems*. London: Sage Publications.

Nielsen, J. (1993). *Usability engineering (Interactive Technologies)*. New York: Academic Press.

Patton, M. Q. (1990). *Qualitative Evaluation and Research Methods* (2nd ed.). London: Sage Publications.

Paul, L., John, I., & Pierre, C. (2003, January). Why do people use information technology, A critical review of the technology acceptance model. *Association for Information Systems*, *40*(3), 191.

Powell, P. L. (1999). Evaluation of Information Technology Investments: Business as usual. In Willcocks, L. P., & Lester, S. (Eds.), *Beyond the IT Productivity Paradox* (pp. 151–182). Chichester, England, UK: John Wiley & Sons.

Presti, S., Butler, M., Leuschel, M., & Booth, C. (2006). Holistic Trust Design of E-Services. In Song, R., Korba, L., & Yee, G. (Eds.), *Trust in E-Services: Technologies, Practices and Challenges* (pp. 113–139). USA: Idea Group Publishing.

Rahimi, B., & Vimarlund, V. (2007). Methods to Evaluate Health information Systems in Healthcare Settings: A Literature Review. *J. Med. Syst.*, *31*, 397–432. Springer Science + Business Media, LLC 2007.

Ray, S. (2007). Development of a framework towards successful implementation of e-governance initiatives in health sector in India. [Emerald Group Publishing Limited.]. *International Journal of Health Care Quality Assurance*, *20*(6), 464–483. doi:10.1108/09526860710819413

Rodrigues, R. (2003). Deploying e-Health Solutions in Latin America and the Caribbean: Development and Policy Issues. *Forum PL11: Workshop on Telemedicine,* Geneva.

Rogers, E. M. (1995). *Diffusion of Innovations* (4th ed.). New York: The Free Press.

Serafeimidis, V., & Smithson, S. (2000). Information Systems Evaluation in Practice: a Case Study of Organizational Change. *Journal of Information Technology*, *15*(2), 93–105. doi:10.1080/026839600344294

Skinner, R. (2003). The value of information technology in healthcare. *Frontiers of Health Services Management*, *19*(3).

Slaymaker, M., Politou, E., Power, D., & Lloyd, S. (2004). E-health security issues: the eDiaMoND perspective. In *Proceedings of the 2004 UK e-Science All Hands Meeting*.

Smaglik, P., Hawkins, R., Pingree, S., & Gustafson, D. (1998). The quality of interactive computer use among HIV infected individuals. *Journal of Health Communication*, *3*, 53–68. doi:10.1080/108107398127508

Steinfeld, E., & Danford, G. S. (1999). *Enabling Environments. Measuring the impact of Environment on Disability and Rehabilitation*. New York: Kluwer Academic.

Stroetmann, K., Jones, T., & Dobrev, A. (2006, May 10-12). Evaluating the economic impact of e-health applications approach and method. *E-health conference 2006,* Malaga, Spain.

Symons, V., & Walsham, G. (1988). The evaluation of information systems: a critique. *Journal of Applied Systems Analysis*, *15*, 119–132.

Terry Ma, H., & Zaphiris, P. (2003). *The Usability and Content Accessibility of the E-government in the UK*. Centre for Human-Computer Interaction Design, City University, London. Available at: http://www.soi.city.ac.uk/~zaphiri/Papers/HCII2003/HCII2003-Accessibility.pdf.

Tornatzky, L., & Klein, K. (1982, February). Innovation characteristics and innovation adoption-implementation: A meta-analysis of findings. *IEEE Transactions on Engineering Management*, *29*(1), 28–45.

Walsham, G. (1993). *Interpreting Information Systems in Organizations*. Chichester: John Wiley & Sons.

Wang, L., Bretschneider, S., & Gant, J. (2005). Evaluating Web-Based E-Government Services with a Citizen-Centric Approach. In *Proceedings of 38th Annual Hawaii International Conference on Systems Sciences,* Big Island, Hawaii.

West, D. (2000). *Assessing E-Government: The Internet, Democracy and Service Delivery by State and Federal Governments*. Brown University. Available at: www.insidepolitics.org/policyreports.html.

Wickramasinghe, N., & Goldberg, S. (2004). How M=EC2 in healthcare. *International Journal of Mobile Commerce*.

Wickramasinghe, N., & Misra, S. (2004). A wireless trust model for healthcare. *International Journal e-Heal*th.

Willcocks, L. (1992). Evaluating Information Technology Investments: Research Findings and Reappraisal. *Journal of Information Systems*, *2*(3), 243–268.

World Markets Research Centre & Brown University. (2001). *Global e-government Survey 2001*. Available at: http://www.worldmarketsanalysis.com/pdf/e-govreport.pdf

Yin, R. K. (2003). *Case study research: Design and Methods* (3rd ed.). Thousand Oaks, CA: Sage Publications.

Zeithaml, V. A., Parasuraman, A., & Malhotra, A. (2000). A Conceptual Framework for Understanding e-Service Quality: Implications for Future Research and Managerial Practice. *Marketing Sciences Institute: Working Paper Series*, (115).

Zeng, X., & Parmanto, B. (2004). Web content accessibility of consumer health information Web sites for people with disabilities: a cross sectional evaluation. *Journal of Medical Internet Research*, *6*(2), e19. doi:10.2196/jmir.6.2.e19

This work was previously published in International Journal of Healthcare Delivery Reform Initiatives, edited by Matthew W. Guah, pp. 1-18, copyright 2009 by IGI Publishing (an imprint of IGI Global).

Chapter 11
Confirmatory Factor Analysis to Establish Determinants of Wireless Technology in the Indian Healthcare

Raj Gururajan
University of Southern Queensland, Australia

Tiana Gurney
University of Southern Queensland, Australia

Abdul Hafeez-Baig
University of Southern Queensland, Australia

ABSTRACT

This study reports the determinants of wireless technology in the Indian healthcare validated by a second order regression model. In order to assert the determinants, a qualitative study was conducted with 30 physicians using interviews to arrive at a set of barriers and drivers. Further analysis of the qualitative data indicated that there is a third component emerging, namely, clinical influence. The interview data was used to develop a survey instrument and this was administered on the Indian clinicians with 200 completed surveys. This data was used to establish the sub-components of the three major determinants as identified in the qualitative study. This is reported in this article.

INTRODUCTION

In the last few years, high expectations, technological developments, and effective and efficient services have been shown to be prerequisites for improvements in the healthcare domain (Rogoski, 2005; Versel, 2008). Latest trends in the healthcare sector include the design of more flexible and efficient service provider frameworks aimed at providing health services to all stakeholders. In order to implement such frameworks, wire-

DOI: 10.4018/978-1-60960-183-6.ch011

less technology is increasingly being used in the healthcare sector. A decrease in the cost of wireless devices and improved awareness of the benefits by using related wireless applications are two of the contributing factors towards the increased use of wireless technology in this sector (Gururajan, Quaddus, Fink, Vuori, & Soar, 2005; R. Gururajan, Hafeez-Baig, & Gururjan, 2008). Even though the future of this technology and its usability is promising, its adoption is still in its infancy, which is attributed to the complex and critical nature of the healthcare environment. In the current competitive and complex business environment, technology developments have played a critical role in delivering high quality of care (Reinecke, 2004). However, there is limited knowledge and empirical research on the effectiveness and adoption of wireless technology in general, and in the Indian healthcare system in particular.

Recent research has established that investment in emerging Information Technology (IT), including Information Systems (IS), can lead to productivity gains only if they are accepted and effectively used by respective stakeholders. Consequently, acceptance and utilization of IT/IS in the healthcare environment have been central themes in the information systems literature. Therefore, the fundamental focus of this research is to investigate and examine the influence of internal and external determinants on the usefulness of wireless technology. Further, this research also assesses how its acceptance contributes to the adoption of wireless technology. We believe that this research is the first of its kind attempted in the Indian healthcare domain and it employs empirical evidence to explore the impact of wireless technology and its usefulness in the Indian healthcare system. The Indian healthcare domain is at the forefront in adopting the latest medical technologies and applications, as evidenced by media reports and, as such, it constitutes an excellent context for validating existing adoption theories and extending them.

The main contribution of this research includes the identification of a set of drivers and barriers to using wireless technology in a given Indian healthcare setting. In addition to this, for the first time, a set of clinical factors influencing the adoption of wireless technology has been identified and validated using a second order regression model.

LITERATURE REVIEW

The concept of wireless technology in healthcare is discussed in many studies (Dyer, 2003; Hu, Chau, & Sheng, 2002; Sausser, 2003; Simpson, 2003; Siracuse, Pharm, & Sowell, 2008; Versel, 2008; Wisnicki, 2002; Wu & Wu, 2007; Zhang, 2007). For example, Wisnicki (2002) provides details of how broadband technology, an essential component of wireless technology, can be used in healthcare. While prior studies agree that wireless applications have the potential to address the endemic problems of healthcare, very limited information can be found about the determinants of such applications (Gururajan, Toleman, & Soar, 2004; Gururajan, Moloney, & Kerr, 2005). In general, the majority of the works reviewed are descriptive about the benefits of wireless handheld devices in healthcare in general, and medicine in particular. There are only a small number of studies that provide evidence-based information concerning these devices in healthcare (Fischer et al., 2003; Sax et al., 2005)(Hafeez-Baig, 2007). Furthermore, five major studies in the area of healthcare (evaluated by (Spil & Schuring, 2006) testing the Technology Acceptance Model (TAM) produced findings which were inconsistent with the body of knowledge in non-healthcare settings. With 'Perceived Ease of Use' and 'Perceived Usefulness' as the major TAM attributes, these studies found that in the health environment, 'Perceived Usefulness' is an important attribute in technology adoption, while 'Perceived Ease of Use' was found to have no effect (Spil & Schuring, 2006). This is different to findings reported in non-health IS studies, where both attributes were found to be reliable technology adoption predictors. Therefore, further empirical investigation is required to explain the reasons why this variation exists in healthcare. In addition, there is a need to explore if further attributes exist which may influence the adoption of wireless applications in the healthcare environment.

TECHNOLOGY ADOPTION IN HEALTHCARE CONTEXT

In healthcare literature, the discussion on wireless technology falls into three periods. For example, studies prior to and including 2000 discussed the status of wireless technology and the possible role the technology can play in healthcare. Studies between 2000 and 2003 discussed how wireless technology can be deployed in healthcare and the potential benefits the technology can bring to healthcare. It should be noted that these studies were only 'discussion' type studies. Majority of these studies did not provide any empirical evidence as to the use or acceptance of wireless technology in healthcare domains. Studies from 2004 till current date have collected data to establish the usefulness of wireless technology in healthcare. These studies, to some extent have focussed on the PDAs as these devices have been found to be useful in nursing domain for clinical data management.

The studies between 2000 and 2003 discussed a number of potentials of wireless technology in clinical domains. For example, how broadband technology can be used in healthcare was discussed by (Wisnicki, 2002), ability to address prevailing healthcare staff crisis by adopting intelligent solutions using agent and wireless technology that can identify the need and match the need with available resources in a timely and efficient manner was outlined by (Davis, 2002), better compliance with the rigorous regulatory framework was highlighted by (Wisnicki, 2002), reduction in medication errors and hence the benefits that can be realised was discussed by (Turisco, 2000), provision for greater flexibility and mobility of healthcare workers in performing their work was portrayed by (Athey & Stern, 2002), effective management of the increasingly complex information challenges and improved access to those information from anywhere at anytime was discussed by (Stuart & Bawany, 2001). Our review clearly identified that all these studies were only implying the potential of wireless technology and did not provide any empirical evidence.

While prior studies agreed that wireless applications have the potential to address the endemic problems of healthcare, very limited information can be found about the determinants of such wireless applications in order to establish the adoption of technology in a given healthcare context (Gururajan et al., 2004; Gururajan et al., 2005). During the period of 2004 – 2006, studies emerged in the area of technology acceptance, specifically focussing on the acceptance of wireless technology in healthcare domains. These studies were empirical in nature and were testing the available models of technology acceptance or a variation in order to ascertain whether previous models hold good for a new technology in a specific domain. These studies were reported in a book titled 'E-Helth Systems Diffusion and Use', published by Idea Group Publishing in 2006 (Spil & Schuring, 2006). These studies are summarised below:

Predicting Internet Use: Applying the Extended Technology Acceptance Model to the Healthcare Environment (Chismar & Wiley-Patton, 2006) – This study empirically established that only perceived usefulness is significant and ease of use was not significant.

The dynamics of IT adoption in a major change process in health delivery (Lapointe, Lamothe, & Fortin, 2006) – This study established that TAM as devised by (Davies, Bagozzi, & Warshaw, 1989) is not adequate for health systems because adoption/resistance factors may be group related as opposed to the fundamental basis of TAM which is individualistic, influence of intra and inter organisational factors, linkages to cultures, environmental factors as well as the complexity of the environment.

Introducing electronic patient records to hospitals: Innovation adoption paths (Suomi, 2006) – This study found that relative advantage, strong network externalities available, rich availability of information through different communication channels are key factors for innovation and adoption. It should be noted that these are not discussed in the TAM models.

User acceptance and diffusion of innovations summarised (Spil & Schuring, 2006) – This summary established that perceived usefulness is a predictor of technology acceptance in healthcare. Ease of use was not found to be significant.

Understanding physicians' use of online systems: an empirical assessment of an electronic disability evaluation system (Horan, Tule, & Hilton, 2006) – This study found that in order to diffuse technology in an organisation, it is important to ascertain physicians' behaviour, their workflow practices and their perceptions regarding the value of specific information systems.

In essence, the recent studies appear to be indicating that the current models of technology acceptance or its derivatives are not suitable to predict the adoption factors of wireless technology in healthcare environment. Strong support can also be derived from three specific studies that have tested TAM models in healthcare. The first study conducted by (Jayasuriya, 1998) established that ease of use was not significant in a clinical domain. The second study by (Chau & Hu, 2002) echoed similar sentiments. The third study by Hu et al. (Hu, Chau, & Tam, 1999) also found similar findings.

Further, recent studies conducted by (Howard, Gururajan, Hafeez-Baig, & Howard, 2006) also established that ease of use was not significant while determining factors of adoption in a clinical domain in regard to wireless technology. Further, (Ivers & Gururajan, 2006) also found that there are other factors beyond the TAM models influencing the acceptance of technology (Versel, 2008).

Interviews conducted with Queensland nursing staff members in Australia (Gururajan, Moloney, & D. Kerr, 2005) revealed that clinical usefulness of wireless technology is far more significant than ease of use factor as established in TAM. Another focus group discussion with the Western Australian senior health managers (R. Gururajan, M. Quaddus et al., 2005) also indicated that aspects of clinical usefulness such as integration of clinical data may be a significant factor than the ease of use factor. (Howard et al., 2006) also identified clinical usefulness is far more influencing than the ease of use factor while determining factors of adoption of wireless technology in the Indian healthcare domain.

However, the recent findings that the ease of use factor not showing strong significance in healthcare domain while determining wireless technology adoption warrants explanation as this is different to many other reported studies in the generic IS domain where both attributes (ease of use and perceived usefulness) were reported to be reliable predictors.

This variation requires further empirical investigation in order to explain the reason behind this variation specific to healthcare. Therefore, there is a need to identify attributes that assist in the adoption of wireless applications in healthcare environment. We argue that the initial validity of many technology acceptance models was predominantly established by testing the model with students as surrogates in a generic software application domain. This environment is very different to the healthcare environment, where the skills are at different levels. Further, the healthcare environment is complex, sensitive and time critical. These could be some of the reasons why TAM did not perform as expected in healthcare settings.

In addition, in the recent variant of technology acceptance, namely, UTAUT, (Venkatesh, Morris, Davis, & Davis, 2003) reviewed eight prominent models of user acceptance and managed to create a unified view. The unified model comprised of seven constructs. The first four – performance expectancy, effort expectancy, social influence and facilitating conditions – were theorised to be direct determinants. The last three – attitude towards technology, self efficacy and anxiety – were theorised to be indirect. All the seven constructs were found to be significant determinants of technology usage by Venkatesh et al ((Venkatesh et al., 2003).

In terms of attitude, Venkatesh et al. (Venkatesh et al., 2003) defined it as an individual's overall affective reaction to using a system. The model depicts four constructs relating to this determinant – attitude towards behaviour, intrinsic motivation, affect towards use and affect. (Spil & Schuring, 2006) verified that in three cases the relation between attitude and behavioural intention is significant. Therefore, this determinant cannot be indirect. If there is significance between attitude and behaviour intention, then there is a direct relationship.

Therefore, there appears to be a basis to identify factors that contribute to the adoption of technologies in healthcare settings. Given that wireless technologies have started making in-roads in healthcare, the overarching purpose of the research is to identify the factors that influence the adoption of wireless technology in the Indian healthcare system. The rationale of the purpose is justified by the fact that India is a leader in software technologies, especially medical applications. Further, India is emerging as 'health tourism', due to the advancement in medical technology and reduction in cost in offering high quality health services—as highlighted by various print media. However, our initial review of available literature indicated that this area is under-researched. Collectively, these aspects led to the following research question:

- What are the determinants for the adoption of wireless technology by physicians in the Indian healthcare system?

The first stage of this study is focused on answering the research question qualitatively and the second stage on answering the research question quantitatively. Details as to how the research question was answered are provided in the research methodology section below.

METHODOLOGY

An examination of existing IS studies indicated that there is a necessity for a suitable research method. Most of the reviewed studies follow a quantitative approach which involves an instrument being administered onto a domain with perhaps a lesser understanding of the domain issues. For this study it was felt that if technology issues are to be studied with respect to a specific domain, then user involvement with the technology issues forms a major part in establishing the adoption (or inhibiting) factors. By necessity, this would occur prior to administering quantitative instruments (e.g. survey). This, in turn, requires an understanding of research philosophy, values of inquiry that would guide the study, and the choice of relevant research techniques required to conduct the investigation in order to answer the research questions.

Further, there appears to be limited information available in the Indian IS domain to guide the principles of this study. This study is relatively new and, hence, requires a rigorous justification as to the choice of research methods employed. We also believe that due to aspects associated with various regulatory issues impacting the Indian health system, unique factors of technology acceptance, as well as usefulness, may emerge. Our initial meetings with Indian physicians also suggested that there is a divide in terms of technology usage between private and public hospitals, where private hospitals are rich in technology use and public hospitals are not. On the other hand, in many traditional studies in IS, either quantitative or, to some lesser extent, qualitative methods are used—but not both. In recent years this has been cited as a weakness (see (Mingers, 2001) for a detailed argument on this). Taking this into account, this study investigates the suitability of both approaches in order to answer the research question.

We recognise that the foundation for any research will be grounded on the researcher's fundamental philosophical view of the world (Myers, 1997). The choice of tools, including research techniques, instruments, and methods such as qualitative and quantitative, are not inherently linked to a particular philosophical position, as these positions are generic in nature. It is the contextual framework within which they are applied that provides consistency to an inquiry. While the choice of tools and methods are not linked to the philosophical view, the articulation—which is commonly the process of explaining choices of research methods and its related choice of research instruments—helps determine the philosophical disposition. This is usually achieved by asking questions on the beliefs, perceptions, experiences, advantages and disadvantages in order to determine this disposition. This may even include a researcher's personal experience within that domain, or their expertise in explicating the information using any approach that may be suitable to that domain. This has prompted us to follow a qualitative approach as the first phase of the study. We argue that this approach facilitates direction to the second phase of the study where quantitative evidence can be collected to establish causality between the dependent and the independent variables.

The research question dictates the need for quantitative research methods, while the behavioural component of the same investigation dictates qualitative research methods. The rationale for this approach is based on the notion that behavioural components require a thorough understanding of how users apply wireless technology in a given setting in order to understand behavioural issues. To extract 'tacit' aspects, this is best accomplished by applying a qualitative approach. A quantitative instrument can then be developed to extract the quantitative aspects, such as the opinion scores.

Health professionals view the term 'wireless technology' in different ways, either as a product or a process. The combined domain of wireless technology and healthcare is relatively new in the Indian IS domain. While IS studies have discussed the impact of Information & Communication Technology (ICT) tools and associated behavioural intentions on healthcare users, limited information can be found as to how the combination of wireless technology and healthcare settings would influence users who are already conversant with novel and advanced medical technologies (Spil & Schuring, 2006). The workplace or organizational factors that influence such combinations are yet to be explored in detail. Such an exploration has close association with the choice of research method as these methods pave the way for proper inquiry into the factors that determine technology acceptance in a given setting. On this basis, the suitability of one research method over another has to be carefully weighed. Consequently, this study identified an exploratory approach to be suitable for the initial investigation. This approach is particularly favourable in confirming the direction of the study, variables chosen for the study, and in helping refine the literature. The exploratory study can also possibly eliminate some variables, while providing opportunities for including emerging variables.

Qualitative Data Collection

As argued, for the first stage of this research the investigators used a qualitative approach to collect initial sets of themes for the adoption of wireless technology in the Indian healthcare system. For this purpose, 30 physicians operating in Indian healthcare were identified randomly. These physicians were interviewed by an independent member (external to the team) who identified the attributes for the adoption of wireless technology by physicians in the Indian healthcare system. This approach was deliberate to address criticisms of 'bias' in the interview process. Further, due to linguistic issues, we required a person with proficiency in both Indian language and English. The interview questions were derived from existing literature. The first stage of the data collection concentrated on Indian hospitals with some form of wireless technology already in use. The physicians were also chosen based on their wireless technology awareness or working experience. They were drawn from both private and government hospitals. The interviews were conducted over a 45-60 minute period and recorded using a digital recorder. Once they were recorded, the interviews were transcribed.

Quantitative Data Collection

This study developed a survey instrument from the interview data. The main reason for this digressed attitude was that previously tested instruments in the technology domain were not relevant to healthcare setting and were found to be inadequate in answering the research question. The data from the interviews were used to develop specific ranges of questions to gather a more detailed view from the wider population. This survey instrument was pilot tested to capture the information reflecting the perceptions and practice of those adopting the wireless technology in the Indian healthcare system. Particularly, it focussed on what internal and external environmental factors affect the adoption of wireless technology and the extent of this influence. The survey was then distributed to over 300 physicians randomly chosen from the telephone book and a total of 200 responses were received. The survey responses were then entered into a spreadsheet file. A Visual Basic interface was written to generate numerical codes for various elements of the survey for data analysis using SPSS. The coded spreadsheet file was then copied onto a SPSS file format.

DATA ANALYSIS

Qualitative data was analysed using the NVivo (version 7) application, which helped identify the initial themes from the interviews. Quantitative data were analysed using SPSS, which helped identify the factors and their correlation for the adoption of wireless technology in the Indian healthcare setting.

Qualitative Data Analysis

Qualitative data was manually coded to extract themes that had an impact on wireless technology acceptance as stated by the physicians. In total, 63 themes were extracted from the interviews. The initial themes include awareness, cost factors, advantages and disadvantages, medical errors, information sharing, current state of technology, usefulness and role of wireless technology, and technology awareness. On the basis of the interviews and the literature review, the themes were classified into drivers and inhibitors as shown in the following table. This list of drivers and inhibitors was expected to provide a direction for the development of the survey instrument for the collection of quantitative data to capture the wider community views and to generalize the outcome of the research. This grouping is presented in Table 1.

The content of the Table 1 is consistent with findings of previous studies conducted by Gururajan et al. (2004; 2005). This prompted conducting a quantitative study in order to establish causality among dependent and independent variables, as well as external validity and generalisability.

Quantitative Data Analyses

In order to ensure statistical reliability, suitable tests were run on the entire instrument, as well as selected group of variables. For example, the reliability test returned a Cronbach alpha value of 0.965 for the instrument indicating high reli-

Table 1. The factors driving and inhibiting wireless technology adoption in healthcare

Drivers	Barriers
Save-time Improve-clinical-workflow Efficiency-in-communication Delivery-of-high-qual-info Better-quality-of-service Save-effort Improve-clinical-performance More-contact-time-with-patients Improved-delivery-of-information Reduce-overall-cost Positive-impact-on-patient-safety Reduce-inaccuracies Improve-public-image Reduce-medical-errors Easy-access-to-data Attract-more-practitioners Reduce-workload	Legal barriers Administrative purpose Communication with physicians Patient education Communication with colleagues Obtain lab results Note taking Electronic medical records Device usage barrier Benefit evaluation barrier Resource barrier Electronic prescribing

Table 2. The factors driving and inhibiting wireless technology adoption in healthcare from data analysis of survey result

Drivers	Loading values	Barriers	Loading values
Improve-clinical-workflow	.798	Poor technology barrier	.605
Tech-support	.764	Time for training barrier	.572
Delivery-of-high-qual-info	.760	Tech expertise barrier	.554
Save-time	.757	Benefit evaluation barrier	.503
Better-quality-of-service	.749	Legal barriers	.465
Save-effort	.743	Solutions barrier	.444
Improved-delivery-of-information	.732	System migration barrier	.442
Efficiency-in-communication	.730	Technical support barrier	.436
More-contact-time-with-patients	.725	Lack of support barrier	.352
Improve-clinical-performance	.702	Device access barrier	.316
More-training	.699	Device comfort barrier	.248
Improve-public-image	.695	Funding barrier	-.225
Easy-access-to-data	.692	Security as barrier	.224
Positive-impact-on-patient-safety	.679	Device usage barrier	.208
Reduce-inaccuracies	.659		
Reduce-workload	.657		
Reduce-medical-errors	.650		
Reduce-overall-cost	.634		
Attract-more-practitioners	.600		
Org-culture	.464		

Table 3. The factors driving wireless technology adoption in healthcare from data analysis of survey result

Descriptions	Organizational	Management	Clinical
Save-effort	.716		
Reduce-overall-cost	.708		
Reduce-inaccuracies	.703		
Save-time	.667		
Easy-access-to-data	.659		
Attract-more-practitioners		.769	
Improve-public-image		.680	
Tech-support		.680	
Reduce-workload			.817
Improve-clinical-performance			.797

ability (Zikmund, 1994). We ran this test because the instrument was generated from the interview data and, hence, it was necessary to establish statistical reliability. In addition, reliability tests were also run for three factor groupings, namely, drivers, inhibitors of adoption and other technology factors. The reliability tests returned values of 0.941, 0.447 and 0.536, respectively, indicating that the data were suitable for factor analysis testing.

As a second step, survey data were analysed for factor analysis using SPSS. It is evident from the table below that two factor component matrix identified drivers and the barriers for the adoption of wireless technology in the Indian healthcare setting. This finding is consistent and aligned with the findings of the qualitative data collection stage (i.e. first stage) of this research.

The drivers were further tested for factor groupings. The analysis resulted in Table 3.

The driving factors of adoption yielded three categories of factors, namely, 'organisational', 'management' and 'clinical'. The organisational components include wireless technology drivers that can generate specific benefits for organisations. The management components represent the

Table 4. The factors inhibiting wireless technology adoption in healthcare from data analysis of survey result

Descriptions	Technology	Resource	Usage
Poor technology barrier	.625		
Time for training barrier	.582		
Solutions barrier	.575		
Benefit evaluation barrier	.528		
Tech expertise barrier	.527		
System migration barrier	.511		
Funding barrier		-.749	
Resource barrier		-.690	
Technical support barrier			.542
Device usage barrier			.519

benefits that healthcare managers can realise using wireless technology. The clinical components encompass clinical drivers of using wireless technology.

A similar factor model was generated for the inhibitors. The model resulted in Table 4.

Similar to the drivers, the inhibitors also resulted in three specific categories. The 'technology' category includes technology factors that inhibit wireless adoption in the Indian healthcare. The 'resource' category encompasses resource barriers that are currently being encountered in the healthcare setting. Finally the 'usage' category is comprised of inhibiting factors, which are associated with usage issues.

In addition to the two factor groups, namely drivers and inhibitors, we also identified a third. We named this 'clinical usefulness' and its components are shown in Table 5.

This factor group yielded three components. The first component deals with the general communication aspects facilitated by wireless technology in healthcare settings. The second component refers to clinical communication using wireless technology. The third component is specific to records management. In summary, the data analyses yielded three specific categories of fac-

Table 5. The factors 'clinical usefulness' of wireless technology adoption in healthcare from data analysis of survey result

Descriptions	General Communication	Clinical Communication	Records Management
Obtain lab results	.837		
Administrative purpose	.770		
Electronic prescribing	.670		
Medical database referral	.632		
Patient education		.727	
Communication with colleagues		.707	
Communication with patients		.676	
Drug administration		.596	
Communication with physicians		.548	
Electronic Medical Records			.764
Generating exception list			.738
Note taking			.617
Disease state management			.563

Figure 1. Initial model

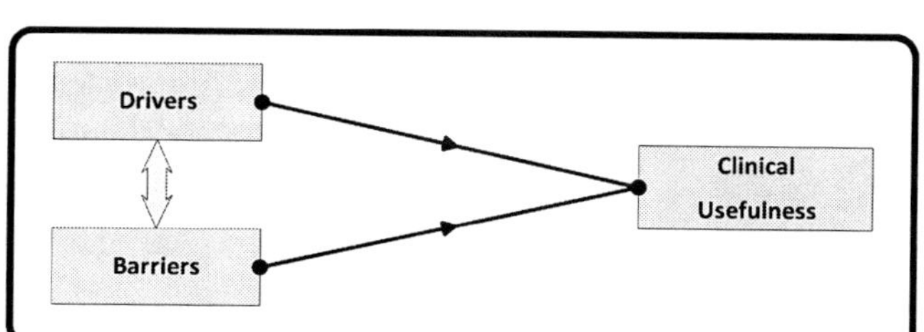

Figure 2. Drivers: $X^2 = 27.5$, $df = 14$, $p = 0.017$, $X^2/df = 1.964$, $GFI = 0.961$, $TLI = .963$

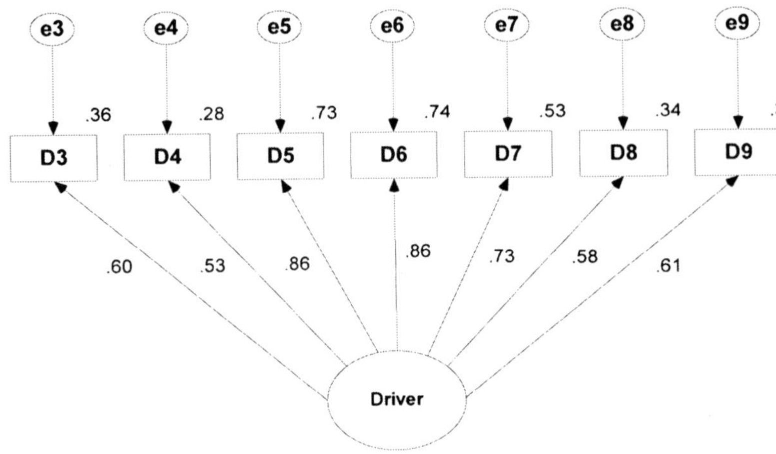

tors which can affect the adoption of wireless technologies in the healthcare setting. These comprise adoption drivers, inhibitors, and clinical usefulness.

Hypotheses Formulation and Testing

Based on the evidence collected, the three sets of factors, namely, drivers, barriers and clinical usefulness, contribute to the acceptance of wireless technology in healthcare. We hypothesise that the drivers positively impact clinical usefulness, whereas the barriers have a negative impact on it. While the drivers and barriers include factors beyond the technology aspects, their respective influences are restricted to the clinical domain as this is where the usefulness of wireless technology can be experienced. Therefore, the following two hypotheses were generated for testing:

H1: Drivers of wireless technology positively impact clinical usefulness.

H2: Barriers to wireless technology negatively impact clinical usefulness.

A "Structural Equaction Modeling (SEM) model was developed in order to test the hypotheses. The rationale for using SEM includes: SEM is used for confirmatory factor analysis (CFA); the pattern of loadings of items on the latent constructs is explicit; SEM provides strong convergent and discriminant validity; p-value of t-value is significant (over 0.50 level) for constructs; and measurement items load highly on theoretically assigned factors and not highly on other factors.

SEM MODEL DEVELOPMENT

In order to develop the SEM model, an AMOS version 16 was used. Initially, the individual drivers, barriers and clinical usefulness were tested for CFA (Confirmatory Factor Analysis) scores and these were found to be reliable. When the CFA was found to be satisfactory, a model was built with clinical influences as dependent variable on drivers and barriers. The final outcome is shown in Figure 8.

Figure 8 shows that the factor loading (the number on the path: for example, for the construct Drivers, has 0.16, 0.21, and .48). The drivers and clinical usefulness load highly (over 0.8 for most of the items), indicating a high reliability. Further, all variables have a t-value of over 2.0 to indicate high convergent validity.

Table 6. Description of items used in building the SEM model and their reliability

Variables	Initial	Descriptions	Reliability
Drivers	D1	Reduce-workload	0.885
	D2	Improve-public-image	
	D3	Improve-clinical-performance	
	D4	Attract-more-practitioners	
	D5	Save-time	
	D6	Save-effort	
	D7	Tech-support	
	D8	Reduce-overall-cost	
	D9	Easy-access-to-data	
Barriers	B1	Funding barrier	0.539
	B2	Resource barrier	
	B3	Solutions barrier	
	B4	System migration barrier	
	B5	Benefit evaluation barrier	
	B6	Time for training barrier	
	B7	Poor technology barrier	
	B8	Tech expertise barrier	
	B9	Technical support barrier	
	B10	Device usage barrier	
Clinical Influences	CI 1	Electronic medical records	0.850
	CI 2	Medical database referral	
	CI 3	Electronic prescribing	
	CI 4	Obtain lab results	
	CI 5	Disease state management	
	CI 6	Adminstrative purpose	
	CI 7	Generating exception list	
	CI 8	Patient education	
	CI 9	Note taking	
	CI 10	Drug administration	
	CI 11	Communiation with physicians	
	CI 12	Communication with colleagues	

Upon construct validation, a simple SEM (consolidated) model was developed to test the hypotheses. The model consists of clinical usefulness as the dependent variable, and drivers ("Organizational" (O), "Clinical" (C), and "Management" (M)) and barriers ("Usage" (U), "Technology" (T), and "Resources" (R)" (M) as independent variables. The model was run with AMOS Graph program and the screenshot shown in Figure 2 displays the values along the link from Drivers to Clinical Usefulness, and Barriers to Clinical Usefulness.

Figure 3. Drivers: $X^2 = 37.3$, $df = 25$, $p = 0.054$, $X^2/df = 1.492$, GFI = 0.959, TLI = .900, RMSEA = 0.050 (Data fit the improved model)

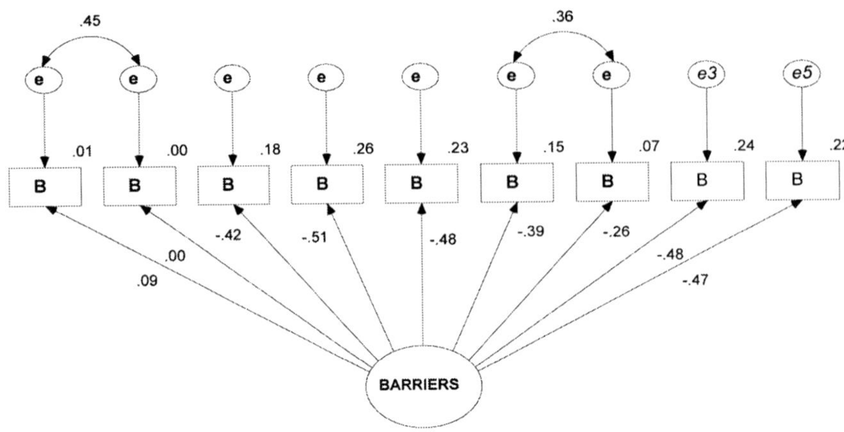

Figure 4. Clinical Usefulness: $X^2 = 30.8$, $df = 12$, $p = 0.054$, $X^2/df = 1.492$, GFI = 0.959, TLI = .900, RMSEA = 0.050 (Data fit the improved model)

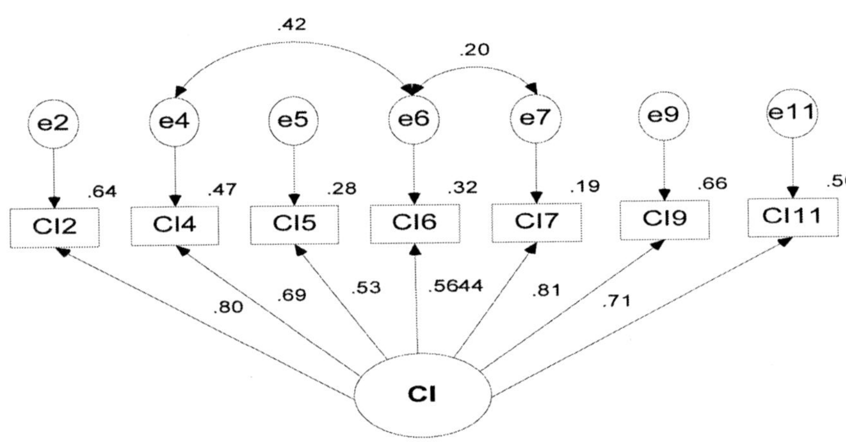

Figure 5. Clinical Usefulness: $X^2 = 9.0$, $df = 7$, $p = 0.252$, $X^2/df = 1.28$, GFI = 0.986, TLI = .992, RMSEA = 0.038 (Data fit the improved model)

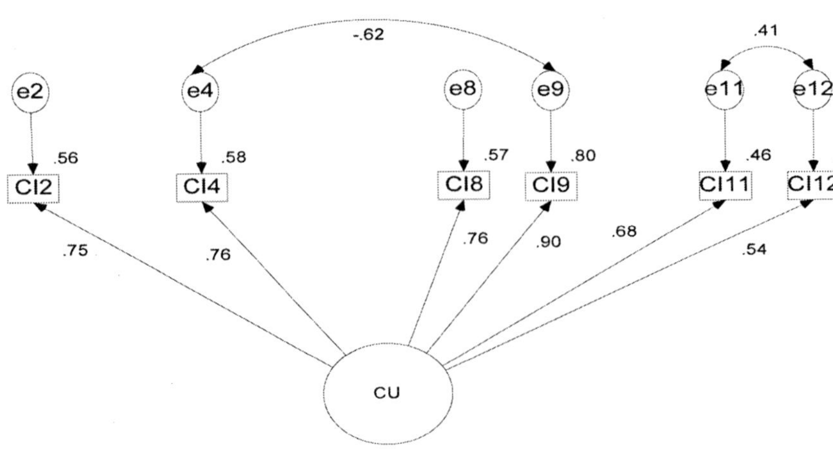

Figure 6. SEM Initial Model: $X^2 = 548.0$, $df = 202$, $p = 0.000$, $X^2/df = 2.713$, GFI = 0.817, TLI = .755, RMSEA = 0.094 (Data did not fit the improved model)

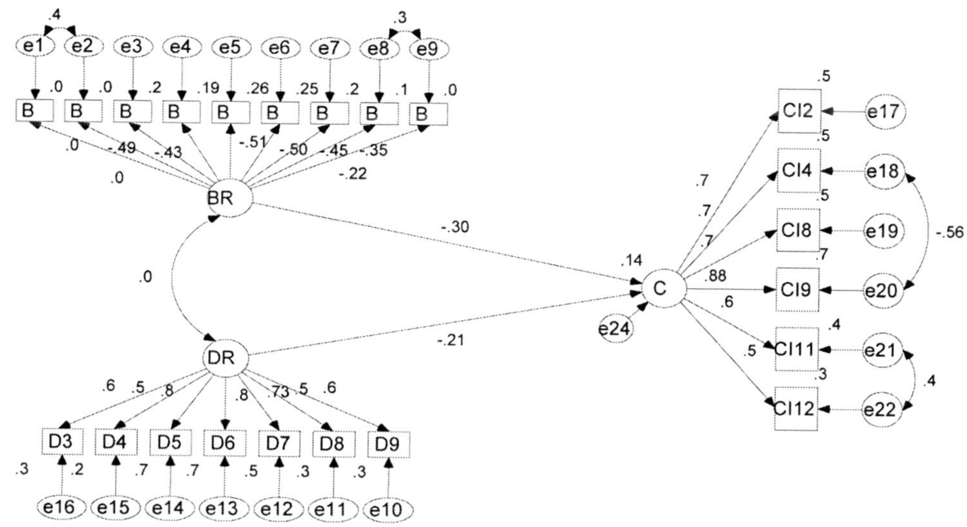

Figure 7. SEM Model: $X^2 = 78.9$, $df = 50$, $p = 0.006$, $X^2/df = 1.577$, GFI = 0.939, TLI = .910, RMSEA = 0.055 (Data fit the improved model)

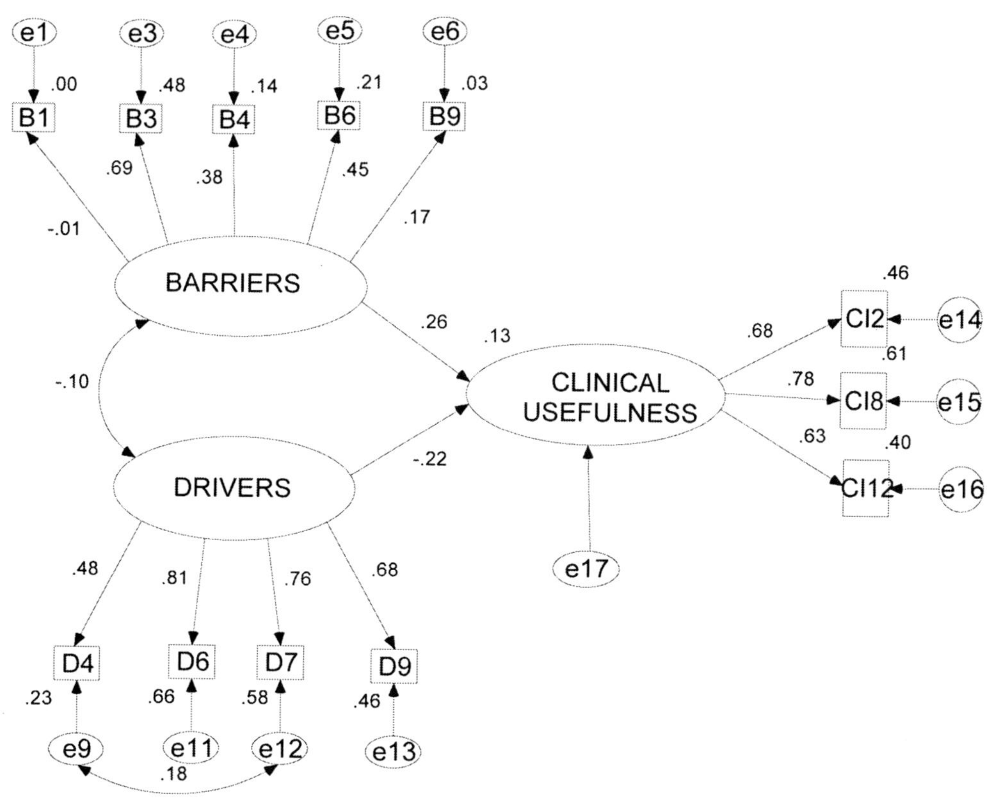

Figure 8. SEM Model: $X^2 = 41.6$, $df = 23$, $p = 0.010$, $X^2/df = 1.810$, GFI = 0.955, TLI = .932, RMSEA = 0.065 (Data fit the improved model)

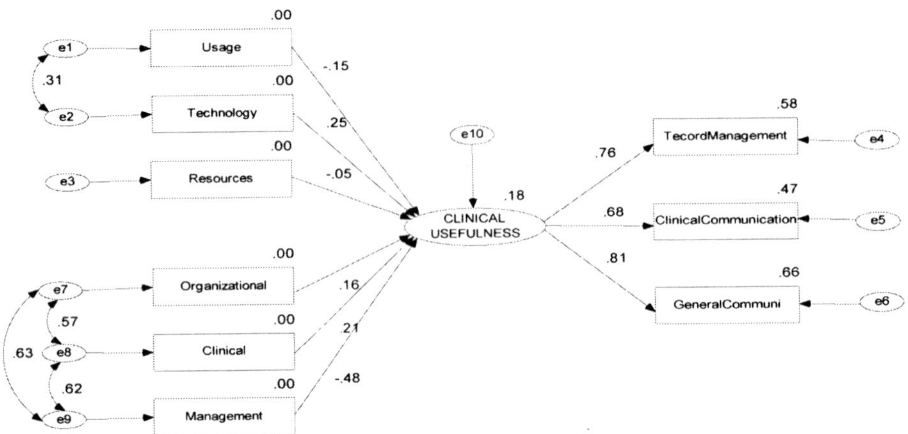

According to (Holmes-Smith, 2000) to analyse a model for the data fit, the following five measurements need to be analysed carefully:

- Chi-square (X^2 acceptable fit: $p > 0.05$)
- Normed Chi-square (X^2/df acceptable fit $1 < X^2/df < 2$)
- Goodness-of-fit index (GFI- acceptable fit value, 0.95<GFI<1, reasonable fit value would be 0.90<GFI<0.95)
- Tucker-Lewis Index (TLI- acceptable value; TLI>0.95; reasonable value of fit 0.9<TLI<0.95 and lack of model parsimony would be TLI>1)
- RootMean-Square Error of Approximation (RMSEA- acceptable fit value: RMSEA<0.05; reasonable level of: 0.05<RMSEA<0.08)

Above criteria was used to analyse the data fit for each of the construct before computing the composite variables. The Figures show the values of each variable separately for initial model and the improved acceptable model for each of the composite model.

Data Reduction and Technique for Compatibility Variable

Diagrams 1, 2 and 3 shows the data fit for the improve model. This was achieved by appropriate after the analysis of the suggestions provided "Modification Indies" provided by SEM along with the analysis of the adequate theoretical support. Objective was to achieve the improved measure of data fit for the empirical data while keeping integrity of the theoretical support. Results shows that changes in the model has resulted all the five indicator showed that empirical data fitted the improve measurement model.

Once the data reduction techniques was used to individual variables and data was found to fit as per (Holmes-Smith, 2000) incies, we draw the initial SEM model with Barriers (B) and Drivers (D) as an independent variables and "clinical Usefulness (CU) as dependent variable in the model.

As can been seen from Figure 4 above five of the popular measured provided by (Holmes-Smith, 2000) is provided under the diagram. First two values (Chi-square, and Normed Chi-square) were not at acceptable level, however values of other three (Goodness-of-fit index, Tucker-Lewis Index, and RootMean-Square Error of Approximation) were not at acceptable level. It was concluded that the data did not adequately fit the model.

Diagram 5 shows the data fit for the improve model. This was achieved by appropriate after the analysis of the suggestions provided "Modification Indies" provided by SEM along with the analysis of the adequate theoretical support. Objective was to achieve the improved measure of data fit for the empirical data while keeping integrity of the theoretical support. Results shows that changes in the model has resulted all the five indicator showed that empirical data fitted the improve measurement model.

The diagram in the above figure provide the visual results of aggregating the items of the measurement model of stage two of the process, which provided the evidence for the data fit the model for the empirical data. As a result we produced a composite variable for "Drivers", "Barriers", and "Clinical Influences" in the complete model for the existing data in order to analyse the influence of drivers and barriers on the clinical influences. Data fit of the model and the indices measures are $X^2 = 41.6$, df = 23, $p = 0.010$, $X^2/df = 1.810$, GFI = 0.955, TLI = .932, and RMSEA = 0.065.

In the above diagram, the latent variable "Clinical Influences" (CI), set of possible predictors, "Usage" (U), "Technology" (T), "Resources" (R), "Organizational" (O), "Clinical" (C), and "Management" (M) are the observed variables. CI is itself indicated by three items, "Technological Management" (TM), "Clinical Communication" (CC), and "General Communication" (GC). As can be seen, the overall structural model fit was good. Criteria used to determined: $X^2 = 41.6$, with 23 df, $X^2/df = 1.810$, CFI = , AIC = , GFI = 0.955, TLI = .932, and RMSEA = 0.065,. Based on these results we proceeded to test the two hypothesis mentioned above (H1, and H2) previously proposed. These hypotheses stated that drivers have positive impact and barrier have negative impact on the clinical usefulness. The result supported theses hypothesis, for example in the case of drivers, "Organizational, ($t=1.56, p>0.01$)", "Clinical, ($t=2.14$, $p < 0.01$)", and "Management, ($t=4.4$, $p < 0.01$)" shows that clinical and management drivers are positively contributing to the clinical usefulness, where as the contribution of organizational is not significant. Whereas barrier have vary limited scope, "Usage, ($t= -1.98, p > 0.01$)", "Technology, ($t=3.13, p<0.01$)", and "Resources, ($t= -0.685$, $p > 0.01$)". Drivers and barriers are the predictive of the clinical usefulness; results indicate that drivers have stronger influence on the clinical usefulness of the wireless technology than the barrier.

DISCUSSIONS

The Confirmatory Factor Analysis agrees with the outcomes derived from the interview qualitative data in that the set of drivers, barriers and clinical influences are indeed the determinants of wireless technology in the Indian healthcare. Within these three determinants, we are able to identify usage, technology and resources influencing the clinical usefulness. The predictor 'usage' is influenced by the usefulness of technology as identified in recent studies. This study also conforms to the notion that 'ease of use' is not a major influence on technology adoption in the Indian healthcare.

In terms of clinical usefulness, we are able to assert that record management, clinical communication and general communication to be the three major aspects. Our qualitative study had already given us some indication to these predictors. Our interviews revealed that the greatest benefits of wireless technology in clinical settings would be records management because it is possible for clinicians to access patient data at the point of care. We also understood that it is possible to use smart phone type technology to send patient conditions to other clinicians in order to get advice. In terms of general communication, our interview transcripts indicate that it si now possible to provide patient education using the wireless technology.

Thus, wireless technology can be used to facilitate access to clinical information and communications between clinicians, maximise clinician time, increase patient safety, and accomplish the strategic and business goals of health organisations. Taken together, these factors have a direct impact on clinical usefulness and its effectiveness. However, achieving clinical usefulness with wireless handheld devices can be a challenge and has several implications.

Firstly, the highest security standards must be achieved. This includes direct end-to-end data encryption, authentication, authorisation, maintenance of audit logs and session management (Chen et al. 2004). While high security standards are essential, their implementation is likely to affect usability. For example, the download and encryption of patient information from the server where it is stored into a wireless handheld device may not be prompt. Sax et al. (2005) argue that clinicians may experience increasingly longer time lags when they carry out increasingly more complex procedures. This is likely to adversely affect clinical usefulness and, hence, decrease user acceptance.

Closely associated with security is also the issue of patient confidentiality, which is of significant importance and concern. Although wireless handheld devices have locking security features and password protection functions which activate during periods of inactivity, the frequent use of these functions during the clinicians' busy daily schedules may have an impact on clinical usefulness.

A crucial lesson learnt in this study was in the use of qualitative and quantitative components. We approached the healthcare professionals to seek their opinions on the benefits of using wireless technology. This stage was followed up with a survey instrument. We conducted a first order regression analysis to regress the 90 or so factors explored into a set of manageable factors. The lesson was quite valuable because as outsiders (coming from an Information Systems background), we were able to appreciate the complexities of healthcare information systems. Similarly, our open minded approach enabled healthcare professionals to appreciate IS related aspects. We also found out through our informal discussions that the study would have been a stereo-type study had we approached a quan-qual type mixed method because we would have been restricted by what was available in the literature to derive our quan part and this would have restricted our qual part.

To our own surprise, we found both IS and health literature to be limited in catching up with wireless technology related attitude and perception data. While the technology literature such as the IEEE provided us with the technical knowledge, human aspects have not yet been discussed in IS and healthcare literature. The results established through a second order regression are consistent with what we found for the Australian Healthcare (published elsewhere).

We measured only perceptions and attitudes in this study. While there is sufficient information available through interviews on the type of savings and benefits that can be attained by using wireless technology in healthcare, it is still not clear as to the exact quantification of these. Therefore, it would be useful to measure this by employing a wireless technology in a clinical setting and then collecting some evidence as to the savings and benefits.

REFERENCES

Athey, S., & Stern, S. (2002). The impact of information technology on emergency health care outcomes. *The Rand Journal of Economics*, *33*, 399–388. doi:10.2307/3087465

Chau, P. Y. K., & Hu, P. J.-H. (2002). Investigating healthcare professionals' decision to accept telemedicine technology: An empirical test of competing theories. *Information & Management*, *39*,297–311. doi:10.1016/S0378-7206(01)00098-2

Chismar, W. R., & Wiley-Patton, S. (2006). Predicting Internet Use: Applying teh Extended Technology Acceptance Model to the Healthcare Environment. In Spil, T. A. M., & Schuring, R. W. (Eds.), *E-Health Systems Diffusion and USe: The Innovation, the USer and the USE IT Model*. Hershey, PA, USA: IGI Global.

Davies, F. D., Bagozzi, R. P., & Warshaw, P. R. (1989). User acceptance of computer technology: A comparison of two theoretical models. *Communications of the ACM, 35*, 982–1003.

Davis, R. (2002). Pursue front end solutions to revenue problems. *Healthcare Financial Management, 56*, 30–36.

Dyer, O. (2003). Patients will be reminded of appointments by text messages. *British Medical Journal, 326*, 281.

Gururajan, R., Hafeez-Baig, A., & Gururjan, V. (2008). Clinical Factors And Technological Barriers As Determinants For The Intention To Use Wireless Handheld Technology In Healthcare Environment: An Indian Case Study. In *16th European Conference on Information Systems*, National University of Ireland, Galway.

Gururajan, R., Moloney, C., & Kerr, D. (2005). Drivers for wireless handheld technology: Views from Queensland nurses. In *Australian Business & Behavioural Sciences Association (ABBSA) Conference,* Cairns, Australia, James Cook University (pp. 258-267).

Gururajan, R., Quaddus, M., Fink, D., et al. (2005). Drivers and Barriers to adoption of wireless handheld system in WA healthcare: Selected views. In *HIC 2005*. Melbourne, HISA.

Gururajan, R., Toleman, M., & Soar, J. (2004, July 25-27). Necessity for a new technology acceptance model to predict adoption of wireless technology in healthcare. In *Let's Make a Difference with Health ICT, HIC Conference*. Health Informatics Society of Australia (HISA).

Hafeez-Baig, A. (2007). Technology Management, Data management, Improved outcomes, Efficiency and Software limitation influencing the use of wireless technology for healthcare in Pakistan. In *6th IEEE/ACIS International Conference on Computer and Information Science (ICIS 2007)* (pp. 1104-1110), Melbourne: IEEE.

Holmes-Smith, P. (2000). *Introduction to Structural Equation Modeling Using AMOS 4.0*. Melbourne: SREAMS.

Horan, T. A., Tule, B., & Hilton, B. N. (2006). Understanding physician use of online systems: An empirical assessment of an electronic disability evaluation system. In Spil, T. A. M., & Schuring, W. R. (Eds.), *E-Health Systems Diffusion and Use: The Innovation, the User and the USE IT Model*. Hershey, PA, USA: IGI Global.

Howard, A., Gururajan, R., Hafeez-Baig, A., et al. (2006). Clinical Usefulness of Wireless Technology in Healthcare: An Indian Study. In *The Australasian Conference on Information Systems*, University of South Australia.

Hu, P. J., Chau, P. Y. K., & Liu, S. O. R. (2002). Adoption of telemedicine technology by health care organisations: An exploratory study. *Journal of Organizational Computing and Electronic Commerce, 12*, 197–222. doi:10.1207/S15327744JOCE1203_01

Hu, P. J., Chau, P. Y. K., & Tam, K. Y. (1999). Examining teh technologya cceptance model using physician acceptance of telemedicine technology. *Journal of Management Information Systems, 16*, 91–112.

Ivers, B., & Gururajan, R. (2006). Management issues in telecommunications: videoconferencing & telehealth. In *International Conference on Recent Trends in Information Systems Proceedings* (pp. 796-806), India: Allied Publishers Pvt Ltd.

Jayasuriya, R. (1998). Determinants of microcomputer technology use: Implications for education and training of health staff. *International Journal of Medical Informatics*, *50*, 187–194. doi:10.1016/S1386-5056(98)00067-7

Lapointe, L., Lamothe, L., & Fortin, J. (2006). The dynamics of IT adoption in a major change process in healthcare delivery. In Spil, T. A. M., & Schuring, R. W. (Eds.), *E-Health Systems Diffusion and Use: The Innovation, the User and the USE IT Model*. Hershey, PA, USA: IGI Global.

Mingers, J. (2001). Combining IS research methods: Towards a pluralist methodology. *Information Systems Research*, *12*, 240–259. doi:10.1287/isre.12.3.240.9709

Myers, M. D. (1997). Qualitative research in Information Systems. *Management Information Systems Quarterly*, *21*, 241–242. doi:10.2307/249422

Reinecke, I. (2004). *Managing Information in Health*. Melbourne National Health Information Summit.

Rogoski, R. (2003). Wireless by Design. *Health Management Technology*, 1–7.

Sausser, G.D. (n.d.). Thin is in: web-based systems enhance security, clinical quality. *Healthcare Financial Management, 57*, 86-88.

Simpson, R. L. (2003). The patient's point of view -- IT matters. *Nursing Administration Quarterly*, *27*, 254–256.

Siracuse, M. V., Pharm, D., & Sowell, J. G. (2008). Doctor of Pharmacy Students' Use of Personal Digital Assistant. *American Journal of Pharmaceutical Education*, *72*, 1–7.

Spil, T. A. M., & Schuring, R. W. (2006). *E-Health system diffusion and use*. Hershey, PA, USA: IGI Global.

Stuart, D., & Bawany, K. (2001). *Wireless Services*. UK: Gartner.

Suomi, R. (2006). Introducing electronic patient records to hospitals: Innovation adoption paths. In Spil, T. A. M., & Schuring, W. R. (Eds.), *E-Health Systems Diffusion and Use: The Innovation, the User and the USE IT Model*. Hershey, PA, USA: IGI Global.

Turisco, F. (2000). Mobile computing is next technology frontier for health providers. *Healthcare Financial Management*, *54*, 78–82.

Venkatesh, V., Morris, M. G., & Davis, G. B. (2003). User Acceptance of Information Technology: Toward A Unified View. *Management Information Systems Quarterly*, *27*, 425–478.

Versel, N. (2008). Use of Mobile and Wireless Technology Jumps in Hospitals. *Digital HealthCare*. Retrieved from http://www.digitalhcp.com/DigitalHealthCare_Content.aspx?id=72018

Wisnicki, H. J. (2002). Wireless networking transforms healthcare: physician's practices better able to handle workflow, increase productivity (The human connection). *Ophthalmology Times*, *27*, 38–41.

Wu, K., & Wu, X. (2007). A Wireless Mobile Monitoring System for Home Healthcare and Community Medical Services. In the 1st International Conference on Bioinformatics and Biomedical Engineering (ICBBE) (pp. 1190-1193).

Zhang, D. (2007). Web content adaptation for mobile handheld devices. *Communications of the ACM*, *50*, 75–79. doi:10.1145/1216016.1216024

Zikmund, W. (1994). *Business research methods* (International Ed. Edition). Orlando, FL: The Dryden Press.

This work was previously published in International Journal of Healthcare Delivery Reform Initiatives, edited by Matthew W. Guah, pp. 19-37, copyright 2009 by IGI Publishing (an imprint of IGI Global).

Chapter 12
Adoption of Mobile Technology by Public Healthcare Doctors:
A Developing Country Perspective

Nesaar Banderker
University of Cape Town, South Africa

Jean-Paul Van Belle
University of Cape Town, South Africa

ABSTRACT

South African doctors working in the public healthcare sector are faced with the unique resource constraints prevalent in a developing country. Mobile information and communication technologies (ICTs) hold the promise of improving the quality of healthcare, but this potential can only be unlocked if individuals decide to adopt the new technologies. Understanding the factors that influence the doctor's adoption of a technology is therefore vital. This article reports on an investigation into the factors influencing the adoption of mobile devices by doctors in the public healthcare sector in the Western Cape, South Africa. The research methodology was shaped by qualitative enquiry and described through thematic analysis. The authors confirmed the key adoption factors identified in prior research: job relevance, usefulness, perceived user resources and device characteristics. However, some additional adoption factors were uncovered in this research, namely patient influence, support structures from national government and hospital administration, and unease in respect of malpractice legal suits.

DOI: 10.4018/978-1-60960-183-6.ch012

BACKGROUND

Healthcare in South Africa

Healthcare is a key component of South African society, socially and economically (Chiasson et al., 2004). Total healthcare spending in South Africa is 8.7% of GDP which is substantially above the norm of 5% recommended for developing countries by the WHO (Chetty, 2007). The *public* healthcare budget alone totalled R47.8 billion (approximately US$ 6.7 billion) in 2006, representing 4.27% of GDP. This represents a substantial growth compared with 1995 when it stood at only 1.84% of GDP. However, despite these efforts by the new democratically elected government, huge inequalities remain. The budget of the private sector, which services less than 8 million people, exceeds that of the public sector servicing 38 million (Chetty, 2007). Much of this remains a legacy of the pre-1994 apartheid era inequalities institutionalised through labour laws and highly unequal provision of services for different racial groups (Department of Health, 2004). There is still a movement of skilled resources from areas of poverty and low socio-economic development to more wealthy areas. Doctors who have recently qualified and completed their compulsory two years working for the public healthcare sector are either moving into private practice or leaving South Africa to work in other countries (Padarath et al., 2003). This results in a scarcity of skilled clinical resources in the public healthcare sector.

Although doctors working in the public healthcare sector are highly skilled, their available time is preciously sliced to try and diagnose and care for as many patients in a day as is possible. 80 to 85% of the South African population has access to public healthcare facilities only (Chetty, 2007). A doctor in the public day hospital environment is expected to diagnose, treat and manage about 40 patients during an 8–hour shift. This means that the doctor spends an average of only 12 minutes with each patient. Doctors in public healthcare also have to work extremely long shifts of sometimes more than 30 hours. Due to this extreme pressure, doctors can easily make an incorrect diagnosis or prescribe the incorrect patient management routine. Patients attending these public hospitals have to wait in long queues to be seen by the doctor. When they finally see the doctor, the visit is rushed. A full examination of the patient is not always possible and this could result in inadequate care of the patient.

ICTs offer tremendous potential in supporting the public healthcare function in the South African society. Although administrative healthcare information systems have been implemented, the shift to systems that support the clinical work performed by healthcare professionals directly has been slow to take off (Andersen, 1997). Better ICT support would, in turn, enable doctors to facilitate the provision of high quality, better informed and cost-effective public healthcare to all the citizens of South Africa.

Mobile Technologies in Healthcare

Mobile technologies can bring immense benefits to the healthcare environment (Varshney, 2006), because it is so information intensive (Li, Chang, Hung & Fu 2005). Doctors do most of their work at the point of care, which is the patient. This means that they move around between wards, outpatient clinics, diagnostic and therapeutic departments and operating theatres. This movement, together with the fact that most South African public hospitals usually only have one central computer terminal per ward, makes it extremely difficult to service all the needs of the doctor. The use of ICTs in support of this point of care activity of the doctor is what is relevant to this research. Mobile device technologies are quite suitable for supporting the doctor at the point of care. They are small, lightweight, can be carried around with the doctor and usually come with some form of networking protocol built into the device (Porn & Patrick, 2002). Mobile devices are also becoming more affordable and offer more processing power and storage capabilities (Varshney, 2006). Mobile technology ranges from cellular telephones, pagers and PDAs, to very sophisticated tablet computers. Key benefits, as summarized from a large number of studies, include a reduction in medical errors, time savings, better quality care and higher productivity (Lu, Xiao, Sears & Jacko, 2005).

A number of studies have looked at adoption of mobile computing devices. An excellent, systematic analysis of surveys of healthcare providers' PDA adoption is given by Garritty & Emam (2006) who found adoption rates in developed countries to vary between 45% and 85%. For instance, in a longitudinal study of mobile technology 33% of Canadian doctors reported use of a mobile device in their clinical practice in 2003, up from 19% in 2001 and 28% 2002 (Martin, 2003). By contrast, a similar study at selected healthcare institutions in Florida revealed that as many as 95% of the respondents to the survey owned a mobile computing device (Joy & Benrubi, 2004). The study also showed a pattern of perceived benefit for using the devices to maintain procedural statistic logs, pharmacology reference manuals and personal clinical protocols; but respondents did not perceive a massive time saving. Both studies also show quite a sharp increase in mobile device technology adoption by doctors.

Porn and Patrick (2002) and Hameed (2003) identify a number of healthcare applications that could be run successfully on a mobile device:

E-Prescription

This allows doctors to access basic patient information and check formulary compliance before writing the prescription. Potentially harmful drug interactions can be determined and often a patient's personal medication history is available. Prescriptions can be printed or transmitted directly to a pharmacy. The main benefits are a reduction in medication errors and less calls from pharmacies due to illegible handwriting (Berkowitz, 2002).

Charge Capture

This application allows a doctor to view schedules, capture patient charges and access or update patient information all at the point of care.

Order Entry

Applications to order certain tests could be scheduled, delivered to a central processing unit and acted upon. This will reduce errors due to misplacement of application forms.

Test Result Reporting

The results of the tests can be delivered directly to the mobile device. This will free doctors from having to refer to a specific PC workstation to retrieve test results.

Medical Information

Access to the latest medication formulary, disease description, symptoms and treatment as well as access to clinical procedures can be provided on a mobile device.

More technical descriptions of how mobile technologies can work in healthcare sector can be found in numerous sources, e.g. (Varshney, 2006)

Adoption Models and Healthcare

In order to realise the full potential and promise of healthcare information systems, technologies and applications, a better understanding of the organisational context as well as people and social issues is required. The adoption of mobile technologies in the healthcare sector involves both an organisational and an individual aspect. The organisational context or motivational factors that drive mobile ICT adoption is a relatively under-researched field; refer to Khoumbati & Themistocleous (2006) for an overview of relevant research and a comprehensive framework.

The focus in this research is on the *individual factors* that drive mobile technology adoption in healthcare, with particularly focus on the doctors.

Because explaining human behaviour in all its complexity is quite a daunting task, a variety of models have been developed to explain and predict user behaviours and intentions. The most widely used of these models are the diffusion of innovation (DOI) theory published by Rogers (1995), the theory of reasoned action (TRA) (Ajzen & Fishbein, 1980), the theory of planned behaviour (TPB) (Ajzen, 1991) and the technology acceptance model (TAM) (Davis, 1989). These models have been well tested, validated and proven to be reliable when used in the evaluation of user acceptance in studies of business organisations, corporations and even students. However, there is less research evaluating technology adoption using TPB, TRA, DOI within a healthcare context.

In validating TAM and its extensions, researchers have determined some key factors that are of significance for use in general technology adoption models. These include perceived ease of use, perceived usefulness, perceived user resources, voluntariness, experience, subjective norm, image and computer self-efficacy. However, doctors are professionals who are particularly highly skilled, knowledgeable, autonomous and pragmatic decision makers. This impacts on the applicability of a number of constructs and causes some of the models not to behave in the way determined by prior research in other contexts. For instance, Hu & Chau & Tam (1999) found that the original TAM did not correlate well with doctor's intentions to use a new technology. When reviewing literature on the adoption of healthcare technologies by medical professionals the majority of the studies found apply to general healthcare systems such as telemedicine, internet health and clinical systems (Chau & Hu 2002, Chismar & Patton, 2003, Horan et al., 2004) while some studies were found that applied specifically to mobile healthcare (Wu, Wang, & Lin, 2005, Harkke, 2005; Li et al., 2005; Lu et al., 2005; Varshney, 2006; Wu, Wang & Lin, 2007).

Overall, however, researchers find the TAM-inspired models to be a successful approach to explaining the adoption of mobile technologies in the healthcare sector, with Wu et al., (2007) purporting to be able to explain up to 70% of the variance in behavioural intention to use mobile healthcare systems. These studies found the following factors to be of relevance when researching adoption in a healthcare setting:

- **Perceived usefulness/Job relevance:** A new technology needs to be useful to its user. Usefulness is defined as causing an increase in the doctor's productivity by being relevant to the doctor.
- **Perceived user resources:** The extent to which an individual believes that they have the personal and organisational support to use the device. This was validated by Horan et al. (2004) and Lu et al. (2005) whose research discovered that workplace compatibility played a more important role in predicting user intentions than the current TAM construct of perceived ease of use.
- **Subjective norm:** People who are close to the doctor could influence the doctor by their opinions of whether the device should be used or not.
- **Image:** Doctors will perceive the use of a mobile technology device as enhancing their status within their working environment. This was validated by Succi and Walter (1999) who state that doctors will more likely be influenced by the impact of the use of the new technology on their professional status. Further research has contested the idea that social processes of subjective norm and image would influence the decision to adopt. This is seen to be a result of the pragmatic nature of doctors in decision making, as well as a reli-

ance on their own assessment rather than that of others. However, in the context of South Africa where being a medical doctor is often seen as a status symbol the two factors of subjective norm and image will be retained to ascertain whether they would play a positively influencing role.

- **Task/technology fit:** A study by Chau & Hu (2002), added this factor – defined as alignment with current work practices – to TAM. It was thought that doctors would more likely adopt a new technology if it aligned closely with their current work practices.
- **Result demonstrability:** The technology should visibly improve the doctor's quality of care provided and enhance his effectiveness thus improving the quality of the doctor's work

Furthermore, in the evaluation of TAM2 (Venkatesh & Davis, 2000) by Chismar and Patton (2003), it was found that the construct of perceived ease of use showed an insignificant effect when used to predict intention of doctors. It has also been found that for technologies that are not mandated for use by the healthcare institutions, the construct of voluntariness can be removed from the model. In studies of a new technology the construct of experience can also be removed, since it was intended to measure the adoption of existing technologies. Due to the high intellectual and cognitive capacity of doctors, they appear to understand new technologies quicker. Doctors are therefore individuals with a high level of self-efficacy. This makes a good argument for the removal of the computer self-efficacy construct from the model. However, due to mobile technologies being relatively new to the South African market and not being widely diffused this factor will be included in the model developed.

The above research reduces the significant factors in the context of doctors' intention to use a mobile technology device to subjective norm, image, task/technology fit, result demonstrability, perceived user resources, computer self-efficacy and the technology device characteristics. These factors are summarized graphically in Figure 1.

The factors listed above formed the starting point for the research interviews.

Figure 1. Significant influencing factors

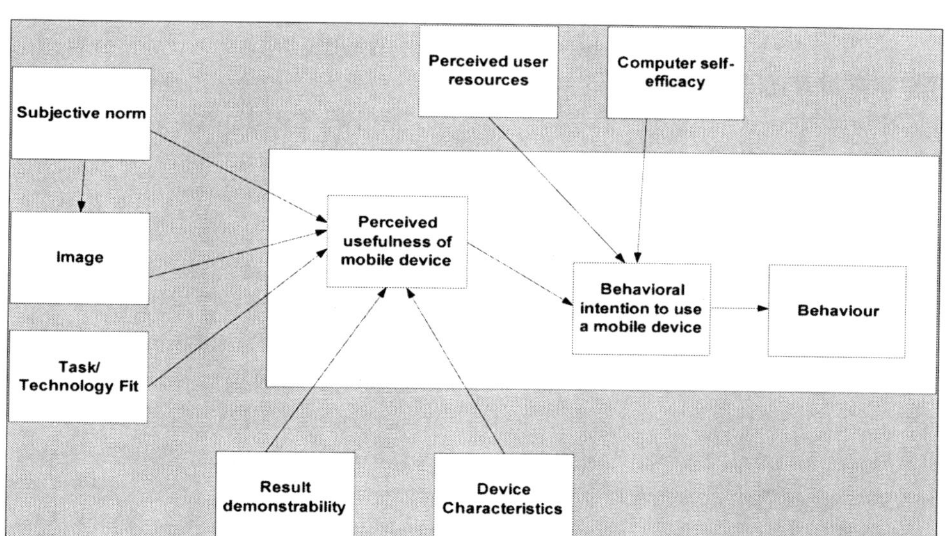

RESEARCH OBJECTIVE

Despite the purported advantages of mobile technology there is a distinct lack of adoption of this technology in the public healthcare sector in developing countries in general, and South Africa in particular. The public healthcare sector is recognized as having lagged behind other South African industries, such as the financial sector, in the use and adoption of new information technologies (Bower, 2005). ICTs encompass a wide range of technologies.

This research hopes to provide a better view as to *what* the significant factors influencing the adoption of innovative mobile technology solutions by public healthcare doctors to support them in their daily clinical activity are. More specifically, the objective of this research is to identify key factors that hinder or assist doctors' adoption of mobile technologies in healthcare.

Identifying these significant factors of influence will hopefully also provide an *insight* into how ICT solutions for healthcare should be developed, marketed, implemented and who the key stakeholders in the adoption process are. This research is particularly relevant because it cannot be assumed that research conducted in developed world contexts is applicable to developing countries.

RESEARCH METHODOLOGY

The factors identified in the literature (see figure 1) forms the basis for the framework that could be tested against public healthcare doctors. This section addresses the problems of *who* to test the framework against and *how* it will be tested.

Strategy

This research follows an exploratory qualitative research design strategy. It is exploratory since it is not directly involved with hypothesis testing and theory evaluation. It is more directly involved with laying a basic descriptive foundation to explain and understand the possible factors influencing adoption of a mobile technology device by doctors. A qualitative study was chosen over a quantitative one since the former allows for a better understanding of the people, and the social and cultural context in which the technology adoption can occur. Also, richer data sets from which factors influencing the possible adoption of mobile technologies can be obtained by discourse between people instead of having them complete a questionnaire. We believe that our specific qualitative approach complements the quantitative approach adopted by (Wu et al., 2007) who summarized a large number of quantitative adoption studies, and the evidence/opinion-based qualitative approach of (Lu et al., 2005) into adoption factors.

Site Selection and Sampling

The study was conducted in the two largest public healthcare facilities in Cape Town, namely the Groote Schuur Hospital (widely known because of the first heart transplant) and Tygerberg Hospital. These hospital are directly associated with the University of Cape Town and the University of Stellenbosch respectively. They are of similar size, offer very similar services, have similar administrative processes and are analogous to the rest of South Africa's academic public hospitals.

Due to time, resource and financial constraints as well as the limited time availability of doctors, a convenience sampling method was used. Possible doctors were identified by two doctors acting as the researcher's contacts in the hospitals and were selected based on their willingness to take part in the research since all participation was voluntary. Although a convenience sample allowed the researcher to skirt many of the resource issues mentioned, this did come at the expense of possibly compromising the generalisability and representativeness (Pare, 2004). In total, twelve doctors were interviewed. The interview sample was made up of doctors from each of the South African racial profiles.

Data Collection

Participant interviews were used as the primary source of gathering data. The interviews were semi-structured, with set questions as well as open-ended questions. Basic demographic data was also collected from the doctors. Key questions were developed around all the significant factors of influence identified during the literature review (Figure 1 above) with additional questions being derived from Chismar and Patton (2003). Questions were not necessarily asked in the order they were set out since the conversation dictated which question would be asked next. The complete list of the questions is available from the authors. A checklist was kept during the interview to ensure that all questions were asked. Interaction and discussion usually led to further follow-up questions of both explanatory and exploratory nature (Ritchie & Lewis, 2003).

The interview was recorded on an audio recording device, freeing up the interviewer to more closely observe the interviewee and possibly gain some further insight from the visual clues provided by the interviewee. A protocol for conducting the interview was established. This ensured that each interview process was consistent. It also helped ensure that standard items like obtaining consent, providing the interviewee with basic information about the research and informing them that the interview would be recorded, would not be forgotten.

As a departure point for starting the discussion, pictures of other mobile technology devices were shown to the interviewees. In addition, the interviewees were also shown a physical Nokia 9300 with a demonstration of some of the medical software obtained for the device, namely a drug formulary program, a fracture analysis program and a nutrition analysis program.

Data Analysis

There are many methods of analysis suggested for the interpretation of the data collected. These include Hermeneutics (Klein & Myers, 1999), Grounded Theory (Sarker & Wells, 2003), Semiotics – which includes content analysis, conversation analysis and discourse analysis – and thematic analysis (Ritchie & Lewis, 2003). However, these modes of analysis work to develop theory in most cases and fit closely with the interpretive paradigm (Fitzgerald & Howcroft, 1998). A thematic analysis of the textual data was performed, as recommended by Ritchie and Lewis (2003).

The analysis process that was followed can be described as follows:

- The recorded data from the interviews was listened to. While listening to the recording, reflective remarks about the interview and the data from the interview were made. This allowed for the visualization of the researcher's perceptions and ideas (Miles & Huberman, 1994).
- A coding scheme that is consistent with the theoretical propositions identified during the literature review was then developed (Hammersley & Atkinson, 1983). Additional codes were created for ideas presented by the interviewee that did not fit into the original coding scheme.
- The coding scheme was used to allow the segmentation of the data into units that are easily mapped to the theoretical propositions identified during the literature review. The scheme also allows for easier organization and retrieval of the data.
- These codes were then grouped together in logical units which formed higher order categories.
- For these categories a response from each interviewee was mapped. This formed the basis of a thematic chart. The visual nature of a thematic chart helped in discover-

ing connections between coded segments (Miles & Huberman, 1994).

- From this thematic chart, themes were developed by checking the occurrence of a certain idea and the language used by the interviewee.
- These themes were then used to answer the objectives of the study.

An important consideration in qualitative research is the reliability of the findings. Although a "mere count" of quotations or mentions is not necessarily an appropriate measure, a strong and consistent pattern across respondents does contribute towards a stronger confidence in the results. It was found that there was indeed a surprising degree of agreement between the various respondents and thus the table with the occurrence frequencies for the various factors has been included (Table 2 in the Appendix).

FINDINGS AND DISCUSSION

The results obtained by the analysis of the interview data as well as a discussion of these results are presented together in order to maintain a logical flow of information. Since the data analysis was done using a thematic analysis, the findings will be presented in the themes identified. These themes can also be referred to as the adoption factors identified.

Postulated Themes

Perceived Usefulness of a Mobile Device

The doctors agreed unanimously that the mobile technology device would be very useful and relevant to them. Two of the older doctors, however, could only conceptualise the device being useful by providing information to them. Even so, the information that they thought the device would be able to provide was of enough importance to warrant them stating that it would help in providing better medical care to their patients. "*I know I would be able to obtain electronic versions of certain reference manuals for such a device and I could use this as a source of information.*"

This use as an information providing tool was confirmed when a doctor emphatically stated that he *"currently carr[ies] 2 to 3 management reference books around with me. I know that there is an electronic version of all 3 books available for the iPaq."*

The younger doctors could conceptualise many other exciting uses for the device. A few of the solutions that really excited the doctors are:

- Making paper records of patients obsolete: *Such a device could make the need for paper records obsolete. All patient information could be stored electronically and accessed from this device and not from the only PC assigned to an entire ward. This will make missing folders and folders not containing up-to-date patient information a thing of the past.*
- Not having to struggle with reading illegible notes and other information: *Doctors handwriting is generally quite poor and illegible. This device could make incorrect prescriptions due to bad writing a thing of the past.*
- Mobility: *Patient information could be delivered to such a device when you walk into the ward. This would alleviate the need to consult the slow, outdated PC assigned to the floor.*
- As a decision support tool: *I will have the latest available patient management information and with this can ensure that the patient is treated correctly.*

However the doctors did strongly indicate that the device would never be able to replace their skill and training and actually make the decision for them.

Most of the imagined uses envisaged by the doctors are a reality in more developed countries. Examples of mobile electronic patient record systems exist (Turisco & Case, 2001). E-prescriptions systems which make the "illegible" handwriting problem of doctors obsolete also exist (Berkowitz 2002). The transmission of real-time patient information using mobile devices and telecommunication infrastructure has been implemented in Sweden and the Netherlands (Wu, Wang, & Lin, 2005). There are also examples of medical reference material on mobile devices being useful in certain situations (Harkke, 2005).

Social Influences

A strong statement *against* the effect of social influences guiding a doctor's decision to use a mobile technology device was made. One of the older doctors hesitated when answering the questions regarding status. When clarifying her hesitation she stated: "*Indian doctors, especially the older ones, were usually recommended by their parents to become a doctor.*" This was usually for the prestige that came with being able to say that one's child is a doctor as well as the desire to have their children "be better off than the parents". This image of the medical profession being one of status was hard to totally avoid for an Indian doctor. The remainder of the doctors did not agree with the statement that status, image or peer influence will have some bearing on their decision to use the device. "*I would not at all be influenced to use this device by my peers nor would I think of it as increasing my status.*"

There was one softly conflicting statement of "*...as more doctors start using these devices you will become the odd one out for not using one...*" but when explored further it developed into the fact that doctors would only use the device when found to be useful and relevant to their daily clinical activity: "*If I see a colleague using such a device and he is able to provide better care to his patients I would most definitely be influenced to get one.*"

Perceived User Resources

When asking the interviewees questions around perceived user resources, they were quite emphatic that they did not believe they would obtain support for the use of a mobile technology device from within the public healthcare environment. There was a feeling of hopelessness when talking about the public hospitals IT support structures. One aspect of the lack of support related to the level of skills: "*I believe that the hospital IT department is not highly skilled and would take some time to adjust to support a more innovative device like this Nokia 9300.*" It was also felt that the hospital IT department was under-resourced and would not be able to cope with the added support required for the mobile technology device:

They barely cope with just running the daily activities of the hospital. How will they cope with the added support required for this device?

Even though doctors felt that public hospitals did not have the resources to support the use of such a device, they would not be negatively influenced by this:

The hospital might not support the device but that still will not stop me from using it.

The doctors also felt they had the necessary personal resources and skill to use the device.

The University [...] needed an online MMed program for family medicine. The university provided a very basic infrastructure to do this and the doctors lecturing in the department did all of the rest to provide this online program."

Computer Self-Efficacy

All the doctors interviewed considered themselves to be highly skilled professionals who had daily interaction with computers. "*I have an interaction with computers throughout my working day.*" The fact that 10 of the 12 doctors did not have much prior experience with mobile technology devices did not scare them away from using the device: "*As a highly skilled professional I think I am capable of learning to use a new technology from a user manual.*"

Device Characteristics

Ten doctors expressed an initial concern that the limited screen size of the handheld devices might make it less useful: "*Perhaps the screen on this device would not be able display information very legibly*" and "*I don't think a web page will display very nice on such a small screen*". However, some were quite surprised at the amount of information displayed with the drug formulary program on the Nokia 9300: "*That displays information in a very comprehensive manner and with one click of page down you can see the rest of the information.*"

There was a surprising request that the device be able to withstand small liquid chemical spills from the pathology doctors. This was due to the fact that they work with chemicals for most of their day and would probably leave the device lying around near chemicals. "*Would the device be able to withstand a chemical spills?*" The fact that it could not withstand substantial liquid spills and therefore liquid chemical spills even less did not detract from their eagerness to use the device. "*Ok, so it can't. I don't think that this will stop me using it*"

Both loss and theft of the device was also a major consideration for the doctors. "*I think such a device would easily be able to get feet.*" However, the two doctors who were high adopters of a mobile technology device said that doctors would have to learn to take care of the device in a similar manner in which they care for their stethoscopes.

The software demonstrated to the doctors was accepted with great enthusiasm. "*That could most definitely help me as a look up when I don't know what the drug does*" and "*You could look up side effects to make certain there will be no complications for the patient.*" The doctors were enthusiastic that the technology would be able to help them deliver better quality care. This is supported by the uses they conceptualised for the device. One of the doctors working in an emergency trauma unit, where rapid diagnosis and accurate patient management are essential, was sure that a mobile device could further ensure that patient management was in line with the diagnosis as well as being the most effective one and aiding in the fight for the patient's life.

Emerging Themes

A number of additional themes were identified during the analysis of the interview data. They do not form part of the original significant factors of influence identified during the literature review and appear to be specific to the healthcare environment.

Patient Influence

An addition to the social influences theme that was not part of the original significant factors was the patients' perceptions of the doctor if they should see the doctor using a mobile technology device. When talking about a patient's perception of the doctor if the patient should see the doctor using a mobile technology device to reference information from, there was a majority consensus that the patient's perception would *not* negatively influence their decision to use the device. This was conveyed strongly through statements like: "*It will help me improve the care and management provided to the patient and result in a much improved patient outcome*"; "*I will not mind at all to use the device to look up information in front of a patient*" or "*Patients should understand or be educated that having the latest information available as a reference tool will be of great benefit to them at the end of the day*".

However, two doctors did say that they would be hesitant to use the device while sitting with the patient: "*The patients might question my competence if they see me looking up information in front of them with this device. The same goes for looking up information from a book.*" However, that would not stop them from using the mobile device to look up information, just that they would not do it while the patient was sitting with them. "*I would most definitely use it when not in front of a patient*" or "*If I needed to look up information then and there I would go to another room and then come back.*"

By contrast, it was also mentioned by one of them that patients are starting to move away from the idea that a doctor should know everything. They are generally starting to ask more questions about the conditions they are diagnosed with. He did say that a mobile device might be useful in explaining conditions graphically to patients, as they would more readily be able to understand a picture than a wordy explanation. "*When patients ask questions about their medical condition, we could perhaps provide a clearer explanation to patients using such a device to display information graphically.*"

Malpractice Legal Suit

Another social influence factor was identified by the pattern of doctors wanting to use the mobile technology device as an information and decision support tool, reflecting the growing unease amongst the doctors of the increasing trend of malpractice legal suits being brought against doctors. This device could help doctors prevent such a situation from arising: "*This will help in action that could be taken against the doctor for incorrect treatment and management.*" If such a device could keep a history of the patient and all decisions made regarding diagnosis and treatment, it could help defend the doctor's decisions: "*An audit of patient information and history, patient management and drugs prescribed could be kept.*"

This unease of legal action being brought against the doctor was also discovered during the discussion on patient influence. So long as the patient knew that the device was being used to make 100% certain that the correct diagnosis and management of the patient takes place, doctors would use the device in front of a patient.

Management and Government Support

Even though these two factors of hospital administration and government help could form part of perceived user resources on a micro-scale it is the macro-scale that was being referred to by the doctors. They were referring to national government and healthcare management and the fact that healthcare could not escape the political reality it found itself in. This is why these two factors are regarded as separate from the de facto definition of perceived user resources.

Support from the managerial structures of the hospital evoked responses tainted with a lot of emotion: "*The people in hospital management have completely forgotten what it is like to be a doctor. They seem to be fighting for some of the wrong things.*" There was a unanimous agreement between all doctors interviewed that absolutely no support would be garnered from the management of public hospitals for the purchase of mobile technology devices: "*Even if we proved to them how useful such a device would be and how it would increase my productivity and improve patient outcomes, I really don't think they would spend money on it.*"

However, this stance is understandable in the context of South Africa as a developing country with more than 70% of working age adults being unemployed, 53% of the population living below the poverty line and 20% of the population being HIV positive (Department of Health, 2004). There are too many needs for the already thinly sliced portion of resources cake provided to the public healthcare sector by the South African government with problems of HIV, TB and inadequate resources deemed to receive more share of the healthcare budget: "*In a developing country like ours we have too many other health concerns to warrant healthcare budgetary expense on such a device*"; "*TB, HIV, infant mortality and cost of health services to the general public all take priority on already scarce financial resources*" and "*Our hospitals are overcrowded and you cannot spend money on a nice-to-have while you do not have beds for patients or doctors to service the patients.*"

When asked whether an external party would not be able to perhaps put some pressure on the hospital management to incorporate a mobile technology device into use in the public hospitals, there was mostly exasperation in the voices of the interviewees. It was said that no such external party exists. Not even the provincial or local government would be able to do this. They set out the budgets for each hospital and stipulate at a very high level what the money should be spent on: "*Government allocates the hospital budget for the year and they stipulate at a very high level where the money should be spent.*"

Even then, these stipulations are guidelines and it is up to the hospital management to decide how this money is spent: "*It is up to the hospital management using the government guidelines to spend the money allocated to the hospital" and "They would not be able to say exactly on what the money should be spent. They will say that so and so an amount is allocated to information technology. It is up to the hospital management to decide what specific IT to spend the money on.*"

This relative freedom to spend the money allocated results in a lot of political battles within the hospital management. This means that sometimes scarce resources are not properly allocated by the hospital management: "*They seem to be fighting for the wrong things*" or "*The management cannot collectively decide what the money should be spent on. This results in this one wanting this and that one wanting that.*"

This results in poor administration of the hospital, as well as poor outdated equipment being used. This also results in poor working conditions for doctors, of which the patient has ultimately to bear the consequences.

These findings show that there is a clear statement being made by the doctors that no support would be given to them by the hospitals in the use of a mobile technology device. However, this lack of support for the adoption of a mobile technology device by the environment doctors find themselves in will not detract from there willingness to use the device. In fact 10 of the 12 said that they would purchase the device from their private funds as they could see many potential uses for the device: "*So long as it does not cost too much and the benefit it will add is quite visible, I will not mind paying for it*"; "*I don't think I would mind paying for such a device out of my own pocket if one can be found for about R3500*" (≈ US$500).

It was mentioned that if the use of the device was privately funded, hospital management would grab the opportunity to use the device in the hospital. "*If a company like HP came and privately funded such a device they would jump at the opportunity.*"

Patient-Doctor Relationship

Two of the doctors mentioned that they rarely worked directly with patients: "*I don't work directly with patients. I perform tests on blood samples from the patient.*"

These doctors did therefore mention that they would not be influenced negatively in the use of a mobile technology device by patients' perception of them. They were also less worried about malpractice legal suits than their colleagues who worked directly with patients: "*Because I don't work with patients, I would be less worried about these legal suits. I would still worry but far less than my other colleagues."*

Another factor that distinguished these doctors from the ones that worked directly with patients was their perception of what the mobile device could offer them. They were less interested in using the device as an information or decision support tool and more interested in having the device act as a workstation for them. They wanted the device to be integrated into the hospital systems they used so that they were not tied down to a desk: *"If we could have the test results delivered directly to this device so I can report on it, it would help me greatly and I would not be tied down to my desk or my outdated computer."*

They did not however fully understand the intricacies of integrating such a device directly into the hospital systems even though they showed some understanding of security concerns that might be raised by this integration: *"I know that with such a device it will have to be very secure since we are dealing with confidential patient information."*

They did however understand that having the device fully integrated into all the hospital systems would be beneficial to them and make them more productive: *"They upgraded our result reporting application this year but to me it is more of a downgrade. This new application is not integrated into anything else. You cannot even export data to Excel and this makes life exceptionally difficult for us."*

SUMMARY AND CONCLUSION

The data analysis revealed that the factors of job relevance, usefulness, task/technology fit, result demonstrability, computer self-efficacy and device characteristics were in agreement with the findings of previous research on ICT adoption in healthcare. The more technically competent doctors are, the more likely their intention to use a mobile technology device. Where doctors found the device relevant and useful to their daily clinical activities, they would use the device. The better the device and its software could support them, the greater would be their intention to use such a device. Table 1 lists the adoption factors identified as significant during this research.

Could these factors form part of a generalised technology acceptance model for innovative technology in the South African public healthcare sector, along the same lines as (Wu, Wang & Lin, 2007)? We suggest that the hospitals from which participants were obtained are comparable to the rest of the South African public hospitals: doctors working in these hospitals face similar working conditions, challenges, administrative tasks and resource shortages. Their opinions could therefore be seen to be fairly representative for the South African public healthcare sector. This would mean that the factors identified could form a revised TAM for South African public hospitals; this could be researched using quantitative means.

In conclusion, the research shows that South African public healthcare doctors are eagerly looking for ways to support themselves in their daily clinical activities. They can conceptualise many uses for a mobile technology device, many of which are already a practical reality in countries like the USA, UK and many countries in Europe. Using the device as an information and decision support tool can be made a reality for public healthcare doctors in South Africa. This will not only provide much needed support to overworked doctors, it will also help improve healthcare outcomes for the majority of the South African public. The key stakeholders involved in the public healthcare function, the government, healthcare management and ICT industry, can help push the adoption of these devices. The ICT industry could get involved by developing strategic partnerships with the public healthcare sector. These partnerships can be used firstly for the showcasing the potential of mobile devices to the public healthcare sector. Once an interest is

Table 1. Adoption factors identified by the research

Factors	Supports the literature?	Comments
Perceived usefulness of a mobile device	Yes	In general a very positive perception of mobile technology devices by doctors was evident even though half of them had never come into contact with one before. They perceived the device being able to provide them with relevant information either via the internet or software for the device. They perceived the device as a reference tool, patient information tool and even contemplated its use as a decision support tool that could help in diagnosis and medication prescription.
Social influences	**No**	Doctors in public healthcare in the Western Cape display a professional maturity that does not allow factors like image or subjective norm to influence them.
Perceived user resources	**No**	Lack of resources to support their use of these devices by the hospitals did not negatively influence their intention to adopt. This could be attributed to the social circumstances South African doctors find themselves in, where they have learnt to cope with limited resources on a daily basis. Despite their extremely pressurised work environments, and poor hospital management and administration, patient care is uppermost in their minds.
Computer self-efficacy	Yes	Concurred with previous research (Chismar & Patton 2003), that due to the high self-efficacy beliefs of doctors this factor can be ignored even when researching an innovative technology in a South African context.
Device characteristics	Yes	Doctors would be negatively influenced by characteristics they regarded as being important for them.
Task/technology fit	Yes	The medical profession is a very information intensive one (Harkke 2005) and doctors realised that this device would be able to help keep abreast of the latest information.
Result demonstrability	Yes	Doctors believed that the technology would be able to help them deliver better quality care to their patients.
Patient influence	New	Doctors did not feel intimidated by possible patient perceptions on their doctor's use of the device. Most doctors did however expect that the patient perception would be positive anyway.
Fear of legal action	New	Underlying doctors' perceptions of the device as an information tool was an unease in respect of malpractice legal suits. It was thought that the technology could aid the decisions made. This could help reduce the possibility of incorrect diagnosis and treatment and perhaps legal action against the doctor.
Management and government support	New	Negative sentiments were expressed about the lack of national healthcare structures and government support for the use of such a device. Nevertheless this did not appear to influence their personal intention to adopt mobile technology. It was however felt that these structures should be providing more impetus for the use of these devices.
Doctor-patient relationship	New	Where doctors do not interact with patients, a number of the above factors are not applicable. Thus this can be seen as a moderating variable or factor on the other factors, especially patient influence and fear of legal action.

shown the partnerships can be used for the development of standards, infrastructure and solutions. Government can involve themselves through e-government initiatives and push the concept of mobile technology and healthcare. Hospital management can become involved by starting to support initiatives to help doctors provide better quality care to patients by using these devices as they have envisaged in this research, as a reference-, decision support- and record keeping tool.

The interpretation of the research results should take into account a number of limitations. Firstly, the sample was quite small and, to an extent, self-selected. Also, other stakeholders, especially hospital management and patients, were not interviewed. Finally, the perceptions of mobile technology are influenced by potential and actual use thus many responses could have been based on incorrect or incomplete conceptualisations of potential mobile technology application(s).

ACKNOWLEDGMENT

This article is a revised and updated version of a paper initially presented at the European Conference on Information Systems and later expanded into a chapter in the Handbook of Research on Advances in Health Informatics and Electronic Healthcare Applications. The feedback of the anonymous reviewers is hereby gratefully acknowledged.

REFERENCES

Ajzen, I. (1991). The theory of planned behaviour. *Organizational Behavior and Human Decision Processes*, *50*, 179–211. doi:10.1016/0749-5978(91)90020-T

Ajzen, I., & Fishbein, M. (1980). *Understanding Attitudes and Predicting Social Behaviour*. Eaglewood Cliffs, NJ: Prentice-Hall.

Andersen, J. G. (1997). Clearing the way for physicians' use of clinical information systems. *Communications of the ACM*, *40*(8), 83–90. doi:10.1145/257874.257895

Berkowitz, L. L. (2002). Clinical informatics tools in physician practice. *Healthcare Informatics*, *19*(4), 41–44.

Bower, A. G. (2005). *The diffusion and value of healthcare information technology*. Santa-Monica, CA: Rand Publishing.

Chau, P. Y. K., & Hu, P. J. (2002). Examining a model of information technology acceptance by individual professionals: An exploratory study. *Management Information Systems*, *18*(4), 191–229.

Chetty, K. S. (2007). *Equity Promoting Health Care Policies in South Africa*. Report to the Health Systems Knowledge Network. Retrieved Jan 10, 2008 from: http://www.wits.ac.za/chp/kn/Chetty%20 2007%20Equity.pdf

Chiasson, M., Davidson, E., Kaplan, B., Lau, F., & Reddy, M. (2004, September). *Interdisciplinary windows for studying information systems in healthcare: Challenges and opportunities*. Paper presented at IT in healthcare: Socio-technical Approaches Second International Conference, Oregon, USA.

Chismar, W. G., & Patton, S. W. (2003). Does the extended technology acceptance model apply to physicians? *36th Hawaii International Conference on System Sciences*, Hawaii.

Davis, F. D. (1989). Perceived usefulness, perceived ease of use, and user acceptance of information technology. *Management Information Systems Quarterly*, *13*(3), 319–340. doi:10.2307/249008

Department of Health. (2004). *National HIV and Syphillis Antenatal Seroprevalence Survey in South Africa 2003*. Retrieved January 10, 2008, from http://www.doh.gov.za/docs/2003hiv-f.html.

Fitzgerald, B., & Howcroft, D. (1998, December). Competing dichotomies in IS research and possible strategies for resolution. *AIS International Conference on Information Systems*, Helsinki, Finland.

Garritty, C., & Emam, K. E. (2006). Who's Using PDAs? Estimates of PDA Use by Health Care Providers: A Systematic Review of Surveys. *Journal of Medical Internet Research*, *8*(2), e7. doi:10.2196/jmir.8.2.e7

Hameed, K. (2003). The application of mobile computing and technology to health care services. *Telematics and Informatics*, *20*, 99–106. doi:10.1016/S0736-5853(02)00018-7

Hammersley, M., & Atkinson, P. (1983). *Ethnography: Principles in Practice*. London: Tavistock.

Harkke, V. (2005). Physicians' usage experiences of a mobile information system. *38th Hawaii International Conference on System Sciences*, Hawaii.

Horan, T. A., Tulu, B., Hilton, B., & Burton, J. (2004). Use of online systems in clinical medical assessments: An analysis of physician acceptance of online disability evaluation systems. *37th Hawaii International Conference on System Sciences*, Hawaii.

Hu, P., Chau, P., & Tam, K. (1999). Examining the technology acceptance model using physician acceptance of telemedicine technology. *Journal of Management Information Systems*, *16*(2), 91–112.

Joy, S., & Benrubi, G. (2004). Personal digital assistant use in Florida in obstetrics and gynaecology residency programs. *Southern Medical Journal*, *97*(5), 430–433. doi:10.1097/00007611-200405000-00002

Khoumbati, K., & Themistocleous, M. (2006). Integrating the IT Infrastructures in Healthcare Organisations: a Proposition of Influential Factors. *The Electronic. Journal of E-Government*, *4*(1), 27–36.

Klein, H. K., & Myers, M. D. (1999). A set of principles for conducting and evaluating interpretive field studies in information systems. *Management Information Systems Quarterly*, *23*(1), 67–94. doi:10.2307/249410

Li, Y. C., Chang, I. C., Hung, W. F., & Fu, H. K. (2005). The critical factors affecting hospital adoption of mobile nursing technologies in Taiwan. *Proceedings of the 38th Hawaii International Conference on System Sciences*, Hawaii, USA.

Lu, Y. C., Xiao, Y., Sears, A., & Jacko, J. A. (2005). A review and a framework of handheld computer adoption in healthcare. *International Journal of Medical Informatics*, *74*(5), 409–422. doi:10.1016/j.ijmedinf.2005.03.001

Martin, S. (2003). More than half of MDs under age 35 now using PDAs. *Canadian Medical Association Journal*, *16*(2), 952–952.

Miles, M. B., & Huberman, A. M. (1994). *Qualitative Data Analysis: An Expanded Sourcebook*. Beverly Hills, CA: Sage.

Padarath, A., Chamberlain, C., McCoy, D., Ntuli, A., Rowson, M., & Loewenson, R. (2003). Health personnel in Southern Africa: Confronting maldistribution and brain drain. *Equinet discussion paper no. 4*. Health Systems Trust, South Africa.

Pare, G. (2004). Investigating information systems with positivist case study research. *Communications of the Association for Information Systems*, *13*, 233–264.

Porn, L. N., & Patrick, K. (2002). Mobile computing acceptance grows as applications evolve. *Healthcare Financial Management*, *56*, 66–70.

Ritchie, J., & Lewis, J. (2003). *Qualitative Research Practice: A Guide for Social Science Students and Researchers*. London: Sage Publications.

Sarker, S., & Wells, J. D. (2003). Understanding mobile handheld device use and adoption. *Communications of the ACM*, *46*(12), 35–40. doi:10.1145/953460.953484

Turisco, F., & Case, J. (2001). *Wireless and Mobile Computing*. Health Reports, California Healthcare Foundation.

Varshney, U. (2006). Using wireless technologies in healthcare. *International Journal of Mobile Communications*, *4*(3), 354–368.

Venkatesh, V., & Davis, F. D. (2000). A theoretical extension of the technology acceptance model: Four longitudinal field studies. *Management Science*, *46*(2), 186–204. doi:10.1287/mnsc.46.2.186.11926

Wu, J. H., Wang, S. C., & Lin, L. M. (2005). *What drives mobile healthcare? An empirical evaluation of technology acceptance. 38th Hawaii International Conference on System Sciences*, Hawaii.

Wu, J. H., Wang, S. C., & Lin, L. M. (2007). Mobile computing acceptance factors in the healthcare industry: A structural equation model. *International Journal of Medical Informatics*, *76*(1), 66–77. doi:10.1016/j.ijmedinf.2006.06.006

APPENDIX: OVERVIEW OF RELATIVE SUPPORT FOR VARIOUS FACTORS

The following table summarizes the relative support for positively influencing factors (✓ = support, ✓✓ = strong support) or inhibiting factors (✗). Blank cells indicate a lack of influence under current conditions.

Table 2. Consistency of support for influencing factors between respondents

Influencing Factor	D1	D2	D3	D4	D5	D6	D7	D8	D9	D10	D11	D12
Device usefulness	✓✓	✓✓	✓✓	✓✓	✓✓	✓✓	✓✓	✓✓	✓✓	✓✓	✓✓	✓✓
Job relevance	✓	✓✓	✓✓	✓	✓✓	✓✓	✓✓	✓✓	✓✓	✓✓	✓✓	✓✓
Status			✓✓									
Image												
Subjective norm				✓								
Perceived user resources												
Computer Literate	✓✓	✓✓	✓✓	✓✓	✓✓	✓✓	✓✓	✓✓	✓✓	✓✓	✓✓	✓✓
User Efficacy	✓✓	✓✓	✓✓	✓✓	✓✓	✓✓	✓✓	✓✓	✓✓	✓✓	✓✓	✓✓
Size of screen	✗	✗	✗	✗	✗			✗	✗	✗	✗	✗
Theft	✗	✗	✗	✗	✗			✗	✗	✗	✗	✗
Task/technology fit		✓✓	✓✓		✓✓	✓✓	✓✓	✓✓	✓✓	✓✓	✓✓	✓✓
Patient Perception		✗	✗									
Fear of legal suit			✓✓		✓	✓✓	✓✓	✓✓	✓✓	✓✓	✓✓	✓✓
Management support												
Government support												

As can be gleaned from the table, there generally seems to be a high degree of correspondence or agreement between doctors. This is therefore a fairly strong indication of the reliability of the research findings, despite the small sample.

This work was previously published in International Journal of Healthcare Delivery Reform Initiatives, edited by Matthew W. Guah, pp. 37-54, copyright 2009 by IGI Publishing (an imprint of IGI Global).

Chapter 13
Telepractice:
A 21st Century Model of Health Care Delivery

Thomas W. Miller
University of Connecticut, USA

Jennifer A. Wood
VA Texas Valley Coastal Bend Health Care System, USA

ABSTRACT

Telehealth is viewed as the removal of time and distance barriers in the provision of health care and patient education to underserved populations. Examined is a twenty first century clinical consultation model of healthcare. Offered are specific applications within a broad spectrum of services utilizing telehealth technology. Important technology shifts for administrative paradigms, clinical models, and educational information technology for healthcare services through telehealth technology are examined. The future of telehealth and its interface with various critical components of society needs to examine the potential benefits over risks in providing healthcare consultations and services through the educational settings available. Addressed is a technology model, which demonstrates the capability of reducing time and distance barriers in the provision of health care and education through telehealth technology. The use of telehealth technology in rural settings is seen as a viable medium for providing needed diagnostic and clinical consultation for underserved and rural.

INTRODUCTION

The purpose of this chapter is to examine contemporary applications of telepractice within a rural community setting.. A brief review of current data regarding the impact of telepractice upon access and satisfaction with clinical care is provided. A clinical telepractice consultation model is outlined along with illustrative vignettes. Readers are also provided with suggested clinical practice guidelines and practical considerations

DOI: 10.4018/978-1-60960-183-6.ch013

for telepractice implementation. Telehealth, or the use of telecommunication technology to provide access to health assessment, diagnosis, intervention, consultation, supervision, education, and information across distance, has become a well recognized vehicle for delivering services and disseminating information to a variety of consumer populations as well as professionals and practitioners (Nickelson, 1998; Miller & Hutchins 2008). Given its ability to transcend many of the economic, cultural, and geographic barriers that often prohibit or restrict the provision of health care, the use of telehealth has reshaped traditional systems of care. Moreover, due to its unique capacity to negate many of the traditional obstacles in service delivery, telehealth is often a desirable option for the provision of health care to rural, confined, underserved or isolated groups (Miller & Holcomb 2007).

As a result, a large proportion of telehealth studies have focused on evaluating the effectiveness of telecommunications technology in delivering health services to rural and specialty populations (Wood, 2000). Numerous studies suggest that telehealth can be successfully utilized to improve access to health care services amongst underserved populations and that the quality of care delivered via telehealth is similar to or surpasses that of face-to-face services (Bischoff, Hollist, Smith, & Frank, 2004; Miller, Miller, Kraus, & Sprang, 2003; Norman, 2006) while maintaining a high degree of satisfaction

Since its inception, one of the primary advantages of telepractice has been its ability to improve access to health care services for people living in rural or remote areas where health care professionals are often scarce or absent. In the words of Nickelson (1998), "Telehealth is simply a tool that...makes it easier to practice already established professional skills across distance and to serve individuals and organizations who may not, but for telehealth, have access to such services" (p. 527). This ability to transcend geographic barriers has been the basis for three decades worth of demonstration projects targeted at rural populations. The use of telepractice to improve access to mental health care has since expanded to include other isolated groups, such as inner city families (Yellowlees, 2005; McLaren, Blunden, Lipsedge, & Summerfield, 1996; Straker, Mostyn, & Marshall, 1976), prison inmates (Ax et al, 2007), and homebound elderly (Maheu, Whitten, & Allen, 2001). Overall, these projects suggest that the use of telepractice is an effective means of improving access to both health care services as well as improving the exchange of information between providers (Blackmon, Kaak, & Ranseen, 1997). Efforts to assess the quality of telepractice care compared to traditional face-to-face services indicate that there is little difference in diagnostic and assessment outcomes across the two treatment modes (Ball & Puffett, 1998; Biggins, 2000; Zarate, et al., 1997 and that telehealth applications may serve to enhance the continuity and efficiency of care (Ghosh, McLaren, & Watson, 1997).

Research assessing patient and provider satisfaction with telecare services reveals uniformly positive results (Miller, 2006; Morgan, Patrick, & Magaletta, 2008; Wood, 2006). In one of the earliest studies of patient satisfaction with telepractice, Solow, Weiss, & Bergen (1971) reported that patient acceptance was impressively high even among highly paranoid patients. Since that time, further research has indicated that satisfaction with telepractce care remains high even when patients are acutely or chronically psychotic or agitated (Kavanagh & Yellowless, 1995). Such data are especially relevant in the public sector where mental health services are often lacking. As a response to service deficits, prison systems (e.g., the Federal Bureau of Prisons, the Texas Department of Criminal Justice) have developed sophisticated telepractice care networks. It is noted that offenders are generally satisfied with mental health services received via telepractice (Leonard, 2004; NIJ, 2002). Of particular importance is that incarcerated mentally ill offenders, historically perceived as resistant to mental health services, reported no significant differences in the working alliance between treatment provider and client, post-session mood or treatment satisfaction when receiving psychiatric services regardless of method of service delivery (i.e., telemedicine vs. face-to-face) (Morgan et al., 2008). Similar findings have been found among parents and children who participate in telepsychiatric consultations (Blackmon, Kaak, & Ranseen, 1997), geriatric clients (Wood, O'Quin, & Eftink, 2004), inner-city families (Straker, Mostyn, & Marshall 1976), active-duty military personnel (Jerome, 1999), veterans (Wood, 2006), and adults with mild to moderate mental retardation and their mental health care providers (Wood & Hargrove, 2006).

TELEPRACTICE CARE MODEL

Realizing its high level of user acceptability and distinct ability to transcend geographic and social barriers, a visionary telehealth model for public education that focuses on the role of psychology and its interdisciplinary partners can be used to create a national, regional, state and local stratified network of health care professionals and other stakeholders engaged in a nationwide public education campaign (Miller, 2007). The Telehealth Intervention Project (TIP) is a proposed model designed to offer teleconferenced psychological and health related informational and demonstrational sessions focused on a broad spectrum of health related topics. Telepractice technology is uniquely suited to reach underserved populations and rural practitioners offering relevant evidence-based psychological information to the community. The telepractice network can be used to educate a range of target populations including clients, service providers, educators and community personnel including children and families, school populations, prison inmates, legislators, public officials, and inpatients and outpatients in various public and private sector programs.

As modeled in Figure 1, telepractice affords a sophisticated medium for reaching these targeted populations (consumers and providers) by making psychology a household word. Outlined below are mechanisms (processes) for successfully implementing the Telehealth Intervention Project, a proposed model for implementing a dimension of the public education campaign to reach underserved target groups in need of health and prevention education information nationally.

USE COMMUNICATION STRATEGICALLY TO IMPROVE HEALTHCARE

Health care communication encompasses the study and use of communication strategies to inform and influence individual and community decisions that enhance health. It links the domains of communication and health and is increasingly recognized as a necessary element of efforts to improve personal and public health (Kreuter, Strecher, & Glassman, 1999). Health care communication can contribute to all aspects of disease prevention and health promotion and is relevant in a number of contexts, including (1) health professional-patient relations, (2) individuals' exposure to, search for, and use of health information, (3) individuals' adherence to clinical recommendations and regimens, (4) the construction of public health messages and campaigns, (5) the dissemination of individual and population health risk information, that is, risk communication, (6) images of health in the mass media and the culture at large, (7) the education of consumers about how to gain access to the public health and health care systems, and (8) the development of telehealth applications (Miller, Burton, & Kraus, 2004; Wood, Miller, & Hargrove, 2005; Miller, 2007)

Utilizing health care communication can help raise awareness of health risks (including physical and psychological) and solutions, provide the motivation and skills needed to reduce these risks, help consumers find support from other people in

Figure 1. A telepractice intervention model for rural health care. Adapted from: Miller, T.W.; Miller, J.M.; Burton, D. (2003). Telehealth: A model for clinical supervision in allied health. The Internet Journal of Allied Health Sciences & Practices, 1(2)

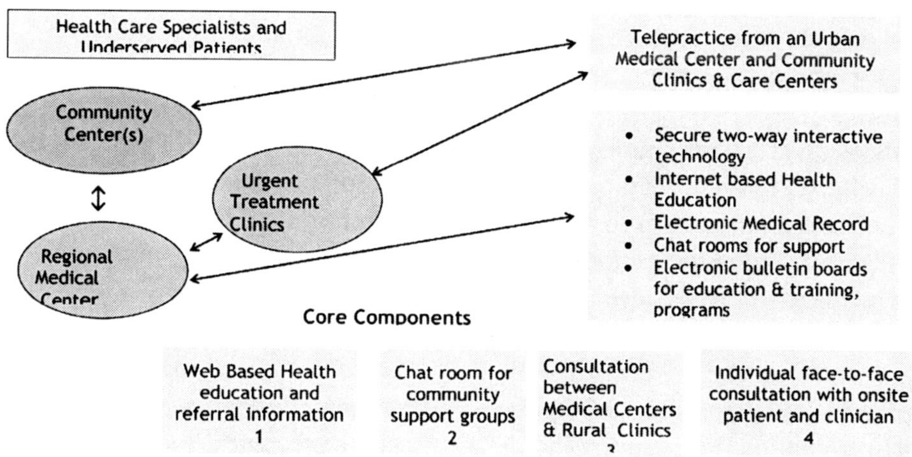

similar situations, and affect or reinforce attitudes. Health care communication also can increase demand for appropriate health services and decrease demand for inappropriate health services. It can make available information to assist in making complex choices, such as selecting health plans, care providers, and treatments. At a macro level, health communication can be used to influence the public agenda, advocate for policies and programs, promote positive changes in the socioeconomic and physical environments, improve the delivery of public health and health care services, and encourage social norms that benefit health and quality of life (Monagan, 2010).

Health care communication may also inform health care providers for improved service delivery. The Institute of Medicine (IOM) criticized current health care training and reported that training of health professionals requires a "major overhaul." Specifically, the IOM stated that health care professionals are not properly trained with regard to changes in patient demographics and health related needs, evolving expectations within health care systems, evolving practice methods and technological advances, or enhanced quality control. Improved health communication among health professionals may alleviate these shortcomings, and telepractice offers a mechanism for improved training that is immediate and accessible. For example, the TIP could be used to offer health professionals an opportunity to discuss physical and psychological issues for targeted populations, interactive education, and face-to-face consultations with specified experts.

PUBLIC EDUCATION VIA THE INTERNET

The environment for communicating about psychology and health has changed significantly. These changes include dramatic increases in the number of communication channels and the number of health issues vying for public attention as well as consumer demands for more and higher quality physical and psychological health information. Psychology has the potential of communicating through the home, the school, and the work environment through group, organizational, community, and the Internet interactive telehealth options (Stamm, 1999). For instance, health care providers can take advantage of digital technologies, such as CD-ROM, World Wide Web,and listservs to target audiences, tailor messages, and engage people in interactive, ongoing exchanges about health. Brief sessions via web-based interactive video can provide easier access to needed information and reduce health care cost, travel time, and expenses.

Research indicates that health communication best supports health promotion when multiple communication channels are used to reach specific audience segments with information that is appropriate and relevant to them. Evidence based decision-making suggests that effective psychological health promotion and communication initiatives adopt an audience-centered perspective, which means that promotion and communication activities reflect audiences' preferred formats, channels, and contexts. Targeting specific segments of a population and tailoring messages for individual use are two methods to make reaching home based health promotion care through telepractice activities relevant to audiences. Advances in health informatics are changing the delivery of health information and services and are likely to have a growing impact on individual and community health. Advantages include (1) improved access to personalized health information, (2) access to health information, support, and services on demand, (3) enhanced ability to distribute psychologically accurate information quickly, and (4) just-in-time expert decision support and advice.

INCREASING ACCESS TO HEALTH INFORMATION THROUGH TELEPRACTICE

The goals of community based and professional organizations should dovetail with *Healthy People 2010* and other similar initiatives worldwide with the focus on using communication strategically to improve health. This can be accomplished through advocacy for: households with Internet access, health literacy, and the quality of Internet health information resources (Zarate, Weinstock, Cukor, Morabito, Leahy, Burns, Baer,

1997); DeLeon, Crimmins, Wolf, 2003; Karlinky, 2004; Hilty, 2004). According to the Computer and Internet Use Supplement to the Current Population Survey, U.S. Department of Commerce, Bureau of the Census (US Department of Commerce, 2002), approximately 26 percent of households had access to the Internet at home. Importantly, the greatest growth in Internet access was for lower income households (approximately 25 percent between 1998 and 2001). Continued growth in household access to the Internet is critical to improve psychological health as technical literacy, or the ability to use electronic technologies and applications, will be essential to gain access to health information. This is particularly important for lower income individuals who may be lacking health insurance or financial means for regular health care. Internet availability in the home is an important indicator of equitable access to health information among targeted populations.

Critical to the success of telepractice technology is literacy level of the consumer. The data regarding health and technology literacy indicate that approximately 90 million adults in the United States have inadequate or marginal literacy skills. Psychology can play a role in the implementation of this initiative by increasing the proportion of health communication activities that include research and evaluation. Effective health communication programs are built on sound research and evaluation (Casper, 2004; Web Based Education Commission, 2000).

Providing counseling about health behaviors could enhance adherence and compliance with healthy behavior (both physical and psychological). Culturally appropriate and linguistically competent community health promotion programs, substance abuse treatment, HIV counseling and testing in prisons, worksite promotion of nutrition education and weight management, public access to information and surveillance data, perception of risk associated with substance abuse and tobacco targeting adolescents and young adults are all potential targets for psychology in the home (Deleon et al., 2003).

DEVELOPING A TELEPRACTICE INTERVENTION PROGRAM

Providers or organizational groups who wish to establish a telepractice service delivery system or network should begin by identifying existing programs and/or local and national technological resources. Organizations such as the Department of Veterans Affairs and the Kentucky Department of Criminal Justice are currently using technology to disseminate health care information and direct patient care. Within the VA, employees have access to an intranet, which contains training modules, informational handouts, clinical guidelines, etc. In addition, employees have the ability to participate in local and national informational broadcasts, videoconferences, and conference calls. With regard to patient care, the VA has developed an Internet-based program called My Health*e*Vet, which serves as a gateway to veteran health benefits and services as well as a tool for enabling veterans to better understand and manage their health. It provides access to trusted health information, links to Federal and VA benefits and resources, a Personal Health Journal, and an online VA prescription refill program. Eventually, veterans will be able to view their appointments, co-pay balances, and access portions of their VA medical records online (My Health*e*Vet, 2006). By examining programs such as these, it is possible to identify the technological resources needed, learn from challenges existing programs have overcome, and to manage various types of informational programs.

In addition to reviewing established programs for implementation strategies, it is important to identify existing technological networks, which might be more effectively used to disseminate health information to consumers and providers. For example, many states now include videoconferencing or cable networks in public school systems, public libraries, health care facilities, and other community facilities for efficient connection capabilities. Such existing networks could be utilized to broadcast health information programs targeted toward specific populations or providers. For providers who may not have access to large-scale telepractice resources, there are simple strategies for utilizing existing resources to obtain and disseminate health information. For example, health care providers who wish to obtain information on evidence-based practice or innovative techniques may consult reputable websites or join one of the many professional listservs designed to promote dissemination of information. Providers may also refer their clients to reputable websites (e.g., National Heart Association, National Center for PTSD Research) in order to assist them in gathering information or obtaining support.

Rural school systems are often faced with providing qualified care to their student population and may not have ready access to needed expertise. Consider the following scenario: A rural school district needs expert consulation to address the needs of a seriously disruptive student. The nearest board certified child psychiatrist is located 500 miles away. To remedy this situation, it was proposed that the needed clinical consultation could be provided to this school system using telepractice technology.

The clinical consultation team included a child psychologist on site working with a school psychologist, an advanced practice nurse, clinical social worker, special education specialist and the consultation of a child psychiatrist by video link from a university based psychiatry clinic through a cost effective model of telepractice. Through the use of this specialized telehealth link using video telephones, the needed interdisciplinary clinical consultation and service was provided to the rural school system and its staff. The services included diagnostic and treatment planning and classroom observation of the student in question with a secure telepractice video link to the care provider.

Illustrated in Figure 1 is the conceptual model that exemplifies a community based telepractice technology system. Telepractice healthcare links in this model exist between health care specialists at the university-based medical center, physicians at the rural community clinic and psychologist, social worker and advanced practice nurse at the rural district. Within this configuration a secure two-way video link exists for interactive staffing of patients and pediatric emergency care. In addition, Internet-based case conferences via video link can provide necessary and essential face-to-face discussions, as well as video images and streaming video of case materials for review. The combined web based and interactive videoconferencing allows for clinicians and school personnel to exchange information that can be to the benefit of both educational and health care planning and consultation. Each of these segments is noted in the model presented in Figure 1. This model provides children with special needs in rural settings the necessary and appropriate consultation to the benefit of client, clinician and families in our society.

This collaborative partnership between educators and clinicians may be enhanced and facilitated by the use of telepractice using video telephones designated for confidential patient care and planning. School personnel may incorporate consultation with a local or regional specialist and may use Internet video technology through a community clinic. In some cases, the need to have specialized psychiatric consultation services from a medical center-based child psychiatric clinic linked to a community clinic and to a school district may be offered through telehealth technology. In this case, patient health information, patient education materials, clinical records can be shared through electronic medical records sent to consulting clinicians, thus providing them with an opportunity to review information individually and then respond to relevant clinical issues. Clinical staffing of the child involving the referring clinician in the rural setting, the community consulting specialists and the university-based specialist can be beneficial and more effective when time and distance barriers are removed via the use of telehealth technology.

The need for telehealth technology is obvious in the face of the obstacles clinicians face in providing a high standard for health care delivery in a time efficient and cost-effective manner (Miller, 1998; Miller, Miller, Kraus, Burton, Sprang & Adams 2003). Emerging systems of managed health care that interface with the educational system have the potential to benefit from the needed services for children as noted in the Young and Iresaon (2003) study. Telehealth is seen as the use of various models of telecommunication, which connect the consumer with the health care provider through live, two-way video transmission, across, distances and which permit diagnosis, treatment, and other health care services. This definition stresses a focus on delivery of services across distances with a sense of concern for ethical provision of services and confidentiality of the health care needs in our society.

Telehealth benefits for clinical health care and for educational settings include: increased access to clinical consultative services and health education programs for school and community organizations and populations; improved and expanded psychiatric health care services to underserved areas in rural communities and areas; provision of a feasible and sustainable system of clinician-directed consultations using telehealth video conferencing; access to current approved education and training programs for health care providers in settings where access to advanced clinical training may be a barrier due to geographic location; reduction of the isolation for educators and health care providers in rural areas through the development of innovative consultation video conferencing systems that enhance clinical support and consultation regarding the diagnostic, treatment, consultative and educational services available to clinicians and other health care providers in certain geographical regions; and use of telepractice technology in rural communities to decrease the time, inconvenience, expense and risks of travel, as well as other associated problems that distance and isolation cause in obtaining psychological and other health care services.

PRACTICE GUIDELINES FOR TELEPRACTICE HEALTHCARE

Community-based telepractice services offer a visionary consultation model for providing standardized and special needs coverage to underserved areas by linking specialists and expert providers with consumers and practitioners in underserved communities. As an alternative way of providing traditional health services, telepractice is considered by some to be a solution to America's toughest health care challenges: increasing access to clinical consultation service and involving health care professionals while decreasing the costs involved in providing quality care (Office of Rural Health Policy, 1994). In order to insure standardization of care, practice guidelines offer a way of incorporating quality care, consistency in educational material and standard models for information technology.

Clinical algorithms and pathways of care are developed and used to provide case management. The goal is to make the client management guideline the accepted professional behavior and a reward in itself. To the extent that this is successful, five components occur: (a) the guideline is widely used and becomes habitual, (b) multidisciplinary professionals can use it to anticipate care events, (c) clinicians can use it as a shorthand or outline to guide their decisions and their communications to others, (d) the logistics for delivering the guideline components are convenient and reliable, and (e) the guideline defines the measure of performance and incorporates information collected that can be used for its evaluation and improvement. The individualized plans clinicians may use also contribute information for guideline revision.

Case management through algorithms presents a systematic perspective. Algorithms try to answer the question, "What is the best way to systematically handle this problematic condition?" Algorithms have a problem solving orientation coupled with functional specific actions or critical pathways to be taken. If desired results are produced, the problem was managed effectively. If the desired results are not produced, adjustments can be made to achieve the desired results.

The point to be made is that in our professional roles, it is important to be a creative problem solver who can translate relevant research into functional interventions. The model practice guideline that appears in Figure 2 outlines a situation in which the clinician recognizes that it would be more efficient if telemedicine had a place in the treatment intervention process. Note that a question is asked as to whether a telecare option exists in the patients' locality. If yes then the clinician begins the review with the client of the differences between tradition and telemedicine delivery of care. Informed consent is provided and compliance with all state and federal laws is to be reviewed. Then the clinician assesses the appropriate needs of the medium dependent upon the clinical nature of the consultation. Appropriately training the patient in the use of telemedicine and the equipment follows this. Risk management options are offered, a practice session is to occur to assure the patient can use the telemedicine option. The use of web based educational programs is provided. Finally there is a review and monitoring process in place so the clinician can monitor its use. Through this configuration, issues related to liability for negligence or liability for abandonment would be considerable reduced and hopefully eliminated.

LIABILITY ISSUES IN THE USE OF TELEPRACTICE TECHNOLOGY

Liability is a primary risk factor for service providers utilizing telepractice models and technology. Risk management strategies should educate psychologists and consumers about telemedicine equipment. It is important to consider who will provide training, what mechanisms will be used to evaluate the effectiveness of training, and how to document deficits in knowledge following completion of initial training. Another concern with respect to liability involves *"liability for abandonment."* Abandonment may occur when the clinician unilaterally terminates the relationship with a client or the relationship was terminated without reasonable notice; and termination occurred when further attention was needed. Practitioners using telepractice technology continuously monitor the patients' ability to participate in telemedicine activities and confirm their understanding of their responsibilities in

Figure 2. Clinical alogorithm for telepratice care

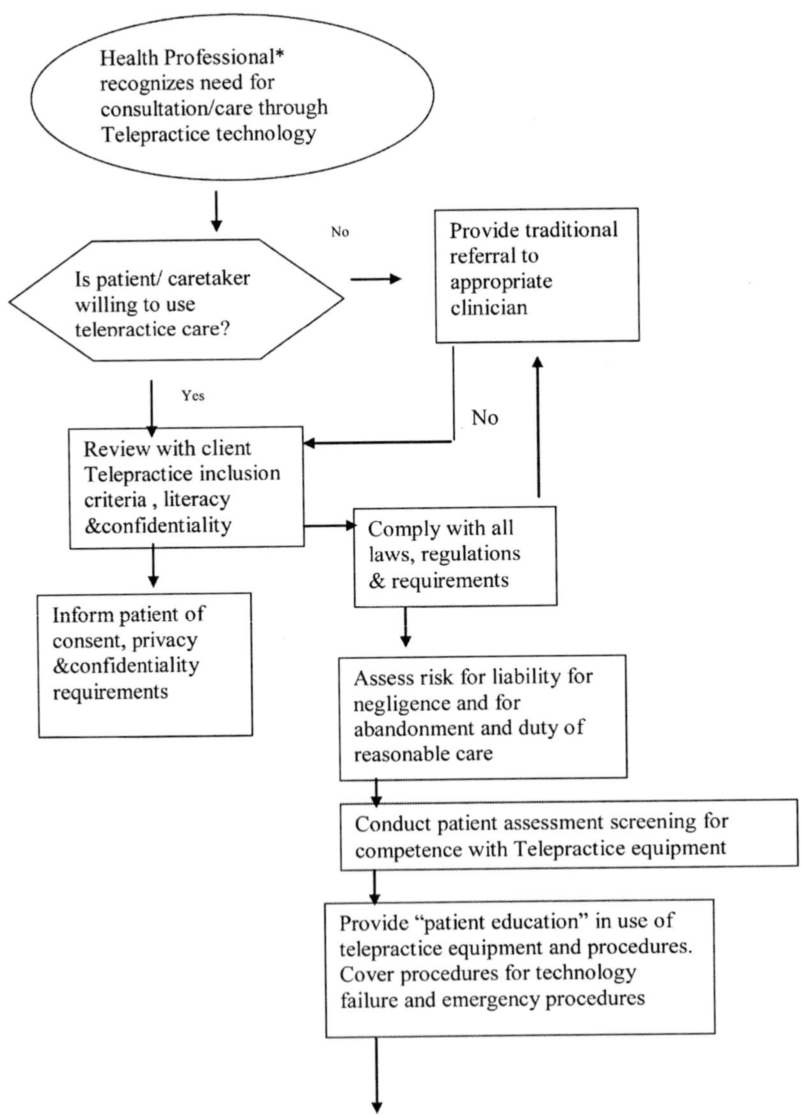

the use of telepractice equipment. While there are certain advantages, telepractice is subject to many of the same shortcomings associated with face-to-face care as well as several technology-specific limitations. Most notably, users should be aware of and attend to the following issues prior to establishing a telepractice network.

Security, Privacy, and Confidentiality. In an electronically mediated society, concerns regarding security, privacy and confidentiality may take on new meaning with telepractice models. One of the most serious compromises to security and to one's privacy is the unauthorized access to confidential patient health and educational information. Fortunately, these risks may be reduced by utilizing secure or closed networks, encryption programs, and by adhering to the standards set forth in the Health Insurance Portability and Accountability Act (HIPAA) which provides national standards to reduce health care inefficiencies by encouraging the use of information technology to better secure and protect patient information. In addition, one must consider technological risks that originate from software or computer systems. For example, computer viruses may be designed to destroy data or disrupt computer systems. To avoid these dangers, system managers must continually update virus scan programs, be alert for system glitches, and work to ensure compatibility of all system components (Stamm, 1999; Striefel, 2000).

Technology Expences. The cost of acquiring and maintaining the necessary technology including maintenance and update expenses) should be considered. With availability of the Internet, e-mail, listservs, and chat rooms may serve as a cost effective, accessible medium of communication. Equipment needs are minimal; requiring only a computer and Internet access at each location. Fortunately, for organizations interested in incorporating technology-mediated face-to-face contact, several types of videoconferencing applications exist. When considering these options, providers must take into account both the clinical demands on the system as well as the type of transmission infrastructure required to reliably support a particular application. Options for videoconferencing applications include, but are not limited to, videophones, PC-based desktop systems, and/or high-quality integrated videoconference units. The speed with which advances in technology, prices for the above equipment vary from a few hundred to several thousand dollars. Ironically, the cost of developing and maintaining telehealth systems tends to be the highest in the regions where telepractice would be most beneficial (e.g., rural areas) (Nickelson, 1998). Fortunately, federal programs such as the Universal Service Program for Rural Health Providers may help to defray the operating costs of such systems (Stamm, 1999).

Transmission quality. Along with variations in the technical infrastructure and expenses required for various telepractice applications, the quality of data transmission also varies accordingly. When considering options for videoconferencing, providers must take into account both the clinical demands on the system as well as the type of transmission infrastructure required to reliably support a particular application. Videoconferencing systems vary in the type of transmission channel required and thus may operate at different bandwidths. As a measure of a communication channel's ability to carry information, bandwidth directly influences the quality of video transmission. In other words, if detecting fine motor movements is critical, a system with higher bandwidth would be most suitable. On the other hand, lower bandwidths might be more appropriate when movement is not an important factor or when the cost of the infrastructure needed to support higher bandwidth is prohibitive. Among telepractice networks in the United States, the most common transmission rate is currently 384-786 Kbps (Mahue, Whitten, & Allen, 2001).

Consumer Satisfaction. Regardless of the specific type of technology implemented, the success of a telecommunications system often hinges on its acceptance among participants. As noted by Young and Irenson (2003), once providers and clients become familiar with telepractice technology, there seems to be an acceptable level of satisfaction with the use of this equipment. Adequate and appropriate training based on the intent of the users of such equipment is essential. Beyond training, it is important to normalize the equipment as part of the environment to desensitize those unfamiliar to telehealth practices and technology.

Scope of Practice. The legal and ethical issue of licensure and scope of practice in the use of telepractice may well extend beyond state boundaries or jurisdictions. Licensure requirements, as a limitation to interstate practice, are often cited as a major barrier to the development of services. As with most health care professionals, licensure is on a state-by-state basis, which requires that a practitioner hold a full, unrestricted license in all states he or she practices. For many professionals, acquiring and maintaining multiple licenses is a significant professional and financial burden, which falls particularly hard on rural health care providers who often experience significant travel, lost work time, and other costs in complying with multiple state regulations.

In anticipation of legislative changes with respect to the use of telecommunication technology, there have been efforts on the part of the medical and nursing professionals to develop alternative licensure models for their professions. For instance, Texas offers a "special purpose license" for out-of-state physicians who provide telepractice services to Texas residents. Similarly, the Joint Commission on the Accreditation of Healthcare Organizations recently revised its Hospital Medical Staff Standards which now state that practitioners who treat patients via telemedicine are subject to the credentialing processes of the organization that receives the telemedicine service (Joint Commission on the Accreditation of Healthcare Organizations, 2003). Utilizing a different approach, the National Council of State Boards of Nursing has developed a mutual license recognition program which allows nurses who hold a valid license in one state to enjoy a "multi-state licensure privilege" to practice in states that are members of the licensure compact (DeLeon, 2003). Legally and ethically the direct and immediate delivery of patient care is always the responsibility of the on-site licensed professional.

APPLICATIONS FOR TELEPRACTICE MODELS IN RURAL EDUCATIONAL SETTINGS

Multiple applications hold significant potential for educational settings seeking to meet the health related needs of patients through telepractice. These include:

1. clinical interview and/or evaluation by a clinician specialist; consultations for crisis stabilization in the healthcare and community settings;
2. Brief screening and assessment prior to comprehensive evaluations for various diagnostic entities;
3. Team assessment and treatment planning may include multiple links with physicians, child psychiatrists, school psychologists, occupational therapists, physical therapists, speech-language pathologists, counselors, nurses, teachers, social workers, and other allied health profesionals;
4. Diagnostic testing with the assistance of a technician on site;
5. Short-term health education and counseling interventions;
6. Vocational assessment, placement and counseling services;
7. Evaluations and diagnostics related to second opinions;
8. Short-term case management for children with special needs;
9. Consultation-liaison services for patients and care givers.

10. Consultation with primary care physicians and/or specialists, clinicians and educators regarding patients with special needs;
11. Continuing medical and health education for administrators, faculty, students, caregivers and others.

CONCLUDING COMMENTS AND LESSONS LEARNED

The future of telepractice healthcare delivery models and their interface with various critical components of society needs to examine the potential benefits over risks in providing healthcare consultations and allied services. The Department of Veterans Affairs, the largest healthcare delivery system in the United States sees telepractice healthcare a critical medium for serving its patients in rural and underserved areas of our country (Monagan 2010) Health care provision through telepractice technology must be vigilant to the challenges and cognizant of the added value when realizing that this technology will reach populations who have been traditionally underserved because of their remote location to needed services.

Examined herein has been a model, which demonstrates the capability of reducing time and distance barriers in the provision of health care and education through telepractice technology. Best practice guidelines have emerged and provide both ethical and legal parameters for practitioners (Miller and Wader, 2002). Vignettes highlighting the usage of this technology through educational settings have been presented as have the advantages and potential disadvantages of its use. Several suggested applications have been noted, as have the changing paradigms in delivery of healthcare through community-based services. When consultation with a needed health care professional is not readily available, the use of telepractice technology in rural settings is a viable medium for providing needed diagnostic and clinical consultation for underserved and rural populations in our society.

ACKNOWLEDGMENT

The authors wish to acknowledge the support and assistance of Rob Sprang Director of University of Kentucky Telecare,, Lon Hays, MD, Charles Lowe, Ph.D. Robert Kraus MD, Patricia Beckenhaupt RN, MS, MPH, Catherine Russell, Jill Livingston MLS, Lane J. Veltkamp MSW, and Brenda Frommer in the preparation of this manuscript.

REFERENCES

Armfield, N., Donovan, T., & Wootton, R. (2005). Real-time video in the neonatal intensive care nursery. *Journal of Telemedicine and Telecare, 11*, 238–245.

Ax, R. K., Fagan, T. J., Magaletta, P. R., Morgan, R. D., Nussbaum, D., & White, T. W. (2007). Innovations in correctional assessment and treatment [Special issue]. *Criminal Justice and Behavior, 34*, 893–905. doi:10.1177/0093854807301555

Ball, C., & Puffet, A. (1998). The assessment f cognitive functioning in the elderly using videoconferencing. *Journal of Telemedicine and Telecare, 4*, 36–38. doi:10.1258/1357633981931362

Bischoff, R. J., Hollist, C. S., Smith, C. W., & Frank, P. (2004). Addressing the mental health needs of the rural underserved: Findings from a multiple case study of a behavioral telehealth project. *Contemporary Family Therapy*, 26.

Blackmon, L. A., Kaak, H. O., & Ranseen, J. (1997). Consumer satisfaction with telemedicine child psychiatry consultation in rural Kentucky. *Psychiatric Services (Washington, D.C.), 48*, 1464–1466.

Casper, E. S. (2004). A formative evaluation of a rent subsidy program for homeless substance abusers. *Journal of Service Research, 31*(2), 25–39.

Casper, L.M., & King, Rosalind, K.B. (2004). Changing families, shifting economic fortunes, and meeting basic needs [Comment/Reply]. *Work Family Challenges for Low-Income Parents and Their Children, 55-79.*

Casper, V. (2004). Beyond feeders and growers: Changing conceptions of care in the Western Cape. *Journal of Child and Adolescent Mental Health, 16*(1), 55–59.

DeLeon, P. H., Crimmins, D. B., & Wolf, A. W. (2003). Afterword-the 21st century has arrived. *Psychotherapy (Chicago, Ill.), 40*(1-2), 164–169. doi:10.1037/0033-3204.40.1-2.164

Ghosh, G. J., McLaren, P. M., & Watson, J. P. (1997). Evaluating the alliance in video-link teletherapy. *Journal of Telehealth, 3*(suppl. 1), 33–35.

Kavanagh, S., & Yellowlees, P. (1995). Telemedicine: Clinical applications in mental health. *Australian Family Physician, 24*, 1242–1246.

Kreuter, M. W., Strecher, V. J., & Glassman, B. (1999). One size does not fit all: The case for tailoring print materials. *Annals of Behavioral Medicine, 21*(4), 276–283. doi:10.1007/BF02895958

Mahue, M., Whitten, P., & Allen, A. (2001). *E-health, telehealth, and telemedicine: A practical guide to start-up and success*. San Francisco: Jossey-Bass.

McLaren, P., Blunden, J., Lipsedge, M., & Summerfield, A. (1996). Telepsychiatry in an innercity community psychiatric service. *Journal of Telemedicine and Telecare, 2*, 57–59. doi:10.1258/1357633961929178

Miller, T. W. (1998). The psychologist with 20/20 vision. *Consulting Psychology Journal: Practice and Research, 50*(1), 25–35. doi:10.1037/1061-4087.50.1.25

Miller, T. W. (2006). Telehealth issues in consulting psychology practice. *Consulting Psychology Journal: Practice and Research, 58*(2), 82–90. doi:10.1037/1065-9293.58.2.82

Miller, T. W. (2007). (Accepted). Telehealth Issues in Consulting Psychology Practice. *Consulting Psychology Journal: Practice and Research.*

Miller, TW, DeLeon, P., Morgan, R., Penk, W. Magaletta, P. (2006) The Public Sector Psychologist with 2020 vision. *Professional Psychology: Research and Practice. 37-2*, 531-538.

Miller, T. W., & Holcomb, T. F. (2007). Telehealth Applications for Counselors in the Schools. *Kentucky Counseling Association Journal, 26*(1), 6–13.

Miller, T. W., & Hutchins, S. A. (2008). (Accepted). 21st Century Teaching technology: Best Practices and Effectiveness in Teaching Psychology. *International Journal of Instructional Media.*

Miller, T. W., & Miller, J. (1999). Telemedicine: New directions for health care delivery in Kentucky schools. *The Journal of the Kentucky Medical Association, 97*(4), 163–166.

Miller, T. W., Miller, J. M., Burton, D., Sprang, R., & Adams, J. M. (2003). A Telehealth Model for Clinical Supervision In Allied Health. *Internet Journal of Allied Health, 2*(1), 1–10.

Miller, T. W., Miller, J. M., Kraus, O. F., & Sprang, R. (2003). Telehealth a clinical application model for rural consultation. *Consulting Psychology Journal, 55*(2), 119–127. doi:10.1037/1061-4087.55.2.119

Miller, T. W., & Wader, B. (2002). Best Practices for Psychologist using 21st Century Technology. Annual Convention Connecticut Psychological Association, November 1-2, 2002. Westbrook, CT.

Monagan, B. (2010) *Telehealth Tools Seen as Key to VA's Rural Health Care Strategy*. Healthcare IT News June 28, 2010. Web Based retrieval at: http://www.ihealthbeat.org/articles/2010/6/24/telehealth-tools-seen-as-key-to-vas-rural-health-care-strategy.aspx

Morgan, R. D., Patrick, A. R., & Magaletta, P. R. (2008). Does the use of telemental health alter the treatment experience?: Inmates' perceptions of telemental health vs. face-to-face treatment modalities. *Journal of Consulting and Clinical Psychology*, *76*, 158–162. doi:10.1037/0022-006X.76.1.158

My Health. *e*Vet. (n.d.). Retrieved June 2, 2006, from https://www.myhealth.va.gov/mhvPortal/anonymous.portal?_nfpb=true&_nfto=false&_pageLabel=mhvHome

National Advisory Committee on Rural Health and Human Services. (2004).*The 2004 Report to the Secretary: Rural Health and Human Services*. Available at: ftp://ftp.hrsa.gov/ruralhealth/NAC04web.pdf

Nickelson, D. (1996). Behavioral telehealth: Emerging practice, research, and policy opportunities. *Behavioral Sciences & the Law*, *14*, 443–457. doi:10.1002/(SICI)1099-0798(199623)14:4<443::AID-BSL256>3.0.CO;2-G

Nickelson, D. W. (1998). Telehealth and the evolving health care system: Strategic opportunities for professional psychology. *Professional Psychology, Research and Practice*, *29*, 527–534. doi:10.1037/0735-7028.29.6.527

Norman, S. (2006). The use of telemedicine in psychiatry. *Journal of Psychiatric and Mental Health Nursing*, *13*, 771–777. doi:10.1111/j.1365-2850.2006.01033.x

Office of Rural Health Policy, Health Resources and Services Administration. (1994). *Reaching: Rural health travel in the telecommunications highway*. Rockville, MD: Federal Office of Rural Health Policy.

Sammons, M. T., & DeLeon, P. H. (2004). Whither online counseling: Conceptualizing the Challenges and promises of distance mental health service provision. In Kraus, R., Zack, J., & Stricker, G. (Eds.), *Online Counseling: A Handbook for Mental Health Professionals*. New York: Elsevier Press.

Sargent, I. (1999). School based mental health in rural Kansas: A novel use for telepsychiatry. [abstract]. *Telemedicine Journal*, *5*(1), 52.

Shaw, P., Goodwin, J., Whitten, P., & Doolittle, G. (1999). Tele-Kid Care: An urban telemedicine service for an underserved pediatric population. [abstract]. *Telemedicine Journal*, *5*(1), 25.

Solow, C., Weiss, R., Bergen, B., & Sanborn, C. (1971). 24-hour psychiatric consultation via TV. *The American Journal of Psychiatry*, *127*, 120–123.

Stamm, B. H. (1999). Creating virtual community: Telehealth and self-care updated. In Stamm, B. H. (Ed.), *Secondary traumatic stress: Self-care issues for clinicians, researchers, and educators* (pp. 179–208). Lutherville, MD: Sidran Press.

Straker, N., Mostyn, P., & Marshall, C. (1976). The use of two-way TV in bringing mental health services to the inner city. *The American Journal of Psychiatry*, *133*, 1202–1205.

Striefel, S. (2000, Summer). Telehealth uses in biofeedback and applied psychophysiology. *Biofeedback*, 28 (2). Retrieved February 4, 2004, from http://www.aapb.org/public/

Whitten, B., Cook, D. J., Shaw, P., Ermer, D., & Goodwin, J. (1998). Telekid Care: Bringing health care into schools. *Telemedicine Journal*, *4*(4), 335–343.

Whitten, P. S., & Cook, D. J. (1999). School-based telemedicine: Using technology to bring health care to inner-city children. [abstract]. *Journal of Telemedicine and Telecare*, *5*(Suppl 1), S23–S25. doi:10.1258/1357633991932423

Wood, J. A. (2000). *The effectiveness of videophone technology in bringing mental healthservices to rural residents.* Unpublished master's thesis, Stephen F. Austin State University, Nacogdoches, TX.

Wood, J. A. (2006, April). *Patient and provider satisfaction with telemental health services.* Poster presented at the VA Psychology Leadership Conference, Dallas, TX.

Wood, J. A. & Hargrove, D. S. (2006). *Use of videoconferencing to deliver mental health services to adults with mental retardation.* Manuscript submitted for publication.

Wood, J. A., Miller, T. W., & Hargrove, D. S. (2005). Clinical supervision in rural settings: A telehealth model. *Professional Psychology, Research and Practice*, *36*(2), 173–179. doi:10.1037/0735-7028.36.2.173

Wood, J. A., O'Quin, J., & Eftink, S. (2004). A preliminary investigation of the use of videophone technology as a training tool for students working with older adults. *Journal of Teaching in Social Work*, *24*, 35–46. doi:10.1300/J067v24n03_03

Yellowlees, P. (2005). Successfully developing a telemedicine system. *Journal of Telemedicine and Telecare*, *11*, 331–335. doi:10.1258/135763305774472024

Young, T., & Irenson, C. (2003). Effectiveness of School based Telehealth Care in Rural Elementary Schools. *Pediatrics*, *112*(5), 1088–1096. doi:10.1542/peds.112.5.1088

Zarate, C. A., Weinstock, L., Cukor, P., Morabito, C., Leahy, L., Burns, C., & Baer, L. (1997). Applicability of telemedicine for assessing patients with schizophrenia: Acceptance and reliability. *The Journal of Clinical Psychiatry*, *58*, 22–25. doi:10.4088/JCP.v58n0104

Chapter 14
Clinical Continuity by Integrated Care

Torben Larsen
University of Southern Denmark, Denmark

ABSTRACT

The fragmented delivery of healthcare and social services was put on the research agenda by WHO in 2002. Integrated Homecare (IHC) combining efficacy with net savings represents a prototype of integrated care for better clinical continuity. Frequent chronic conditions as stroke, heart failure and chronic obstructive pulmonary disease exhibit parallel results as explained by a common neuroeconomic framework. A SWOT analysis of IHC emphasizes: 1) Strength: health economic dominance; 2) Weakness: fragmented financial conditions; 3) Opportunity: low-tech patient benefits affordable to European countries facing tight finances as the elder share grows; 3) Threat: low levels of trust across professions and settings. A meso-strategy for EU recommends: 1) A health technology assessment (HTA) of IHC by multidisciplinary teamwork across the hospital and primary care interface synthesizes existing research for health care decision-makers. 2)Dissemination focuses on a regional level with direct contact between the clinical and financial level, see information on practical implementation guides at www.integratedhomecare.eu.

INTRODUCTION

A number of studies from the 1990s focused on healthcare problems related to the lack of clinical continuity. The fragmented delivery of healthcare and social services was put on the agenda as a major problem by WHO (Gröne, 2002) and was followed up by the European Commission and Council (Joint Report, 2003, p.15). However, a FP5 project on integrated health and social care for older persons (Leischenring, 2004) concludes that 'Integrated care (IC) 'by law' as a top-down implementation will certainly not suffice, and market mechanisms as bottom-up approaches

DOI: 10.4018/978-1-60960-183-6.ch014

are less likely to improve joint working and the development of shared visions'. What could then be done to overcome the problems of a fragmented delivery of healthcare?

Fragmented delivery and lack of clinical continuity is more relevant to chronic conditions (CC) than to time limited acute episodic care (Holman, 2004).

This chapter aims to review the present state of research on integrated care (IC) specific to chronic conditions (CC) focusing on the efficacy regarding Activities of Daily Living (ADL) in order to develop an effective and economic strategy for clinical continuity.

METHODS AND MATERIALS

General Strategy of Evaluation

The essence of IC is 'overlapping' services in the secondary/primary interface after discharge in contrast to coordination at the management level alone (Gröne, 2002, p. 2). IC should apply only as far as quality outcomes are improved with the overall aim to improve equitably distributed population health (Gröne, 2002, p. 3). He illustrates the causal relationships derived from IC as reproduced in figure 1.

Operational quality outcomes are crucial for the design of IC. Mortality is seldom a major indicator for IC. Typically, studies of effectiveness on IC address activities of daily living (ADL) as:

1. Referrals to permanent institutional care (i.e. nursing homes)
2. Independence in ADL as indicated by functional indices as Barthel Index (BI) or Functional Independence Measure (FIM)
3. Shortened length-of-stay at hospitals / less readmissions

Evaluation of the relationship between IC and outcomes will follow best international practice as formalised in the international operation of Health Technology Assessment (HTA). According to the definition of HTA by EUnetHTA:

Health technology assessment (HTA) is a multidisciplinary process that summarises information about the medical, social, economic and ethical issues related to the use of a health technology in a systematic, transparent, unbiased, robust manner. It aims to inform the formulation of safe and

Figure 1. Action model for integrated care (IC)

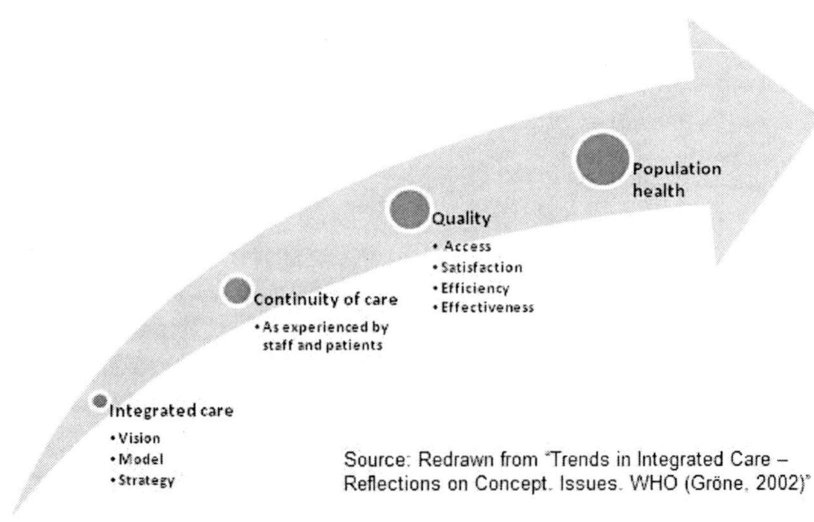

Source: Redrawn from "Trends in Integrated Care – Reflections on Concept. Issues. WHO (Gröne, 2002)"

effective health policies that are patient focused and seek best value.

HTA may address direct and intended consequences of technologies as well as indirect and unintended consequences. The main purpose of an HTA is to assist informed technology-based policymaking in health care. Most health professionals and many decision-makers in health care might comply with the conclusions from an HTA as far as it investigates all of the following aspects:

1. Effectiveness regarding the physiologic outcome of the intervention
2. Patient safety and satisfaction, solicited i.e. by focus group interviews
3. Economic efficiency based on the principle of alternative costs
4. Organizational implementation of the intervention

Review Findings on Integrated Care

Searching Medline ultimo 2007 identifies many trials on IC wherefore the selection of literature is based on reviews of 'clinical continuity' and 'integrated care' which are closely related concepts in this study. A 'review of reviews' (Servellen, 2006, p. 186) focuses on the definition of clinical continuity and the significance to quality outcomes. Servellen identifies three categories of continuity which is used in a number of other studies of continuity, too:

1. *informational* continuity on past events and personal circumstances
2. *management* continuity across settings with several providers
3. *relational* continuity between a patient and one or more providers

Management continuity corresponds to the continuity across the secondary/primary care interface and relational continuity to the longitudinal or provider continuity defined by WHO (Gröne, 2003). Management continuity is the focus of most continuity studies while only a few studies focus all three categories of continuity. According to Servellen et al. the relationship between continuity of care for CC and quality outcomes relies on the impact of three values of social patient psychology:

- Perceived control over their care (*feeling safe*)
- Great involvement in decision-making (*participation*)
- Knowledge about their illness and its treatment (*primary health feedback*)

The three psychological factors stated above seem more relevant to CC where patients have limited capacity of self-care i.e. stroke patients. Half of the studies in clinical continuity focus on the transition from hospital to home care (Servellen, 2006, p. 192). In all, the action mechanism of IC might be conceived as a human relations management effect in the care for CC parallel to the *Hawthorne-effect* discovered in industrial work organisation (Mayo, 1949).

Reviewing 36 reviews focusing on the management aspect of clinical continuity or organisational interventions to improve outcome a total of five different types of organisational interventions are identified (Wensing, 2006):

- Revision of professional roles i.e. delegation of responsibility from physicians to nurses
- Multidisciplinary teams i.e. clinical teams of physicians, nurses and other health professionals
- Integrated care delivery services as disease management programs, integrated care pathways or case management overlaps to patients with specific CC receiving care according to a protocol

- Knowledge management defined as the optimal organisation of knowledge within an organisation. It mainly refers to the use of information and communication technology i.e. computerized medical records
- Quality management focusing on customers, continuous efforts to improve measurement and analysis of performance and supportive management

It is concluded that general reviews of clinical continuity are too heterogeneous for quantitative analysis. However, patient outcomes were generally improved by multidisciplinary teams, integrated care services and computer systems. Also, cost savings were reported from integrated care services appearing as dominant interventions in the health economic sense of this term. Another review of reviews with an overlap of authors focuses on IC (Ouwens, 2005). Ouwens concludes that IC seemed to have positive effects on the quality of care. However, to compare IC programmes and clarify cost-effectiveness, more consistent definitions must be used and component interventions must be well described.

Figure 2. Neuropsychological Model

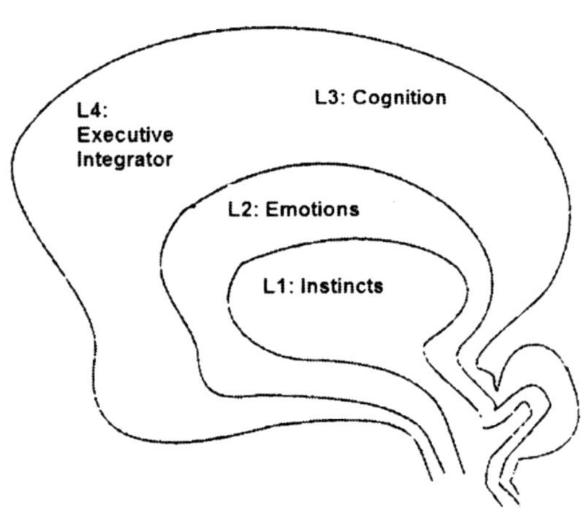

Clinical Trials on IC

Focusing directly on clinical trials on IC specific to major CC it appears that home health interventions are the most frequent type of IC (Servellen, 2006). Further, this type of IC favours relevant psychological conditions of the patient as 1) feeling safe, 2) participation and 3) primary health feedback i.e. when measured at home a patient's blood pressure is significantly lower compared to when this is measured at a medical clinic (Verberk et al, 2005). The home rehabilitation effect is explained by neuropsychology as illustrated in Figure 2 (Larsen, 2008):

As L1-2 becomes more relaxed by home rehabilitation the integration of L2-4 (Learning/recovery) is facilitated.

Such interventions might be dominant (Wensing, 2006) wherefore they represent a synergy of interests between the political/administrative and health professional levels of decision-making relevant to rapid dissemination in the health care sector. Accordingly, trials with home health intervention focusing on IC have been identified from the reviews mentioned above as well as from additional systematic searches in Medline for 'trials' and 'clinical continuity' or 'integrated care' or 'home training'. From these searches the following trials on home interventions for major CC have been extracted setting the priorities. Review results as complemented by midway results from the FP7-Homecare 222954 granted by the European Commission is summarized below. Further information on www.integratedhomecare.eu .

MIDWAY RESULTS FROM FP7-HOMECARE 222954

Early Home-Supported Discharge of Stroke Patients as Prototype of Integrated Care

Early supported discharge (ESD) is claimed to be a promising alternative to conventional stroke rehabilitation by the ESD Trialists in 2002. The ESD Trialists have published an extended study demonstrating a significant effect on poor outcomes and length of stay (Langhorne et al, 2005). In 2006 these results were elaborated in a HTA of EHSD where the added 'H' specifies that this intervention has to be delivered at the domicile of the patient (Larsen, 2006). This implicates that purely municipal alternatives without domiciliary training are excluded. The HTA concludes that EHSD is a dominant intervention in comparison to conventional stroke unit rehabilitation due to shorter hospital stay and less referral to nursing homes. The net saving by EHSD is calculated to 800 EURO per patient. This applies to about 40% of all newly diagnosed strokes or about 1 pro mille of the total population in industrialized countries with a life expectancy of about 80 years. From an EU perspective such savings address about 500.000 new stroke patients per year with a potential net saving of around 400 million Euro each year.

Within Homecare 222954 these results are object to further investigation by randomized controlled trials (RCT) in both a high-income country (Denmark) and a middle-income country (Portugal). Midway in the project the INFO-sheet shown in Table 1 has been released for local teams aiming to implement IHC Stroke (ESD):

For IHC-Stroke, FIM is the preferred indicator of ADL as it, unlike BI, includes cognitive aspects which provides useful information for internal communication in the multidisciplinary team as well as communication across the secondary/primary interface. The prognostic efficacy regarding recovery of independence in ADL is about the same for BI and FIM (Hobart, 2001).

It should be emphasized that EHSD is not considered an alternative to a stroke unit. IHC-STROKE is considered an extension of stroke unit services. A study of IHC-STROKE (Langhorne, 2007) reports an illustrative example of the psychological values associated with training at home (safety, motivation and transference) producing the extra recovery. Accordingly, IHC-STROKE might serve as prototype of excellence in IC.

The potential of IHC-STROKE expands to some degree to other related neurological CC as Traumatic Brain Injury (TBI) and Multiple Sclerosis (MS). In all, Stroke, TBI and MS represent a burden to society in terms of prevalence, morbidity, mortality and economic costs that rank in top 3 among CC.

EFFICACY OF INTEGRATED CARE FOR CHRONIC CONDITIONS OTHER THAN STROKE

Home Support to Patients with Heart Failure (HF)

Continuity of cardiac care is considered an integrated part of secondary prevention and improved health outcomes. A significant positive relationship between continuity of cardiac care, rehabilitation participation, greater tangible support and less serious perception of illness consequences is evidenced in a 9 months post discharge survey in Canada (Riley, 2007).

A quasi experimental American pilot study of a structured home health intervention with many similarities to IHC-STROKE indicates decreased rehospitalisation, decreased symptoms of Heart Failure (HF) and increased quality of life (Quinn, 2006). However, more empirical research is required for evaluation of the effectiveness of this type of home intervention. Regarding the cost-effectiveness a study (Taylor, 2007) concludes that the costs per patient of running the home-based rehabilitation programme was just slightly lower than that of the hospital- based programme. Supposing that a better structured home health intervention improves outcomes – as indicated by the Quinn pilot study – such intervention would be as preferable for HF as homecare for stroke patients.

A survey on HF management programmes in Europe (Jaarsma, 2006) concludes that only

Table 1.

Information sheet on Early Supported Discharge for stroke patients
Background
Recently services have been developed that challenge the traditional emphasis on rehabilitation in hospital, in particular Early Supported Discharge (ESD) services. ESD services aim at accelerating the patients' discharge home providing an equivalent level of rehabilitation input in the patient's own home – with less poor outcomes at follow-up 6-12 months after discharge.
Intervention services
ESD services comprises a multidisciplinary team which coordinates discharge from hospital, post discharge care and provides rehabilitation in the patient's home. In particular, beneficial effects of ESD services have been seen in those that are provided by an expert coordinated multidisciplinary team who meet on a regular basis to coordinate patient care. The organisational base for the ESD team is usually either a hospital or a community base.
The multidisciplinary team comprises physiotherapy, occupational therapy, speech and language therapy with medical nursing and social support. Typical teams have approximately 3.0 whole time equivalents (WTE) staff to manage a notional hundred patients per year, as follows: physiotherapy 1.1, occupational therapy 1.0, speech and language therapy 0 – 0.5, medical 0.1, nursing 0 – 1.2, assistant 0.2.
Patient characteristics
Patients tend to be elderly (average ranges from 66 – 78 years) with a clinical diagnosis of stroke. Selection of patients is normally based on need (persisting disability), stability of their medical condition and practicality (living within the local area). The typical initial Barthel Index at the time of recruitment ranges from 10/20 to 17/20 with a lower interquartile limit of 6/20 and upper limit of 19/20. The Barthel Index at the time of discharge is typically between 12/20 to 17/20.
Illustration of patient pathway
The typical patient pathway includes the following: In hospital, there is an early identification of the patient in hospital and a visit from the key worker from the ESD team. The key worker makes contact with the patient and carer, carries out a patient assessment and arranges a home assessment. A home assessment is carried out either with the patient (home visit or home training session) or without the patient (environmental visit). Thereafter discharge home is planned with agreement of rehabilitation goals.
After discharge home, the ESD team implements the rehabilitation plan usually beginning on the day of discharge or the following day. In some trials part of the home rehabilitation is placed before discharge to soften the transition from hospital to home. The rehabilitation plan includes accessing relevant services (e.g. community services) and multidisciplinary team review of progress. There will then be a negotiated withdrawal of the ESD service within 1-3 months and a late review of ongoing needs or problems.
978-1-60960-183-6.ch014.f01
Rehabilitation programme
Home rehabilitation programmes vary in terms of length and frequency of visits in accordance with individual patient needs. In terms of content, the focus is usually on activities of daily living (ADL), ambulation and speech and communication. Typically, a key worker of the ESD team is responsible for coordinating services with the hospital, local community services, primary care or other relevant general care services.
The IHC STROKE info-sheet is available at www.integratedhomecare.eu

in the UK, a combination of hospital and home-based programmes is common (present in 75% of the HF programmes in UK). So, evidence-based guidelines on HF home interventions for improvement of outcome might be very useful as it tops the list of health burden to society in terms of economic costs. To structure the IHC HF-intervention a query has been made to about 100 European heart centres.

Midway in the Homecare 222954 project, the INFO-sheet shown in Table 2 has been released for local teams aiming at implementing IHC Stroke HF services:

Home-Support to Patients with Chronic Obstructive Pulmonary Disease

In recent years, more trials on IC for patients with chronic obstructive pulmonary disease (COPD) have been reported. An RCT reports an intervention with an individually tailored care plan at discharge combined with a primary care team and access to a specialized case manager nurse through a web-based call centre including a joint home visit of the specialized nurse and the primary care team (physician, nurse and social worker) within 72 hours after discharge (Garcia-Aymerich, 2007). Non-scheduled home visits could be triggered through the call centre. This IC improved disease knowledge and treatment adherence after one year treatment. The improvement in lung function compared to usual treatment was only border-significant in this rather small trial.

A combined Spanish-Belgian RCT (Casa, 2006) reported a similar intervention which demonstrated a significant reduction in both

Table 2.

Information sheet on Home Care for heart failure patients
Background
Patients with chronic heart failure often have complex care needs due to old age, poor social support, cognitive decline, co-morbidities and poly-pharmacy. Prognosis of heart failure is poor and half of the patients die within 4-5 years after their diagnosis (Dickstein et al. 2008). A growing number of HF patients will be in need of lifelong care with regular follow up to optimize treatment and educate and support self-care management. Ideally, long term follow-up should be integrating primary-secondary care and organize care around the patient and his family.
Intervention services
An integrated heart failure disease management program provides care to patient either in the hospital or at home. The homecare should include a patient centered collaboration between primary-secondary care, community care and the patient/family.
Team: The team members are a cardiologist, GP, heart failure nurse, home care nurse. If possible the team could also include a physical therapist, occupational therapist, dietician, psychologist, social worker, administrator on a regular or consultative basis
Meeting: Organization of collaboration between team members with regular meetings may be face to face or remotely via telephone/ video conferencing. In some instants this might be daily meetings, while in other situations a weekly meeting might be sufficient
Care plans: Care is planned in collaboration between the patient/family and the care team. First a structured assessment is performed with the possibility to triage patients to different care pathways related to the stage of the disease trajectory, including pathways related to palliation and end of life care.
Optimised treatment according to guidelines: Ongoing assessment of optimal pharmacological and non-pharmacological treatment in the individual. This can be done either in the hospital during admission, during the HF clinic time or at home. Drug titration to the highest tolerable doses of appropriate heart failure drugs. Self-care management should be evaluated with special emphasis on symptom- recognition and adherence to treatment.
Educational strategies for patients/families/caregivers: Verbal information in combination with written materials or other approaches such as CD roms or www.heartfailurematters.org should be provided and repeated. Families should be involved. Patients should also be advice and instructed on diet and physical activity/exercise training.
Increased accessibility to care: The hospital or the homecare service will provide:
Telephone access to a specified health care provider/team, home visits and have a mechanism in place to react to emergencies including out of office hours. The possibility to provide telemonitoring is evaluated
Patient characteristics
Patients tend to be elderly (average ranges from 65 – 80 years) with a clinical diagnosis of heart failure. Selection of patients is normally based on need (persisting symptoms, deterioration), stability of their medical condition and practicality (living within the local area). Patient are mostly in NYHA class II-IV
Illustration of patient pathway The typical patient pathway includes the following:
In hospital, patient will be identified by a nurse to be in need for a multidisciplinary integrated approach, with the main focus from the heart failure clinic, the home care team or both.
The heart failure nurse contacts the patient and carer, carries out a patient assessment and contacts the relevant professionals and makes a care plan.
Three options after discharge are: 1) Follow up at the heart failure clinic only, 2) Follow up at heart failure clinic first and transfer to home care, 3) Follow up at home care only.
1. If the main focus of care is given from the heart failure clinic, home care will not be informed at first stage, but the GP will receive a letter with information on the patient condition. All components will be provided at the HF clinic
2. After hospitalization the patient will be seen for first follow-up in the heart failure clinic. Medication is optimized, first education provided at the HF clinic in the hospital. The heart failure nurse will assess the patient during each visit and will contact the home care and GP as soon is the patient ready to be transferred. A joint care plan is made and used.
3. If the main focus of care in home care, the heart failure nurse contacts the home care organization and transfers the patient to their care. The home care organization contacts the patient and carer and makes a appointment and assessment and plans care. All components will be provided in home care, with additional possibility to consult to the cardiology clinic, the heart failure clinic.
Preparation:
The team needs to have competencies to deliver optimal HF care. The knowledge and skills on heart failure care in the team members should be sufficient (for nurses part of the "European curriculum for clinical expertise in heart failure" can be used). (Depending on the health care system modules on prescribing and assessment of non medical health care providers might be added). The education should have team-based educational activities
The IHC HF info-sheet is available at www.integratedhomecare.eu

hospitalisation and readmission rates related to exacerbations in COPD patients.

In all, the findings regarding the efficacy of IC for COPD patients seem parallel to the findings for stroke patients. As the burden of COPD in terms of prevalence, morbidity, mortality and economic costs is in top 5 of CC, improved outcomes by IC should be prioritised. However, from a healthcare provider perspective further studies of this IC application must include cost-effectiveness as well as effectiveness in older disabled patients with COPD. Midway in the FP7 Homecare 222954 project, the INFO-sheet shown in Table 3 has been released for local teams aiming at implementing IHC COPD services:

Table 3.

Information sheet on Integrated Homecare for COPD patients
Background
Chronic Obstructive Pulmonary Disease (COPD) is a prevailing chronic condition worldwide. As in the case of heart failure and type II diabetes, management of COPD patients should not be limited to pharmacological treatment. A more comprehensive approach is preferable and has proved to be more successful. Aspects like active life-style, addressing co-morbidities and coping with social needs are important. Traditional health care systems have failed in providing an adequate framework for this alternative approach. New home based integrated care models are demonstrating better efficacy.
Intervention services
The name 'home hospitalisation' originally referred to a service modality designed to keep the patient in his/her own environment, thus reducing the risk of hospital acquired infections and decreasing the occupancy of hospital beds by chronically ill patients. In COPD, home hospitalisation is a short-term high-intensity intervention mainly applied to severe exacerbated patients discharged from emergency room or after a short hospital stay. It is carried out by specialised personnel as an alternative to conventional admission. It has been proved to be safe and to have a comparable efficacy and reduced costs.
However, from a patient-centric perspective, best results can only be achieved if an integrated care strategy is adopted. This typically involves a multidisciplinary team of professionals from different institutions / levels of care that are coordinated by a case manager. Patients and their carers play a more active role in this model. Quite often, the level of coordination required is supported by information and communication technologies. This integrated care strategy for COPD patients hold the potential to move care beyond the management of crisis to early detection and prevention.
Patient characteristics
It is estimated that COPD affects 10% of the population older than 40. Spirometry is a reliable diagnostic test for COPD and easy to perform, but in spite of this the condition typically remains undiagnosed during early stages. As a result, patients tend to be elderly. In those ones with a mild-to-moderate condition diagnosed, the survival is 13.9 years. If airway obstruction is severe then survival is reduced to 10 years. Severe exacerbations are common in patients in advanced stages of the disease leading to frequent visits to emergency care departments and/or admissions at hospitals and progressive deterioration.
Illustration of patient pathway
The following graph illustrates a characteristic integrated care (home hospitalisation) pathway for a COPD patient. Albeit the described building blocks can be generalised, local customisation is important and can notably affect relevant details (i.e. who is the responsible professional and what task is allocated to whom)
978-1-60960-183-6.ch014.f02
Case identification: eligible patients can be identified at conventional facilities such as acute & emergency department, hospital wards, outpatient departments, day-case areas. Ideally, professionals working in these areas should be aware of the basic inclusion criteria to the programme to consider referring the patient.
Case evaluation: Patients referred to the programme are assessed by the case manager, and if required with the concurrence of other professionals (e.g. doctors or social workers) Special attention is paid to co-morbidities, social aspects, patient education and informal carer support. In addition to regular clinical information, instruments monitoring quality of life and dependence are applied at this stage.
Work plan definition: The case manager coordinates the multidisciplinary team that elaborates the individual care plan for the patient. The plan includes the regime of visits by nurses and/or doctors, the need for education sessions, frequency and type or monitoring sessions (if needed) and other logistics (i.e. oxygen at home)
Follow-up: Corresponds to the actual execution of the individual plan and may vary in duration. During this spell, the case manager coordinates any unexpected demand of the patient. Adequate facilities (call centre, ICT supported team work) should be made available to guarantee timely reactions.
Discharge: Discharge occurs when the patient does not longer meet the inclusion criteria. This can be the result of a change in the health or social condition (i.e. stroke episode, change of carer) or other causes (i.e. patient moving to another area).
The IHC COPD info-sheet is available at www.integratedhomecare.eu

TeleRehab as Supplement to Direct Home Intervention

A systematic review of home telemonitoring for CC concludes that it produces accurate and reliable data, empowers patients, influences their attitude and behaviours, and potentially improves their medical conditions (Paré, 2007). An RCT on telerehabilitation for stroke patients (Piron, 2005) indicates that telerehabilitation might be as effective as home rehabilitation to improve motor deficits. More research in the substitution between direct personal home interventions and the use of telerehabilitation is recommended i.e. regarding telerehab as a complement in cases of

- A long distance between patient and hospital
- Special needs for acute home monitoring of the patient
- Needs for training by virtual reality programmes

Midway in the Homecare 222954 project, a systematic review has been conducted to summarize the state of the evidences on telerehabilitation and telemedicine homecare approaches. The major conclusions of the review are shown in Table 4:

Based on this review three pilot-studies on the use of Tele-facilities in IHC HF are conducted within the Homecare project. Also, a pilot on virtual motor rehabilitation pilot is carried out as a supplement to IHC Stroke.

Long Term Community-Based Domicile for Patients with Mental Disease

IC for patients with mental disorders might represent the same psychological values of safety, participation and transference as evidenced by IHC-STROKE. Actually, the net benefits of IC were evidenced for the first time for patients with mental disorders in the London TAPS Study (Leff, 1997). This five year follow-up on 95% of 670 non-demented, long-stay psychiatric patients discharged to community-based domicile gave the following encouraging results:

- Two out of three were still living in their original residences after five years
- Less than 1 of 100 patients became homeless, and no patient from a staffed home was lost to follow-up
- More than one third of the patients were readmitted during the five years follow-up, but at the end of the period only 10% were in hospital
- Overall, the patients quality of life was greatly improved by the move to the com-

Table 4.

Results of systematic review of Tele-support to IHC interventions
The state of the evidence emerging from this overview appears to be in favour of HF rather than COPD and STROKE patients, due both to differences in the literature available and to a longer experience in the field of remote monitoring of patients discharged after heart failure.
This general finding should be considered in planning trials on tele-applications in homecare, with the consequent need to adopt different objectives and strategies for the three different populations.
Moreover, it should be considered that the few indications emerging from the extracted data are not so strong.
In both HF and COPD patients, interventions should be targeted to a telemonitoring (automated or not) more than to a telephone follow-up application. Transferring this finding to STROKE patients, an on-line interactive device (allowing also videoconference) should be preferred rather than a store and forward device to provide the tele-intervention.
Outcomes like "overall mortality" and "hospital admission" should be included to prove the effectiveness of interventions. Moreover variables like "QoL, "cost", "adherence" and "patient acceptability" should be taken into consideration to perform a complete analysis of the telecare approach choices.
Regarding the systematic analysis of the literature, the gap in the COPD and the STROKE population should be filled in order to obtain a more complete framework of the effectiveness of telemedicine as a useful intervention in the homecare of chronic conditions.

munity, but their disabilities remained (due to the nature of severe psychotic illness)
- There was little overall difference between hospital and community costs, but economic evaluation suggests that community care is more cost-effective than long term stay hospital care because effectiveness had improved

In practice, long term stay community residential care can be divided into three categories (Chilvers, 2003):

- 24-hour staffed residential care which are well-staffed hostels like nursing homes
- Day-staffed residential places which are hostels that works fixed hours
- Accommodations with low levels of staff support only

As emphasized in the review of community-based mental healthcare by Thornicroft and Tansella, mental disorders account for more than 30% of all years lived with disability wherefore improvements have the most extensive impact on daily life (HEN, 2003). However, as the implementation of this line of research seems to be taken care of within psychiatry, the Homecare 222954 focuses on major 'somatic' CC, only.

DISCUSSION OF PATIENT SCHOOLS AND INTEGRATED CARE

Essentially, IC depends on the interdependence and potential synergy of behavioural and somatic health (LaBrie, 2007). The most direct use of this synergy might be patient training empowering and educating patients for better self-management of CC or even life style modification (Helene, 2000). For more CC such patient education is evidenced as both effective and efficient:

The prototype in this field might be diabetes schools which are that well-established that national guidelines already exist in a number of countries i.e. USA (Mensing, 2005). Also, the effectiveness of patient education on low back pain is evidenced (Tavafian, 2007). As evidenced by Guevara et al educational programmes for self-management of asthma in children and adolescents to improve lung function and the feeling of self-control reduce absenteeism from school, number of days with restricted activity, number of visits to an emergency department, and possibly the number of disturbed nights (Guevara, 2003).

Another heavy CC is rheumatism where patient education is evidenced to lead to both better and more cost-effective management (Lind-Albrecht, 2006).

However, as Homecare 222954 highlights CC where interventions at home are effective, the CC where patient schools are sufficient, are not included in the project.

CONCLUSIONS ON THE POTENTIAL IMPACT OF IHC

1. Homecare 222954 aims at a systematic approach to clinical continuity across the secondary/primary interface for CC by integrated homecare (IHC).
2. IHC interventions is found to be an excellent form of IC as our domicile is the place where we *feel safe, participate most and have direct feedback* from ADL training (An obvious parallel in rehabilitation to the Hawthorne effect discovered in industrial work group management). Community-based interventions might to some degree give patients the same psychological advantages. Telerehabilitation is an economic form of reproducing the values of direct home health interventions when patients are not too weakened mentally i.e. for HF-patients, or when distance and time spent make transport and weariness from travel important extra costs.

3. Research has been reviewed on IHC on major CC representing the better part of the burden to society in terms of prevalence, morbidity, mortality and costs:
   - 1) Stroke, 2) COPD and 3) HF are all diseases which (due to the Hawthorne effect) would benefit from giving priority to home health interventions measured by a comprehensive assessment of effectiveness, efficiency and quality of life
   - Regarding diabetes, asthma, low back pain and rheumatism, patient education for better self-management is assessed as an excellent strategy for clinical continuity for patients that are already independent in ADL. Consequently, these CC are excluded from the present study
   - The focus on the specific medical diagnosis should not be overemphasized as most patients in the target group typically is elderly persons suffering from co-morbidities
4. The potential outcomes from IHC focus on 'Poor outcome' as a composite of mortality and disability. Disability outcomes i.e. including prevention of readmissions or referrals to institution might be priced in accordance with their savings in health care and social services on activities of daily living (ADL). Accordingly, cost-effectiveness analysis is an important tool for decision-makers having to set priorities for a variety of alternative IHC interventions. Regarding IHC, priorities are facilitated by a synergy between effectiveness and efficiency which should enable a relatively rapid dissemination. Moreover, these benefits are relevant to a majority of the population suffering from one or more CC from some point in their life.
5. However, in practice the realization of the potential benefits of IHC have to overcome serious barriers as stated in an Australian report (Jordan, 2007):
   - Fragmented health service delivery due to funding complexities between national and local government
   - Recruitment of a sufficient number of patients to document effects as RCT on ADL outcomes often requires inclusion of several hundred patients
   - Low status of low-tech approaches in IHC within the healthcare sector
   - Lack of knowledge within the healthcare sector of the psychological factors relevant to IHC
   - Lack of mutual trust between health care professionals across the secondary/primary interface. Even between physicians in different settings distinct differences in values have been identified (Pettersen and Johnsen, 2007). IHC requires much more than collaboration of physicians across the secondary/primary interface, it requires a multidisciplinary collaboration across the secondary/primary interface

SWOT ANALYSIS OF IHC

In order to design an appropriate strategy for the dissemination of IHC to harvest the potential benefit, it is necessary to clarify the true character. For this purpose, a comprehensive analysis of the relative Strengths, Weaknesses, Opportunities and Threats (SWOT analysis) regarding IHC is appropriate. For the sake of simplicity only the three most important aspects of each of the dimensions as listed in Table 5 are described.

Strengths

Normally, health economic choices are about how much to pay extra for some specific health

Table 5. SWOT analysis of Integrated Homeare (IHC)

Strengths • Dominant interventions creating synergy • Based on a neuro-psychological holism shared by more health professions • Job enrichment to therapists and nurses	**Opportunities** • Potential benefits for a majority of people • Low-Tech interventions are a special opportunity to low-income countries • General improvement of organisational quality in public health
Weaknesses • Lack of trust across the secondary/primary interface • Relative low medical research priority • Moderate improvements on a day-to-day basis	**Threats** • Fragmented financial conditions • Mono-disciplinary strategies • Mediocre implementations without effect

improvement. This might involve tough negotiations between the involved parties representing different interests: professionals representing their specialty, administrators having budget restraints and politicians representing the population as both potential patients and tax payers in the type of national healthcare organisations which are characteristic for EU. In comparison to the typical conditions of healthcare decisions, dominant healthcare interventions are characterized by synergy between the interests of healthcare professionals and the economic interest of society. For example, the HTA of IHC-STROKE concludes two things: Firstly, quality is increased as demonstrated by the increased share of patients living in their own home one year after the intervention. Secondly, economic net savings due to the positive net value of the following three factors:

1) Fewer bed-days at the hospital plus 2) saving nursing home beds minus 3) the costs of doing therapeutic home sessions. In this situation alliances across disciplines are facilitated to the benefit of a relatively quick dissemination of dominant interventions as IHC for major groups of CC. The specific economic evaluation of IHC-STROKE calculates a net saving of 800 EURO per patient compared to conventional rehabilitation at hospital. The impact of this result might be illustrated extrapolating the net benefit from IHC-STROKE as well as HF, COPD and mental disease to a significant share of the 500 million people in the extended EU. Furthermore, this result might be accentuated by a comparison to modest marginal improvement of effectiveness increasing costs by mono-disciplinary research.

Further, the promising results as outlined above rest on specified psychological values in IHC which are rooted in a neuroeconomic model [Larsen, 2010], i.e.:

- The evidence of 'feeling more safe at home' is well known from the clinic as the blood pressure of a patient is lower when measured at home compared to at the hospital
- The motivational effect of 'increased participation' is well known from sociological trials
- The learning effect of primary feedback is well known from learning in general and especially as better transference in rehabilitation

IHC represents a unique option for job enrichment to subordinated health professionals at the hospital, i.e. nurses and therapists. Home health interventions from the hospital by an outgoing multidisciplinary team result in team members – who are often nurses and therapists – becoming more independent of the formal line of authority in hospitals. Visiting the home of the patient means that much extra information about the patient is collected. It is important for the outgoing team members to consider the individual conditions of the patient and take responsibility to act on these. For example, if a stroke patient with motor problems is used to have his exercise by cycling, the final objective for his rehabilitation should be to modify his cycle in a way that enables him to restart cycling. If his rehabilitation is limited to a standardised hospital walking test implemented as being able to walk around in his house, the real benefit from home health is lost. To nurses and therapists, especially, this kind of development of their services from a level of standardisation to a level of individualised creativity may represent a lift from the ordinary towards excellence in professional performance which represents a strong motivator to these professions [Larsen, 2006].

Weaknesses

It is evident e.g. from qualitative interviews related to IHC that lack of mutual trust across settings represent a barrier to specific IHC initiatives. However, this kind of emotional resistance is not specific to IHC. It is a general obstacle to change which should be overcome by the benefits from IHC. Actually, professionals in both healthcare and social services report better mutual understanding and collaboration as an independent staff benefit from IHC besides the specific improvements to the patients and carers. Also within the hospital, the same benefit may arise as nurses and therapists become better integrated.

The present focus on IHC is driven by the expected rise of the share of elderly as life expectancy rises in the industrialised countries. However, this means on the other hand that a majority of patients needing IHC are old age pensioners who, in general, hold a low status in politics compared to people in the work active age. In reality, pressures exist for short termed down-sizing of social services disregarding long term benefits as indicated by Leichsenring. This represents an obstacle to the development of IHC that has to be taken into account. This is, however, slightly moderated by the growing significance of elderly voters in democratic societies. Also, among physicians IC may have a relative low professional status compared to specialist research augmenting the peer status.

Opportunities

Besides being dominant IHC addresses the majority of the population as most people, especially the elderly, are exposed to high risk of suffering from stroke, HF, COPD or mental disease. This means that IHC represents a unique opportunity for EU to demonstrate population health which in turn should provide a lot of goodwill.

In EU, IHC exhibits a special opportunity to support healthcare improvements in low and middle income countries because this kind of low-tech intervention is relatively cheap compared to its effectiveness. However, as the benefits of IHC presuppose a relatively high level of organisational competence, it might be relatively difficult to implement IHC in low and middle income countries without additional special support from EU as a whole.

As IHC aims to utilise the potential synergy between medicine and behavioural science, remarkable results regarding CC might point in the direction of general health promotion as a dominant intervention: IHC in the format of a Life Style Modification Program at the Kaiser Permanente in USA comprises involvement of the participants over a 3-6 months period in 1) a low-fat vegetarian diet, 2) participation in yoga classes and 3) weekly exercise sessions monitored by a physiologist followed by individualized home exercise programs and 4) weekly educational classes and support groups. Statistical analysis of before and after program tests revealed improved physical and mental health among individuals who reported chronic disorders as well as reduced healthcare utilisation (Guevara et al, 2003).

Threats

Fragmented financial systems are obvious threats to IHC. In the case of IHC-STROKE, hospitals have to take on the extra costs of an outgoing team while the primary sector harvests the major part of savings from reduced use of nursing homes. Despite the expected net savings for society as a whole, the separation of the finance systems for hospitals and primary care means that the dissemination of IHC-STROKE is very difficult before some redistribution of savings is accomplished between the financial authorities in hospitals and primary care. Local cash-flow-incentives might easily block IHC initiatives that are health economic dominant from a full societal point of view.

A special threat to IHC arises from the hierarchical organisation of power characteristic to hospitals. As the leading physician is the health professional in charge of establishing IHC, he might be biased in favour of core issues to physicians instead of IHC initiatives involving mainly subordinated nurses and therapists. In the case of IHC-STROKE, an anti-hypertension programme for stroke patients preventing readmission might get priority compared to IHC-STROKE, as treatment of hypertension is a core competence for physicians and young physicians in particular aiming to promote their professional career by research. In this case, it is not necessarily decisive when choosing between these interventions at the same level of costs that the anti-hypertension programme requires about 50 patients to treat to prevent one bad outcome while the parallel level for IHC-STROKE is about 15. To expect physicians to give priority to interventions benefiting other health professionals means to expect some kind of altruism from physicians that you could not expect from other professionals. The solution to this dilemma might be to educate leading physicians to a level where they identify themselves more as open-minded managers rather than as specialists. A framework for such training is the HTA methodology which is the general framework of this project. However, for clinical implementation a better management education for interdisciplinary integration is requested.

A special threat to the dissemination of IHC is too many mediocre projects without intended outcomes. Once again referring to experiences from stroke rehabilitation, it is characteristic that a number of home training projects have been launched in relatively good scientific settings as an RCT with a poor understanding of the psychological nature of the intervention as this is outside the central scope of the physicians planning the trial. In such cases, the outcome of the project might be disappointing. The lesson to be learned from these experiences is that the results from RCT on IHC are not automatically replicated in implementations as the ordination of a new pharmaceutical. RCT results on IHC should be considered as potential benefits that might be replicated by best practice as we deal with psychological values. Probably, a practical solution to this problem is an equalization of the scientific and the therapeutic/nursing settings in the planning and execution of the RCT. Such planning is implemented in a Danish as well as a Portuguese RCT on IHC-STROKE which is part of the Homecare 222954 project.

A MESO-STRATEGY FOR DISSEMINATION OF INTEGRATED CARE IN THE EUROPEAN UNION

Micro, Meso or Macro Strategy

A basic strategic question is whether the anticipated dissemination of IHC should rely on the micro level with bottom-up developments from the care level or on the macro level with top-down legislation from national levels of health authority or on some meso level related to organisations somewhere between the micro and macro levels? (Gröne and Garcia-Barbero, 2002). According to a description and comparison of IHC in Finland, Sweden, Austria, Spain, The Netherlands and Great Britain the actual situation is the following (van Raak et al, 2003):

It is a common feature by the countries in the study that they have collective financed healthcare systems. Some are based on taxes and political control of health authorities (Beveridge System) others are based on compulsory social insurance funded by legal private organisations, i.e. sickness funds and commercial insurers making agreements with care providers on service and payments (Bismarck System). So, the European variants of collective financed and controlled healthcare contrast the commercial US-model of healthcare organisation (Semashko System). However, some new states in Eastern Europe (not represented in the 2003 description) have adapted the Semashko System.

- Within the collective healthcare systems Great Britain represents the most top-down macro approach as the British government has produced legislation, policy documents, obligatory measures and control mechanisms to both encourage and compel integrated care delivery
- Austria represents the most distinct bottom-up micro policy as the establishment of a commission responsible for preparing integrated care delivery was the only action taken at the time of the 2003 description. Along this line, an interesting Vienna initiative was established 2004 to explore challenges and possible solutions to realized problems of fragmentation by more patient orientation in a bottom-up learning process
- The Netherlands and the Scandinavian countries are somewhere in the middle of these more extreme positions representing a meso approach. They emphasize stimulating and supporting measures as well as encouraging inter-professional working and patient empowerment as well as providing subsidies to integrated care initiatives, stimulating the development of ICT and reallocation of staff

Further, van Raak evaluates the macro, meso and micro strategies as follows:

> At first glance, the macro approach in Britain looks attractive because a tight co-ordination of cross sector decision-making is assured and supervised by one national centre. However, in practice such centralisation has a number of shortcomings. Firstly, central decisions tend to develop over bureaucratic procedures. Secondly, not all centrally made decisions are comprehensible to those working on the care level. Thirdly, the central reaction time to problems focused at a local care level tends to become very long and often out of contact with the real context. Fourthly – but not least – centralisation tends to kill motivation at the care level.

Decentralisation on the other hand, has a number of disadvantages, too. Firstly, too many decision-makers and too many decision procedures slow down decision-making. Secondly, it hinders more radical changes because too many different points of view and interests have to be included in vague compromises.

Decentralized systems are inherently incremental decision making systems!

Recent assessments of IC-strategies confirm the criticisms of existing implementation strategies, e.g. a national survey study among professional stakeholders in Denmark reports where several initiatives have been implemented to integrate care:

Conclusion of Survey among Danish Stakeholders in Healthcare

Most physicians agree that only half of all patients experience well coordinated pathways. Clinical integration is a strategic priority at the managerial levels, but this is not visible at the functional levels. Financial incentives are not used to encourage coordination. The information communication technology to facilitate clinical integration is perceived to be inadequate.

The scope for improvement is high due to the structural composition of the system. Increased managerial stewardship, alignment of the financial incentives, and expanded use of information communication technology to link sub-organizations will be a way to move the system forward to meet its explicit goal of providing an integrated delivery of services [Strandberg-Larsen and Krasnik, 2008].

All in all, the advantages and disadvantages of more centralisation or decentralisation, respectively, are not relevant for the kind of problems in integrated care development and delivery. Instead of focusing on the distribution of power the core issue is upgrading the professionalism from the present level of professional defensiveness to a more advanced level of open-minded professionalism. In practice this means some meso approach developing from monodisciplinary towards multidisciplinary decision-making models which is accomplished in HTA aiming at a synthesis of physiological, psychological, economic and organisational knowledge.

Elements of a European Meso-Strategy Towards Clinical Continuity

1. The health economic dominance of IHC enables focus at a regional instead of a national level of decision-making in health care

Health economic dominance of an intervention means that better effectiveness and satisfaction of the patient goes hand in hand with societal economic net-savings. This means that the disadvantages of a centralized implementation strategy might be minimized at a regional level with some direct communication between budget authorities and clinical management about 1) how to share savings and costs in a fair way and 2) how to assure good quality in the execution of IHC. Such direct negotiations as a cornerstone of a new meso-strategy of execution should enable an adaptation of the prototypes of IHC to local conditions with significant local involvement and motivation.

In order to develop such meso-strategy, Homecare 222954 offers local teams aiming to execute an IHC-pilot including 40 patients practical planning support in the way that 2-3 representatives from the team are invited to present their project at INIC11 (www.integratedcare.org) and have the latest research news from the field including a practical start guide and membership of an international network with peer-groups in other EU-countries. Besides the practical guides for executive teams the project makes a comprehensive HTA-report of IHC to the regional top-level of decision-makers.

2. Neuroeconomic teaching of IHC key staff

IHC represents the special case of inter-organizational collaboration. In this case horizontal communication and interaction with a minimum of vertical interference is crucial to the over-all effectiveness of the intervention [Alter and Hage, 1993].

On this background a number of studies are done on training for inter-professional collaboration (IPC) in health care. A Cochrane review concludes that practice-based IPC-interventions can lead to positive changes in health care, but further studies are needed to have a better understanding of the range of possible interventions and their effectiveness, how they affect inter-professional collaboration and lead to changes in health care, and in what circumstances these interventions may not be useful [Zwarenstein et al, 2009]. On this background we conclude that the development of inter-organizational collaboration where each member has both horizontal and vertical obligations demands more than practice-based multidisciplinary meetings and discussion. We suppose that inter-organizational collaboration calls for better self-management skills than simpler organizations. In order to strengthen the self-management of members of a multidisciplinary IHC-team, the basics of the new interdisciplinary science "neuroeconomics" is a common knowledge [Larsen, 2010].

CONCLUSION

In summary of the research, IHC is found to be an excellent form of rehabilitation as our domicile is the place where we *feel safe, participate most and have direct feedback* from ADL training. The effectiveness of such integrated homecare has a solid theoretical foundation in the finding that our blood pressure on average is 5-7 mmHg lower at home than in a hospital setting which facilitates limbic activity (L2). Summary-sheets on IHC for patients suffering from Stroke, HF and COPD, respectively, are presented above. Moreover, tele-facilities are economic substitutes for home health interventions when patients are not too weakened mentally, or when distance and time spent make transport and weariness from travel important extra costs. For HF and COPD patients Telemonitoring has a complementary effect on the top of traditional hospital care.

Instead of focusing on either the micro or macro levels of health care organisations, the Homecare-strategy of implementation focuses on an intermediate meso level of direct negotiation between health professional organisations and health finance authorities in order to strengthen the integration of the micro and macro levels, respectively. Such strategy might be implemented forming local multidisciplinary interest groups on IHC specific to member states (MS). This includes the formation and maintenance of an e-mail list of resource persons in IHC specific to MS with a confirmed interest in organising the IHC demo projects. The construction of this network is initiated by invitation of representatives for local IHC-teams to present their executive pilot-project at INIC11. The ultimate indicator of the impact of the project is the number of implementation projects this network establishes within a five year period.

Regarding IHC, the specific medical diagnosis should not be overemphasized as most patients in the target group – the elderly people – suffer from co-morbidities. However, CC where schools for patients that are already independent in ADL are relevant, i.e. diabetes, asthma, low back pain and rheumatism, are not considered in this study.

The potential outcomes from IHC in general and home health interventions in particular focus on ADL-indicators as alternative to or in combination with mortality. Such outcomes, i.e. prevention of readmissions or referrals to institution, might be priced in accordance with their savings in health care and social services. Accordingly, cost-effectiveness analysis is an important tool for decision-makers having to set priorities for a variety of alternative IHC interventions. Moreover, the health risks that are envisaged by IHC are relevant to a majority of elder people. Alone in the EU27 about 2 million new patients each year may benefit from IHC for the three selected CC. This is seldom in a modern specialised health care sector where improvements of care often address small, specific groups of patients, only.

REFERENCES

Alter, C., & Hage, J. (1993). *Organisations working together*. Newbury Park, CA: Sage Publications.

Casa, A., Troosters, T., & Garcia-Aymerich, J. (2006). Integrated care prevents hospitalisations for exacerbations in COPD patients. *The European Respiratory Journal*, *28*, 1–8.

Chilvers, R. & Macdonald, G. & Hayes A (2003). Supported housing for people with severe mental disorders. Cochrane Library.

Garcia-Aymerich, J. & Hernandez, C. & Alonso A. (2007). Effects of an integrated care intervention on risk factors of COPD readmission. *Respiratory Medicine*, 10.1016.

Gröne, O., & Garcia-Barbero, M. (2002). Trends in Integrated Care – Reflections on Conceptual Issues. WHO, Copenhagen, EUR/02/5037864.

Guevara, J. P., Wolf, F. M., & Grum, C. M. (2003). Effects of educational Interventions for self management of asthma in children and adolescents: systematic review and meta-analysis. *BMJ (Clinical Research Ed.)*, *326*, doi:10.1136/bmj.326.7402.1308

Helene, B., & Ford, P. (2000). Mind-body Innovations, an Integrative Care Approach. *Psych Quart*, *71*(1), 47–58. doi:10.1023/A:1004614717641

Hobart, J. C., Lamping, D. L., & Freeman, J. A. (2001). Evidence-based measurement. Which disability scale for neurologic rehabilitation? *Neurology*, *2001*, 57.

Holman, H. (2004). Chronic disease – the need for a new clinical education. *Journal of the American Medical Association*, *292*, 1057–1059. doi:10.1001/jama.292.9.1057

Hutton, P., Trueman, P., & Henshall, C. (2007). Coverage with Evidence Development. *International Journal of Technology Assessment in Health Care*, *23*(4), 425–435.

Jaarsma, T., Strömberg, A., & De Geest, S. (2006). Heart failure management programmes in Europe. *European Journal of Cardiovascular Nursing*, *5*, 197–205. doi:10.1016/j.ejcnurse.2006.04.002

Joint Report by the Commission and the Council on supporting national strategies for the future health care and care for the elderly. EU 7166/03 SOC 116 ECOFIN 77 SAN 41.

LaBrie, R. A., LaPlante, D. A., & Peller, A. J. (2007). The interdependence of behavioural and somatic health: implications for conceptualizing health and measuring treatment outcomes. [May.]. *International Journal of Integrated Care*, *7*, 16.

Langhorne, P., & Taylor, G. (2005). Early supported discharge services for stroke patients: an individual patient data meta-analysis. *Lancet*, *365*, 501–506.

Langhorne, P., & Widén-Holmquist, L. (2007). Early Supported Discharge after Stroke. *Journal of Rehabilitation Medicine*, *39*, 103–108. doi:10.2340/16501977-0042

Larsen, T. (2010). Neuroeconomics and Public Health. *Acta Systemica*, *X*(1).

Larsen, T., Olsen, T. S., & Sorensen, J. (2006). Early Home-supported Discharge of Stroke Patients: a Health Technology Assessment. *International Journal of Technology Assessment in Health Care*, *22*(3), 313–320. doi:10.1017/S0266462306051208

Leff, J. (1997). *Care in the community: illusion or reality*. London: Wiley.

Leichsenring, K. (2004). Developing integrated health and social care services for older persons in Europe. *International Journal of Integrated Care*, 4.

Lind-Albrecht, G. (2006). Patientenschulung in der Rheumatologie: Ein Weg zum besseren Krankheitsmanagement durch Kompetenzsteigerung bei den Betroffenen. *Wiener Medizinische Wochenschrift*, *156*(21–22), 583–586. doi:10.1007/s10354-006-0350-1

Mayo, E. (1949). *Hawthorne and the Western Electric Company, the Social Problems of an Industrial Civilization*. Routledge.

Ouwens, M., Wollersheim, H., & Hermens, R. (2005). Integrated care programmes for chronically ill patients: a review of systematic reviews. *International Journal for Quality in Health Care*, *17*(2). doi:10.1093/intqhc/mzi016

Paré, G., Jaana, M., & Sicotte, C. (2007). Systematic review of home telemonitoring for chronic diseases: the evidence base. *Journal of the American Medical Informatics Association*, *14*(3), 269–277. doi:10.1197/jamia.M2270

Pettersen B, Johnsen R (2007). Legers oppfatning av samhandlingen mellom nivåene i helsetjenesten. *Tidsskr Nor Lægeforen nr. 5, 2007; 127: 565–8*.

Piron, L., & Tonin, P. (2004). Motor telerehabilitation in post-stroke patients. *Medical Informatics and the Internet in Medicine*, *29*, 119–125. doi:10.1080/14639230410001723428

Quinn, C. (2006). Low-technology Heart Failure Care in Home Health Improving Patient Outcomes. *Home Healthcare Nurse*, *24*(8), 533–540. doi:10.1097/00004045-200609000-00012

Riley, D.L. & Stewart, D.E. & Grace, S.L. (2007). Continuity of cardiac care: Cardiac rehabilitation participation and other correlated. *Int J Cardiology*, doi:10.1016.

Servellen, G., Fongwa, M., & Errico, E. M. (2006). Continuity of care and quality care outcomes for people experiencing chronic conditions: A literature review. *Nursing & Health Sciences*, *8*, 185–195. doi:10.1111/j.1442-2018.2006.00278.x

Strandberg-Larsen, M., & Krasnik, A. (2008). *Does a public single payer system deliver integrated care? A national survey study among professional stakeholders in Denmark* (*Vol. 8*). IJIC.

Tavafian, S. S., Jamshidi, A., & Mohammad, A. (2007). Low back pain education and short term quality of life: a randomized trial. *BMC Muscul. Disorder*, *8*, 21.

Taylor, R. S., Watt, A., & Dalal, H. M. (2007). Home-based cardiac rehabilitation versus hospital-based rehabilitation: A cost-effectiveness analysis. *International Journal of Cardiology*, *119*, 196–201. doi:10.1016/j.ijcard.2006.07.218

Van Raak, A., Mur-Veeman, I., & Hardy, B. (2003). *Integrated Care in Europe*. Elsevier Gezondheidszorg.

Verberk, W. J., Kroon, A. A., & Kessels, A. G. H. (2005). Home Blood Pressure Measurement - A Systematic Review. *Journal of the American College of Cardiology*, *46*(5), 743–751. doi:10.1016/j.jacc.2005.05.058

Wensing, M., Wollersheim, H., & Grol, R. (2006). Organisational interventions to implement improvements in patient care: a structured review of reviews. *Implementation Science; IS*, *1*, 2. doi:10.1186/1748-5908-1-2

What are the arguments for community-based mental health care? (2003). *WHO/HEN*.

Zwarenstein M, Goldman J, Reeves S (2009). Interprofessional collaboration: effects of practice-based interventions on professional practice and healthcare outcomes (Review). *Cochr Lib*, Issue 3.

Chapter 15
SMART: Mobile Patient Monitoring in an Emergency Department

Esteban Pino
Universidad de Concepción, Chile

Dorothy Curtis
Massachusetts Institute of Technology, USA

Thomas Stair
Brigham and Women's Hospital, USA

Lucila Ohno-Machado
University of California San Diego, USA

ABSTRACT

Patient monitoring is important in many contexts: at mass-casualty disaster sites, in improvised emergency wards, and in emergency room waiting areas. Given the positive history of use of monitoring systems in the hospital during surgery, in the recovery room, or in an intensive care unit, the authors sought to use recent technological advances to enable patient monitoring in more diverse circumstances: at home, while traveling, and in some less well-monitored areas of a hospital. This paper presents the authors' experiences designing, implementing and deploying a wireless disaster management system prototype in a real hospital environment. In addition to a review of related systems, the sensors, algorithms and infrastructure used in our implementation are presented. Finally, general guidelines for ubiquitous methodologies and tools are shared based on the lessons learned from the actual implementation.

DOI: 10.4018/978-1-60960-183-6.ch015

INTRODUCTION

As technology advances, there are more options available for pervasive monitoring. Sensor miniaturization, wireless communication and increasing processing power in smaller packages allow more efficient, reliable and convenient systems, at least from the end-user perspective. In healthcare, one of the main driving forces behind ubiquitous computing is the increasing need to move patient care from the hospital to non-standard settings such as homes, nursing homes, improvised waiting areas, hazardous locations or the battlefield. For at-risk patients, such as those with chronic diseases or the increasingly aging population, being able to live in a familiar and comfortable environment improves quality of life and frees hospital resources. In disaster situations or during seasonal or regional disease outbreaks, response teams move from the hospitals to improvised settings to care for multiple casualties with varying levels of urgency. Firefighters, hazmat teams and soldiers need real-time, ubiquitous monitoring to detect life threatening events. Existing solutions from industry, academia and the military share the same goal of developing unobtrusive, reliable and pervasive monitoring systems.

Powerful, disposable computers, wireless technologies, sensors and energy storage have made possible the development of Body Sensor Networks (BSN) (Aziz et al., 2008). These networks are ubiquitous, allowing patient supervision wherever they may go. Personalized health care is a natural extension of these BSN. Future challenges are user acceptance (from both patients and practitioners), ease of use, and avoiding data flooding with little information.

This paper presents a particular experience of embedding a pervasive system in a healthcare setting and the steps required in the design and test of such a system in the hospital. We show benefits from fusing information from different sensors, the complications that arise when dealing with untethered subjects and finally the evaluation in a real environment. We also show how the implementation of this system required the skills of a multi-disciplinary team.

BACKGROUND

Pervasive Systems in Healthcare

In healthcare, the main technological components in pervasive systems are sensors and network technologies. The most frequently used physiological sensors measure ECG, SpO_2, temperature, acceleration, sound, and non-invasive blood pressure (BP). Since most physiologic variables present slow variations, networks are usually low bandwidth, adequate to handle the low data rates. Many of these networks are also characterized by short range transmissions, such as in Body Sensor Networks (BSN) or Personal Area Networks (PAN). These low bandwidth, short range networks are usually implemented using ZigBee or Bluetooth networks (Table 1). As the system aggregates data and forwards it to central servers, higher bandwidth is required. Local Area Networks (LAN) use the widely adopted WiFi networks for their wireless requirements. For larger ranges, cellular networks and WiMAX provide a reasonable solution (Fourty, Val, Fraisse, & Mercier, 2005; Kavas, 2007). Currently, cellular networks are the preferred method to relay data from ambulances and other fast moving patients due to its hand-over capability. WiMAX is being updated to allow roaming but its main strength is its suitability to provide wireless Metropolitan Area Network (MAN) capability to rural, low density areas where cellular networks are not economically viable. Naturally, wired networks provide much better bandwidth and reliability and are used at the earliest opportunity.

Location information is also highly desirable. In a distributed system, finding the patient who has a problem is not easy and a location system should be deployed to solve this problem. Posi-

Table 1. Wireless technologies for data transmission

	Standard	Max. Bandwidth	Use	Frequency	Range
Short range					
ZigBee	IEEE 802.15.4	250 Kbps	PAN	ISM 2.4 GHz	100 m
Bluetooth	IEEE 802.15.1	1 Mbps	PAN	ISM 2.4 GHz	10 m
WiFi (b)	IEEE 802.11b	11 Mbps	LAN	ISM 2.4 GHz	30 m
WiFi (g)	IEEE 802.11g	54 Mbps	LAN	ISM 2.4 GHz	100 m
WiFi (n)	IEEE 802.11n	300 Mbps	LAN	ISM 2.4 GHz	300 m
Long range					
Cellular (3G)	UMTS	3 Mbps	MAN	Licensed: 1.95 GHz, 2.14 GHz	~ 40 km
WiMAX	IEEE 802.16	70 Mbps	MAN	Licensed: 10-66 GHz Unlicensed: 2-11 GHz	50 km

Table 2. Location technologies

	Use	Advantages	Disadvantages
GPS	Outdoors	Easy to compute position on a map, works anywhere on the planet.	Is obstructed by high buildings, expensive, does not work indoors.
Cell tower	Outdoors	Uses existing cell tower network.	Accuracy depends on tower density.
RFID	Indoors	Unobstructed by clothing, walls, people.	Requires expensive archway detectors for unattended operation.
Ultrasound	Indoors	Excellent room level accuracy, inexpensive.	Tags can be obstructed, low transmission speed limits simultaneous tags in one location.
Infrared	Indoors	Excellent room level accuracy.	Easily obstructed by clothing, people. Requires line of sight with detectors.

tioning technologies range from GPS or cellular tower referencing used outdoors to RFID, ultrasound or infrared used indoors (Table 2). Sometimes the data network infrastructure acts as a location system by using received signal strength to infer positioning. Some solutions offer a combination of technologies in order to improve their performance.

Korhonen and Bardram (2004) review pervasive healthcare as a multidisciplinary field. It involves hardware, software, sensors, embedded systems, human-computer interfaces, wireless communications and distributed systems among others. In healthcare, this multidisciplinary nature is further extended to cope with medical aspects: physiologic sensors, location systems, resource management and intelligent systems. Further, deploying such a system inside a hospital requires collaborating with caregivers, as well as working with the institutional review board, to make sure that patient safety is protected.

Orwat, Graefe, and Faulwasser (2008) present a literature review on pervasive computing in health care. It provides a thorough analysis of 69 articles published from 2002 to 2006. They call for more reports on implementations that evaluate actual acceptance and problems. Privacy concerns are a priority for both patients and caregivers and need to be addressed properly for a wide acceptance of pervasive monitoring. Saranummi and Wactlar (2008) agree with this view of the current problems in the emerging field of pervasive healthcare.

There is a need for more clinical evidence of solution feasibility and user acceptance. Most works are research projects but few present real-world implementation and results.

Regarding networks, Varshney (2003) proposes wireless technology solutions to solve a wide range of challenges in the healthcare industry, including reducing costs, decreasing medical errors and improving service in under-staffed areas. Triantafyllidis, Koutkias, Chouvarda, and Maglaveras, (2008) propose an open and reconfigurable wireless sensor network architecture with emphasis on facilitating the addition of new sensors via a sensor modeling language. Wade and Asada (2007) present a cable-free Body Area Network (BAN) that uses a conductive-fabric garment with both signal and power. It facilitates pervasive monitoring by providing support for multiple sensors per patient.

Commercial monitoring systems range from complete embedded systems that alarm on thresholds and have more than one sensor to a simple SpO2, blood pressure or ECG sensor for occasional self-checking. A few examples are: Welch Allyn Micropaq Monitor (Welch Allyn, n.d.) provides an ECG and SpO2 patient monitoring solution, Cleveland Medical Devices (CleveMed, n.d.) provides general acquisition hardware and an assortment of physiological sensors, and Crossbow wireless sensor network (Crossbow), which supplies low level mesh network hardware to support BAN.

The United States military has developed and tested several systems. Originally, they were only used by physicians in the field but later systems recorded soldier data and were able to alert on critical conditions such as low thresholds or soldier unresponsiveness to medics and unit commanders. BMIST-J (Battlefield Medical Information System Tactical – Joint, n.d.) (now AHLTA-Mobile) and the ARTEMIS system (McGrath et al., 2003) are examples of such military systems.

In the Hospital

Pervasive technologies in a hospital have different requirements than in other settings, such as serving highly mobile personnel, implementing patient-specific management protocols and supporting diverse monitoring goals. Meeting these needs improves monitoring in these complex environments. In 2007, Bardram and Christensen explore Activity-Based Computing (ABC) in hospitals, based on pervasive computing, supporting the naturally collaborative nature of hospital work. Sanchez, Tentori, and Favela (2008) present an activity recognition system for the smart hospital, specific to hospital worker activities. In a different publication, Tentori and Favela (2008) present a set of tools for activity aware computing in a hospital. Pervasive healthcare systems must be prepared for highly mobile caregivers. This study shows the variety of tasks that are performed during a typical shift. The proposed solution involves a mobile activity monitor that is configured to alert based on patient actions or status. Coronato and Esposito (2008) discuss a localization system that combines two sources of information (RFID and WiFi) to obtain a reliable location in a hospital.

Mass Casualty Response Systems

Several prototypes of mass casualty response systems, built in academia, are good examples of pervasive systems in healthcare. The basic goal of monitoring a large number of patients with varying degrees of urgency is best served designing a supervisory system that collects physiological data, analyses and provides some decision support to respond to critical patient conditions. In these cases, where patients far outnumber caregivers, a supervisory system that aids in detecting critical patients among many "walking-wounded" is of great value to first responders and caregivers in overcrowded settings.

Lin et al. (2004) implement wireless PDAs to monitor patients during transport. The physiological variables acquired are heart rate (HR), ECG and SpO2. Real-time data transmissions allow a central management unit to supervise patient status and detect deteriorating conditions. A prototype was tested for intra-hospital transport. Lenert, Palmer, Chan, and Rao (2005) propose an "intelligent triage tag" for their Wireless Internet Information System for Medical Response in Disasters (WIISARD) architecture. Location is estimated from received signal strength using the same wireless data network to send data. Only general location is inferred. When the care providers are in the vicinity, the tag can identify itself and stand out among several injured in close proximity. Electronic Tags have bi-directional communication, can display triage status via LEDs and have sensors to determine patient status. Arisoylu, Mishra, Rao, and Lenert (2005) propose a "one switch" wireless access point with access to multiple cellular backhauls for internet connectivity, for use by the WIISARD system. Killeen, Chan, Buono, Griswold, & Lenert (2006) present the caregiver's wireless handheld device for WIISARD. It provides an electronic medical record that replicates the rapidity and ease of use of a standard paper triage tag. Malan, Fulford-Jones, Welsh, & Moulton (2004) present CodeBlue, a sensor network infrastructure to report vital signs and location and seamlessly transmit this data among caregivers. It is meant to enhance responders' ability to triage patients on scene and allocate hospital resources. The network is designed to scale from sparse to very dense deployments, covering a range of settings, from clinics or hospitals to mass casualty response sites. It features encryption, mesh networks, a flexible security model to grants access rights to arriving EMTs and a flexible infrastructure for connecting medical devices and routing physiological data to a central server or hospital information system. In the Advanced Health and Disaster Aid Network (AID-N) project, Massey, Gao, Welsh, Sharp, and Sarrafzadeh (2006) present a low-power electronic triage system with SpO2, blood pressure, ECG and location sensor capability. This work is an extension on the CodeBlue project. Gao, Kim, White, & Alm (2006) present the patient monitoring system for AID-N. The wearable devices use a SpO2 sensor as the primary sensor and implement GPS and MoteTrack location systems for outdoors and indoors positioning respectively. Monitoring is done at a central computer, where location and physiologic data can be seen simultaneously. In the event of requiring assistance, the operator may activate an audible alarm on the patient tag to facilitate aid. Finally, Gao et al. (2007) present the complete AID-N project. In a mass casualty incident a large number of embedded physiologic and location capable electronics report real-time data to a central station where response efforts can be coordinated. Sensor data is transmitted in three different network layers. A ZigBee-like ad hoc network is used to form a body-area network, connecting each Mote-based embedded system with that patient's SpO2, ECG and/or BP sensors. The ZigBee ad hoc network also provides location data. The second layer connects the embedded system to the Internet backbone. The third layer is the central server at the hospital or with public health authorities. Results from a disaster drill are presented. The large number of small distributed sensors facilitates inferring the actual state of a mass casualty site. Gao et al. (2008) present the latest version of their original project, this time using miTags with an assortment of possible sensors and a ZigBee based mesh network for data transport. The miTags are based on motes, originally developed at University of California, Berkley and are low power, low bandwidth devices.

All of these pervasive healthcare proposals share some key elements: They implement patient centered, low power, wireless computers (mostly PDAs) to acquire and forward location and physiological data. The most recurring physiological variables monitored are SpO2 and ECG. HR is derived from one or the other of these sensors or is directly reported by one of them. The data are transmitted wirelessly to a central station to supervise patients and coordinate efforts. Data are also transmitted back to caregivers in the field to notify them of events requiring special attention or to provide them with updated patient information. In all proposals, there is an agreement that location and patient status are the basic data required to guide caregiver's efforts.

SMART

The Scalable Medical Alert and Response Technology (SMART) project is a good example of a pervasive healthcare monitoring system. A prototype was implemented from June 2006 to December 2007 in the waiting area of the Emergency Department at the Brigham and Women's Hospital in Boston, USA. Originally devised as a disaster management response system, its goal is to monitor, alert and facilitate reprioritization of multiple untethered patients (Waterman et al., 2005; Pino, Ohno-Machado, Wiechmann, & Curtis, 2005; Curtis et al., 2008).

From the point of view of pervasive technology, SMART turns an improvised site or otherwise regular waiting room into an enhanced ambient where subjects can be monitored and located from a central station with low impact in their regular activities. For such a healthcare application, the two main aspects to consider are: (1) physiologic monitoring of key parameters and (2) location of individuals. Such a location system does not need to be of a high precision. Generally, a small room-sized area is enough to select the closest caregivers and to direct them to find the affected patient promptly.

The steps considered in designing SMART were:

1. Selecting physiological sensors and a location technology that can be implemented using low-power and low-cost components
2. Selecting a platform to integrate sensor electronics and wireless data transmission
3. Devising a physical packaging comfortable to the end users
4. Making sure the wireless system can support all the patients
5. Analyzing collected data and presenting aggregated data in a usable way
6. Integrating all components into an easy to set-up, scalable and easy to use system

SMART shares the key elements of other pervasive monitoring systems: distributed patient data collection, location information, central server data aggregation for multiple patient supervision and alarm generation on abnormal conditions. However, SMART incorporates new concepts that allow higher integration into the environment and thus differentiates itself from related projects. Compared to Lin et al. (2004), SMART uses a similar set of patient sensors, but provides a central management infrastructure to aid in patient categorization and a location system to track patient positions. WIISARD (Lenert, Palmer, Chan, & Rao, 2005) and SMART share a similar architecture, the main difference being the intended use. SMART can be implemented in different settings using commercially available equipment. It is envisioned as a pervasive and ubiquitous system that can be deployed in disaster sites, nursing homes, hospital waiting rooms or even adapted for home use. In an emergency situation, first respondents will be already familiar with the system due to its presence in multiple environments. CodeBlue (Malan, Fulford-Jones, Welsh, & Moulton, 2004) focus more on hardware and network requirements. They propose custom-made, low-power sensors using motes as radio transceivers, while SMART is based on off the shelf equipment and provides a software platform for data analysis, classification and alarm. AID-N (Gao et al., 2007), the follow up project from CodeBlue, is very similar to SMART, both in monitored variables, architecture and intended goal. SMART, however, has several possible deployment scenarios and tries to accommodate patients in a variety of conditions, the most difficult ones being those with higher mobility. Special algorithms that combine sensor information from ECG and SpO2 sources try to minimize false alarms, while keeping the algorithm simple to allow scaling. In sum, SMART is based on three concepts. First, the positioning system can be used for locating patients, caregivers and equipment, thus facilitating resource allocation based on proximity to the point of care. Second, a Logistics module is in charge of alarm handling, selecting the closest available caregiver, re-alarming if ignored or escalating the alarm to other caregivers if necessary. Third, a diagnosis suggestion is presented along physiologic data to facilitate supervision of a larger number of patients. The classification algorithm aggregates sensor information to minimize false alarms and allow a supervisor to focus on particular patients. This is a first approximation to automatic triage, which will be critical in a future unattended, fully automatic, triage system for mass casualty incidents.

System Description

The design considers off-the-shelf parts as primary components. It involves physiologic sensors for patients, a room-level location system, a wireless network infrastructure to cover a waiting area, a central station running software to fuse sensor information and an alarm subsystem for diagnosis support, with the ability to wirelessly notify roaming caregivers.

Figure 1 shows a patient wearing a commercial SpO2 sensor with serial communication and 3 ECG leads (1 signal, monitoring quality). The ECG instrumentation amplifier and serial data board are the only custom made elements in the project. Both data streams are sent to an HP iPaq 5510 PDA running Familiar Linux. A standard 802.11b wireless network (WiFi) carries the data packets to the main server. The location subsystem is implemented via ultrasound (US). An emitter attached to the patient sends its tag number to stationary receivers. The receivers forward the tag id and its signal strength to the main server, where a simple algorithm associates the tag with the closest detector position. The required bandwidth is less than 50 kbps per patient, considering ECG, SpO2, location and battery data. Power consumption is high due to our requirement for live ECG data that has to be transmitted wirelessly. To this end, an iPaq backpack providing additional battery is used, giving the system 3 to 4 hours of monitoring on a single charge. This autonomy proved enough for our pilot study but has to be addressed in future deployments.

The main server is called SMART Central, a regular commodity PC running Fedora Core Linux. It is wired to a wireless access point that provides 802.11b coverage for the patient and caregiver PDAs and for the US receivers. At SMART Central, the SMART operator is in charge of supervising the system and notifying triage personnel when a patient needs further assistance. The user

Figure 1. Patient with location tag and sensor box

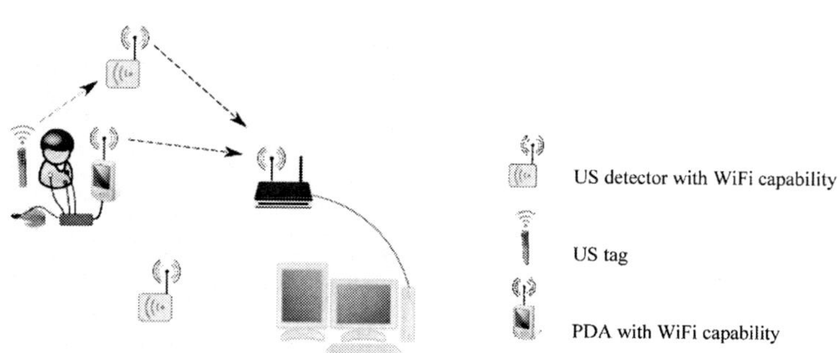

Figure 2. Main user interface and map in SMART central

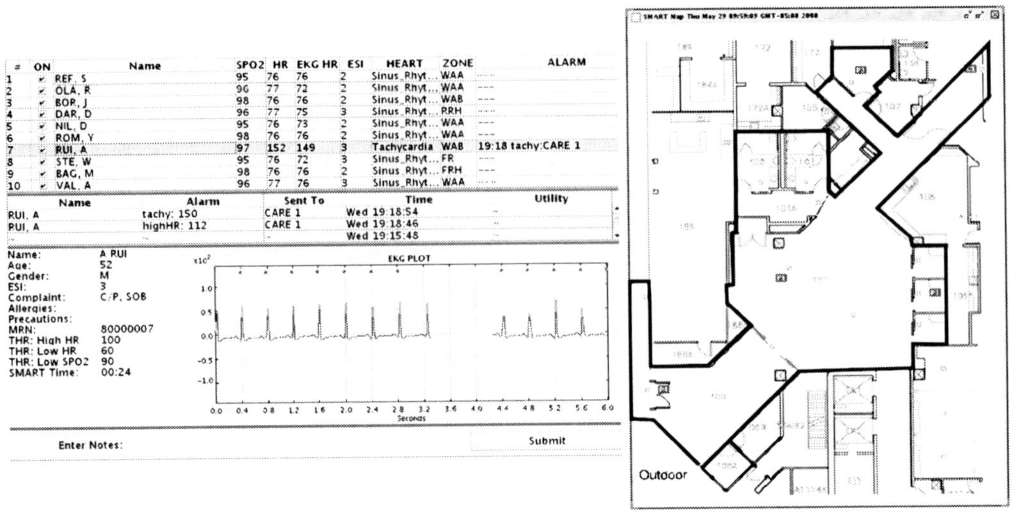

Figure 3. Caregiver view of patient and alarms

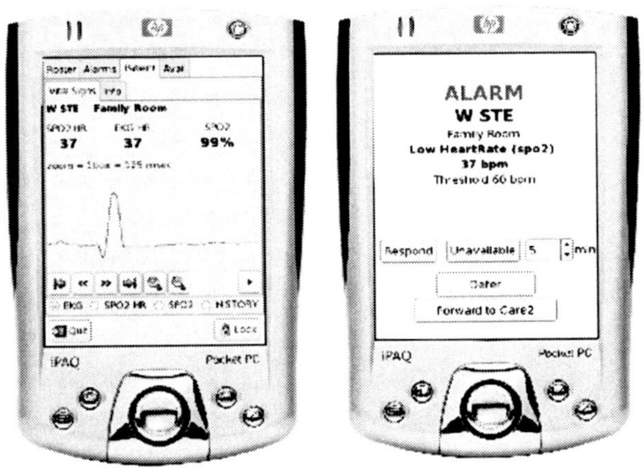

interface consists of a main display with a patient roster, alarms and real-time physiological data, as shown in Figure 2. A secondary display shows the position of all tagged patients, caregivers and eventually equipment.

The roaming caregiver equipment has the US tag for location purposes and a handheld PDA to receive alarms, review monitored patient information and indicate busy/available status to SMART Central. With his (or her) PDA, the caregiver can review clinical data of a patient, real time SpO2 data and ECG tracing. A live ECG and an alarm screen are shown in Figure 3. All communications to and from these PDAs are encrypted because they contain identifiable patient information.

Due to restrictions from the hospital's Institutional Review Board, we could not deploy or test the caregiver subsystem, but a prototype was implemented and used by the SMART operator while away from the main station.

The US location system is shared by all indoor assets that require tracking. Receivers on the walls listen to the US tags and report signal strength to determine the closest known location.

Figure 4. Component software and data paths in SMART

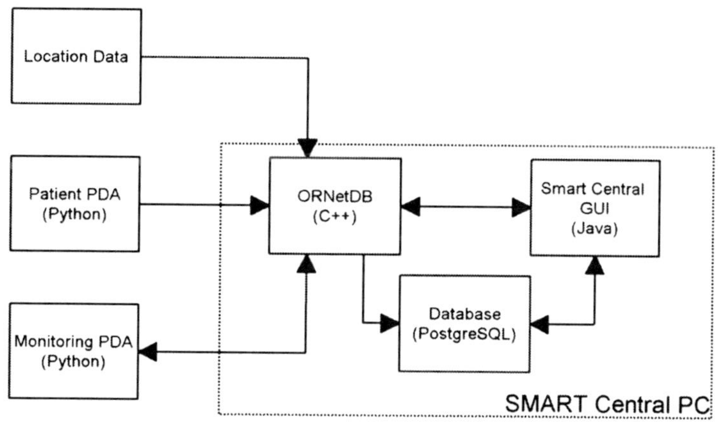

For SMART, room area accuracy was enough, and allowed caregivers to quickly find a patient or resource when approaching the area. An added benefit of US is that it is blocked by walls, thus getting a wrong location is highly unlikely. Among the alternatives listed in Table 2, US was also the least intrusive in any setting, only requiring affixing detectors in the walls. For outdoor location, such as tracking a patient in an ambulance, a setup with a GPS in lieu of the US for location and the cellular network instead of WiFi for data transmission is used.

Core Software

All of the software was developed using open source tools, with the goal of producing a flexible system that could accommodate other sensors, subsystems or outputs. Depending on the platform, different programming languages are used, as shown in Figure 4. The PDAs are programmed in Python with GTK. In SMART Central, C and C++ are used in ORNetDB, an engine for streaming databases. The main Graphical User Interface (GUI) is written in Java and the underlying database is implemented in PostgreSQL. Auxiliary GUIs are web–based and implemented as python scripts which have database access.

ORNetDB can accommodate a variable number of connections of various data. Every time a new patient is registered, a new connection is generated for the location, and the ECG and SpO2 data streams. ECG data are fed into a QRS detection node that generates a new stream that contains time-stamped QRS detections in noisy environments. All raw and computed data streams are saved in PostgreSQL databases. The caregiver PDAs have two-way connections to ORNetDB. They receive the patient roster with general information or live streams for a specific patient and send busy/responding notifications when an alarm is issued. SMART Central implements several GUIs, a Decision Support Module and a Logistics Support Module. The SMART Operator interacts with the GUIs to register, monitor and un-register patients. The Decision Module uses real-time information to suggest a classification among 7 medical conditions (bradycardia, sinus rhythm, tachycardia, ventricular tachycardia, ventricular fibrillation, irregular beats, asystole) and 3 technical conditions (noise, leads off, sensor mismatch). Other straightforward technical alarms are: no ECG signal, no SpO2 signal, no communication from PDA and low battery. When an alarm is due, the Logistics Module is in charge of selecting the closest available caregiver based on the location information, handling re-alarming

Figure 5. Diagnosis suggestions for two different patients in SMART

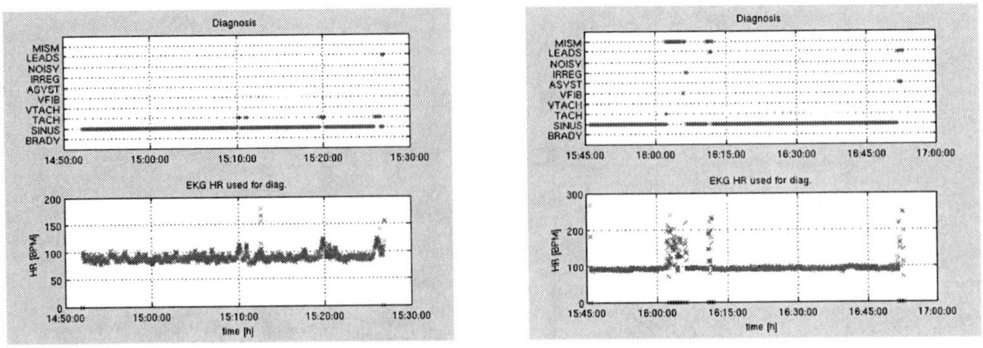

and escalating alarms to other caregivers if there is no response. As mentioned earlier, administrative restrictions prevented us from fully testing the alarm escalation algorithms, but a prototype showed that it is feasible. This integrated system behavior is possible due to the information fusion from location, physiologic and caregiver status information.

Results

In general the system performed well. The SMART system was able to monitor multiple roaming patients in the waiting room area for the Emergency Department (ED) at the Brigham and Women's hospital in Boston, MA. The pilot test was conducted from June 2006 to October 2007, monitoring 145 patients or 6815 minutes of data. Patients with shortness of breath and patients with chest pain were invited to participate in the trial. The system is set up after the patient underwent triage with a nurse. The SMART Operator initiated the process by obtaining consent, handling the hardware pouch, and checking that standard lead II ECG and SpO2 were being recorded. Particular results varied according to the subjects being monitored. In Figure 5, the first patient produced a sinus rhythm alternating only with sinus tachycardia when its HR was consistently over 100 BPM. On the other hand, we also had cases where episodes of highly noisy signals generated false alarms such as ventricular fibrillation or irregular beats. These episodes were always correlated with patient movement, when the beat detection algorithm did not identify the segment as noise and produces false beat annotations. The technical alarms mismatch (when SpO2 HR was normal, but ECG data looked like asystole or ventricular fibrillation) and leads off (when leads act as antennas and ECG data fluctuated among all possible values) were more appropriate, but we had expected more "NOISY" classifications. The LEADS (leads off) or ASYST (asystole) diagnoses at the end of the record are generated when the SMART operator removes the equipment from the patient.

The alarms positive predictability fell from over 0.95 in simulated patients to 0.71 in real patients. This decrease was due to inaccurate detection of noise produced by movement and muscle artifacts in the ECG. SpO2 data were used to cross-validate the results and disregard contradictory classifications. Another attempt at improving the noise detection was made using the US tags, but they proved too sensitive to be of practical use. In any case, the incidence of alarms was low, averaging 1 every 12 minutes. During the pilot study, 3 patients were reprioritized and admitted sooner to the ED due to findings while being monitored.

Figure 6. User acceptance

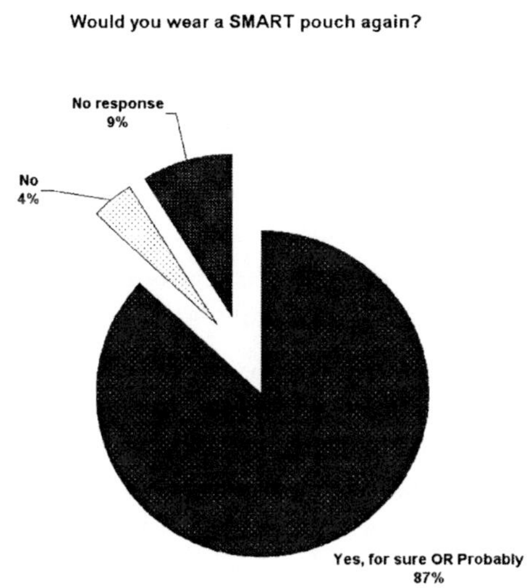

Figure 7. User acceptance. Perceived safety.

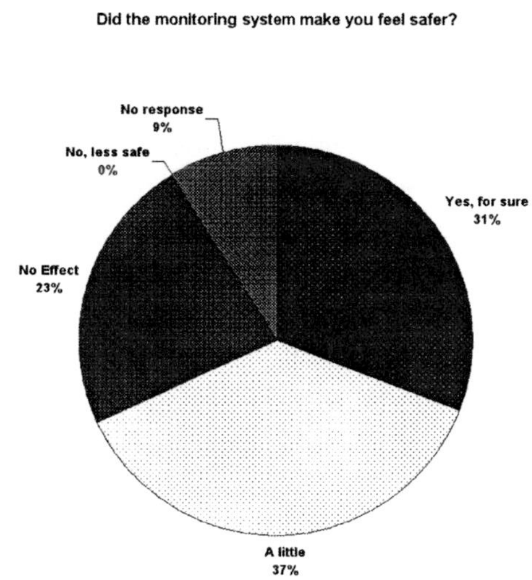

User Acceptance

A survey conducted for patients who volunteered to participate in the study shows that the system had a very good acceptance. Out of 91 respondents, 87% said that they would probably or likely use such a system again and 68% felt at least a little safer by being monitored. Finally, 38% answered that it improved the care, even though it had been explained to them that it wouldn't (see Figures 6, 7 and 8).

Figure 8. User acceptance. Perceived effect of monitoring on care.

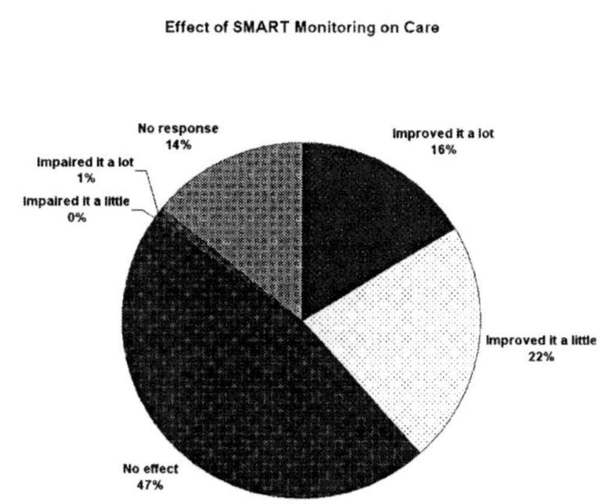

FUTURE RESEARCH DIRECTIONS

With increasing miniaturization, improved low-power electronics and further development of algorithms to deal with noisy data, we expect the development and deployment of pervasive health monitoring systems to increase. However, we feel that the first step towards implementing a robust pervasive healthcare system for mass casualty response or for multiple untethered patient monitoring system must be improvement of alarm rates. As the alarms become more trustworthy, it will be possible to augment human resources in a crowded environment with automated supervision. This has to be accomplished by lowering false alarms without sacrificing true alarms. Patient monitoring systems are bound to be biased towards detecting true positives because the cost of missing a real alarm is much higher than the cost of dealing with a false alarm.

From the lessons learned in SMART, the first step to improve alarm generation is enhancing noise detection. In a real environment with ambulatory patients, noise plays a fundamental role in confusing beat detection and diagnosis algorithms that otherwise performs satisfactorily. Movement artifacts and muscle noise, especially when walking, are easily confused with abnormal rhythms. The two possible approaches are via software detection, directly on the noisy signal, or via hardware, incorporating other sensors such as accelerometers, to identify regions of low data quality. SMART's approach is based on software detection, via "leads off", "noisy" and "asystole" classifications. Redmond, Lovell, Basilakis, & Celler (2008) propose an ECG quality measurement based on similar ECG signal characteristics, detecting zones with signal saturation, high frequency noise or lack of signal, and marking unusable ECG with a dilated mask, comparable to SMART's voting mechanism. When the alarm management has matured, we look forward to a future deployment where we can also study the physician acceptance of the system.

Location tracking performed adequately. When patients were transitioning between areas, we could see that sometimes intermediate areas were not occupied. However, this was not deemed important, as the location system's goal was to inform of patient's last location in order to find and treat him. A future research direction is associating movement with probable noise presence in physiological data.

Power requirements allow 3 to 4 hours monitoring on a single charge. In the future, we will try to lower power consumption in order to increase monitoring length. This can be accomplished by changing to a lower power data transmission such as ZigBee or Bluetooth (Paksuniemi, Sorvoja, Alasaarela, & Myllyla, 2006) and/or by changing the iPaqs as the mobile platform.

CONCLUSION

We have presented the SMART system, a pervasive health monitoring system for mass casualty emergencies but also useful in waiting areas of emergency rooms and other ad hoc patient monitoring sites. The system prototype was deployed in a hospital and evaluated over an eighteen month period. Both the implementation and deployment of this system were facilitated by having a multidisciplinary team; computer science researchers and physicians worked together to produce a system that could effectively monitor ambulatory patients awaiting treatment.

From our experience, we conclude that building an acceptable pervasive health monitoring systems requires the interaction of many people: engineers, hospital personnel and patients. Data from real patients allow algorithm designers to produce effective algorithms. While we tested our algorithms on data from various sources, including healthy volunteers and a synthetic patient and web repository of signals, it turned out that data from real patients was qualitatively different, because we monitored them for longer periods of time and even normal patients' ECGs displayed unexpected features. Interacting with hospital personnel makes sure that the system does not adversely affect current standards of patient care. In particular, doctors should not be subjected to excessive false alarms and the nursing staff should not be burdened with additional duties related to prototype systems. The deployment of the networking and location equipment should be done in such a way that the patients are not bothered by it.

Patients in unmonitored areas can benefit from pervasive monitoring systems. These monitoring systems are effective when they do not interfere with patients' normal activities. Systems such as SMART allow a limited number of healthcare personnel to oversee a large number of people with minimal effort. As shown, a wireless system providing simple physiological and location data can be of great help in both improvised and regular settings, and patients evaluate these efforts positively.

ACKNOWLEDGMENT

We would like to thank the National Library of Medicine for supporting this work through contract number N01LM33509. We would also like to thank our colleagues who provided essential assistance in building the SMART prototype and in deploying and evaluating it: From the Brigham and Women's Hospital Emergency Department: Jacob Bailey, the SMART Operator; from MIT: Jason Waterman, Eugene Shih, and John Guttag; from the Decision Systems Group at Brigham and Women's Hospital: Staal Vinterbo, Rosa Figueroa, and Robert A. Greenes. Terry Aasen and the Sonitor® team provided essential assistance with the deployment of the indoor location system.

REFERENCES

Allyn, W. (n.d.). *Welch Allyn Micropaq Monitor model Micropaq 404 Monitor (ECG/SpO$_2$) Directions for use*. Retrieved February 13, 2009, from http://www.welchallyn.com/documents/Patient%20Monitoring/Continuous%20Monitoring/Micropaq/usermanual_20070615_402_404_micropaq.pdf

Arisoylu, M., Mishra, R., Rao, R., & Lenert, L. A. (2005). 802.11 wireless infrastructure to enhance medical response to disasters. In *Proceedings of the AMIA Annual Symposium* (pp. 1-5).

Aziz, O., Lo, B., Pansiot, J., Atallah, L., Yang, G.-Z., & Darzi, A. (2008, Oct). From computers to ubiquitous computing by 2010: Health Care. *Philosophical Transactions of the Royal Society A, 366*(1881), 3805-3811.

Bardram, J. E., & Christensen, H. B. (2007). Pervasive computing support for hospitals: An overview of the activity-based computing project. *IEEE Pervasive Computing / IEEE Computer Society [and] IEEE Communications Society, 6*(1), 44–51. doi:10.1109/MPRV.2007.19

Battlefield Medical Information System Tactical - Joint. (n.d.). *BMIST-J home page*. Retrieved February 13, 2009, from http://www.mc4.army.mil/AHLTA-Mobile_CBT.asp#

CleveMed. (n.d.). *Home page*. Retrieved February 13, 2009, from http://www.clevemed.com/

Coronato, A., & Esposito, M. (2008). Towards an implementation of smart hospital: A localization system for mobile users and devices. In *Proceedings of the Sixth Annual IEEE International Conference on Pervasive Computing and Communications PERCOM 2008* (pp. 715-719).

Crossbow. (n.d.). *Home page*. Retrieved February 13, 2009, from http://www.xbow.com

Curtis, D. W., Pino, E. J., Bailey, J. M., Shih, E. I., Waterman, J., & Vinterbo, S. A. (2008). SMART - An Integrated Wireless System for Monitoring Unattended Patients. *Journal of the American Medical Informatics Association, 15*(1), 44–53. doi:10.1197/jamia.M2016

Fourty, N., Val, T., Fraisse, P., & Mercier, J.-J. (2005). Comparative analysis of new high data rate wireless communication technologies "from Wi-Fi to WiMAX". In. *Proceedings of the Joint International Conference on Autonomic and Autonomous Systems and International Conference on Networking and Services, ICAS-ICNS, 2005*, 66–71. doi:10.1109/ICAS-ICNS.2005.34

Gao, T., Kim, M. I., White, D., & Alm, A. M. (2006). Iterative user-centered design of a next generation patient monitoring system for emergency medical response. In *Proceedings of the AMIA Annual Symposium* (pp. 284-288).

Gao, T., Massey, T., Selavo, L., Crawford, D., Chen, B., & Lorincz, K. (2007). The advanced health and disaster aid network: A light-weight wireless medical system for triage. *IEEE Transactions on Biomedical Circuits and Systems, 1*(3), 203–216. doi:10.1109/TBCAS.2007.910901

Gao, T., Pesto, C., Selavo, L., Chen, Y., Ko, J. G., Lim, J. H., et al. (2008) Wireless Medical Sensor Networks in Emergency Response: Implementation and Pilot Results. In *Proceedings of the 2008 IEEE Conference on Technologies for Homeland Security* (pp. 187-192).

Kavas, A. (2007). Comparative analysis of WLAN, WiMAX and UMTS Technologies. In *Proceedings of the Progress In Electromagnetics Research Symposium 2007,* Prague, Czech Republic (pp. 140-144).

Killeen, J. P., Chan, T. C., Buono, C., Griswold, W. G., & Lenert, L. A. (2006). A wireless first responder handheld device for rapid triage, patient assessment and documentation during mass casualty incidents. In *Proceedings of the AMIA Annual Symposium* (pp. 429-433).

Korhonen, I., & Bardram, J. E. (2004). Guest editorial introduction to the special section on pervasive healthcare. *IEEE Transactions on Information Technology in Biomedicine*, *8*(3), 229–234. doi:10.1109/TITB.2004.835337

Lenert, L., Palmer, D., Chan, T., & Rao, R. (2005). An intelligent 802.11 triage tag for medical response to disasters. In *Proceedings of the AMIA Annual Symposium* (pp. 440-444).

Lin, Y.-H., Jan, I.-C., Ko, P. C.-I., Chen, Y.-Y., Wong, J.-M., & Jan, G.-J. (2004). A wireless PDA-based physiological monitoring system for patient transport. *IEEE Transactions on Information Technology in Biomedicine*, *8*(4), 439–447. doi:10.1109/TITB.2004.837829

Malan, D., Fulford-Jones, T., Welsh, M., & Moulton, S. (2004). *Codeblue: An ad hoc sensor network infrastructure for emergency medical care*. Paper presented at the International Workshop on Wearable and Implantable Body Sensor Networks.

Massey, T., Gao, T., Welsh, M., Sharp, J. H., & Sarrafzadeh, M. (2006). The design of a decentralized electronic triage system. In *Proceedings of the AMIA Annual Symposium* (pp. 544-548).

McGrath, S., Grigg, E., Wendelken, S., Blike, G., Rosa, M. D., Fiske, A., et al. (2003, November). *ARTEMIS: A vision for remote triage and emergency management information integration*. Hanover, NH: Dartmouth University.

Orwat, C., Graefe, A., & Faulwasser, T. (2008). Towards pervasive computing in health care - a literature review. *BMC Medical Informatics and Decision Making*, *8*, 26. doi:10.1186/1472-6947-8-26

Paksuniemi, M., Sorvoja, H., Alasaarela, E., & Myllyla, R. (2006). Wireless sensor and data transmission needs and technologies for patient monitoring in the operating room and intensive care unit. In *Proceedings of the 27th Annual International IEEE EMBS05 Conference* (pp. 5182-5185).

Pino, E., Ohno-Machado, L., Wiechmann, E., & Curtis, D. (2005). Real-Time ECG Algorithms for Ambulatory Patient Monitoring. In *Proceedings of the AMIA Annual Symposium* (pp. 604-608).

Redmond, S. J., Lovell, N. H., Basilakis, J., & Celler, B. G. (2008, August 20-24). ECG Quality measures in telecare monitoring. In *Proceedings of the 30th Annual International IEEE EMBC08 Conference* Vancouver, BC, Canada (pp. 2869-2872).

Sanchez, D., Tentori, M., & Favela, J. (2008, March-April). Activity recognition for the smart hospital. *IEEE Intelligent Systems*, *23*(2), 50–57. doi:10.1109/MIS.2008.18

Saranummi, N., & Wactlar, H. (2008). Editorial: Pervasive Healthcare. Selected papers from the pervasive healthcare 2008 conference, Tampere, Finland. *Methods of Information in Medicine*, *47*(3), 175–177.

Tentori, M., & Favela, J. (2008, April-June). Activity-aware computing for healthcare. *IEEE Pervasive Computing / IEEE Computer Society [and] IEEE Communications Society*, *7*(2), 51–57. doi:10.1109/MPRV.2008.24

Triantafyllidis, A., Koutkias, V., Chouvarda, I., & Maglaveras, N. (2008). An open and reconfigurable wireless sensor network for pervasive health monitoring. In *Proceedings of the Second International Conference on Pervasive Computing Technologies for Healthcare PervasiveHealth 2008* (pp. 112-115).

Varshney, U. (2003). Pervasive healthcare. *Computer*, *36*(12), 138–140. doi:10.1109/MC.2003.1250897

Wade, E., & Asada, H. (2007, Jan.-March). Conductive fabric garment for a cable-free body area network. *IEEE Pervasive Computing / IEEE Computer Society [and] IEEE Communications Society*, *6*(1), 52–58. doi:10.1109/MPRV.2007.8

Waterman, J., Curtis, D., Goraczko, M., Shih, E., Sarin, P., Pino, E., et al. (2005). *Demonstration of SMART (Scalable Medical Alert Response Technology)*. Paper presented at the AMIA 2005 Annual Symposium.

This work was previously published in International Journal of Healthcare Delivery Reform Initiatives, edited by Matthew W. Guah, pp. 1-16, copyright 2009 by IGI Publishing (an imprint of IGI Global).

Chapter 16
A Transaction Cost Economics Assessment of a Diabetes Self-Management Solution

Indrit Troshani
University of Adelaide Business School, Australia

Nilmini Wickramasinghe
RMIT University, Australia

Steve Goldberg
INET International Inc., Canada

ABSTRACT

Diabetes is one of the leading chronic diseases affecting Australians and is increasingly becoming a serious challenge and threat for both the quality of healthcare while increasing cost pressures on the Australian healthcare system. The goal of this study is to provide a transaction cost economics framework which can be used as a tool for high-level assessments of the economic viability of a pervasive technology solution developed by INET in the form of a wireless enabled mobile solution to facilitate superior diabetes self-management. In doing so, we prepare the inroads for proposing an approach for refined quantifiable assessments of a pervasive IT-enabled healthcare solution.

INTRODUCTION

Diabetes is one of the leading chronic diseases affecting Australians and its prevalence continues to rise with an estimated 275 Australians developing diabetes daily (DiabetesAustralia, 2008). Evidence shows that diabetes and its complications are incurring significant costs for the healthcare system in Australia including costs incurred by patients, carers, government, and the entire health system. Only in 2004-05 direct healthcare ex-

DOI: 10.4018/978-1-60960-183-6.ch016

penditure on diabetes was A$907 million which constituted approximately 2% of the allocatable recurrent health expenditure in that year (AIHW, 2008). Further costs include societal costs that represent productivity losses for both patients and carers. Diabetes can, therefore, have considerable social, human, and economic impacts and tackling these requires solutions that substantially enhance the existing fragmented and uncoordinated capacity for effective prevention, early detection and management (VictorianGovernment, 2007).

Furthermore, there are many deficiencies that are rooted the Australian health system setup (Wickramasinghe, Troshani, & Goldberg, 2009, 2010). Based on fee-for-service episodic doctor-patient consultation, the current Australian healthcare system can handle short-term illnesses involving a limited range of interventions including their diagnosis and treatment (Hunt, 2007). However, this system is comprised of a mixture of fragmented private and public healthcare subsystems that provide both healthcare funding and delivery. Largely uncoordinated, these subsystems are deemed to be unsuitable for the treatment of long-term chronic diseases including diabetes (Dixon & Webbie, 2006; Sprivulis, et al., 2007). In particular, diabetes requires teams of various health professionals and long-term support to help sufferers make effective healthy lifestyle changes and constantly maintain them (Hunt, 2007). This has the potential to substantially increase costs while potentially adversely affecting diabetes treatment effectiveness.

Since diabetes is and is expected to be a major challenge for the Australian healthcare system in both providing quality healthcare and in incurring increasing expenditures (Swerissen & Taylor, 2008), a treatment imperative is required that provides patients with appropriate levels of monitoring ensuring diabetes containment and prevention of further complications (AIHW, 2008). A pervasive technology solution would offer the necessary monitoring that is cost-effective and convenient to both patients and clinicians and least disruptive to patient lifestyle. The goal of this chapter is to investigate the application of a pervasive technology solution developed by INET International in the form of a mobile phone to facilitate superior diabetes self-management in Australia. Moreover, this chapter provides a transaction cost economics framework and uses it for a preliminary assessment of the proposed solution.

CURRENT TRENDS IN DIABETES SELF-MANAGEMENT RESEARCH

As there is no cure for diabetes, non-medical approaches are used jointly with medical approaches so that patients can have a life which is as normal as possible. However, non-medical approaches can be challenging as they require effective lifestyle management and meticulous attention and monitoring by both patients and healthcare professionals (Britt, et al., 2007). Particularly, to be successful, patients need to be both informed and active in their treatment regimen (AIHW, 2007, 2008). This can be achieved by effective self-management which is a non-medical approach and which constitutes the focus of this chapter.

Self-management is important as it empowers diabetes patients while acknowledging their central role and responsibility for managing their healthcare (ICIC, 2008). Extant research indicates that active participation of diabetes patients in self-management is a key strategy for managing their condition and reaching improved treatment outcomes (Colagiuri, Colagiuri, & Ward, 1998; Poulton, 1999; Rasmussen, Wellard, & Nankervis, 2001; Wellard, Rennie, & King, 2008). However, self-management is constantly time-consuming and requires significant self-discipline (Russell, Churl Suh, & Safford, 2005) and support strategies including assessment, goal-setting, action-planning, problem-solving and follow-up (ICIC, 2008). Moreover, because effective self-management may require patient interaction with various healthcare professionals, including general practitioners, diabetes educators, dieticians, and community nurses (Knuiman, Welborn, & Bartholomew, 1996), difficulties can arise when diabetes patients encounter problems ranging from making appointments to needing to travel to many locations (Van Eyk & Baum, 2002; Wellard, Rennie, & King, 2008; Zigbor & Songer, 2001).

Current methods used in Australia for achieving patient self management include various types of training and education and support options including peer-led, generic and tailored chronic disease self-management planning, training and support, telephone coaching etc. (Francis, Feyer, & Smith, 2007; Harvey, et al., 2008). Although these were found to be effective to various extents, they are also resource-intensive and their long-term sustainability is questionable (Francis, Feyer, & Smith, 2007). Additionally, current research shows that quality improvement factors including cost-effectiveness remain elusive in the ambit of chronic disease services including diabetes (Tabrizi, et al., 2008). In attempting to address these issues, we borrow from the transaction cost economics literature and provide a framework that can be used for the assessment of pervasive wireless technology solutions.

A TRANSACTION COST ECONOMICS ASSESSMENT FRAMEWORK

Transactions cost economics (TCE) theory constitutes a natural and logical theoretical setting for guiding the evaluation of actor interactions in a diabetes monitoring healthcare setting (Hesterly, Liebeskind, & Zenger, 1990; Hesterly & Zenger, 1993; Jones, Hesterly, & Borgatti, 1997; Williamson, 1991). That is, TCE focuses on economic exchange relations amongst actors, including diabetes patients and healthcare providers that are typically involved in interactions. Using the TCE extensions proposed by Jones, Hesterly, and Borgatti (1997) as a basis, the interactions of these actors are comprised of economic exchanges the efficiency of which is jointly determined by four conditions, namely, 1) demand uncertainty, 2) complexity, 3) asset specificity, and 4) frequency. We explain these in turn.

Demand uncertainty is defined as the inability of an actor to predict future events concerning the success or failure of new product offerings, such as a diabetes monitoring solution (Milliken, 1987). It can be caused by many sources including rapid changes in knowledge and technology or even by the actors themselves. Understanding potential sources of demand uncertainty is important because it helps control it and reduce the magnitude of associated risks. Task complexity refers to the number of different specialized behavioral inputs that are required to fully develop and distribute a product or service (Jones, Hesterly, & Borgatti, 1997). Task complexity creates behavioral interdependencies while increasing the need for coordinating actors involved in related processes (Pfeffer & Salancik, 1978).

Asset-specific exchanges can be based on both unique human (e.g. unique processes and knowledge developed by various actors) and non-human assets (e.g. unique equipment) which actors can use to enable exchanges. Asset-specific exchanges create dependencies which can in turn require enhanced cooperation, coordination, and proximity for the effective transfer of both assets or their deliverables among actors (Jones, Hesterly, & Borgatti, 1997; Williamson, 1991). Frequency concerns how often actors are involved in exchanges with one another (Jones, Hesterly, & Borgatti, 1997; Williamson, 1985b). Jones, Hesterly, and Borgatti (1997) argue that "frequency allows human asset specificity to develop from learning-by-doing and to "deepen" through continued interaction; this creates exchanges where the "identity" of the other [actors] matters and enhances the transfer of tacit knowledge…" (p. 922) while also maximizing the cost efficiencies of existing interaction structures (Williamson, 1985a).

A PERVASIVE MOBILE SOLUTION FOR DIABETES SELF-MANAGEMENT

We contend that a possible solution is to apply the INET pervasive technology solution which has proved successful in Canada and in a pilot in Chicago (Goldberg, 2002a, 2002b, 2002c, 2002d, 2002e; Wickramasinghe & Goldberg, 2003, 2004). Integral to this approach is the incorporation of a wireless enabled mobile phone that facilitates the ubiquitous monitoring of an individual's diabetes, thereby, contributing to diabetes self-management. The journey began by realizing that the traditional System Development Lifecycle (SDLC) is fundamentally flawed for healthcare initiatives. Mainly, this is due to the length of time it would take to realize the final application and the structures and inflexible stages that had to be traversed. Thus, INET developed a refocused SDLC model (Figure 1a) and delivery framework (Figure 1b) making it possible to keep the strengths of SDLC while moving from start to finish in a relatively more compressed timeframe (Table 1).

The research goal is to use a standardized mobile Internet (wireless) environment to improve patient outcomes with immediate access to patient data and provide the best available clinical evidence at the point of care. To achieve this, INET International Inc.'s research (Goldberg, 2002a, 2002b, 2002c, 2002d, 2002e; Wickramasinghe & Goldberg, 2003, 2004) starts with a 30-day e-business acceleration project in collaboration with many key actors in hospitals, such as clinicians, medical units, administration, and I.T. departments. Together, they follow a rigorous procedure that refocuses the traditional 1-5-year SDLC into concurrent 30-day projects to accelerate healthcare delivery improvements. At completion, an e-business acceleration project delivers a scope document to develop a handheld technology application (HTA) proof-of-concept specific to the unique needs of a particular environment. The proof-of-concept is a virtual lab case scenario which operates within a mobile Internet (wireless) environment by working with hospitals and technology vendors. The final step is the collection of additional data with clinical HTA trials consisting of two-week hospital evaluations.

With the refocused SDLC model it was then possible to design a robust and rigorous web-based business model, the INET web-based business model (Figure 2). This business model provides the necessary components to enable the delivery framework to be positioned in the best possible manner so it can indeed facilitate enacting the

Figure 1. a) Re-focused SDLD Model, b) Components of the Delivery Framework

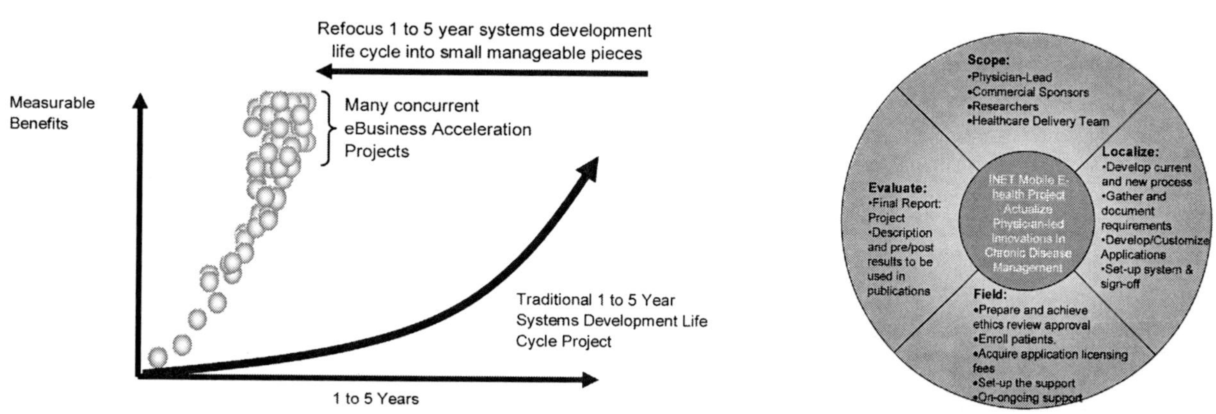

a b

Table 1 INET Practice Framework – Compressing the SDLC

SDLC (waterfall)	INET Mobile e-Health Project			
	Scope	Localize	Field	Evaluate
I.T. Role & Responsibility	Project Management Business Analysis	Data Analysis Technical Tools Expert Programmer Data Administrator Network Architect Database Administrator Network Administrator	Technical Support	Account Manager
Investigation	Problem Definition Feasibility Study – can objectives be met at a reasonable cost. Project Definition			Document Solution, Data analysis of outcomes, benefits and Next Steps
Analysis (Logical Design)		Define what the IS must do to fix the problem Less temptation to follow existing practices which may not be best Define the user's requirements and priorities Analyze existing system Develop logical design for the new system		
Design (Physical Design)		Define how the new system will work Detail Schedule and budget Produce a physical design showing system inputs, outputs, user interfaces.		
Implementation		Research technology Product Acquisitions Test programs, sub-systems and systems acquire or develop software Code programs Software developer manual System operators manual Purchase and Install hardware and software package	User's Manual People Changeover Tasks Data Conversion. Technical Changeover Tasks	
Maintenance		Fix Problem/Solution Determination	Fix Database, Network and 3rd Party Products Fix security and access problems Fix learning curve time disruptions Fix collaboration problems	

key components of the chronic disease model successfully (Table 2). The model is positioned to suit the complex nature of healthcare environments by iteratively, systematically, and rigorously incorporating lessons learnt from data to healthcare processes for ensuring superior healthcare delivery. This does not only maximize the value of past data and organizational learning but it also

Figure 2. INET-web-based-business model

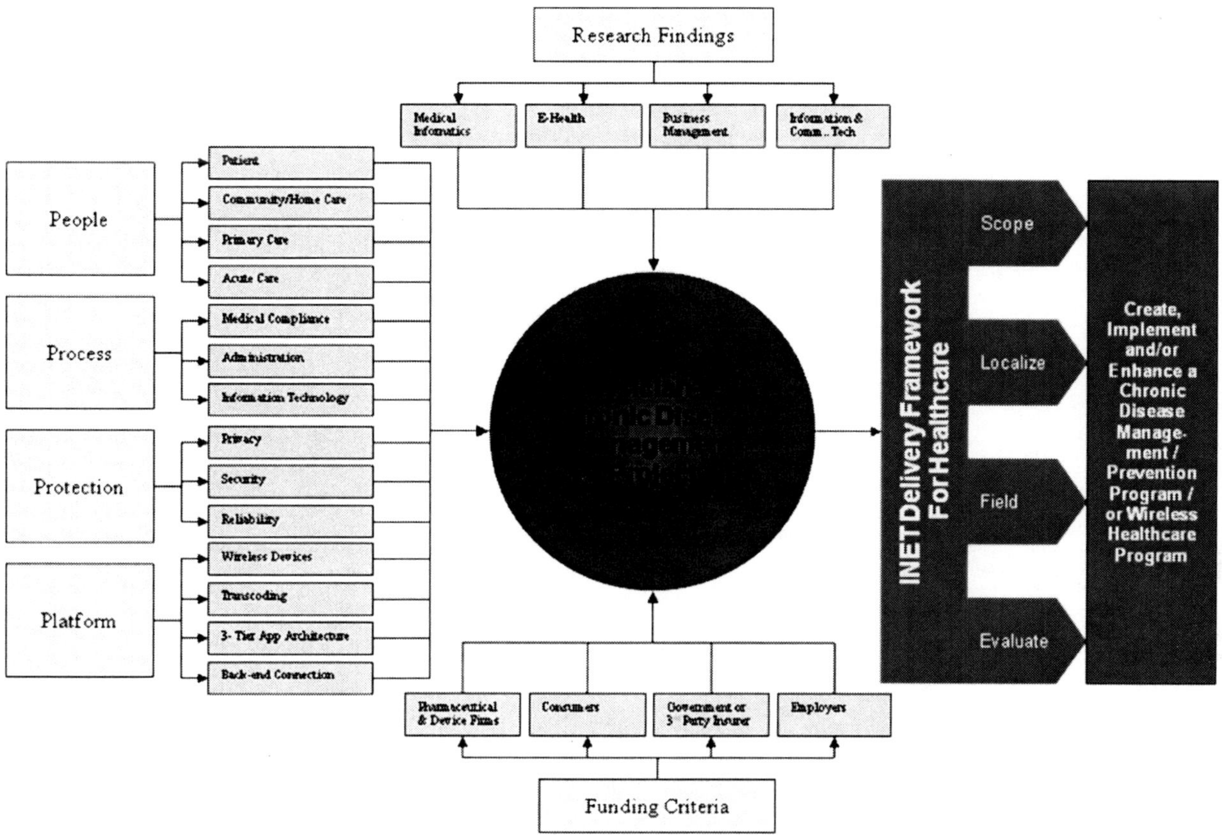

makes processes amendable as complex needs and requirements evolve.

It is important to note that in this business model the three key areas of risk, namely, people, processes and technology, are minimized through the use of pervasive technology which we believe is a unique benefit of the INET solution. Specifically, since the proposed solution is an application that is compatible with any mobile phone or wireless device (e.g. a PDA) data transfers occur between patients and providers on a well vetted model. Therefore, the learning curve for patients may be minimal as they are likely to be in possession of mobile devices.

Successful web-based projects in healthcare require the consideration of many components. Figure 2 provides an integrative model for all key success factors that we have identified through our research (Goldberg, 2002a, 2002b, 2002c, 2002d, 2002e; Wickramasinghe & Goldberg, 2004; Wickramasinghe, Schaffer, & Geisler, 2005). What makes this model unique and most beneficial is its focus on enabling and supporting all areas necessary for the actualization of ICT initiatives in healthcare. By design, the model identifies the inputs necessary to bring an innovative chronic disease management solution to market. These solutions are developed and implemented through a physician-led mobile e-health project which is the heart of the model that bridges the needs and requirements of many different players into a final deliverable, a "Wireless Healthcare Program". To accomplish this, the model is continually updated to identify, select and prioritize the ICT project inputs that will:

Table 2 Components of Chronic Care Model (Rachlis, 2006)

Component	Description
Organisation of Health System	• Leadership in chronic disease management (CDM) • Goals for CDM • Improvement strategy for CDM • Incentives and regulations for CDM • Benefits
Self-management support	• Assessment and documentation of needs and activities • Addressing concerns of patients • Effective behaviour change interventions
Decision Support	• Evidence-based guidelines • Involvement of specialists in improving primary care • Providing education for CDM • Informing patients about guidelines
Delivery System design	• Practice team functioning • Practice team leadership • Appointment system • Follow-up • Planned visits for CDM • Continuity of Care
Clinical Information Systems	• Registry • Reminders to providers • Feedback • Information about relevant subgroups of patients needing services • Patient treatment plans
Community	• Linkages for patients to resources • Partnerships with community organizations • Policy and plan development

- Accelerate healthcare system enhancements and achieve rapid healthcare benefits. The model identifies key healthcare system inputs with the four Ps: 1) **People** that deliver healthcare, 2) **Process** to define the current healthcare delivery tasks, 3) **Platform** used in the healthcare technology infrastructure, and 4) **Protection** of patient data.
- Close the timing gaps between information research studies and their application in operational healthcare settings.
- Shorten the time cycle to fund ICT projects and receive adequate returns on investments.

Together the components of the model will help in actualizing physician-led solutions for the management of chronic diseases in general and of diabetes in particular. The delivery framework activities (Figure 1a and 2) are ongoing and represent a continuous improvement cyclical approach towards a given wireless healthcare program. These activities, however, require the relevant and complete inputs from the healthcare system if they are to be carried out successfully. With the refocused SDLC in constructing mobile e-health solutions, both the healthcare inputs (i.e. the four Ps) and the delivery framework may require funding from various sources in return for healthcare improvements and the building up of intelligence in terms of relevant research findings.

To successfully implement the business model described above it was, however, necessary to have an appropriate methodology. Based on this need the adaptive mapping to realization methodology (AMR) was developed (figure 3). The methodology applies a systematic rigorous

Figure 3 AMR Methodology

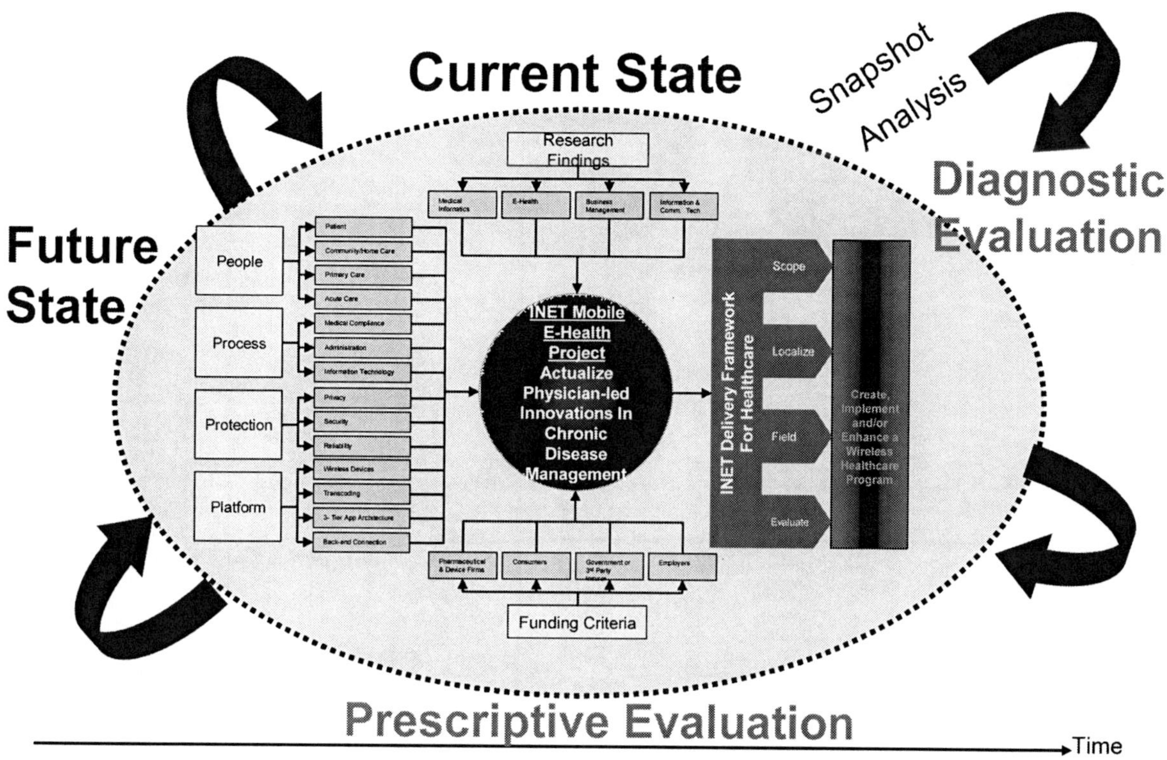

set of predetermined protocols to each business case and then maps the post-prior results back to the model. Thus, it was possible to compare and contrast both a priori and post priori findings. From such comparisons a diagnosis of the current state was made and then prescriptions were derived for the next business case. Hence, each pilot study incorporated the lessons learnt from the previous one and the model was adapted in real time.

By applying the tools and techniques of today's knowledge economy as presented in the intelligence continuum (IC) it is possible to make the AMR methodology into a very powerful knowledge-based systems development model (figure 4). The IC was developed by Wickramasinghe and Schaffer (2006) to enable the application of tools and technologies of the knowledge economy to be applied to healthcare processes in a systematic and rigorous fashion and thereby ensure superior healthcare delivery. The collection of key tools, techniques and processes that make up the IC include but are not limited to data mining, business intelligence/analytics and knowledge management (Wickramasinghe & Schaffer, 2006). These represent a very powerful system for refining the raw data stored in data marts and/or data warehouses and thereby maximizing the value and utility of these data assets for any organization. To maximize the value of the data generated through specific healthcare processes and then use this to improve processes, IC techniques and tools must be applied in a systematic manner. Once applied, the results become part of the data set that are subsequently reintroduced into the system and combined with other inputs of people, processes, and technology to develop an improvement continuum. Thus, the IC includes the generation of data, the analysis of these data to provide a "diagnosis", and their reintroduction into the cycle as a "prescriptive" solution. Therefore, the

Figure 4. Knowledge-based Systems Development Model

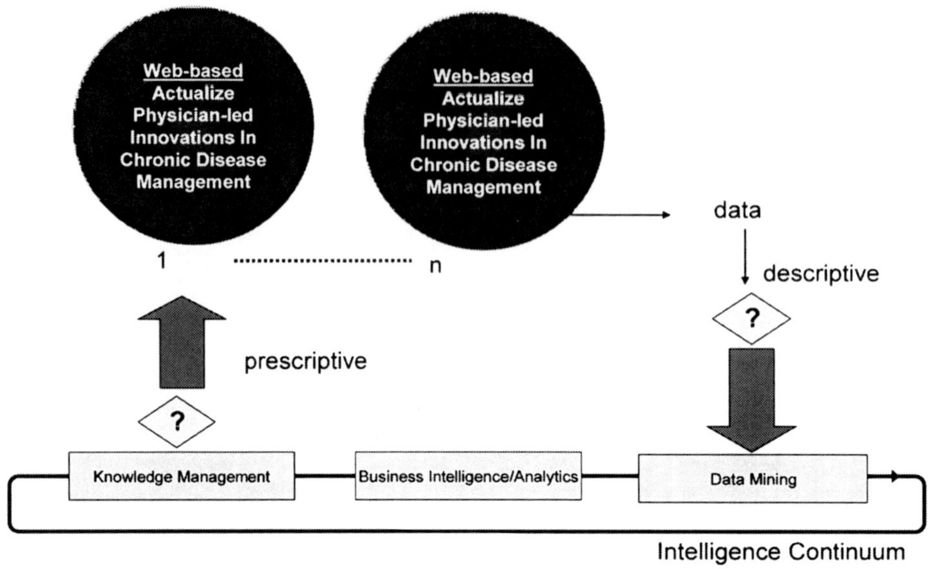

IC is well suited to the dynamic and complex nature of healthcare environments and ensures that the future state is always built upon the extant knowledge-base of the preceding state. Through the incorporation of the IC with the AMR methodology we then have a knowledge-based systems development model that can be applied to any setting, including chronic disease management. The power of this model is that it brings best practices and the best available germane knowledge to each iteration and is both flexible and robust.

From this process, pervasive ICT enabled solution results which while not exorbitantly expensive, it facilitates the superior monitoring of diabetes (Figure 5). It enables patient empowerment by way of enhancing self-management. This is desirable as it allows patients to become equal partners with their clinicians in the management of their own healthcare (Opie, 1998; Radin, 2006) by enhancing the traditional clinical-patient interactions (Mirza, Norris, & Stockdale, 2008).

A PRELIMINARY ASSESSMENT OF THE SOLUTION

Demand uncertainty. Given the growing incidences of diabetes sufferers and the relative ineffectiveness of existing non-medical approaches (Reach, et al., 2005), it is anticipated that upon being made available there will be demand for the proposed solution. Additionally, costs incurred by diabetes patients to operate the solution, that is, to systematically send glucose readings to their diabetes healthcare professionals (Figure 5), are likely to be negligible. Hence, it is not expected to adversely affect demand for the solution.

Complexity. We argue that the proposed solution is easy to use and useful for both diabetes patients and healthcare professionals. As shown in Figure 5, the solution requires diabetes sufferers to input their glucose readings systematically via a simple user interface before sending them for processing. In fact, the solution is very similar to Short Message Service (SMS) applications which are renown for their popularity (Mackay & Weidlich, 2007; O'Doherty, et al., 2010; Oh, et al., 2008). It is, therefore, anticipated that diabetes

Figure 5. ICT Support for Diabetes

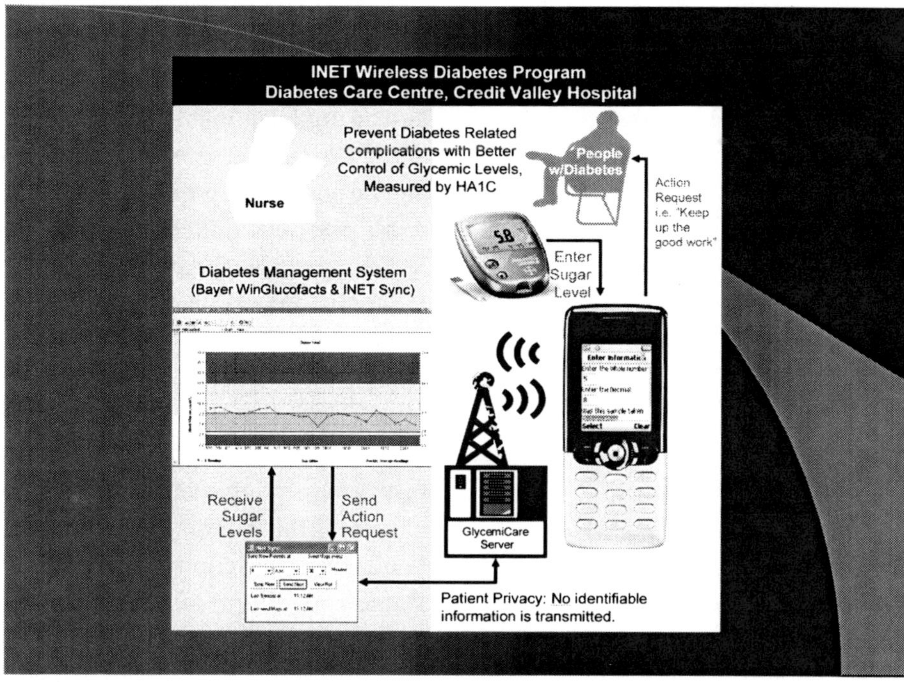

sufferers will find the solution easy to use and useful as also supported in preliminary studies and assessments in previous trials both in the US and Canada (Wickramasinghe & Goldberg, 2004, 2007a; Wickramasinghe, Goldberg, & Bali, 2007; Wickramasinghe, Goldberg, & Bali, 2008). Additionally, as research evidence from the US and Canada and preliminary anecdotal evidence from Australia show, healthcare professionals that have used the proposed solution have indicated that the functionality that concerns them (see Figure 5) is also easy to use and useful (Wickramasinghe & Goldberg, 2004, 2007a; Wickramasinghe, Goldberg, & Bali, 2007; Wickramasinghe, Goldberg, & Bali, 2008). That is, the solution enables healthcare professionals to both monitor diabetes trends and interact with patients relatively easily, inexpensively, and pervasively.

Asset specificity. We anticipate that asset specificity will not constitute an obstacle for both diabetes patients and healthcare professionals. From the patients' viewpoint, operating the proposed solution entails a mobile handset and a data plan. Current evidence shows that in many countries worldwide, including Australia, mobile penetration rates exceed 100% (Netsize, 2009; Rao & Troshani, 2006). Evidence also shows increasing trends of usage of mobile data services suggesting that a growing number of mobile phone users are subscribed to mobile data plans (Informa, 2005a, 2005b, 2006a; Netsize, 2009; Rao & Troshani, 2006). Therefore, the proposed mobile diabetes self-management solution can be run on assets, i.e. mobile handset, which diabetes patients are likely to already have in their possession. Similar arguments can be made for healthcare professionals and their organization. It is anticipated that aside from software upgrades in existing servers and corresponding license fees, upgrades to new assets including computer hardware, are not necessary.

Frequency. We anticipate that interaction frequency between diabetes patients and healthcare providers using the proposed mobile solution will be high, though dictated by the treatment regimen that healthcare professionals prescribe to patients. For example, some patients may be required send their glucose readings to their healthcare professional six times daily, i.e. three times daily before and after each meal, while other patients may be required to fulfill different patterns. We argue that interaction frequency is only a means of maximizing cost efficiencies, but also as a way of strengthening and complementing long term patient-healthcare professional relationships thereby improving the overall quality of healthcare services offered.

DRIVERS AND INHIBITORS

Although successful in proof-of-concept settings in Canada and Chicago, we also identify some critical success factors (table 3) that we anticipate might affect the adoption of the proposed solution in Australia (Gururajan & Murugesan, 2005; Mirza, Norris, & Stockdale, 2008).

DISCUSSION

Given the general global consensus that effective and efficient healthcare delivery will only occur through the judicious application of ICTs (Frost & Sullivan, 2004; Kulkarni & Nathanson, 2005; Lacroix, 1999; Porter & Tiesberg, 2006; Wickramasinghe, 2007), it is inevitable that, as we move into the second decade of the 21st century, the prevalence of ICTs to facilitate the delivery of value driven healthcare will increase. We believe in such a climate our proposed solution will be even more appropriate not only because it utilizes ICTs to provide superior healthcare delivery in the case of diabetic patients but it is also simple to implement and use and cost effective both at the micro and macro levels. These levels include both individual patients and clinicians and organizations including public and private healthcare providers. Nevertheless, it is anticipated that increased adoption and diffusion of chronic disease mobile self-care solutions may depend increasingly less on technology and increasingly more on acceptability by both patients and clinicians on the one hand and on organizational healthcare providers on the other. Clearly, these mobile solutions need to suit and be consistent with both patient lifestyles and work practices undertaken by clinicians within healthcare provider organizations. This may be indicative that education programs and promotional campaigns may need to be undertaken for enhancing awareness and incentivizing adoption.

We argue that one of the most important aspects the will drive the adoption of a diabetes self-management solution such as the one proposed in this chapter is the extent to which it is cost-effective. While the transaction cost economics assessment framework discussed previously suggests that costs associated with operating the proposed solution will be minimal, it does not quantify its costs or benefits. In fact, further research is required to investigating the economic impact of using pervasive healthcare solutions of this nature (eHealthImpact, 2006). We propose that preliminary transaction cost economics assessments need be used jointly with cost benefit analysis (CBA) to investigate the economic feasibility of the proposed solution. Accordingly all costs and benefits should be identified in a comprehensive manner for all actors involved, including diabetes sufferers, healthcare providers, and third party payers. CBA can subsequently compute net economic gains as the difference between the economic value of benefits and identified costs (eHealthImpact, 2006).

Using past research as a starting point, it is anticipated that costs will include investment costs, software setup and installation, process changes costs. Benefits are identified from all actors related to quality of service, access, and efficiency. We propose that monetary values be assigned to all benefits in order to enable quantifiable economic assessments to be made. We also propose using sensitivity analysis in order to assess the relative importance of both cost and benefit variables and

Table 3 Anticipated drivers and inhibitors in Australia

Issue	Description
Potential to reduce face-to-face interaction between patients and their clinicians	While this may be favourable for some patients, it may impact on the social needs of others for human interaction. This may lead to resistance or even rejection for adopting the proposed solution at both conscious and subconscious levels (Vanjara, 2006). However, our solution incorporates mobile phones which are perceived to confer a social status amongst some segments of society which may well become an adoption facilitator. Furthermore, usage of mobile phones may also help eliminate the social stigma that can occur with alternative obvious devices that are used for monitoring chronic diseases (Mirza, Norris, & Stockdale, 2008).
Mobile phones are location-independent making healthcare monitoring both flexible and ubiquitous, that is, not confined to specific settings, such as hospitals (Istepanian, Jovanov, & Zhang, 2004; Istepanian & Lacal, 2003).	While also generating potentially significant cost savings (e.g. by reducing false positive or non serious hospitalisations) for managing the care of non-critical diabetes sufferers our solution will also improve their quality of life (Istepanian, Jovanov, & Zhang, 2004; Istepanian & Lacal, 2003; Mirza, Norris, & Stockdale, 2008; Norris, 2002). This may, thus, facilitate adoption of the proposed solution.
The ageing population in Australia combined with the fragmented nature of the Australian healthcare system that is designed to treat episodic conditions, and the generally poor awareness of life style implications will increase the pressure on this system for better chronic disease treatment standards over longer periods (ABS, 2003; Rowland, 2003).	The pervasive nature of our solution combined with its ability to offer targeted and tailored health messages can contribute to ease that pressure, and consequently, become a facilitator for its adoption in Australia(Neville, et al., 2002).
There is evidence suggesting that to date, some sectors of the healthcare system in Australia have not been convinced of the benefits of ICT in general and pervasive mobile solutions in particular (Yu, Li, & Gagnon, 2008).	At least partially, this is due clinicians' preference and bias towards traditional face-to-face forms of interactions with their patients (Skulimowski, 2006). Furthermore, in a recent study, Australian nurses and clinicians considered that the vast majority of employers did not encourage ICT training, and for those for whom training was available, heavy workloads were considered to be major barriers for training uptake (Eley, et al., 2008). Taken together, these factors are expected to become barriers for the adoption of the proposed solution. Organisational changes, including establishment or awareness and training are, thus, required for extended adoption and diffusion (Mirza, Norris, & Stockdale, 2008).
Proposed wireless solution is expected to be highly cost-effective for people with diabetes.	Costs to patients are estimated to be confined to data transfer charges which include the systematic texting (e.g. by SMS) of glycemic levels (measured by HA1C readings). With increasing competition amongst Australian operators, data transfer charges are expected to decrease in the future (Troshani & Rao Hill, 2009; Troshani & Rao, 2007a). Another possible cost to patients may include mobile handset acquisition. However, with a very high mobile penetration rate in Australia, diabetes patients are likely to already be in possession of mobile phones (Rao & Troshani, 2007a, 2007b). Nevertheless, our proposed solution may require investment outlays from health providers. Initial setup, operational, and supporting infrastructure costs may be barriers for the smooth adoption of our solution in Australia (Khambati, et al., 2008).
Perceptions of security and privacy are likely to have a strong bearing on the successful adoption of the proposed solution.	Although the proposed model accounts for protection of patient information in terms of privacy, security, and reliability, both individual and organisational adopters are expected to require solid guarantees that continuous security improvements will reliably safeguard the privacy of patient data. Nevertheless, extant research shows that these concerns may dissipate overtime as mobile technology matures and benefits and convenience begin to be experienced on a wide scale (Mirza, Norris, & Stockdale, 2008).
General inhibitors	Other factors that, in various forms, may become barriers for the adoption or our solution in Australia include existing disparate legacy systems and possible integration costs, lack of standards and limited bandwidth[34]. Additionally, prioritisation and decision-making processes concerning the introduction and diffusion of new health technologies in some areas in Australia are described to be 'ad-hoc' (Gallego, Fowler, & van Gool, 2008). Budgetary constrains often drive uptake and diffusion of new technologies (Gallego, Fowler, & van Gool, 2008).

the manner in which they affect the cost/benefit outcomes of the proposed solution. We argue that this approach can make important inroads in showing how solutions such as the one proposed in this chapter can be adopted to accomplish e-health sustainability (Wickramasinghe, et al., 2006).

CONCLUSION

In this chapter we set out to present a case for the need to embrace a pervasive technology solution for the superior monitoring of diabetes self-management in Australia. We proffered the INET wireless solution as a suitable solution, for many reasons including that it is equally successful in controlling both type I and type II diabetes, is as effective irrespective of patient's age, socio economic standing or location and has minimal risks and a slight learning curve (if at all). We contend that if such a model were to be incorporated into the Australian context, the growing segment of the population suffering from diabetes would have a convenient, cost effective and superior means of monitoring and controlling their diabetes while enjoying a better quality of life. A transaction cost economics framework was provided for high-level assessments of the economic viability of the proposed pervasive technology diabetes self-management solution.

The INET wireless diabetes solution can facilitate the work of all healthcare stakeholders including government, healthcare providers that are looking for improved and measurable outcomes among diabetes patients. Specific benefits range from decreasing diabetes related complications to reducing the economic burden on the health system. We realize that further research is required to test the proposed solution in Australia. However, we conclude by warning that if a pervasive technology solution is not sought for the monitoring and support of diabetes self-management not only will this chronic disease become a silent epidemic but it will also be a very costly burden for both the healthcare sector and the community at large. In the future, we also believe that the proposed solution can be extended and adapted to provide the necessary monitoring and self-care to other chronic diseases including but not limited to hypertension, cardiac conditions and obesity. Diseases of this nature require daily tests and continuous monitoring which are typically essential to recommended treatment. However, widespread adoption and diffusion of mobile self-care solutions for chronic disease management also implies that practical steps may need to be undertaken in the future concerning the development, implementation, and evaluation of information standards as well as subsequent integration with healthcare legacy systems.

REFERENCES

ABS. (2003). *Population Projections, Australia, 2002-2011, Cat. No. 3222.0.* Canberra: Australian Bureau of Statistics.

AIHW. (2007). *National Indicators for Monitoring Diabetes: Report of the Diabetes Indicators Review Subcommittee of the National Diabetes Data Working Group: AIHW cat. no. CVD 38.* Canberra: AIHW.

AIHW. (2008). *Diabetes: Australian Facts 2008.* Canberra: Australian Institute of Health and Welfare.

Britt, H., Miller, G. C., Charles, J., Pan, Y., Valenti, L., & Henderson, J. (2007). *General Practice Activity in Australia 2005-06, Cat. no. GEP 16.* Canberra: AIHW.

Colagiuri, S., Colagiuri, R., & Ward, J. (1998). *National Diabetes Strategy and Implementation Plan.* Canberra: Diabetes Australia.

DiabetesAustralia. (2008). *Diabetes in Australia.* Retrieved from http://www.diabetesaustralia.com.au/Understanding-Diabetes/Diabetes-in-Australia/

Dixon, T., & Webbie, K. (2006). *The National System for Monitoring Diabetes in Australia (AIHW Cat. No. CVD 32). Canberra: Australian Institute of Health and Wealfare. eHealthImpact. (2006). Study on Economic Impact of eHealth: Developing an evidence-based context-adaptive method of evaluation for eHealth*. Bonn: Information Society and Media.

Eley, R., Fallon, T., Soar, J., Buikstra, E., & Hegney, D. (2008). The status of training and education in information and computer technology of Australian nurses: a national survey. *Journal of Clinical Nursing*, *17*, 2758–2767. doi:10.1111/j.1365-2702.2008.02285.x

Francis, C. F., Feyer, A.-M., & Smith, B. J. (2007). Implementing chronic disease self-management in community settings: lessons from Australian demonstration projects. *Australian Health Review*, *31*(4), 499–509. doi:10.1071/AH070499

Frost, & Sullivan. (2004). Frost and Sullivan Country Industry Forecast - European Union Healthcare Industry, May 11, 2004. http://www.news-mdical.net/print_article.asp? id=1405.

Gallego, G., Fowler, S., & van Gool, K. (2008). Decision makers' perceptions of health technology decision making and priority setting at the institutional level. *Australian Health Review*, *32*(3), 520–526. doi:10.1071/AH080520

Goldberg, S. a. (2002a). *Building the Evidence for a standardized Mobile Internet (wireless) Environment in Ontario, Canada, January Update, Internal INET Documentation*. Ontario, Canada: INET.

Goldberg, S. a. (2002b). *HTA Presentational Selection and Aggregation Component Summary. Internal INET Documentation*. Ontario, Canada: INET.

Goldberg, S. a. (2002c). *Wireless POC Device Component Summary, Internal INET documentation*. Ontario, Canada: INET.

Goldberg, S. a. (2002d). *HTA Presentation Rendering Component Summary, Internal INET documentation*. Ontario, Canada: INET.

Goldberg, S. a. (2002e). *HTA Quality Assurance Component Summary, Internal INET documentation*. Ontario, Canada: INET.

Gururajan, R., & Murugesan, S. (2005). *Wireless solutions developed for the Australian healthcare: A review.* Paper presented at the 4th International Conference on Mobile Business, Sydney, Australia.

Harvey, P. W., Petkov, J. N., Misan, G., Fuller, J., Battersby, M. W., & Cayetano, T. N. (2008). Self-management support and training for patients with chronic and complex conditions improves health-related behaviour and health outcomes. *Australian Health Review*, *32*(2), 330–338. doi:10.1071/AH080330

Hesterly, W. S., Liebeskind, J., & Zenger, T. R. (1990). Organizational economics: an impeding revolution in organizational theory. *Academy of Management Review*, *15*(3), 402–420. doi:10.2307/258016

Hesterly, W. S., & Zenger, T. R. (1993). The myth of a monolithic economics: Fundamental assumptions and the use of economic models in policy and strategy research. *Organization Science*, *4*, 496–510. doi:10.1287/orsc.4.3.496

Hunt, D. (2007). *Urgent health system reform needed to tackle disease epidemic, says head of new University of Melbourne centre*. Retrieved 25 November, 2008, from http://uninews.unimelb.edu.au/view.php?articleID=4615

ICIC. (2008). *Improving Chronic Illness Care: The Chronic Care Model*. Retrieved from http://www.improvingchroniccare.org/indix.php?p=The_Chronic_Care_Model&s=2

Informa. (2005a). *Mobile Content and Services: Worldwide Market Analysis & Strategic Outlook*. London: Informa Telecoms & Media.

Informa. (2005b). *Global Mobile Forecasts to 2010: Worldwide Market Analysis & Strategic Outlook 2005-2010* (5th ed.). London: Informa Telecoms & Media.

Informa. (2006a). *Global Mobile: The International Business Newsletter of Mobile Communications Markets. 13*(6).

Istepanian, R. S. H., Jovanov, E., & Zhang, Y. T. (2004). Guest Editorial: Introduction to the special section on m-health: beyond seamless mobility and global wireless healthcare connectivity. *IEEE Transactions on Information Technology in Biomedicine*, *8*(4), 405–414. doi:10.1109/TITB.2004.840019

Istepanian, R. S. H., & Lacal, J. C. (2003). *Emerging mobile communication technologies for health: some imperative notes on m-health.* Paper presented at the 25th Annual International Conference of the IEEE EMBS, New York.

Jones, C., Hesterly, W. S., & Borgatti, S. P. (1997). A general theory of network governance: exchange conditions and social mechanisms. *Academy of Management Review*, *22*(4), 911–945. doi:10.2307/259249

Khambati, A., Warren, J., Grundy, J., & Hosking, J. (2008). *A model driven approach to care planning systems for consumer engagement in chronic disease management.* Paper presented at the HIC 2008 Australia's Health Informatics Conference, Health Informatics Society of Australia Ltd (HISA).

Knuiman, M. W., Welborn, T. A., & Bartholomew, H. C. (1996). Self-reported health and use of health services: a comparison of diabetic and nondiabetic persons from a national sample. *Australian and New Zealand Journal of Public Health*, *20*(3), 241–247. doi:10.1111/j.1467-842X.1996.tb01023.x

Kulkarni, R., & Nathanson, L. A. (2005). *Medicine Informatics in Medicine. Available:*http://www.emedicine.com/emerg/topic879.htm.

Lacroix, A. (1999). International concerted action on collaboration in telemedicine: G8sub-project 4. *Studies in Health Technology and Informatics*, *64*, 12–19.

Mackay, M. M., & Weidlich, O. (2007, March 2007). *Australian Mobile Phone Lifestyle Index, 3rd Edition, Australian Interactive Media Industry Association (AIMIA), Mobile Content Industry Development Group (MCIDG).* Retrieved 8 April, 2007, from http://www.aimia.com.au/mobile

Milliken, F. J. (1987). Three types of perceived uncertainty about the environment: state, effect, and response uncertainty. *Academy of Management Review*, *12*(1), 133–143. doi:10.2307/257999

Mirza, F., Norris, T., & Stockdale, R. (2008). Mobile technologies and the holistic management of chronic diseases. *Health Informatics Journal*, *14*(4), 309–321. doi:10.1177/1460458208096559

Netsize. (2009). *Netsize Guide 2009 Edition: Mobile Society and Me: When worlds combine.* Levallois-Perret: Netsize.

Neville, G., Greene, A., McLeod, J., & Tracy, A. (2002). Mobile phone text messaging can help young people with asthma. *British Medical Journal*, *325*, 600. doi:10.1136/bmj.325.7364.600/a

Norris, A. C. (2002). *Essentials of Telemedicine and Telecare*. Chichester, UK: Wiley.

O'Doherty, K., Rao Hill, S., Mackay, M. M., & McPherson, J. (2010). Mobile Data Service usage and preference: an investigation of Australian consumers. *International Journal of Mobile Communications*, *8*(1), 106–127. doi:10.1504/IJMC.2010.030523

Oh, S., Yang, S., Kurnia, S., Lee, H., Mackay, M. M., & O'Doherty, K. (2008). The characteristics of mobile data users in Australia. *International Journal of Mobile Communications*, *8*(2), 217–230. doi:10.1504/IJMC.2008.016578

Opie, A. (1998). Nobody's asked me for my view: users' empowerment by multidisciplinary health teams. *Qualitative Health Research*, *18*, 188–206. doi:10.1177/104973239800800204

Pfeffer, J., & Salancik, G. R. (1978). *The external control of organizations: a resource dependence perspective*. New York: Harper & Row.

Porter, M., & Tiesberg, E. (2006). *Re-defining health care delivery*. Boston: Harvard Business Press.

Poulton, B. C. (1999). User involvement in identifying health needs and shaping and evaluating services: is it being raised? *Journal of Advanced Nursing*, *30*(6), 1289–1296. doi:10.1046/j.1365-2648.1999.01224.x

Rachlis, M. (2006). Key to sustainable healthcare system. Retrieved 21 June, 2008, from http://www.improveinchroniccare.org

Radin, P. (2006). To me, it's my life: medical communication, trust, and activism in cyberspace. *Social Science & Medicine*, *6*, 591–601. doi:10.1016/j.socscimed.2005.06.022

Rao, S., & Troshani, I. (2006). *AMC-ER Preliminary Research Report: Understanding Market and Mobile Content Selection for Distribution*. Adelaide, South Australia: Australian Mobile Content – Export Research Initiative, m.Net Corporation Ltd.

Rao, S., & Troshani, I. (2007a). *AMC-ER Challenges and Rewards: Experiences of Australian Content Exporters*. Adelaide, South Australia: Australian Mobile Content – Export Research Initiative, m.Net Corporation Ltd.

Rao, S., & Troshani, I. (2007b). *AMC-ER Initial Selection of Content, Markets, and Distribution Channels for the Australian Mobile Content – Export Research Initiative*. Adelaide, South Australia: m.Net Corporation Ltd.

Rasmussen, B., Wellard, S., & Nankervis, A. (2001). Consumer issues in navigating health care services for type I diabetes. *Journal of Clinical Nursing*, *10*, 628–634. doi:10.1046/j.1365-2702.2001.00550.x

Reach, G., Zerrouki, D., Leclercq, D., & d'Ivernois, J. F. (2005). Adjusting insulin doses: from knowledge to decision. *Patient Education and Counseling*, *56*(1), 98–103. doi:10.1016/j.pec.2004.01.001

Rowland, D. (2003). An ageing population: emergence of a new stage of life? In Khoo, S., & McDonald, P. (Eds.), *The Transformation of Australia's Population: 1970-2030* (pp. 239–265). Sydney, Australia: UNSW Press.

Russell, L. B., Churl Suh, D., & Safford, M. M. (2005). Time requirements for diabetes management: too much for many? *The Journal of Family Practice*, *54*(1), 52–56.

Skulimowski, A. M. (2006). The Challenges to the Medical Decision Making System posed by mHealth. Centre for Decision Sciences and Forecasting, Progress & Business Foundation, Institute for Prospective Technological Studies (IPTS). Retrieved 21 June, 2008, from http://ipts.jrc.ec.europa.eu/home/report/english/articles/vol81/ICT1E816.htm

Sprivulis, P., Walker, J., Johnston, D., Pan, E., Adler-Milstein, J., & Middleton, B. (2007). The economic benefits of health information exchange interoperability. *Australian Health Review*, *31*(4), 531–539. doi:10.1071/AH070531

Swerissen, H., & Taylor, M. J. (2008). Reforming funding for chronic illness: Medicare-CDM. *Australian Health Review*, *32*(1), 76–84. doi:10.1071/AH080076

Tabrizi, J. S., Wilson, A. J., Coyne, E. T., & O'Rourke, P. K. (2008). Review of patient-reported type 2 diabetes service quality. *Australian Health Review*, *32*(1), 23–33. doi:10.1071/AH080023

Troshani, I., & Rao, S. (2007a). The diffusion of mobile services in Australia: an evaluation using stakeholder and transaction cost economics theories. *IADIS International Journal of WWW/Internet*, *5*(2), 40-57.

Troshani, I., & Rao Hill, S. (2009). Linking stakeholder salience with mobile services diffusion. *International Journal of Mobile Communications*, *7*(3), 269–289. doi:10.1504/IJMC.2009.023672

Van Eyk, H., & Baum, F. (2002). Learning about interagency collaboration: Trialling collaborative projects between hospitals and community health services. *Health & Social Care in the Community*, *10*(4), 262–269. doi:10.1046/j.1365-2524.2002.00369.x

Vanjara, P. (2006). Application of mobile technologies in healthcare diagnostics and administration. In Lazakidou, A. (Ed.), *Handbook of Research on Informatics in Healthcare and Medicine* (pp. 113–130). Hershey, PA: Idea Group.

VictorianGovernment. (2007). *Diabetes Prevention and Management: A Strategic Framework for Victoria 1007-2010*. Melbourne: Victorian Government, Department of Human Services.

Wellard, S. J., Rennie, S., & King, R. (2008). Perceptions of people with type 2 diabetes about self-management and the efficiency of community based services. *Contemporary Nurse*, *29*(2), 218–226. doi:10.5172/conu.673.29.2.218

Wickramasinghe, N. (2007). Fostering knowledge assets in healthcare with the KMI model. *International Journal of Management and Enterprise Development*, *4*(1), 52–65. doi:10.1504/IJMED.2007.011455

Wickramasinghe, N., & Goldberg, S. (2003). *The wireless panacea for healthcare.* Paper presented at the 36th Hawaii International Conference on System Sciences, Hawaii, 6-10 January, IEEE.

Wickramasinghe, N., & Goldberg, S. (2004). How M=EC2 in healthcare. *International Journal of Mobile Communications*, *2*(2), 140–156. doi:10.1504/IJMC.2004.004664

Wickramasinghe, N., & Goldberg, S. (2007a). Adaptive mapping to realisation methodology (AMR) to facilitate mobile initiatives in healthcare. *International Journal of Mobile Communications*, *5*(3), 300–318. doi:10.1504/IJMC.2007.012396

Wickramasinghe, N., Goldberg, S., & Bali, R. (2007). Enabling superior m-health project success: a tri-country validation. *International Journal of Services and Standards*, *4*(1), 97–117. doi:10.1504/IJSS.2008.016087

Wickramasinghe, N., Goldberg, S., & Bali, S. (2008). Enabling superior m-health project success: a tri-country validation. *International Journal of Services and Standards*, *4*(1), 97–117. doi:10.1504/IJSS.2008.016087

Wickramasinghe, N., Misra, S., Jenkins, A., & Vogel, D. R. (2006). The Competitive Forces Facing E-Health. *International Journal of Healthcare Information Systems and Informatics*, *1*(4), 68–81.

Wickramasinghe, N., & Schaffer, J. (2006). Creating knowledge driven healthcare processes with the intelligence continuum. *International Journal of Electronic Healthcare*, *2*(2), 164–174.

Wickramasinghe, N., Schaffer, J., & Geisler, E. (2005). Assessing e-health. In Spil, T., & Schuring, R. (Eds.), *E-Health Systems Diffusion and Use: The Innovation, The User, and The User IT Model*. Hershey, PA: Idea Group.

Wickramasinghe, N., Troshani, I., & Goldberg, S. (2009). Supporting diabetes self-management with pervasive wireless technology solutions. *International Journal of Healthcare Delivery Reform Initiatives*, *1*(4), 17–31.

Wickramasinghe, N., Troshani, I., & Goldberg, S. (2010). An investigation into the use of pervasive wireless technologies to support diabetes healthcare. In Coronato, A., & De Pietro, G. (Eds.), *Pervasive and Smart Technologies for Healthcare: Ubiquitous Methodologies and Tools* (*Vol. 114-129*). New York: IGI Global. doi:10.4018/978-1-61520-765-7.ch006

Williamson, O. E. (1985a). *The Economic Institutions of Capitalism: Firms, Markets and Relational Contracting*. New York: Free Press.

Williamson, O. E. (1985b). *The Economic Institutions of Capitalism: Firms, Markets, and Relational Contracting*. New York: Free Press.

Williamson, O. E. (1991). Comparative economic organization: The analysis of discrete structural alternatives. *Administrative Science Quarterly*, *36*, 269–296. doi:10.2307/2393356

Yu, P., Li, H., & Gagnon, M.-P. (2008). (in press). Health IT acceptance factors i n long-term care facilities: a cross-sectional survey. *International Journal of Health Informatics*. doi:.doi:10.1016/j.ijmedinf.2008.07.006

Zigbor, J. C., & Songer, T. J. (2001). External barriers to diabetes care: addressing personal and health systems issues. *Diabetes Spectrum*, *14*, 23–28. doi:10.2337/diaspect.14.1.23

ADDITIONAL READING

Al Hakim, L. (2007). *Web Mobile-Based Applications for Healthcare Management*. Hershey, PA: IGI Global Publishing.

Spil, T., & Schuring, R. (2006). *E-Health Systems Diffusion and Use*. Hershey, PA: IGI Global Publishing.

Wickramasinghe, N. (2009). *Healthcare Knowledge Management*. Primer, New York: Routledge.

Chapter 17
A Review of Wireless Sensor Networks for Wellness Monitoring in Residential Aged Care

Leroy Lai Yu Chan
University of New South Wales, Australia

Branko George Celler
University of New South Wales, Australia

James Zhaonan Zhang
University of New South Wales, Australia

Nigel Hamilton Lovell
University of New South Wales, Australia

ABSTRACT

With the increasing shift in the population profile to the older demographic and rising healthcare costs, it is more critical for developed countries to deliver long-term and financially sustainable healthcare services, especially in the area of residential aged care. A consensus exists that innovations in the area of Wireless Sensor Networks (WSNs) are key enabling technologies for reaching this goal. The major focus of this article is WSN design considerations for ubiquitous wellness monitoring systems in residential aged care facilities. Major enabling technologies for building a pervasive WSN will be detailed, including descriptions on sensor design, wireless communication protocols and network topologies. Also examined are data processing methods and knowledge management tools to support the collection of sensor data and their subsequent analysis for health assessment. To introduce future healthcare reform in residential aged care, two aspects of wellness monitoring, vital signs and activities of daily living (ADL) monitoring, will be discussed.

DOI: 10.4018/978-1-60960-183-6.ch017

Healthcare Delivery Reform and New Technologies:

Organizational Initiatives

A Review of Wireless Sensor Networks for Wellness Monitoring in Residential Aged Care

A Review of Wireless Sensor Networks for Wellness Monitoring in Residential Aged Care

INTRODUCTION

In developed countries the lifespan of the population is lengthening and the elderly group constitutes an increasingly significant portion of the world population. In 2007, statistics from Australia, the European Union, Japan and the United States showed that people aged 65 years and above made up from 13% to 21% of the population in these areas (Australian Bureau of Statistics, 2008; Eurostat/US Bureau of the Census, 2008; Japan Statistics Bureau & Statistics Center, 2008; US Census Bureau, 2008). Assuming the current trends of fertility and mortality rates, the population in this age bracket is expected to grow to between 20% and 36% by 2050. Taking Australia as an example, the number of people aged 65 and over totals 2.75 million (or 13%). However, the more alarming statistic is that more than half the people in this group suffer from at least one chronic disease (Australian Bureau of Statistics, 2006) and as a result about 25% of the annual government spending on healthcare services was used to provide corresponding treatment. Over the next 30 years, the estimated government healthcare expenditure will increase by 127%, amongst which spending on residential aged care is expected to experience the strongest growth (Australian Institute of Health and Welfare, 2008). This prediction coincides with Golant's (2008) view that "a large increase in the numbers of older persons at risk of needing the supportive services offered in assisted living residences is relatively certain" (p. 12) as he assessed the growth demographic factors affecting the future of residential aged care in the United States. These statistics and trends lead to the conclusion that provision of long-term support for the healthcare needs of the elderly, especially in terms of residential aged care services, is needed but burgeoning costs also mean that such services must be provided in a more financially sustainable way.

Recent innovations in the areas of sensor devices, wireless communication protocols and knowledge management are potential enabling information technologies for delivering future residential aged care services in an economic way. In fact the Commonwealth Government of Australia has recognized the promising benefits of these rising information technologies by piloting several key trial projects related to telehealth. These projects targeted the application areas of medication management (Australian Government, 2007a) and clinical well-being monitoring (Australian Government, 2007b; Celler, Basilakis, Budge, & Lovell, 2006).

In simple terms, telehealth refers to the delivery of healthcare over distance. It covers a wide range of medical applications from remote surgery in a hospital to chronic disease management that takes place in a residential setting. This article is centered on a discussion of how wireless sensor networks (WSNs) can be deployed pervasively in a residential aged care facility to achieve ubiquitous monitoring so that the functional health status of the residents can be assessed. It is organized into several inter-related sections. In the background section, existing models of residential aged care are presented, as well as how the research effort in wellness monitoring can potentially revolutionize care approaches. This is followed by a systems architecture description of WSN technologies and a discussion on how these technologies can change the way residential aged care is delivered. Future trends in this area will then be illustrated through analysis of data taken from a simulated residential aged care environment conducted within the authors' laboratories.

BACKGROUND

In the past, healthcare systems were dominated by the so called "medical" model. In this model, the healthcare providers took the primary role in deciding what the patients' needs were and what clinical interventions would be undertaken. Elderly people with chronic conditions were either looked after by their families and carers in their own homes or in nursing homes. In the latter case there have been many reported incidents in which patients were deprived of choice, autonomy and even dignity.

More recently a "social healthcare" model has emerged as a result of changes in societal values, increased demand in the quality and choice of aged care services and a generally more educated public. In contrast to the medical model, the social healthcare model places its emphasis on the person receiving healthcare services, incorporating the "person's medical, psychological, social, and personal needs, as well as strengths, abilities, interests, and preferences – thereby recognizing a person's distinctive life history and set of experiences" (Hyde, Perez, & Reed, 2008, p. 48). In the context of residential aged care, the social healthcare model encourages the patients, if still capable, to make appropriate choices about how they live and the type of services they require. It also fosters an environment in which social interactions with other patients, visiting families and friends are seen to have positive therapeutic values.

As a result, modern residential aged care facilities need to change, both in terms of their environment and the services they provide, to cope with these new demands. The rate by which the residential aged care facilities can respond is largely dependent on overcoming some of the existing challenges. These include current, possibly out-of-date, government regulations and policies that restrict the growth of facilities such as those leading to funding deficiencies outlined in a report assessing the Australian market (Hogan, 2007). Staffing issues also contribute to the delivery of modern residential aged care services. For instance, the shortage of nursing staff is a major issue faced by the American healthcare system and the contributing factors are increased demand, retiring work force, inadequate trainers and alternative career options. Another major concern of the work force is the lack of appropriate training that empowers staff to respond to changing care demands (Hyde et al., 2008, pp.71, 74). Another important challenge to be resolved is the reluctance of the elderly and nursing staff in adopting and using new technologies in the healthcare delivery process, largely due to fear and misunderstanding that machines will gradually outcast human interactions.

"Technologies are likely to help enhance the quality of the living environment and improve service delivery in the coming years" (Wylde, 2008, p. 179). Technology adoption in residential aged care must proceed with caution. The aim of implementing new technologies in aged care facilities should focus on how to assist staff to provide better and more cost-effective care instead of replacing personal relationships with robotic tools that simply perform a set task faster and cheaper. Assistive technologies showcase a diverse spectrum of devices ranging from low-end items such as wheelchairs and walking-aids, to high-end sophisticated electro-mechanical devices such as robotic bathtubs (Popular Mechanics, 2004). New types of devices—for example, sensors that detect falls, or computers that monitor adherence to medication regimens—are continually being introduced (Wolf & Jenkins, 2008, p. 207).

Broadly speaking, assistive technologies can be divided into categories according to their functional applications: (1) computer-based rehabilitation, cognitive stimulation, entertainment, and interpersonal communication systems; (2) resident assessment, data, and medical record software; (3) traditional emergency call systems; (4) passively-activated call systems; (5) wandering prevention and tracking systems; (6) vital signs monitoring;

(7) fall detectors; and (8) more comprehensive activity monitoring systems (Kutzik, Glascock, Lundberg, & York, 2008, p. 224). In this article, the specific research area of wellness monitoring as a tool for functional health assessment in residential aged care settings using assisted technologies will be examined. Essentially, wellness monitoring draws on the collaboration of two of the aforementioned assistive technology categories, namely vital signs monitoring and comprehensive activity monitoring.

The objectives of wellness monitoring is threefold; to discover the onset of certain conditions before obvious symptoms develop in an otherwise reasonably healthy person (Srovnal & Penhaker, 2007); to provide the tools and training to promote self care; and to ensure early hospital admission of chronically ill patients when the condition requires immediate treatment. The first two objectives focus on the growing importance of prevention or early detection of a medical condition while the latter focuses on the urgency in providing necessary therapies to minimize patient morbidity crises and medical costs.

Vital signs monitoring, whether real time or periodic, provide an insight into essential statistics about the patient including heart rate and rhythm disturbances, blood oxygen content, respiratory rate, blood pressure, body temperature, etc.. Taken collectively these clinical measurements can be skillfully combined by an experienced caregiver to infer the well-being of the patient. An elevated body temperature in a normally healthy subject may signal the onset of influenza or gradual weight gain in a congestive heart failure patient may indicate edema related to a failing heart. For a diabetic patient, a steady and uncontrollable increase in blood glucose level above the target range warrants immediate treatment. A conventional vital signs recording session involves the health worker who manually measures a patient's body temperature, records the result and enters the data into the patient health record database. Drawbacks of this approach are numerous and include errors and delays in data entry, lost data records, and clinicians being unable to concurrently access the latest patient health data.

Due to the importance of physiological measurements, vital signs monitoring technology research has proliferated over the past decade. One approach for collecting a patient's physiological data is by means of a home clinical workstation located in a common area, such as the lounge, within an aged care facility. Residents can, and are encouraged to, visit the workstation periodically to have their vital signs checked. Collected data can be stored locally, transferred to an on-site database to be reviewed by staff later, or even transmitted to a remote clinician's site for assessment. The communication protocols that can be used vary from wired platforms such as Ethernet, traditional phone line or Asymmetric Digital Subscriber Line (ADSL) to wireless technologies that are becoming more commonplace such as Wireless Local Area Network (WLAN), Bluetooth, ZigBee, Global System for Mobile communications (GSM), General Packet Radio Service (GPRS) or Universal Mobile Telecommunications System (UMTS). The major advantage of using such a shared system is the reduction in cost since there is no need for an individual monitoring system for each patient. However, as with all other types of shared computers, data security and privacy is an issue not to be overlooked.

One successful example of such a system is the TeleMedCare Home Monitoring System (TeleMedCare, Sydney, Australia) (Figure 1) developed at the University of New South Wales, Sydney Australia (Celler, Basilakis, Budge, & Lovell, 2006; Lovell et al., 2002). The system has features to measure a single lead electrocardiogram (ECG), arterial blood oxygen saturation, body temperature, body weight and spirometry. It also provides an interface for medication management, patient education and secure staff access for patient medical records and service provision history. Other systems that have been in clinical use throughout the world include the

Figure 1. The TeleMedCare Home Monitoring System is capable of recording multiple clinical measurements, including single lead ECG, blood pressure, spirometry and pulse oximetry. A touch screen interface allows recent results to be viewed as longitudinal graphs as well as medication and measurement alerts to be delivered via a remote scheduler.

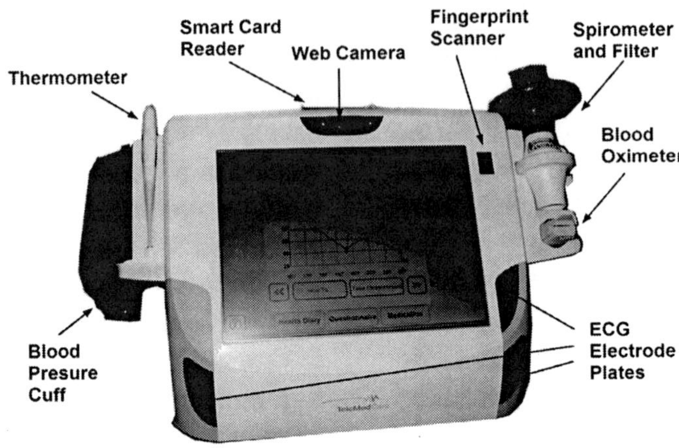

HomMed system (Honeywell, Milwaukee, USA) and doc@Home (Docobo Ltd., Bookham, UK). Figure 1. The TeleMedCare Home Monitoring System is capable of recording multiple clinical measurements, including single lead ECG, blood pressure, spirometry and pulse oximetry. A touch screen interface allows recent results to be viewed as longitudinal graphs as well as medication and measurement alerts to be delivered via a remote scheduler.

Unfortunately in a residential aged care setting, it is often infeasible for the elderly to self-perform routine vital signs monitoring due to their immobility and the lack of necessary motor and cognitive skills to interact with the devices. Therefore, in contrast with the shared workstation method for vital signs monitoring, recently there has been significant progress into using pervasive and ubiquitous networks of sensors for physiological parameter measurements. For example, sensors can be located within the environment such as load sensors installed to the bed frame for weight measurement (Elite Care, 2008). Others can be attached to the patient when required (Chan, Celler, & Lovell, 2006; Warren, Yao, & Barnes, 2002; Wilson et al., 2001) while others are designed to integrate into a wearable garment for long term and continuous monitoring (Pentland, 2004) of a diverse array of body parameters. So far, vital signs monitoring using this distributed computing approach is restricted to development in the laboratory and large scale clinical deployments are yet to occur. Data privacy, mobility and continuous monitoring are characteristic features of this approach. With the remaining technical challenges such as data transfer security, sensor link reliability, system cost and sensor battery life all expected to be resolved or contained in the future, this sensor network approach is expected to prevail as the dominant choice for vital sign monitoring due to the benefits it potentially offers.

Comprehensive activity monitoring is often referred to as activities of daily living (ADL) monitoring in the literature. ADL monitoring systems contribute to wellness monitoring by building and profiling the daily activity pattern of a subject and using it as a baseline for comparison against irregular patterns. Such systems are useful in detecting the onset of problems that are only revealed over a longer period of time. For instance, gradual and unintentional changes in appetite in an otherwise healthy patient may suggest a digestive disease, while increased episodes of wandering can be signs of the onset of dementia.

According to Kutzik, Glascock, Lundberg and York (2008), ADL monitoring systems can take on two distinct design approaches: maximalist and minimalist. The maximalist approach aims to build an infrastructure which supports a diverse network of hardware devices such as sensors, data repeaters, network coordinators and data sinks. This extensive network of devices is designed to collect as complete a data set as possible related to the daily activities of patients. These data are then processed by algorithms and translated into useful information for caregivers such as sleeping patterns, usage of toilet and bathroom facilities, eating patterns, social interaction, time spent with care-givers, activity level, etc.. Most often these can be combined with the vital sign monitoring results in order to design the best care plan tailored for the individual patient. The minimalist approach, on the other hand, employs hardware and software that are designed to monitor specific tasks and/or disease conditions.

Research in this area in terms of impact of ADL monitoring on health status remains embryonic. One of the first technology demonstrators of remote monitoring of the free-living elderly occurred in the early 1990s in Australia as a result of research at UNSW (Celler et al., 1995). More recently a single-subject study was conducted in Japan (Suzuki et al., 2004) to first build up the daily living pattern of the subject by a network of wired sensors that measured movement, human presence, door and window openings, stove usage, television and washing machine usage and sleep occurrence. Subsequent daily patterns were compared with a normal template and any dramatic change in behavior could be ascertained. Similarly, the PlaceLab at the Massachusetts Institute of Technology (Massachusetts Institute of Technology, 2003) is an apartment-style research facility hosting a rich sensing infrastructure of over 300 sensor types and is another typical example of the maximalist approach. ADL-related parameters that can be detected include light, air quality, ambient temperature and humidity, sound, motion, identity, use of appliances, door movements, etc. Some of these parameters may not immediately find their place in providing care to patients but the philosophy of the maximalist approach is to perform excessive measurements. Another study (Philipose et al., 2004) tested the detection of fourteen different ADL by placing over 100 radio frequency identification (RFID) tags in a test house. The subjects were made to wear a specifically designed glove containing an RFID reader and a radio front-end for data transmission to a data sink. When an activity was performed, the subject interacted by touching different RFID-tagged objects, thus providing a record of the time and sequence of the objects used. A probabilistic inference engine was used to estimate the different ADLs performed.

Perhaps the project largest in scale that applied ADL monitoring technologies to residential aged care was the Oatfield Estates project by Elite Care (Stanford, 2002). Each resident and staff on the estate wore an identification badge that could be tracked by embedded readers throughout the buildings. In other words, location tracking and wandering prevention became part of the ADL monitoring system. Residents were also monitored for weight and sleeping pattern changes by specially designed load cells placed under each bed leg. The system also allowed staff and residents to manually enter other activity information into the database.

It can be seen that the main challenge of ADL monitoring systems is the appropriate use of collected data to produce useful information. Technologies and approaches related to this area include data mining, machine learning, artificial intelligence and knowledge management. It may also be obvious to the reader that ADL monitoring systems share similar infrastructure to smart home systems. Research has shown that there are a many positives in blending the two systems. This will be addressed in the section on future research directions.

WIRELESS SENSOR NETWORKS FOR WELLNESS MONITORING

Wireless sensor technologies provide a ubiquitous, non-invasive and cost effective way to continuously and autonomously monitor one's physiological parameters as well as ADL. While these systems may not replace every aspect of the conventional wellness monitoring approach, they allow data to be collected from areas previously inaccessible such as location information with room-level granularity. There are three major subsystems in a wireless sensor, technology-based, wellness monitoring system:

- **WSNs:** collects relevant data from the subject and the subject's interaction with their environment. These data are wirelessly transmitted in either raw or processed format back to a central server for further conditioning, classification and knowledge inference.
- **Data conditioning, feature extraction and data fusion:** Continuous data streaming from multiple sensors over the network means there is flood of information. Data cleaning and noise reduction is critical to ensure only data with an acceptable level of noise and quality is processed to extract waveform features. This sub-system acts on individual data channels to extract relevant information. It also applies data fusion techniques across multiple channels to identify signal interactions. For example, with RFID locator technology, signal interaction can be used to infer the length of time spent toileting, the time spent dispensing medications to a particular subject, etc.
- **Data fusion, knowledge management and decision support:** This sub-system is heavily based on advanced software modeling of the subject data. Based on a normal pattern of ADL for a particular subject, the system will be able to identify consistent discrepancies from this template and from these deviations infer changes in functional health state.

This section will focus on describing the first sub-system, the architectural design of WSNs. As described in the previous section, this is the most advanced area in terms of research and development. The latter two areas are relatively embryonic due to the lack of appropriate hardware systems to acquire the necessary signals and build the necessary knowledge bases.

Sensor and Wireless Network Design

A sensor network system is comprised of wireless sensor nodes, which contain one or more sensor types used to collect data from either a person or the surrounding environment. The collected data is firstly processed locally, such as digital filtering, formatting, noise cleaning, etc.. Data is then transmitted via the RF section of the sensor. There are a number of features to be considered when implementing the wireless network, the most significant being the network protocol; various options exist including WLAN (IEEE 802.11 b/g), Bluetooth (IEEE 802.15.1) and ZigBee (based on IEEE 802.15.4).

Design and deployment of multiple types of low-cost sensors heavily impacts the utility of the monitoring system. In the next section we introduce a range of sensor types, discussing usage implications, size, power, cost and longevity.

Types of Sensors

In one common classification approach, sensors can be categorized into three groupings; ambient environmental sensors, body area network (BAN) sensors, and location and usage sensors. Ambient environmental sensors are used to monitor the ambient condition of a given geographical environment. Some of the widely used sensors are:

- Passive Infrared (PIR) sensors are used commonly to detect the presence of moving infrared emitters. They are very reliable in terms of detecting heat sources (therefore human presence) but cannot recognize the identity of the subject present in the environment, nor are they accurate enough to detect the presence of multiple persons (Ohta, Nakamoto, Shinagawa, & Tanikawa, 2002).
- Ambient light sensors can be used to correlate the sleeping behavior of the subject in reference to circadian rhythms.
- Ambient temperature sensors provide a reference reading of the current temperature settings. Room temperatures could be used for example to build up the temperature preference for an individual subject over a period of time.

The second category of sensors is BAN sensors. These sensors include various types of monitoring transducers with wireless communication capability. The main differentiating point of these sensors is that they must be worn by the subject. They include:

- **Triaxial-accelerometry:** a sensor that measures the acceleration of the body in three-dimensions. Performing continuous acceleration measurements can be used to determine the ambulation and activity-level of a subject, as well as falls propensity and falls risk. It has been demonstrated that such technologies can classify postural orientation (sitting, standing, lying) with a reasonable accuracy (Mathie, Coster, Lovell, & Celler, 2004; Mathie, Coster, Lovell, Celler et al., 2004). Also the signal magnitude area of the acceleration signals can be used as an estimate of energy expenditure (activity level) (Voon, Celler, & Lovell, 2008). Determining activity level of the monitored subject provides an indication of both physical and cognitive health status (Virone et al., 2008). Moreover, we have demonstrated that such algorithms can be effectively coded in real-time, thus relieving the need to transmit large continuous streams of data over a WSN for further processing (Karantonis, Narayanan, Mathie, Lovell, & Celler, 2006).
- **ECG sensing:** it is commonly accepted that in order to accurately diagnose cardiac disease that a 12-lead ECG recording is mandated. However this is only possible in a clinical setting. As a compromise, ECG systems used in the WSN environment are normally single lead recordings using 2 or 3 attached electrodes. By applying advanced signal processing techniques, various types of arrhythmias and conduction abnormalities can be determined (Tsipouras, Fotiadis, & Sideris, 2005) even from a single lead recording.
- **Body temperature:** continual monitoring of the body temperature of an elderly patient can provide timely and accurate information that reflects the onset of infection and/or disease. In hospital wards and nursing homes this manual task is both repetitive and time consuming, so a WSN approach is beneficial.

The third category of sensors relate to location detection. These types of sensors are developed to track the location and specific movements of a subject, including their interaction with other objects, people or resources:

- **Location sensor:** Location tracking is one of the most important sensor types as it

Figure 2. A generic sensor block diagram illustrates the major sub-systems used in a wireless sensor.

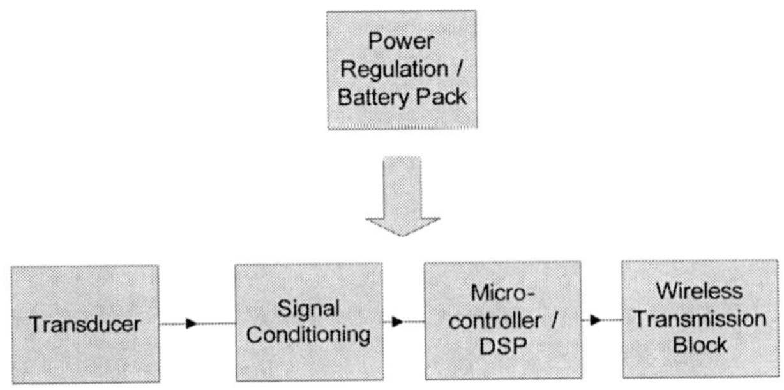

generates useful data for assessing functional health. An example is the social activity level, where the times of interaction between subject, health professionals and care givers can be tracked. One common technique adapted by wireless sensor networks is to implement a set of reference nodes around the target area, for example a nursing home environment. These nodes form a reference grid and a mobile location sensor determines the Received Signal Strength Indicator (RSSI) value from the reference nodes. It is assumed by the mobile sensor that the strongest signal it receives from the reference node is the closest therefore approximating its location within the reference grid via triangulation (Adamodt, 2006). In this instance the subject must wear the mobile sensor and in a similar way, health care professionals and other important objects (medication and meal trolleys) must also have mobile sensors attached. Another way of monitoring location is to implement a grid of pressure sensors on the floor. The advantage is that a very accurate movement path of the subject can be determined. Disadvantages include cost, difficulty of installation and handling the presence of multiple persons in the same area (Mori, Noguchi, Takada, & Sato, 2004).

- **Usage sensors:** Many of these devices are ON/OFF switches or passive RFID tags. They are installed on major objects such as the toilet, shower, fridge, stove, cabin doors, etc. and directly monitor the use of various facilities.

Sensor Design Architecture

The block diagram in Figure 2 illustrates a typical architecture of a wireless sensor. As an illustrative example, a wireless single-lead ECG wireless sensor will be presented.

- **Power regulation/battery:** In a wireless patient monitoring environment, power regulation has to be as efficient as possible to avoid undue power wastage. The voltage regulator has to provide either 5V and/or 3.3V to the different integrated circuits. Also because most of the current-generation wireless sensors use single cell Lithium-ion rechargeable batteries, overcharge and over-discharge protection circuitry has to be implemented to ensure optimal battery life.
- **Transducer:** The transducer acts as the interface between the environment and the sensor. Possibly the biggest barrier to adoption and usage of physiological measurement devices involves the usability and compliance issues associated with at-

taching sensor to the body to transducer the biological phenomena into electrical signals that can then be further processed. In the case of an ECG, ionic currents (carried by ions in solution) in physiological media (tissues and organs of the body) must be converted into electronic currents (carried by electrons) in metallic conductor. Conventional biopotential electrodes in use today consist of a metallic conductor in contact with the tissue of interest (e.g., the skin, when recording body surface potentials such as the ECG) via an electrolyte solution. Due to the presence of the electrolyte solution, such electrodes are sometimes referred to as "wet electrodes" to distinguish them from the less conventional "dry electrodes" which make contact with the tissue without the aid of an electrolyte solution. In nearly all cases of ambulatory ECG monitoring, these conventional or wet electrodes are used, with a pre-gelled disposable Ag/AgCl pellet attached by an adhesive pad.

- **Signal conditioning:** This module is used amplify, filter and perform feature extraction and artifact rejection on the signal. For a single-lead ECG in an ambulatory subject, it is expected that the recorded signal will be severely compromised by artefacts introduced by muscle activity, movement and electrical noise (Redmond, Lovell, Basilakis, & Celler, 2008). Typically the QRS events within the ECG will be detected using a real-time algorithm in order to derive the heart rate. One common approach in the literature is to use a sliding window technique based to derive the heart rate and hence classify the heart arrhythmia status (Raju, 2007; Tsipouras et al., 2005).
- **Wireless transmission:** This module contains the wireless RF transceiver (processor) and antenna. The wireless transceiver handles lower level RF packet formation and transmission. The microcontroller typically communicates with the RF transceiver via an I2C or SPI protocol and transmits data via a program interface provided by the chip vendor.

FUTURE RESEARCH DIRECTIONS

Based on the current literature, nearly all wellness monitoring systems, whether commercial or research, focus on either vital signs monitoring or ADL monitoring. It is becoming clear that to adequately support the needs of health monitoring in residential aged care both elements need to be integrated.

A continuous wellness monitoring system (SensorNet@BSL) currently under further development at University of New South Wales is built with this goal in mind. The initial version of the system operates on a three-layer architecture, consisting of a central server controlling multiple WLANs with each WLAN coordinating multiple Zigbee-based WSNs. The three-layer architecture system design offers flexibility in terms of expanding the sensor network almost indefinitely to suit the facility area and need. It can be applied equally efficiently to a single household and a well-established, multi-storey residential aged care facility. Its complete wireless nature means that the system can be installed into places with minimal building structural change and with maximal ease. Vital signs monitoring is performed via the collection of physiological parameters such as ECG, heart rate, postural orientation, energy expenditure and body temperature. ADL information is obtained by analyzing unobtrusive data such as the resident's interaction with the environment, usage of facilities, interaction with caregivers, time spent on certain activities, etc.. Currently, the system is undergoing additional technology modifications to prepare for major clinical evaluations in several commercial residential aged care facilities around Australia. Figure 3 illustrates a typical deployment

Figure 3. A mock living environment of an Australian aged care facility and the operation of SensorNet@ BSL. The end server, the bridge units and the sensor units form the three-level architecture. The end server communicates with the bridge units via WLAN while the WSN connections between the bridge units and sensor units are ZigBee-based. Sensor units are either placed in the environment (static) or can be carried around (mobile). As a mobile sensor unit moves to a new geographical area served by a different bridge unit, the control of the sensor unit is handed over to the new bridge unit such that the room-level location of the mobile unit at any time is known to the end server.

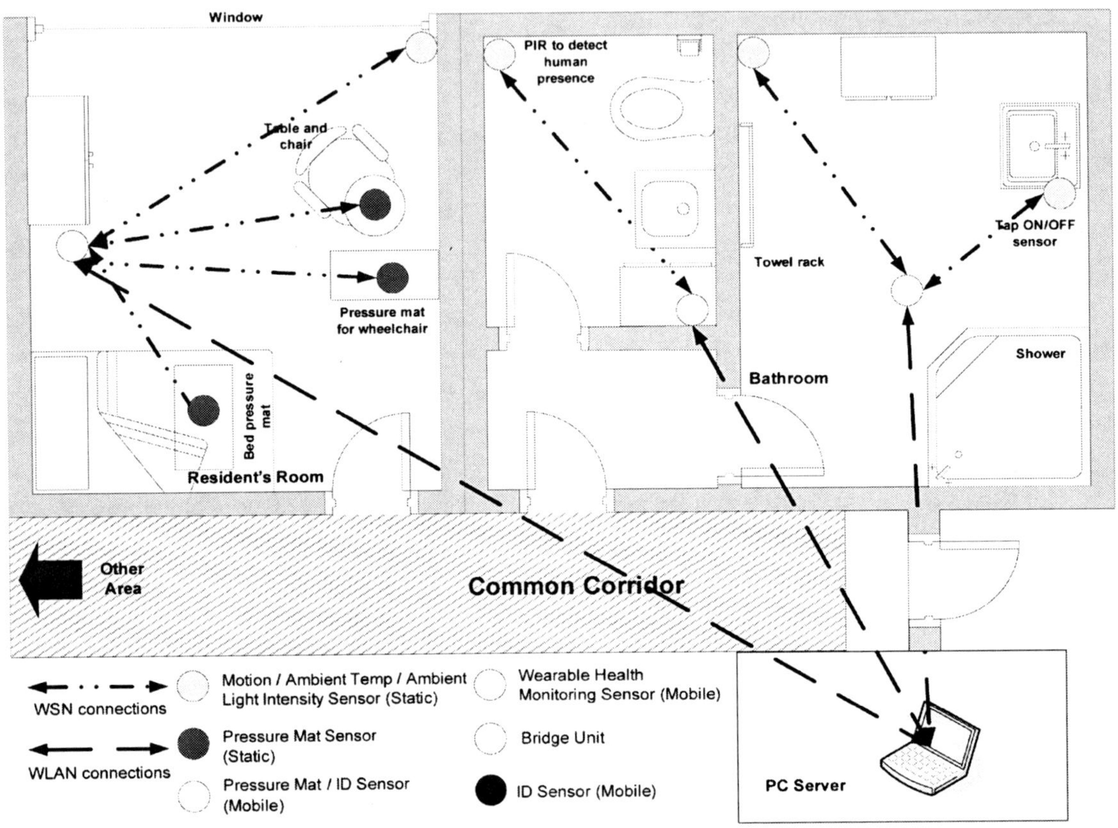

of the SensorNet@BSL project. Figure 4 shows hardware layouts of the various WSN components while Figure 5 shows sample data collected from this deployment.

Similar wellness monitoring systems developed around the world over the last decade include the House_n Group project (Intille, 2002; Tapia, Intille, & Larson, 2004) which studied the qualitative and quantitative relationships between users and surrounding objects. Based on collected data the system was trained to build a Bayesian network model for residential monitoring. The Welfare Techno-Houses project in Japan (Tamura, Togawa, Ogawa, & Yoda, 1998; Yamaguchi, Ogawa, Tamura, & Togawa, 1998) consisted of thirteen houses equipped with infrared sensors and magnetic switches on the doors to monitor both physical activity and physiological signals with the goal of improving the quality of life for both the elderly and their caregivers. The CareNet project in the United Kingdom (Williams, Doughty, & Bradley, 1998) provided the "Hospital at Home" service by collecting the patient's physiological data as well as analyzing the lifestyle

Figure 4. The SensorNet@BSL hardware platform. Left: the modular design of the universal sensor mother board to which different sensor daughter boards can be attached to modify functionality. Middle: the middle layer ZigBee / WLAN bridge acts as the super node. Right: a sensor daughter board attached to the mother board. The illustrated daughter board has a PIR, a temperature and a light intensity sensor incorporated into the printed circuit board.

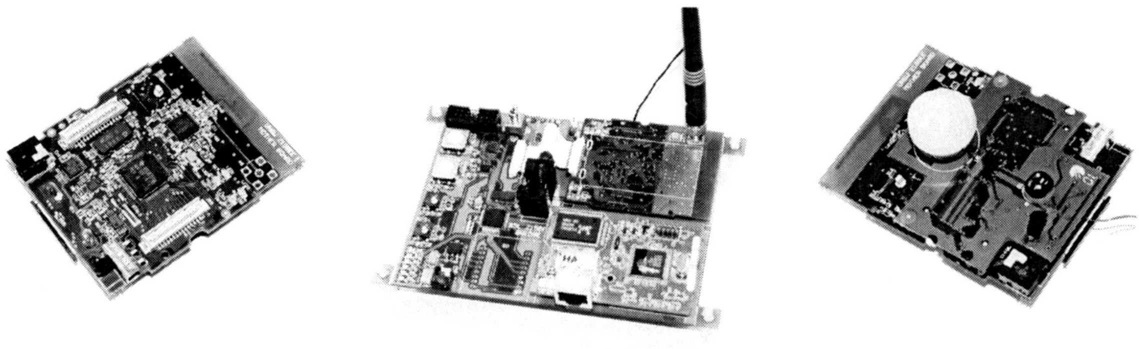

Figure 5. Sample data from tri-accelerometry sensor with derived energy expenditure level.

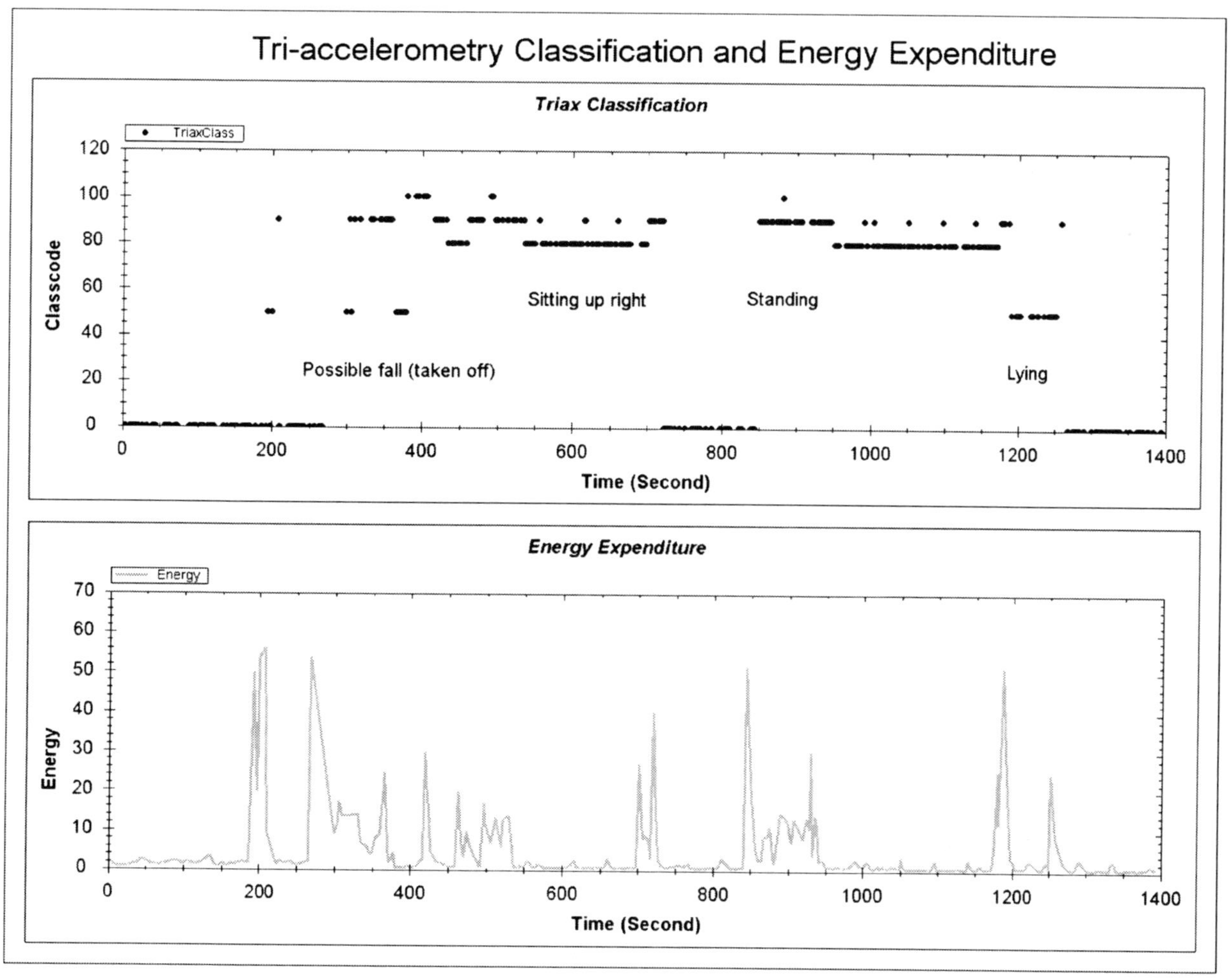

of the patient by sensors embedded in their environment.

Another anticipated trend of wellness monitoring systems for residential aged care is the possible integration with smart home systems. Both systems can leverage on the data collected by a single sensor network to achieve separate outcomes. For instance, a light sensor detecting the light intensity of a room can be used by the smart home system to decide if lighting in a particular area should be adjusted. The same piece of information can be used by a wellness monitoring system to record the number of times a patient wakes up at night to use the bathroom and infer the health status of the patient.

A limited number of larger scale smart home projects implemented in North America and Europe over the past decade have factored in their design a wellness monitoring component. An example of such is the Aware Home Research Initiative at the Georgia Institute of Technology (Kidd et al., 1999) which involved a three-storey smart home to support elderly occupants with context awareness and ubiquitous sensing, location tracking and lost object tracking capabilities. The Millennium House project pioneered by British Telecom and the Anchor Trust (Perry, Dowdall, Lines, & Hone, 2004) used infrared sensors and magnetic switches on doors to study the behavior pattern of the occupant and alert the caregiver should an abnormality be detected. This intelligent system also supported independent living of the elderly by warning them about dangerous events, or checking if they need external assistance.

CONCLUSION

Statistics highlight the fact that the world population is ageing, and this phenomenon is becoming an issue for developed countries. To maintain and improve quality and continuity of care, extra resources must be allocated for maintaining elderly health. The rise of information technologies carries the promise of providing ubiquitous wellness monitoring for functional health assessment in residential aged care facilities with higher quality and at a reduced cost. Among these, the technologies involved in constructing pervasive WSNs have been shown to improve the diversity of the parameters that can be measured in vital signs monitoring and enhance data availability to authorized healthcare personnel. WSNs are also proved to be beneficial in ADL management by monitoring residents' interaction with their environment and alert caregivers when abnormal living patterns are detected.

When designing a WSN for wellness monitoring purposes, many factors need to be considered. Each sensor type has its specific area of application such as ambient environmental monitoring, body signal measurement or location tracking. Sensors must be chosen to fit the type and environment of use while at the same time satisfy requirements such as size, power consumption, cost and longevity for a particular application. In general, a wireless sensor node consists of a transducer unit managed by a microprocessor which provides signal preconditioning capability and acts as an interface to the wireless transceiver front-end. The whole sensor node is most likely powered by a rechargeable battery that enhances mobility of the node. The wireless communication protocol and network topology must also be chosen carefully to optimize battery life, transmission range, throughput and scalability.

Raw data collected by the sensors are often pre-processed, either by the sensor node or the data sink, before further transmissions to optimize limited bandwidth usage and enhance network availability. Data must also be processed to detect and alert for corruption and artifact.

Perhaps the biggest future challenge that has only started to be addressed is the need for data fusion from multiple sensors. These data must feed into knowledge management systems that by way of machine learning and other inference methods can compare changes against normal templates for particular subjects and thus identify a decline in functional health status. The current state of research is that WSN are only now being deployed to provide the necessary baseline data from which the knowledge management systems can be developed.

It is envisioned that future wellness monitoring systems will not only incorporate capabilities to monitor both vital signs and ADL but also integrate seamlessly with smart home systems to provide a truly intelligent environment to cater for all aspects of daily living.

REFERENCES

Adamodt, K. (2006). [Location Engine]. *Application Note, AN042*, CC2431.

Australian Bureau of Statistics. (2006). *4102.0 - Australian Social Trends, 2006*. Retrieved from http://www.abs.gov.au/ausstats/abs@.nsf/Latestproducts/6F443192D27B9360CA2571B00013D954?opendocument

Australian Bureau of Statistics. (2008). *3222.0 - Population Projections, Australia, 2006 to 2101*. Retrieved from http://www.abs.gov.au/ausstats/abs@.nsf/mf/3222.0

Australian Government. (2007a). *Clinical IT in Aged Care Product Trial - Trial of a Medication Management System - Report*. Retrieved from http://www.health.gov.au/internet/main/publishing.nsf/Content/ageing-rescare-econnect-med-mgt-trial.htm

Australian Government. (2007b). *Clinical IT in Aged Care Product Trial - Trial of a System for Monitoring Clinical Well-Being - Report*. Retrieved from http://www.health.gov.au/internet/main/publishing.nsf/Content/1E896B258E583DF8CA2573B5007C788D/$File/Clinical%20Monitoring.pdf

Australian Institute of Health and Welfare. (2008). *Australia's health 2008*. Retrieved from http://www.aihw.gov.au/publications/index.cfm/title/10585

Celler, B. G., Basilakis, J., Budge, M., & Lovell, N. H. (2006). A Clinical Monitoring and Management System for Residential Aged Care Facilities. In *Proceedings of the 28th IEEE EMBS Annual International Conference* (pp. 3301).

Celler, B. G., Earnshaw, W., Ilsar, E. D., Betbeder-Matibet, L., Harris, M., & Clark, R. (1995). Remote monitoring of the elderly at home. A multidisciplinary project on aging at the University of New South Wales. *International Journal of Bio-Medical Computing*, *40*, 147–155. doi:10.1016/0020-7101(95)01139-6

Chan, L. L., Zhang, J. Z., Narayanan, M. R., Celler, B. G., & Lovell, N. H. (2008, February 13-15). *A Health Monitoring and Evaluation System for Assessing Care Needs of Residents in Aged-Care Facilities*. Paper presented at the IASTED Biomed. Eng., Innsbruck, Austria.

Elite Care. (2008). *Elite Care*. Retrieved from http://www.elitecare.com/

Eurostat/US Bureau of the Census. (2008). *People by age classes*. Retrieved January 28, 2009, from http://epp.eurostat.ec.europa.eu/portal/page?_pageid=1996,39140985&_dad=portal&_schema=PORTAL&screen=detailref&language=en&product=REF_TB_population&root=REF_TB_population/t_popula/t_pop/t_demo_pop/tps00010

Golant, S. M. (2008). The Future of Assisted Living Residences. In S. M. Golant & J. Hyde (Eds.), *The Assisted Living Residence* (pp. 3-45). Baltimore, MD: John Hopkins University Press.

Hogan, W. (2007). *The Organisation of Residential Aged Care for an Ageing Population*. St. Leonards, NSW, Australia: The Centre of Independent Studies.

Hyde, J., Perez, R., & Reed, P. S. (2008). The Old Road Is Rapidly Aging. In S. M. Golant & J. Hyde (Eds.), *The Assisted Living Residence* (pp. 46-85). Baltimore, MD: Johns Hopkins University Press.

Intille, S. S. (2002). Designing a Home of the Future. *IEEE Pervasive Computing / IEEE Computer Society [and] IEEE Communications Society*, *1*(2), 76–82. doi:10.1109/MPRV.2002.1012340

Japan Statistics Bureau & Statistics Center. (2008, April 15). *Population by Age (Single Year), Sex and Sex ratio - Total population, Japanese population*. Retrieved January 28, 2009, from http://www.e-stat.go.jp/SG1/estat/ListE.do?lid=000001026128

Karantonis, D. M., Narayanan, M. R., Mathie, M., Lovell, N. H., & Celler, B. G. (2006). Implementation of a Real-Time Human Movement Classifier Using a Triaxial Accelerometer for Ambulatory Monitoring. *IEEE Transactions on Information Technology in Biomedicine*, *10*(1), 156–167. doi:10.1109/TITB.2005.856864

Kidd, C. D., Orr, R., Abowd, G. D., Atkeson, C. G., Essa, I. A., MacIntyre, B., et al. (1999). *The Aware Home: A Living Laboratory for Ubiquitous Computing Research*. Paper presented at the Second International Workshop on Cooperative Buildings, Integrating Information, Organization, and Architecture.

Kutzik, D. M., Glascock, A. P., Lundberg, L., & York, J. (2008). Technological Tools of the Future. In S. M. Golant & J. Hyde (Eds.), *The Assisted Living Residence*. Baltimore, MD: Johns Hopkins University Press.

Labiod, H., Afifi, H., & De Santis, C. (2007). *Wi-Fi Bluetooth Zigbee and WiMax*. Dordrecht, The Netherlands: Springer.

Lovell, N. H., Celler, B. G., Basilakis, J., Magrabi, F., Huynh, K., & Mathie, M. (2002). *Managing chronic disease with home telecare: a system architecture and case study*. Paper presented at the Proceedings of the Second Joint EMBS/BMES Conference.

Massachusetts Institute of Technology. (2003). *PlaceLab: A House_n + TIAX Initiative*. Cambridge, MA: Author. Retrieved from http://architecture.mit.edu/house_n/placelab.html

Mathie, M. J., Coster, A. C., Lovell, N. H., & Celler, B. G. (2004). Accelerometry: Providing an integrated, practical method for long-term, ambulatory monitoring of human movement. *Physiological Measurement*, *25*(2), R1–R20. doi:10.1088/0967-3334/25/2/R01

Mathie, M. J., Coster, A. C., Lovell, N. H., Celler, B. G., Lord, S. R., & Tiedemann, A. (2004). A pilot study of long-term monitoring of human movements in the home using accelerometry. *Journal of Telemedicine and Telecare*, *10*(3), 144–151. doi:10.1258/135763304323070788

Mori, T., Noguchi, H., Takada, A., & Sato, T. (2004). Sensing Room: Distributed Sensor Environment for Measurement of Human Daily Behavior. In *Proceedings of the First International Workshop on Networked Sensing Systems (INSS2004)* (pp. 40-43).

Ohta, S., Nakamoto, H., Shinagawa, Y., & Tanikawa, T. (2002). A health monitoring system for elderly people living alone. *Journal of Telemedicine and Telecare*, *8*(3), 151–156. doi:10.1258/135763302320118997

Pentland, A. (2004). Healthwear: Medical technology becomes wearable. *Computer*, *37*(5), 42–49. doi:10.1109/MC.2004.1297238

Perry, M., Dowdall, A., Lines, L., & Hone, K. (2004). Multimodal and ubiquitous computing systems: supporting independent-living older users. *IEEE Transactions on Information Technology in Biomedicine*, *8*(3), 258–270. doi:10.1109/TITB.2004.835533

Philipose, M., Fishkin, K. P., Perkowitz, M., Patterson, D. J., Fox, D., & Kautz, H. (2004). Inferring activities from interactions with objects. *IEEE Pervasive Computing / IEEE Computer Society [and] IEEE Communications Society*, *3*(4), 50–57. doi:10.1109/MPRV.2004.7

Popular Mechanics. (2004, June). Robots Help Japan Care for Its Elderly. Retrieved January 30, 2009, from http://www.popularmechanics.com/science/technology_watch/1288241.html

Raju, M. (2007). *Heart-Rate and EKG Monitor Using the MSP430FG439* [Electronic Version].

Redmond, S. J., Lovell, N. H., Basilakis, J., & Celler, B. G. (2008, August 20-24). *ECG quality measures in telecare monitoring*. Paper presented at EMBC08, Vancouver, BC, Canada.

Srovnal, V., & Penhaker, M. (2007). *Health Maintenance Embedded Systems in Home Care Applications*. Paper presented at ICONS 2007.

Stanford, V. (2002). Using Pervasive Computing to Deliver Elder Care. *IEEE Pervasive Computing / IEEE Computer Society [and] IEEE Communications Society*, 10–13. doi:10.1109/MPRV.2002.993139

Suzuki, R., Ogawa, M., Otake, S., Izutsu, T., Tobimatsu, Y., & Izumi, S. (2004). Analysis of activities of daily living in elderly people living alone: Single-subject feasibility study. *Telemedicine Journal and e-Health*, *10*(2), 260–276. doi:10.1089/tmj.2004.10.260

Tamura, T., Togawa, T., Ogawa, M., & Yoda, M. (1998). Fully automated health monitoring system in the home. *Medical Engineering & Physics*, *20*, 573–579. doi:10.1016/S1350-4533(98)00064-2

Tapia, E., Intille, S. S., & Larson, K. (2004). Activity Recognition in the Home Using Simple and Ubiquitous Sensors. In *Pervasive Computing* (pp. 158-175).

Tsipouras, M. G., Fotiadis, D. I., & Sideris, D. (2005). An arrhythmia classification system based on the RR-interval signal. *Artificial Intelligence in Medicine*, *33*(3), 237–250. doi:10.1016/j.artmed.2004.03.007

US Census Bureau. (2008). *Projected Population by Single Year of Age, Sex, Race, and Hispanic Origin for the United States: July 1, 2000 to July 1, 2050*. Retrieved January 27, 2009, from http://www.census.gov/population/www/projections/downloadablefiles.html

Virone, G., Alwan, M., Dalal, S., Kell, S. W., Turner, B., & Stankovic, J. A. (2008). Behavioral Patterns of Older Adults in Assisted Living. *IEEE Transactions on Information Technology in Biomedicine*, *12*(3), 12. doi:10.1109/TITB.2007.904157

Voon, R., Celler, B. G., & Lovell, N. H. (2008). The use of an energy monitor in the management of diabetes: A pilot study. *Diabetes Technology and Therapeutics*.

Warren, S., Yao, J., & Barnes, G. E. (2002). Wearable sensors and component-based design for home health care. In. *Proceedings of the Annual International Conference of IEEE Engineering in Medicine and Biology*, *3*, 1871–1872.

Williams, G., Doughty, K., & Bradley, D. A. (1998). A systems approach to achieving CarerNet-an integrated and intelligent telecare system. *IEEE Transactions on Information Technology in Biomedicine*, *2*(1), 1–9. doi:10.1109/4233.678527

Wilson, L. S., Ho, P., Bengston, K. J., Dadd, M. J., Chen, C. F., Huynh, C., et al. (2001). *The CSIRO hospital without walls home telecare system*. Paper presented at the Seventh Australian and New Zealand Intelligent Information Systems Conference.

Wolf, D. A., & Jenkins, C. (2008). Family Care and Assisted Living. In S. M. Golant & J. Hyde (Eds.), *The Assisted Living Residence*. Baltimore, MD: Johns Hopkins University Press.

Wylde, M. A. (2008). The Future of Assisted Living: Residents' Perspectives 2006-2026. In S. M. Golant & J. Hyde (Eds.), *The Assisted Living Residence*. Baltimore, MD: Johns Hopkins University Press.

Yamaguchi, A., Ogawa, M., Tamura, T., & Togawa, T. (1998). *Monitoring behavior in the home using positioning sensors*. Paper presented at the 20th Annual International Conference of the IEEE Engineering in Medicine and Biology Society.

This work was previously published in International Journal of Healthcare Delivery Reform Initiatives, edited by Matthew W. Guah, pp. 32-47, copyright 2009 by IGI Publishing (an imprint of IGI Global).

Chapter 18
Nursing Homes and E-Health

Shuyan Xie
University of Alabama, USA

Yang Xiao
University of Alabama, USA

Hsiao-Hwa Chen
National Cheng Kung University, Taiwan

ABSTRACT

A nursing home provides skilled nursing care and rehabilitation services to people with illnesses, injuries or functional disabilities, but most facilities serve the elderly. Nursing homes provide various services for different residents' needs, including daily care, assistance for the mentally disabled, and drug rehabilitation. The levels of care and quality of care provided by nursing homes have increased significantly over the past decade. The trend is toward continuous quality development and resident satisfaction; therefore, healthcare technology plays a significant role in nursing home operations. This article discusses general information about current nursing home conditions and systems in the United States and explores how technology and e-health help improve the nursing home development based on the present needs and trends. The authors also report on Thomasville Nursing Home, discussing current trends in nursing home technologies.

INTRODUCTION

Nursing home is a significant part of long-term care in the health care system. Nursing homes provide a broad range of long-term care services—personal, social, and medical services designed to assist people who have functional or cognitive limitations in their ability to perform self-care and other activities necessary to live independently. This survey releases some information about nursing homes, including general introduction

DOI: 10.4018/978-1-60960-183-6.ch018

of nursing homes in USA, resident information, quality of life, services that are providing, governmental regulations, and developing trends. Objectives of this paper are providing the broad information about current nursing homes in the United States to help understand the positive and negative situations that confront to nursing homes. Furthermore, our nursing home visiting report points out the real residents' experience and opinions on their life qualities, needs and attitudes on technologies. Based on this information we introduce more technological innovations to improve nursing home development.

PARTI: NURSING HOMES IN THE UNITED STATES

General Information

A nursing home, a facility for the care of individuals who do not require hospitalization and who cannot be cared for at home, is a type of care of residents. It is a place of residence of people who require constant nursing care and have significant deficiencies with activity of daily living (NNHS, 2004).

People enter nursing homes for a variety of reasons. Some may enter for a brief time when they leave the hospital because they need subacute care, such as skilled nursing care, medical services, and therapies (NNHS, 2004). Others, however, need long-term care (LTC). LTC is generally defined as a broad range of personal, social, and medical services that assist people who have functional or cognitive limitations in their ability to perform self-care and other activities necessary to live independently (NNHS, 2004).

In the United States, nursing homes are required to have a licensed nurse on duty 24 hours a day, and during at least one shift each day, one of those nurses must be a Register Nurse (RN) (NNHS, 2004). A RN is a health care professional responsible for implementing the practice of nursing in concert with other health care professionals (American Nurses Association, 2006).

In Apr., 2005, there were a total of 16,094 nursing homes in the United States. Some states having nursing homes that are called nursing facilities (NF), which do not have beds certified for Medicare patients, but can only treat patients whose payments sources is Private Payment, Private Insurance, or Medicaid (U.S. Department of Health and Human Services, 2008). Medicare is a social insurance program administered by the U.S. government, providing health insurance coverage to people who are aged 65 and over, or who meet other special criteria (Castle, 2008). Medicaid is the U.S. health program for eligible individuals and families with low incomes and resources. It is a means-tested program that is jointly funded by the states and federal government, and is managed by the states. Among the groups of people served by Medicaid are eligible low-income parents, children, seniors, and people with disabilities. Being poor, or even very poor, does not necessarily qualify an individual for Medicaid (U.S. Department of Health and Human Services, 2006a).

SERVICES

Baseline Services

Those services included in the daily rate. The following basic services should be made available to all the residents (U.S. Department of Health and Human Services, 2006b; U.S. Department of Health and Human Services, 2003):

- Lodging-a clean, healthful, sheltered environment, proper outfitted;
- Dietary services;
- 24-hour-per-day nursing care;
- Pharmacy services;
- Diagnostic services;

- The use of all equipment, medical supplies and modalities used in the care of nursing home residents, including but not limited to catheters, hypodermic syringes and needles, irrigation outfits, dressings and pads, etc.
- General household medicine cabinet supplies, including but not limited nonprescription medications, materials for routine skin care, dental hygiene, care of hair, etc., except when specific items are medically indicated and prescribed for exceptional use for a specific resident.
- Assistance and/or supervision, when required, with activities of daily living, including but not limited to toileting, bathing, feeding and assistance with getting from place to place.
- Use of customarily stocked equipment, including but not limited to crutches, walkers, wheelchairs or other supportive equipments, including training in their use when necessary, unless such items are prescribed by a doctor for regular and sole use by a specific resident.
- Activities program, including but not limited to a planned schedule of recreational, motivational, social and other activities together with the necessary materials and supplies to make the resident's life more meaningful.
- Social services as needed;
- Provision of optician and optometrist services.
- Physical therapy, occupational therapy, speech pathology services, audiology services and dental services, on either a staff or fee-for-services basis, as prescribed by a doctor, administered by or under the direct supervision of a licensed and currently registered physical therapist, occupational therapist, speech pathologist, qualified audiologist or registered dentist.

Adult Day Health Care (ADHC)

ADHC program provides the health care services and activities provided to a group of persons, who are not residents of a residential health care facility, but are functionally impaired and not home bounded (Castle, 2008). Require supervision, monitoring, preventive, diagnostic, therapeutic, rehabilitative or palliative care or services but not require continuous 24-hour-a-day inpatient care and services to maintain their health status and enable them to remain in the community (Castle, 2008; U.S. Department of Health and Human Services, 2003; Xie et al., in press).

QUALITY OF LIFE

Resident-Oriented Care

Resident oriented care is designed as the place that nurses are assigned to particular patients and have the ability to develop relationships with individuals (Shields, 2005). Patients are treated more as family members. Using resident-oriented care, nurses are able to become familiar with each patient and cater more to their specific needs, both in emotional and medical aspects (District of Columbia Department of Human Services, n.d.). According to various findings residents who receive resident-oriented are experience a higher quality of life, in respect to attention and time spent with patients and the number of fault reports (Boumans, 2005). Although resident-oriented nursing does not lengthen life, nursing home residents may dispel many feelings of loneliness and discontent (Boumans, 2005).

Task-Oriented Care

Task oriented care is where nurses are assigned specific tasks to perform for numerous residents on a specific ward (Shields, 2005). Residents in this particular situation are exposed to multiple nurses at any given time. Because of the random disbursement of tasks, nurses are declined the ability to develop more in depth relations with any particular resident (Shields, 2005). Various findings suggest that task-oriented care produces less satisfied residents (Shields, 2005). In many cases, residents are disoriented and unsure of whom to disclose information to and as a result decide not to share information at all (Shields, 2005). Patients usually complain of loneliness and feelings of displacement.

Resident Characteristics

Nursing home residents are among the frailest Americans. In 2005, nearly half of all residents had dementia, and more than half were confined to a bed or wheelchair. In 2004, nearly 80 percent of residents needed help with 4 or 5 activities of daily living (bed mobility, transferring, dressing, eating, and toileting) (NNHS, 2004). Most nursing home residents are female, especially at older ages (Carrillo, 2006). Widowhood is a key predictor of nursing home use—at time of admission, over half of nursing home residents were widowed, and only 1 in 5 was married or living with a partner (Carrillo, 2006).

CONCERNS ON NURSING HOME QUALITY

Nursing Home Abuse

It seems that a lot of information that we have received are positive and promising; however, negative news would never too small to negligent. From New York Times, nursing home inspectors routinely overlook or minimize problems that pose a serious, immediate threat to patients, said by congressional investigators in a new report (Pear, 2008a). More than 1.5 million people live in nursing homes. Nationwide, about one-fifth of the homes were cited for serious deficiencies last year (Pear, 2008a).

Nursing homes are typically inspected once a year by state employees working under a contract with the federal government, which sets stringent standards (Pear, 2008b). Federal officials try to validate the work of state inspectors by accompanying them or doing follow-up surveys within a few weeks (Xie et al., in press).

Daily Activities

It has been proven that when people move into nursing homes they lose a sense of control and feel a sense of isolation. Activities are one the best ways to fight these feelings and give a sense of empowerment back to the people. The variety of programs available in any nursing home depends on the health and interests of the residents.

A broad range of programs is directed by the activities coordinator (SeniorsSite.com, 2008). A home certified for Medicare and Medicaid must have someone designated as an activities coordinator (SeniorsSite.com, 2008). The planning and implementation of activities comes from requests by residents, families, staff, and volunteers (SeniorsSite.com, 2008). The activities are usually posted on a calendar of events that is available to each resident. Through the web reveal, here are some of the examples (SeniorsSite.com, 2008; Golden Living Centers, 2008; Harding Nursing Home, 2008): monthly birthday parties, celebrations of various holidays, musical events (passively such as concerts, or actively such as singing-along or with friends and family), games, outdoor activities, trips and tours, nursing home newsletter, resident discussion groups, exercise fun and physical fitness, books, coffee/cocktail hours, arts and crafts programs, religious services, etc.

CURRENT PROBLEMS FOR NURSING HOMES

Funding Shortfalls

The majority of nursing home income comes from government reimbursement (Polit & Beck, 2004). The industry claims that many of its nursing homes are losing money on government payments causing yearly net business losses. For those homes that make profit, there's not margin enough for improving infrastructure or hiring more or better qualified staff to improve quality of care (Polit & Beck, 2004).

Staffing

A recent report from the U.S. Government General Accountability Office cites widespread understaffing by nursing homes both in levels of nurses and certified nurse's assistants (Mukamel & Spector, 2000). Staffing in these cases is below government-recommended adequate standards (Mukamel & Spector, 2000).

Shortage of Nurses

There is currently a nationwide shortage of nurses. Nursing homes are willing to pay the salary to attract nurses but in many areas there aren't enough nurses to meet demand (Peter, 2001).

Elder Abuse and Lawsuits

It shouldn't come as a surprise with the problems of funding and staffing that reported incidents of patient neglect and abuse are on the rise (Williams, 2003). Of particular concern is the more frequent occurrence of abuse. Abuse is not only just physical assault or threats but it can also be such things as improper use of restraints, failure to feed or give water, failure to bathe, improper care resulting in pressure sores or allowing a patient to lie too long in a soiled diaper or bed linen. Lawsuits are increasing in number. (Williams, 2003; Webb, 2001)

PARTII: E-HEALTH AND NURSING HOMES

E-health is a type of telemedicine that encompasses any "e-thing" in health field; that is, any database or encyclopedia containing information pertinent to health, medicine, or pharmacy that is accessible via internet (Breen & Zhang, 2008).

It is a typical form commonly referenced and understood as that consists of internet-based services such as WebMD.com, Medlineplus.gov, and Mentalhelp.net. Telemedicine involves the use of telecommunications technologies to facilitate clinical healthcare delivery and exchange at a distance (Thompson, Dorsey, Miller, & Parrott, 2003).

Because of the distance barrier that telemedicine and e-health services are able to transcend, the authors in (Breen & Matusitz, 2007) believed that telemedicine would be particularly beneficial in secluded towns and communities deficient in adequate healthcare services, such as bucolic regions, in mountains, on islands, and in locations of arctic climate (Breen & Zhang, 2008).

E-health provides a faster and easier alternative, as well as a more cost-effective means, to accessing healthcare information, as opposed to more traditional and costly physical interactions between doctors and patients (Breen & Matusitz, 2007).

Health IT Acceptance in Long-Term Care

Nursing homes are often depicted as laggards when it comes to embracing technology tools. But an analysis by the American Association of Homes and Services for the Aging shows that they are more than holding their own.

Nearly all nursing homes at the time had electronic information systems for MDS data collection and billing, and 43% maintained electronic health record systems, according to analysts, who studied data from the 2004 National Nursing Home Survey. By comparison, 25% of doctor offices and 59% of hospitals handled electronic health records (EHRs) (O'Connor, 2008).

Health Information Technology in Nursing Homes

Information technology (IT) has a significant potential to reduce error and improve the quality and efficiency of health care (Bates et al., 2001; Institute of Medicine, 2001). Some researchers also believe that computer systems can be used to reduce error and improve the reporting of adverse incidents in health care settings (Wald & Shojania, 2001). Since October 1998, all state licensed nursing homes have been required to electronically transmit data generated by the federally mandated Resident Assessment Instrument (RAI) via state public health agencies to the Centers for Medicare and Medicaid Services (CMS) (Mor et al., 2003). Advanced features in the software were available to most (87% to 98%) of the facilities; however, most features were not being used all the time. There are huge potentials addressing the technology applications with various aspects such as enhancing the administrator's ability to manage the facility, tracking quality, and monitoring multiple performance indicators.

HIT is used to collect, store, retrieve, and transfer clinical, administrative, and financial health information electronically (U.S. Government General Accountability Office, 2004). The Institute of Medicine publication To Err is Human (Kohn, Corrigan, & Donaldson, 1999) drew attention to the potential for HIT to improve quality of care and prevent medical errors across the health care system. The focus of HIT development and implementation has been mainly on acute and ambulatory care settings (American Health Information Management Association [AHIMA], 2005; Hamilton, 2006; Kramer et al., 2004).

Commonly found HIT systems provide computerized physician order entry (CPOE), EHRs, and point of care (POC) to access data for entry and retrieval (e.g., reviewing records, entering orders at the bedside or in the examination room) (Hamilton, 2006). In addition, electronic systems for management operations such as patient scheduling and reimbursement have been available for longer and are used frequently (AHIMA, 2005; Baron, Fabens, Schiffman, & Wolf, 2005; Poon et al., 2006). An EHR is an electronic formatting of medical records documenting the patient's medical history, written orders, and progress notes. CPOE is a system making information available for physicians at the time an order is entered (Bates et al., 1998; Bates et al., 1999). POC is a technology automating the care provider's procedure, visit notes, and educational materials at the place of care (Anderson & Wittwer, 2004). Although the implementation of HIT in the long-term care sector is recognized to be lagging behind the acute and ambulatory settings (AHIMA, 2005; Hamilton, 2006), there is a wide range potentials for nursing homes such as functions covering domains such as financial management, administration, ancillary care, support, and resident care (McKnight's LTC News, 2005).

Technology Streamlines Long-Term Care Operations

Technology's role in nursing homes has been greater importance as these types of facilities serve much older adults. Most of them are expanding their focus on the best ways to deploy technology to improve residents' quality of care. In this section, we explored some equipments/devices that favor nursing homes, skilled nursing facilities (SNFs), and assisted living facilities.

Fall Management

This care issue includes technologies aimed at decreasing the occurrence of resident falls, as well as technologies that alert caregivers and reduce injury when falls occur (Burland, 2008). Products include grab bars, non slips mats and socks, and different types of alarms. According to Gillespie SM, Friedman SM (2007), the major two categories are as following: *(1) Technologies aimed at reducing the risk of a fall:* a) anti-slip footwears (socks and slippers), (b) anti-slip matting and materials on in slippery areas such as tubs and bathroom floors, (c) grab bars for stability and support, wheelchair anti-rollback devices, alarm signals of chair, bed, and toilet when a resident is at risk for falling attempts, rehabilitation equipment and programs, etc. (2) *Technologies aimed at reducing the risk of injury when falls occur:* (a) hip protectors, (b) bedside cushions, and (c) technologies that notify caregivers when a resident has fallen: Fall detection devices use technologies that sense a change in body position, body altitude, and the force of impact to determine when a fall has occurred.

Medication Management

Products geared toward enabling residents to manage and adhere to their medication regime with greater independence (Field, 2008; Lilley, Lambden, & Gillies, 2006; Wolfstadt, 2008; McGraw, 2004): (1) medication applicators enable the user to apply lotions and ointments on hard to reach areas such as the back and feet; (2) medication reminder software provides reminders to take or administer medication at predetermined time; (3) pill organizers keep dry medications and vitamins arranged in compartments labeled for weekly or daily dosage frequencies; (4) multi-alarm medication reminders and watches remind the user to take medications at predetermined time schedules; (5) multi-alarm pill boxes store medication and provide reminder alerts to take medications at prescribed time; (6) personal automatic medication dispensers automatically dispense a dose of dry medications at predetermined time; etc.

Assistance Call

This care issue, also known as nurse call or emergency call, includes technologies that enable a resident to summon assistance by means of a transmitter that they can carry with them or access from somewhere in their living area (Alexander, 2008; Michael, 2000; Holmes, 2007): (1) wired systems rely on wires for communication and allow for the addition of wireless features; (2) wireless systems require no wiring for installation; and (3) telephone based systems use telephone lines to alert caregivers to a resident need.

Bathing

This care issue includes products that focus on bath safety, enable residents to be more independent with bathing tasks, and that make bathing tasks easier for caregivers (Barrick, 2008).

Concern of Standards

In terms of other challenges, the issue of standards creates a concern. According to Andrews (2009), the technology integration has been a challenge mostly because there are standards out there, but they give the implementers of them great flexibility in how to go about using them. It enables to improve the monthly nursing summary that shared between the nurses and doctors by providing an electronic exchange between our two clinical systems. This has improved access to information and hopefully influenced decision making properly.

"Many nursing homes are adopting a wait-and-see approach until software products are certified by the Certification Commission for Healthcare Information Technology (CCHIT) using the Health Level Seven (HL7)-approved LTC

EHR-S functional profile", says Eileen T. Doll, RN, BS, NHA, president of Efficiency Driven Healthcare Consulting, Inc. in Baltimore. HL7 is an American National Standards Institute standard for healthcare-specific data exchange between computer applications (Sloane, 2006).

Proper integration of technology is essential. True streamlining occurs when the clinical and administrative sides are fully integrated in all aspects—no duplicate entry, no data inconsistency, and integrated processes. Duplications are reduced or eliminated when common information is shared among care settings and information systems (Sloane, 2006). Reduced duplication also improves accuracy, with less likelihood that the same piece of information is different in other systems.

One thing that helps with standardization is the LTC HIT Collaborative. CAST, the American Association of Homes and Services for the Aging, the NCAL, and the AHCA are partners in ensuring that the LTC sector is represented and the national HIT standards cater to the unique requirements of LTC applications (Sloane, 2006).

Nursing Home Size

How large must nursing homes be to make various technologies cost-effective? What can be done for smaller homes interested in technology but unable to invest as much as larger operations? According to Majd Alwan, PhD, director of the Center for Aging Services Technologies (CAST) in Washington, DC, and a member of the LTC HIT Summit, "It really depends on the size of the facility, where they are in the process, whether they have the basic infrastructure in place or not, whether they are part of a chain or not, the management's position, etc. Generally speaking, if shown a return on investment potential, including return in terms of quality and competitive advantage, providers should be willing to invest," Even so, smaller homes should not be discouraged. "The best approach is to have a plan and to take EHR implementation in stages," he says. "Plan one application or module at a time based on the organization's tolerance for change, leadership, and financial resources. If resources are limited, start with one or two smaller applications that will make an impact, such as the nursing assistant documentation/kiosk touchpad, and keep building."

For smaller homes interested in technology, Alwan explains that most companies price technology based on usage, so smaller providers pay less than larger providers. "Many smaller homes choose not to host and manage their software and data," he says. "With software as a service, even the smallest [nursing home] providers can benefit."

The Future of Technology

After thorough research work, we believe that resident access to the electronic documentation will continue to be an area providers will eventually offer for their residents. We think that technologies that connect the resident and family closer together will continue to be the most requested items. Innovative technology enables residents and their families to access basic information such as lists of problems, medications, allergies, contact information, and lab reports. The ability to make this easy to use for all will be the challenge but we see an opportunity with telehealth devices that are coming onto the market today for other uses that will eventually be extended to the SNF environment ("Telehealth can improve quality of life," 2009).

As mentioned earlier, a variety of exciting technologies are on the drawing board, including advanced total quality systems that integrate several basic components already in existence, such as nurse call, wandering management, fall prevention, resident tracking, resident assessment, electronic medication administration record, and electronic treatment administration record systems. Also in the works are advanced fall prevention systems, advanced beds with embedded sensors, and comprehensive interoperable EHRs

Figure 1. Thomasville nursing home (a), (b)

(a) *(b)*

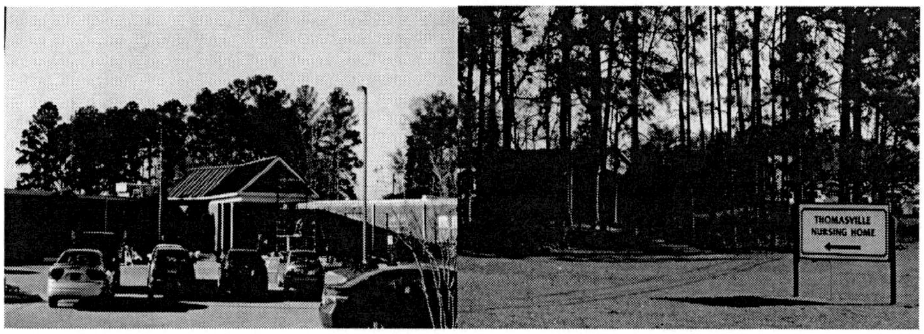

that allow sharing health information securely across different settings.

Resistance to change presents one of the biggest challenges to technology integration in the nursing home environment. The industry has been manual and paper-based for so long, it requires a cultural shift to a technology base. We believe that communication is the key to overcoming this challenge. We look forward to seeing technology beyond EHR systems. According to CosmoCom (2009), in the near future, we will see current high-tech devices integrated with EHRs. Telehealth is an emerging and important technology for the future. Technology is needed to upgrade all equipment used in SNFs as well as changing the homes to meet the cultural change required for a higher quality of life.

PART III: REPORT ON THOMASVILLE NURSING HOME VISITING

In this part, we will report our visiting a nursing home in south Alabama.

Background

Thomasville Nursing Home is a well known nursing home in south Alabama, which is equipped with standardized facilities. It is a religious nonmedical health care institution with SNF/NF (dually certificated). Five residents are interviewed and four filled out the questionnaire. Three nurses, two social workers, and the administrator are also interviewed by giving out some brief opinions on the technology involved in the nursing home daily bases. Figures 1 (a) and (b) shows the outside photos of the nursing home.

Research Purpose

Know the actual conditions in Nursing Home in Alabama rural areas. Research are specific in the residents room decoration, overall quality on the residents' living conditions, residents satisfaction on Nursing Home care, and staff, residents' attitudes about technology applying.

Outcomes

In Thomasville nursing home, what makes residents happy or unhappy? What are their special wishes? In this report, three themes emerged from resident responses: community, care, supportive relationships. In addition to residents' daily happiness in nursing homes, quality life includes another great factor: technology involvement.

Figure 2. Residents' bed room with her Toy Kitty and TV (a), (b)

(a) (b)

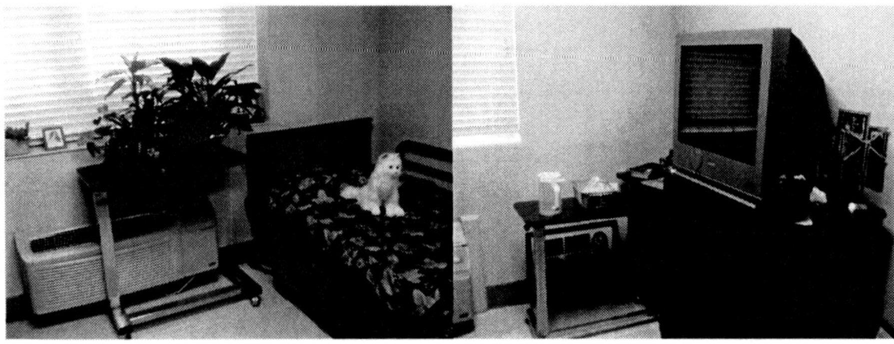

Community

As in any community, nursing home residents focus on their living space, neighbors, and what is happening. For some residents, having others around affords conversation and companionship, especially when their roommate is or becomes a friend. The nursing home provides a sense of "fellowship, friendship, and care." In contrast, other residents may be uncomfortable with the number of people and the amount of activity level within the environment. These residents are unhappy because they "always have someone around," and wish for "a private room" or "a lot of space like I had at home." So that in Thomasville Nursing Home, they offer different types of rooms for their residents, though it is more demanding on the single rooms, all of the interviewed residents are somewhat satisfied with their accommodations. Figures 2(a) and (b) shows the single- room pictures. To some residents, there is a sensor pad underneath the bed sheet to secure residents' safety. Though pets are not allowed, some of the patients still feel like to have a kitty or puppy toy around with them. "TV is another important accompanier to stay away from lonely, which helps us kill time and catch up with the everyday ongoing" said couple of the residents. In the single room, some of the residents feel that they have their own privacy and their own time.

Residents enjoy going to the dining room and visiting with their tablemates. They are happy when the food is good, there are snacks at night, and they celebrate birthdays together. They are unhappy when the coffee is not freshly brewed, the same foods are served too often, or the food is not cooked to their personal taste. Residents' special wishes include "to have food and meat like I had on the farm," "for someone to bring food from outside for my birthday," and "to have a Residents enjoy going to the dining room and visiting with their tablemates. They are happy when the food is good, there are snacks at night, and they celebrate birthdays together. They are unhappy when the coffee is not freshly brewed, the same foods are served too often, or the food is not cooked to their personal taste". Residents' special wishes include "to have food and meat like I had on the farm," "for someone to bring food from outside for my birthday," and "to have a martini once in a while." The dining room (Figure 3) and activity room (Figure 4) play a significant role in their daily life in the nursing home.

The planned activities provided by nursing homes are an important part of the community. Residents like to be busy and enjoy "the chance to play bingo and laugh." Some are happy because church services are offered in their home. One of the residents says that many residents want to get into town and see new sights, and others simply

Figure 3. Dining room for the residents

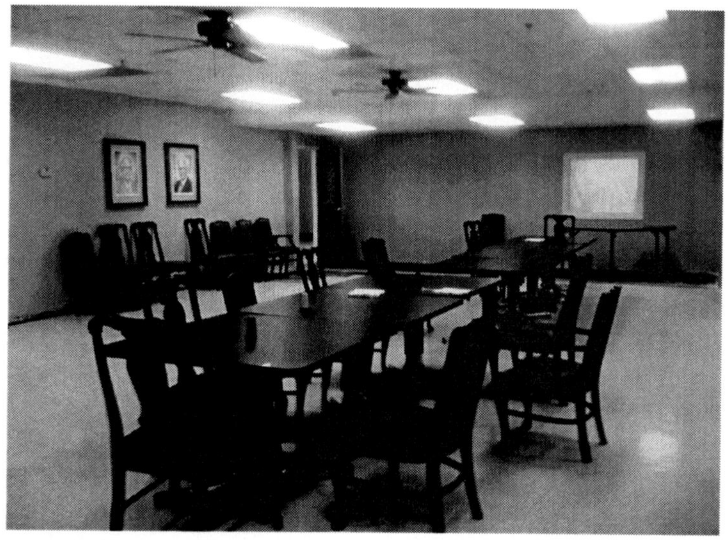

Figure 4. Activity scene: Inauguration day

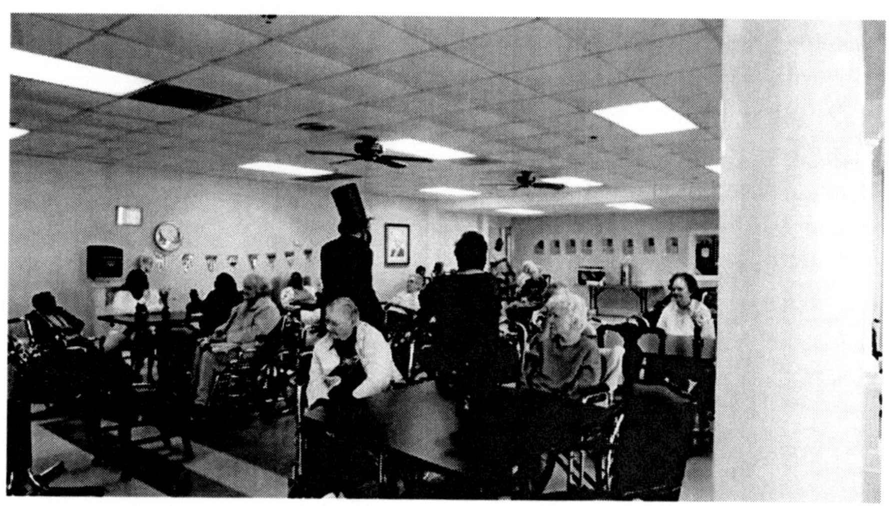

would like to "get out more and see flowers and trees." Others want to go shopping or go out to lunch. Most residents are elders, and the nursing home community may be less satisfying for younger residents. A younger resident says, "There's a bunch of old people here instead of people my own age." In Thomasville, the nursing home staffs also say that they understand the different demands on the their residents, however, it is hard to satisfy everyone, say, it's a complicated process to bring the elders to the shopping in terms of their safety concern; because of the small portion of young residents in the nursing home, considering of the budget concern, it is not realistic to arrange activities for couple of them only.

Fulfilling residents' special wishes could increase their sense of community. According to the administrator, Dania, she says that one approach would be for the care planning coordinator or social worker to ask residents about special wishes when completing the quarterly or annual Myelodysplastic syndromes (MDS), a group of diseases that affect the bone marrow and blood, assessment. Many of the wishes are easy to grant through staff or family members, and that special treat could be added to the respective resident's care plan as an onetime event. Using the MDS assessment process ensures that residents with limiting physical or mental impairments would be included. Other actions to increase residents' sense of community might include providing quiet places where they can go to be alone or arranging activities targeted for younger residents that offer interactions with age-mates. Access to the Internet, with assistance in learning to use that technology, could facilitate participation in chat rooms and, perhaps, cyber friendships with peers in other facilities.

The "Miss Nursing Home", shown in Figure 5, who 90 years old, told me with a big smile and proud that she has rewarded as the Miss Nursing Home last year, which brings her a lot of confidence and self-esteem. Such rewarding games and programs are consistently held by Thomasville Nursing Home, which bring all the residents get into their fun daily life.

Figure 5. "Miss Nursing Home" wears her crown

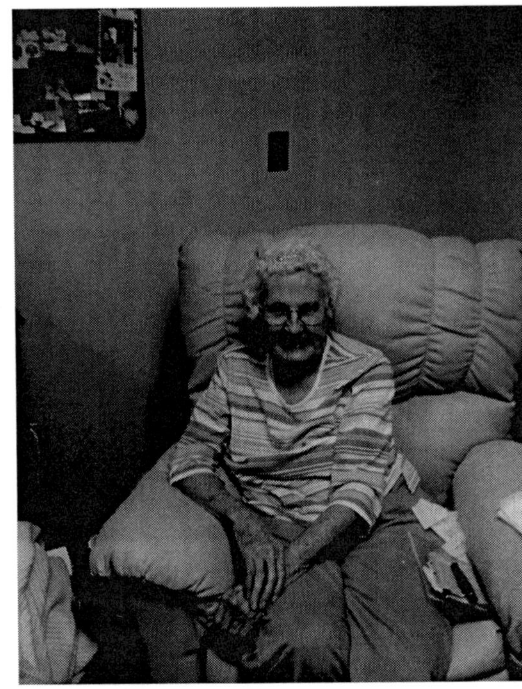

Care

Residents come to nursing homes because they need help with basic activities of daily life. Many residents are happy because someone else does the housework, prepares the meals, washes the dishes, and does the laundry. They like having someone who pays attention to them and helps them meet their needs.

Having things go the resident's way is important. Residents appreciate special attention to unique interests or needs, such as having staff communicate with sign language, being able to listen to music of their choice, and having coffee with the chaplain. They need flexibility; for instance, too many baths make one resident unhappy, whereas another's special wish is to have more baths.

Residents are happy when they are satisfied with staff and believe they receive good care. They describe good care as having staff listen to what they say, having someone respond quickly to the call light, being handled gently by staff during care, receiving proper medications and treatments, and having the doctor visit. Personal cleanliness is valued--being kept clean, having clean clothes, and having clean teeth.

Good care depends on the facility having enough qualified staff to meet resident needs. Long waits—for meals to be served, for help to the bathroom, or for the nurse—make residents unhappy, which has been changed in Thomasville Nursing Home after getting feedbacks from their residents. One of the residents says that sometimes busy staff save time by doing things residents could do for themselves. It may be faster to change a resident's briefs than to take him to the bathroom, or to push a resident's wheelchair to the dining room rather than letting her use a walker.

High staff turnover also creates problems. One resident says, "The people who help me change all the time; they don't know what they're supposed to do."

Some residents are more vulnerable than others because of cognitive impairment, hearing or vision loss, or limited mobility. A touching special wish is that everybody be treated the same. A resident observes, "Some people who don't know where they are get left behind on answering call lights."

According to the nursing home staffs and Diane, It is important that staff seek input from residents and family members about care. Feedback about how their concerns are addressed reinforces a need for their participation. Although maintaining independence is desirable, a resident's ability to do a task warrants careful evaluation. For example, vision and fine motor skills must be considered in deciding how a resident participates in an insulin injection.

Employee recognition programs should emphasize specific staff behaviors that make a difference for residents. They saw a program in another facility where residents and family members nominate staff for a "STAR" award based on outstanding performance, and a star is attached to the employee's name tag.

Supportive Relationships

Establishing new relationships with staff and other residents is part of settling into a nursing home community. Support from family, friends, and staff is critical to new residents' successful transition and adaptation. Family and friends, "Being with those you love", make residents happy. Their hearts will be warmed may be just by receiving a small gift, and services from family and friends, such as a cassette player from a nephew, a fish fillet from a friend, and dresses laundered with a daughter's special touch. Residents who are unhappy about relationships with family most often feel greater separation because of distance or a perceived lack of concern. Special wishes regarding family and friends usually relate to having more contact. However, one man feels that there is too much pressure on his wife and wishes for someone to help her take care of him. Another man wishes that staff would watch his wife, a resident in the same facility, more closely.

Staff members make residents happy through interactions based on respect, kindness, and concern, and by taking time to help, listen, and share their lives. Residents are happy when staff are attentive, but without fuss; when they invite them to events, but also allow them to be alone; and, in general, when they try to make things better for them. Residents appreciate a pat on the shoulder and staff coming to tell them goodbye. It is important for them to have something in common with staff; for example, boosting the same sports team. Shared laughter is a crucial happiness factor. For some residents, teasing staff and being teased, kidding, telling jokes, playing tricks on each other, and "picking on" staff add spice to the day.

In addition to the resident council, residents need an opportunity to voice concerns privately to someone who can do something about them. Residents may feel powerless or threatened by abandonment in conflicts with staff, and may need support from a family member or friend in voicing their concerns. Family members and friends who do support residents and add quality to their daily lives deserve recognition. Examples of uncomplicated acknowledgments include feedback from staff about how much a resident enjoyed a special outing or a snapshot of a resident wearing a new sweater sent by a brother in another town.

Technology

The overall quality is satisfying, and the Thomasville nursing home has already been switch to home-like style, which makes the residents more comfortable to live than that of traditional style.

From the interviews on the residents, it reveals that most of the patients are willing to accept the new technology equipments. The overall attitudes on their nursing home quality is fairly satisfied, including the hygiene, food, daily activities, and nursing home services. Two of them feel it is too hard to communicate with others, and lonely is the major issue they do not want to stay in the nursing home. All of them think that it is safer to have the advanced facilities to assist their livings, and they feel secured to have the sitting pad on the wheel chair, alarm sleeping sheet on the bed, but they reject the clips connect the cloth and the chair, which makes them feel like being framed and controlled by a string.

"Tech-Bed" is another favorite assistant at Thomasville Home. It looks and feels the same as other normal beds, so that the residents do not take it as a weird stuff. The nurses absolutely love those tech beds. "It truly is like another pair of eyes." Sensors in the zip-on, washable mattress cover provide continuous heart and respiratory rate data. Nothing attaches to the patient. A monitor sits next to the bed and picks up the signals. Hoana presets defaults, but nurses can easily program the sensors to alarm at rates specific to their patients. "We have caught someone going into atrial fibrillation, that we had checked vital signs on an hour before," Diane, the administrator, said. "It's an early warning system." Nurses at Thomasville have also picked up respiratory depression in patients receiving patient- controlled narcotics. The nursing home has monitored nurse and residents satisfaction, fall rates and cardiac arrests. Diane notes positive trends in the preliminary data.

The nurses felt that the covers provided a valuable service and they found the device easy to use, said Valerie Martinez, RN, BSN. "It's a great tool for the nurse, to help them monitor the patients when they can't be in there," Martinez said. "You can go back and trend things." The nurse can assess what the alert was for and how many times it activated.

"It allows the nurse to be more involved in the early recognition of patients that are starting to fail," said Heather Long, RN, chief operating officer of Thomasville. "It provides data that brings the nurse to the bedside."

The Tech-Bed also has a bed exit alarm, with three push-button settings for patients at different fall risks. At high risk, the bed will alert if the patient lifts his or her head or shoulders off the bed. For moderate risk patients, it waits until the patient sits up and for low risk it delays issuing an alarm until the patient actually exits the bed. Loved ones or the nurse can program the device to play a personalized, prerecorded message to get back into bed and wait for the nurse.

"It's very helpful for the elderly," Diane said. "They hear a human voice, saying 'I'm coming to get you,' and they will stop and wait."

Heather said that patients do not feel or see the sensors. Once the patient understands the system, she said, "It makes them feel more secure and safe."

All of the being interviewed are holding a positive attitudes to have made the nursing home computerized, such as EMR, monitoring equipments, and alarm system. Technology makes their work a lot easier, though it took a while to get used to it. It is useful and powerful tool to make the working place more organized. Dianesays though it is getting harder to get funds from the state or federal government, the government is still supporting the ideas of keeping getting technology into long-term care, because it worth investing by thinking of saving money in a long run. She also points out that the facilities usages are not from patients' expenses, but from the nursing homes.

As for the e-prescribing which is another revolution for healthcare industry, Diane said lots of concerns. "Standards for e-prescribing have recently been developed, so this isn't an area of widespread adoption yet," says Diane, the administrator of Thomasville Nursing Home, "This is a complex undertaking for long-term care facilities because it requires standards to communicate between three parties: the facility, the pharmacy, and the physician."

To date, cost has been a primary inhibitor. "We as an industry have not compiled and communicated enough quantitative ROI [return on investment] data," Diane adds. "I believe that technology can improve the quality of care, reduce risk, save time, and grow the business. These data will continue to be made available and will definitively show providers that technology is good for business and good for resident care."

Thomasville nursing home has been successfully implementing electronic records management: nurses' use of clinical notes, clinical assessments, orders, and electronic medication administration records. For nursing aides, the company has implemented electronic activities of daily living documentation. "We are in the process of implementing electronic lab and integration with our Doc EMR [electronic medical record] to allow for even better communication between the teams," says Diane.

"The biggest improvements have been on the management side of the implementation," she says. "We have been able to provide greater insight into the amount and frequency of the documentation that we have never had before. We are able to monitor more efficiently the documentation process by providing reporting capabilities that are not feasible with paper." The concern for the Thomasville Home is financial support, "we hope that either the federal government or states will come up with more money to fund general high-tech operation and HIT efforts"

It is a great visiting to Thomasville Nursing Home, which allowed us to approach the residents' real life in the southern United States. Those three themes are the major concern for the residents in this specific nursing home. Additionally, it is a promising future to have technology involve into the nursing homes, because the demanding is still growing, because a lot of facilities in the homes are not greatly developed, however, the residents numbers are still growing. According to the personal visiting and research, it reveals that the elders are willing to accept the new technologies for the sake of their life quality. The staffs as well as the government are taking a positive attitude in considering of long term benefits.

CONCLUSION

This paper provides broad information on the current and future views of nursing home in USA, in terms of the condition and management level, residents' satisfactions and demands, government regulation and influence. The ability of e-health technology enables nursing homes to improve their quality to meet residents' needs, though there are challenges. The visiting report about Thomasville Nursing Home reaches the depth of the consideration to how to catch the trends by implementing the technologies.

ACKNOWLEDGMENT

This work is supported in part by the U.S. National Science Foundation (NSF) under the grant number CNS-0716211, as well as RGC (Research Grants Committee) award at the University of Alabama 2008.

REFERENCES

Alexander, G. L. (2008). A Descriptive Analysis of a Nursing Home Clinical Information System with Decision Support. *Perspectives in Health Information Management / AHIMA, American Health Information Management Association, 5*(12).

American Association of Homes and Services for the Aging. (2007). *Staff Turnover and Retention*. Washington, DC: Author.

American Health Information Management Association. (2005). *A road map for health IT in long-term care.* Chicago: Author.

Anderson, R., Issel, L. M., & McDaniel, R. R. (2003). Nursing homes as complex adaptive systems: relationship between management practice and resident outcomes. *Nursing Research*, *52*(1), 12–21. doi:10.1097/00006199-200301000-00003

Anderson, S., & Wittwer, W. (2004). Using barcode point-of-care technology for patient safety. *Journal for Healthcare Quality*, *26*(6), 5–11.

Andrews, J. (2009). Keeping record: long-term care may not deserve its reputation as a tech laggard. But more could be done to prepare for the electronic health record. *McKnight's Long-Term Care News*, *30*(1), 42–43.

Baron, R. J., Fabens, E. L., Schiffman, M., & Wolf, E. (2005). Electronic health records: Just around the corner? Or over the cliff? *Annals of Internal Medicine*, *143*(3), 222–226.

Barrick, A., & Rader, J. (2008). *Bathing without a battle: Person-directed care of individuals with dementia.* New York: Springer.

Bates, D. W., Cohen, M., Leape, L. L., Overhage, J. M., Shabot, M. M., & Sheridan, T. (2001). Reducing the frequency of errors in medicine using information technology. *Journal of the American Medical Informatics Association*, *8*(4), 299–308.

Bates, D. W., Leape, L. L., Cullen, D. J., Laird, N., Petersen, L. A., & Teich, J. M. (1998). Effect of computerized physician order entry and a team intervention on prevention of serious medication errors. *Journal of the American Medical Association*, *280*(15), 1311–1316. doi:10.1001/jama.280.15.1311

Bates, D. W., Teich, J. M., Lee, J., Seger, D., & Kuperman, G. J., Ma'Luf, N., et al. (1999). The impact of computerized physician order entry on medication error prevention. *Journal of the American Medical Informatics Association*, *6*(4), 313–321.

Berger, L. (2006, January 13). Information technology feature: The IT payback. *McKnight's Long-Term Care News*, 34-37.

Boumans, N., Berkhout, A., & Landeweerd, A. (2005). Efforts of resident-oriented care on quality of care, wellbeing and satisfaction with care. *Scandinavian Journal of Caring Sciences*, *19*(3), 11–15. doi:10.1111/j.1471-6712.2005.00351.x

Breen, G., & Zhang, N. (2008). Theoretical Analysis of Improving Resident Care. *Journal of Medical Systems*, *32*(2), 18–23. doi:10.1007/s10916-007-9121-9

Breen, G. M., & Matusitz, J. (2007). An interpersonal examination of telemedicine: Applying relevant communication theories. *E-health. International Journal (Toronto, Ont.)*, *3*(1), 187–192.

Burland, E. M. J. (2008). An Evaluation of a Fall Management Program in a Personal Care Home Population. *Healthcare Quaterly*, *11*(3), 137–140.

Carrillo, H., & Harrington, C. (2006). *Cross the States 2006: Profiles of Long-Term Care and Independent Living.* Washington, DC: AARP.

Castle, N. G. (2008). Nursing Home Evacuation Plans. *American Journal of Public Health*, *98*(7), 1235–1241. doi:10.2105/AJPH.2006.107532

CosmoCom. (2009). *CosmoCom Showcases Telehealth at World Health Care Congress*. Melville, NY: Author.

David, P. (1994). *A revolution in seating - Nursing Home Technology*. Retrieved November 3, 2008, from http://findarticles.com/p/articles/mi_m3830/is_n9_v43/ai_16539882/

Debra, O., & Brain, H. (2006). A promising Technology to Reduce Social Isolation of Nursing Home Residents. *Journal of Nursing Care Quality*, *21*(4), 302–306.

Demiris, G., Speedie, S. M., & Finkelstein, S. (2001). Change of patients' perceptions of TeleHomeCare. *Telemedicine & E-Health*, *7*(3), 241–249. doi:10.1089/153056201316970948

District of Columbia Department of Human Services. (n.d.). *Home Care and Nursing Home Services*. Retrieved December 12, 2008, from http://dhs.dc.gov/dhs/cwp/view,a,3,Q,613301.asp

ELJAY. LCC. (2006). *A Report on Shortfalls in Medicaid Funding for Nursing Home Care*. Washington, DC: American Health Care Association.

Field, T. S., Rochon, P., Lee, M., Gavendo, L., Subramanian, S., & Hoover, S. (2008). Costs associated with developing and implementing a computerized clinical decision support system for medication dosing for patients with renal insufficiency in the long-term care setting. *Journal of the American Medical Informatics Association*, *15*(4), 466–472. doi:10.1197/jamia.M2589

Finnema, E., de Lange, J., Droes, R. M., Ribbe, M., & Tilburg, W. (2001). The quality of nursing home care: Do the opinions of family members change after implementation of emotion-oriented care? *Journal of Advanced Nursing*, *35*(5), 728–732. doi:10.1046/j.1365-2648.2001.01905.x

Gill, T. M., Allore, H. G., & Han, L. (2006). Bathing disability and the risk of long-term admission to a nursing home. *Journal of Gerontology*, *61*(8), 821–825.

Golden Living Centers. (2008). *Fun Times*. Retrieved October 20, 2008, from http://www.goldenlivingcenters.com/GGNSC

Greenly, M., & Gugerty, B. (2002). How bar coding reduces medication errors. *Nursing*, *32*(5), 70.

Hamilton, B. (2006). *Evaluation design of the business case of health information technology in long-term care (Final report)*. Baltimore: Centers for Medicare and Medicaid Services. Harding Nursing Home. (n.d.) *Activities*. Retrieved October 20, 2008, from http://www.hardingnh.com/

Harris, Y., & Clauser, S. B. (2002). Achieving improvement through nursing home quality measurement. *Health Care Financing Review*, *23*(4), 13.

Harrison, S. (2002). Telehealth skills hailed as answer to discharge delays: Costs of high-tech monitoring systems compare favourably with long-term care. *Nursing Standard*, *17*(12), 7.

Hoban, S. (2003). Activities plus at Montgomery Place: The "new" active senior wants to be entertained, enlightened, and engaged--and will let you know how. *Nursing Homes*, *52*(6), 52–56.

Holmes, D. (2007). An evaluation of a monitoring system intervention: falls, injuries, and affect in nursing homes. *Clinical Nursing Research*, *16*(4), 317–335. doi:10.1177/1054773807307870

Institute of Medicine. (2001). *Crossing the quality chasm: A new health system for 21st century.* Washington, DC: National Academy Press.

Johnson, B., Wheeler, L., Dueser, J., & Sousa, K. (2000). Outcomes of the Kaiser Permanente Tele-Home Health Research Project. *Archives of Family Medicine*, *9*(4), 40–45. doi:10.1001/archfami.9.1.40

Kemper, P., Komisar, H. L., & Alecixh, L. (2005). Long-Term Care over what can Current Retirees Expect? *Inquiry*, *42*, 15.

King, W. R., & He, J. (2006). A meta-analysis of the technology acceptance model. *Information & Management*, *43*(6), 740–755. doi:10.1016/j.im.2006.05.003

Kohn, L. T., Corrigan, J. M., & Donaldson, M. S. (1999). *To err is human: Building a safer human system*. Washington, DC: National Academy Press.

Kramer, A., Bennett, R., Fish, R., Lin, C. T., Floersch, N., Conway, K., et al. (2004). *Case studies of electronic health records in post-acute and long-term care*. Washington, DC: U.S. Department of Health and Human Services.

Lilley, R., Lambden, P., & Gillies, A. (2006). *Medicines management for residential and nursing homes: A toolkit for best practice and accredited learning*. Seattle, WA: Radcliffe.

MacLaughlin, E. J. (2005). Assessing medication adherence in the elderly: which tools to use in clinical practice? *Drugs & Aging*, *22*(3), 55–231. doi:10.2165/00002512-200522030-00005

Matusitz, J., & Breen, G. M. (2007). Telemedicine: Its effects on health communication. *Health Communication*, *21*(1), 10–21.

McGraw, C. (2004). Multi-compartment medication devices and patient compliance. *British Journal of Community Nursing*, *9*(7), 90–285.

McKnight's LTC News. (2005, July). 2005 software. *McKnight's Long-Term Care News,* 43.

Michael, S. J. C. (2000). Wireless clinical alerts for physiologic, laboratory and medication data. In *Proceedings of the AMIA 2000 Annual Symposium* (pp. 789-793).

Mitka, M. (2003). Telemedicine eyed for mental health services. Approach could widen access for older patients. *Journal of the American Medical Association*, *290*(14), 22–25.

Moller, J., & Renegar, C. (2003). Bathing as a wellness experience. *Nursing Homes Long Term Care Management*, *52*(10), 108.

Mor, V., Berg, K., Angelelli, J., Gifford, D., Morris, J., & Moore, T. (2003). The quality of quality measurement in U.S. nursing homes. *The Gerontologist*, *43*(2), 37–46.

Mukamel, B. D., & Spector, D. W. (2000). Nursing home Costs and Risk-Adjusted Outcome Measures of Quality. *Medical Care*, *38*(1), 32–35. doi:10.1097/00005650-200001000-00009

NNHS. (2004). *Analysis of the National Nursing Home Survey.* Washington, DC: AARP Public Policy Institute.

O'Connor, J. (2005). Feds provide info on LTC tech products on market. *McKnight's Long-Term Care News, 14*(11).

O'Connor, J. (2008). Nursing homes up on technology. *McKnight's Long-Term Care News*, *29*(12), 3.

Otis, P. (1997). Don't worry, The Carpet is Keep Watching. *Business Week*, 1.

Parker, O. D., Demiris, G., Day, M., Courtney, K. L., & Porock, D. (2006). Tele-hospice support for elder caregivers of hospice patients: two case studies. *Journal of Palliative Medicine*, *9*(2), 54–59.

Pear, R. (2008a). Serious Deficiencies in Nursing Homes Are Often Missed. *New York Times*.

Pear, R. (2008b). Violations Reported at 94% of Nursing Homes. *New York Times*.

Peter, D. (2001). *The Nurse Shortage: Perspectives from Current Direct Care Nurses and Former Direct Care Nurses*. Washington, DC: Federation of Nurses and Health Professionals.

Polit, F. D., & Beck, T. C. (2004). *Nursing Research: Principles and Methods.* Wickford, RI: Lippincott-Raven Publishers.

Poon, E. G., Jha, A. K., Christino, M., Honour, M. M., Fernandopulle, R., & Middleton, B. (2006). Assessing the level of healthcare information technology adoption in the United States: A snapshot. *BMC Medical Informatics and Decision Making*, *6*, 1. doi:10.1186/1472-6947-6-1

Redfern, S., Hannan, S., Norman, I., & Martin, F. (2002). Work satisfaction, stress, quality of care and morale of older people in a nursing home. *Health & Social Care in the Community*, *10*(6), 17–35. doi:10.1046/j.1365-2524.2002.00396.x

Reilly, J., & Bischoff, J. (2008). Remote Monitoring Tested. *Technology and Health Care*, *34*(9), 12–14.

Schepers, J., & Wetzels, M. (2007). A meta-analysis of the technology acceptance model: Investigating subjective norm and moderation effects. *Information & Management*, *44*(1), 90–103. doi:10.1016/j.im.2006.10.007

SeniorsSite.com. (2008). *Daily Activities*. Retrieved October 20, 2008, from http://seniors-site.com/nursingm/index.html

Shields, S. (2005, March 23). Culture Change in Nursing homes. *The Commonwealth Fund*.

Sloan, F., & Shayne, M. (1993). Long-Term Care, Medicaid, and the Impoverishment of the Elderly. *The Milbank Quarterly*, *70*(4), 19.

Sloane, E. B. (2006). The emerging health care IT infrastructure. *24x7, 11*(12), 42-43.

Sloane, E. B. (2009). Regulatory overview.(Networking). *24x7, 14*(4), 22-24.

Telehealth can improve quality of life. (2009). *Nursing Standard, 23*(24), 21.

Thompson, L. T., Dorsey, M. A., Miller, I. K., & Parrott, R. (Eds.). (2003). *Handbook of Health Communication.* Mahwah, NJ: Lawrence Earlbaum.

U.S. Census Bureau. (2000). *The 65 and Over Population: 2000*. Washington, DC: Author.

U.S. Department of Health and Human Services. (2003). Home Health Service. In *Code of Federal Regulations* (Sect. 484.30).

U.S. Department of Health and Human Services. (2006a). *Overview Medicaid Program: General Information*. Washington, DC: Author.

U.S. Department of Health and Human Services. (2006b). Durable medical equipment: Scope and conditions. In *Code of Federal Regulations* (Sect. 410.38).

U.S. Department of Health and Human Services. (2008). *Medical & You handbook*. Washington, DC: Author.

U.S. Government General Accountability Office. (2002). *More Can Be Done to Protect Residents from Abuse*. Washington, DC: Author.

U.S. Government General Accountability Office. (2004). *HS's efforts to promote health information technology and legal barriers to its adoption.* Washington, DC: Author

U.S. Government General Accountability Office. (2008a). *NURSING HOMES: Federal Monitoring Surveys Demonstrate Continued Understatement of Serious Care Problems and CMS Oversight Weaknesses*. Washington, DC: Author.

U.S. Government General Accountability Office. (2008b). *Inspectors Often Overlook Serious Deficiencies at U.S. Nursing Homes*. Washington, DC: Author.

Virginia Department of Social Services. (2007). Assisted Living Facilities (ALF). Richmond, VA: Author.

Wald, H., & Shojania, K. G. (2001). Incident reporting. In K. G. Shojania, B. W. Ducan, K. M. McDonald, & R. M. Wachter (Eds.), *Making health care safer: A critical analysis of patient safety practices* (pp. 41-47). Rockville, MD: Agency for Healthcare Research and Quality.

Webb, A. (2001). *The Impact of the Cost of Long-Term Care on the Saving of the Elderly*. New York: International Longevity Center.

Whitten, P., Doolittle, G., & Heilmich, S. (2001). Telehospice: using telecommunication technology for terminally ill patients. *Computer-Mediated Communications*, *6*(4), 43–47.

Williams, L. (2003). Medication-Monitoring Lawsuit: Case Study and Lessons Learned. *Nursing Homes/Long Term Care Management*, 3.

Wolf, A. (2003). Behind Closed Doors. *NFPA Journal*.

Wolfstadt, J. (2008). The effect of computerized physician order entry with clinical decision support on the rates of adverse drug events: A systematic review. *Journal of General Internal Medicine*, *23*(4), 451–458. doi:10.1007/s11606-008-0504-5

Wootton, R. (2001). Telemedicine. *British Medical Journal*, *323*, 4. doi:10.1136/bmj.323.7303.4

Wunderlich, G. S., & Kohler, P. O. (2001). *Improving the quality of long-term care: Information systems for monitoring quality*. Washington, DC: National Academy Press.

Xie, S., Xiao, Y., & Chen, H.-H. (in press). Nursing Home. In A. Coronato & G. De Pietro (Eds.), *Pervasive and Smart Technologies for Healthcare: Ubiquitous Methodologies and Tools*. Hershey, PA: IGI Global.

Yu, P., Li, H., & Gagnon, M.-P. (2009). Health IT acceptance factors in long-term care facilities: A cross-sectional survey. *International Journal of Medical Informatics*, *78*(4), 219–229. doi:10.1016/j.ijmedinf.2008.07.006

This work was previously published in International Journal of Healthcare Delivery Reform Initiatives, edited by Matthew W. Guah, pp. 48-67, copyright 2009 by IGI Publishing (an imprint of IGI Global).

Chapter 19
Medical Data Visualization via a Pervasive Multi-Agent Platform

Antonio Coronato
ICAR-CNR, Italy

Luigi Gallo
ICAR-CNR, Italy

Giuseppe De Pietro
ICAR-CNR, Italy

ABSTRACT

Pervasive healthcare is the field of application emerging from the combination of healthcare with pervasive computing, which is the computing paradigm that provides users with access to services in a transparent way, wherever they are and whichever their interacting device is. In this paper, a software infrastructure for pervasive healthcare is presented. Such an infrastructure aims at supporting medical practitioners with advanced pervasive access to medical data, which is also context-aware in the sense that the modality to fruit data depends on the device used by the operator and on his or her physical position within the environment. The paper also describes a service for high quality 3D rendering of medical volume data, which takes advantage of the software infrastructure to distribute the computational load upon the devices available in the environment in a completely transparent way to users.

INTRODUCTION

Pervasive computing and ambient intelligence technologies are more and more frequently adopted to develop innovative solutions in the field of healthcare. As a matter of fact, pervasive healthcare is the emerging computing paradigm that appears to be able to provide both solutions to many existing healthcare problems and new opportunities for better healthcare services.

DOI: 10.4018/978-1-60960-183-6.ch019

Pervasive healthcare aims to provide healthcare to anyone, anytime, and anywhere, in a transparent way, by means of innovative interaction metaphors. It is opening a wide range of innovative applications, from remote monitoring of elder people or ill patients, to new environments like advanced surgery rooms, smart spaces for doctor consulting, assisted living homes, and smart hospitals, which relies on the application of ambient intelligence technologies. Generally speaking, ambient intelligence concerns the ability of a software system to be sensitive, adaptive and responsive to the change of status of the physical environment (Cook, Augusto & Jakkula, 2009). As a specialization of ambient intelligence, Ambient Assisted Living (AAL) regards the realization of smart environments to monitor elderly and ill people. A generic definition for AAL can be found in (Steg, 2006): "AAL aims to prolong the time people can live in decent way in their own home by increasing their autonomy and self-confidence, the discharge of activities of daily living, to monitor and care for the elderly or ill person, to enhance the security and to save resources". The development of such a kind of applications presents new criticalities depending on their intrinsic characteristics, as for an example the dependency of the system behavior from the user and resources location and movements. It has been emphasized the need of having a formal methodology and the advantage of adopting a structured approach to design in (Coronato & De Pietro, in press) and (Lee, Chen, Hsiao & Tseng, 2007). It is also clear the need of tools for rapid integration of technologies and prototyping AAL applications (Cook & Das, 2007).

In this paper, a software infrastructure for a smart medical environment is presented. Specifically, such an environment aims at supporting medical staff with advanced pervasive access to medical data, which is also context-aware in the sense that the modality to fruit data depends on the device used by the operator and his physical position within the environment. As a specific case study, it is presented a service for high-quality volume ray casting of large medical datasets. This service: i) identifies the kind of device that is used by the operator to issue the request; ii) locates the operator to know if a better visualization device is in the proximity of him (e.g. a wall monitor); iii) customizes the service depending on the user location and the visualization device; and, iv) exploits the software infrastructure to distribute the rendering load among the common resources available in a completely transparent way to users.

What about the underling agent-based middleware infrastructure, it is able to transparently handle the distribution of inherently parallelizable tasks in a networked grid of both fixed and mobile devices. This infrastructure can conveniently be applied in scenarios like hospitals, in which a large number of personal computers and mobile devices are available and typically only partially used. In this kind of scenario, users want to execute intensive computing tasks, but they are neither expert nor willing of being aware about task distribution among the available resources. With the approach we describe in this paper, both wired PCs and wireless mobile devices can participate the computing platform in a quite simple and transparent way. Volunteers have just to download and install a lightweight middleware bundle. Users do not have to select, reserve and coordinate any resource. The software infrastructure realizes a P2P network over which tasks can be executed after having been embedded in mobile agents, which, in their turn, chose where to start the execution of the encapsulated task, migrate in order to balance the load, or try to recover in case of failures. Main characteristics of the infrastructure are:

- **Transparent integration of mobile devices as active resources:** This feature grants that, whenever a mobile device enters the environment, it becomes an active resource for the community;

- **Self-execution of tasks:** The environment takes care of executing tasks without any user control. This means that the user is freed of requiring resources, launching execution, controlling it, picking up results and releasing resources;
- **Reliable execution of tasks:** Thanks to cloning mechanisms for agents and heartbeat protocols for devices and tasks, the environment is able to recover from several kinds of failures.

The rest of the paper is organized as follows. Next section introduces some related work. After that, the middleware infrastructure is described. Next, a specific application for high quality volume rendering of 3D medical data is described. Finally, some conclusions are reported.

RELATED WORK

Several infrastructures and services for healthcare, which are based on ambient intelligence technologies, have been proposed.

PERSONA (Perceptive Spaces prOmoting iNdepentent Aging), an ongoing project funded by the European Commission, aims at developing a scalable open standard technological platform for building a broad range of ambient assisted living services (Tazari, Furfari, Ramos & Ferro, 2009). The main technical challenge is the design of a self-organizing middleware infrastructure allowing the extensibility of component/device ensembles. The communication patterns of the infrastructure are based on distributed coordination strategies for service discovery and utilization. Unlike the PERSONA project, which mainly concerns the prevention of chronic conditions of elderly people and represents an environment for ambient assisted living, our middleware infrastructure aims at providing medical staff with pervasive and context-aware access to clinic data to realize a smart medical environment.

One remarkable related work is described in (Jara, Zamora & Skarmeta, 2009). It regards a software infrastructure that concerns the interoperability of heterogeneous devices with the patient electronic health record.

What about the problem of distributing high intensive computations among processors, large communities of researchers and academics have worked on projects aimed at providing novel mechanisms for sharing computing power. Together with fully featured grid solutions like Condor (Thain, Tannenbaum & Livny, 2003) and Globus (Foster & Kesselman, 1997), also lightweight solutions have been proposed. BOINC (Anderson, 2004) is a middleware that harnesses hundreds and thousands of PCs across the Internet to process a massive amount of data from different scientific computing problems, including radio telescope data analysis, protein shapes analysis, and searching for spinning neutron stars. XtremWeb (Fedak, Germain, Neri & Cappello, 2001) is a light-weight Grid that consists of three kinds of peers: the coordinator, the workers, and the clients. Compared to some other platforms, it allows multiple coordinators and clients (workers keep a collection of coordinators' and clients' IP addresses). Entropia (Chien, Calder, Elbert & Bhatia, 2003) is a Windows P2P computing system for enterprise networks. It distinguishes from the solutions cited above for its sandboxed task execution. Binary modification is used to intercept all important Windows API calls. JNGI (Verbeke, Nadgir, Ruetsch, & Sharapov, 2002) is a framework for large-scale computations for problems that feature coarse-grained parallelization. It exploits the JXTA (Maibaum & Mundt, 2002) peer-to-peer communication protocol to construct the overlay network.

More recently, many higher-level programming abstractions have been proposed to simplify the use of distributed computing for application developers. The Simple API for Grid Applications (SAGA) (Sirvent, Merzky, Badia, & Kielmann, 2005) is an example of such abstractions. It insulates applications from technological and other low-level implementation details that regularly occur in the lower layers of the software stack. These new tools simplify the developing of distributed scientific applications. Lazarus (El-Khamra & Jha, 2009) is a framework built upon SAGA that provides a general, extensible approach for developing autonomic computational scientific applications.

Such services and systems allow to share computing power and to coordinate the process of data. Nonetheless, most of them are not completely transparent to users, and do not allow to integrate mobile devices. They usually require that users reserve resources, allocate tasks on them, launch execution, pick up results, and finally, release resources. Obviously, this practice gives almost full control to users on resources. Moreover, these systems require to install many software packages, which may discourage from using them. These systems do not fit the scenario we concern: the one in which users are almost completely inexpert of handling computing resources and a large number of common facilities (personal computers, laptops, tablet PCs, etc.) are available. In this case, the process of task distribution should be completely transparent to users. Our implementation is just aimed at achieving this goal.

With respect to previously published works (Coronato, De Pietro, & Gallo, 2007a, 2007b, 2008; Coronato & De Pietro, 2008), in this paper the whole middleware infrastructure has been completely decentralized. Moreover, we have developed a service for volume rendering that exploits the middleware for distributing the rendering load across the network in a transparent way to users.

Differently from other works on rendering load distribution over a multi-agent platform (see Rangel-Kuoppa, Aviles-Cruz, & Mould, 2003; Gonzalez-Morcillo, Weiss, Jiménez, & Vallejo, 2007), in this work the emphasis is on the autonomic properties of the whole system. In the proposed middleware, rather than communicate with a central entity, mobile agents communicate with each other to configure and optimize the task execution, and to recover from some common failures without human manual configuration operations.

THE SOFTWARE INFRASTRUCTURE

The software infrastructure consists of a set of components that aim at providing medical staff with access to pervasive services. Access is grant by means of heterogeneous devices either mobile (e.g. PDA, mini notebook, laptop) or fixed (PCs and workstations).

The main services, as shown in Figure 1, are:

- The *Event Service,* which enables asynchronous messages dispatching;
- The *Topology Service,* which provides a unique and uniform representation for the topology of the environment. In particular, locations are classified as semantic locations (buildings, floors, rooms, an area in front of a wall monitor, etc) and physical locations (the area sensed by an RFID antenna, the area covered by a WiFi access point, etc.). This service enables functionalities offered by other services like context, location and tracking;
- The *Location Service,* which is in charge of handling global location information for mobile resources and users. In particular, it locates mobile users by means of the RFID technology and WiFi enabled mobile devices by means of classic location techniques;
- The *Resource Service,* which is in charge of registering and monitoring resources;
- The *User Service,* which provides basic authentication mechanisms for users and handles the list of all users active in the environment; the *Resource Service,* which extends standard mechanisms for register-

Figure 1. High level middleware services view

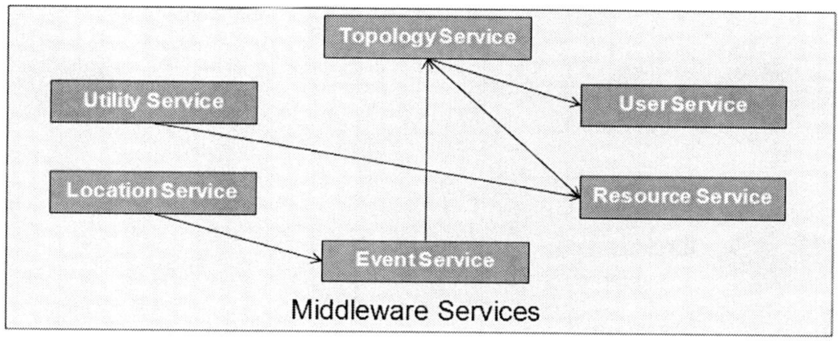

ing and monitoring resources, like laptops, PDAs and sensors;

- The *Utility Service,* which provides mechanisms for distributing computation in a transparent way to users.

In the following, we describe main features of the core services.

Event Service

This is the core of the communication layer that offers asynchronous messages dispatching. This service provides an interaction mechanism based on the event publish-subscribe paradigm. It implements the WSBrokeredNotification specifications (OASIS, n.d.) but extends them. As a matter of fact, the WSBrokeredNotification specifications neither support hierarchies of classes nor simple classes, but require that a consumer subscribe to every specific event for which it is willing of being notified.

The event service extends such specifications with the possibility of publishing and subscribing hierarchies of classes of events. In particular, a class of events is a collection of events that are logically related. In such a case, rather than subscribing every event of the class, a consumer can make just one operation of subscription for the entire class and be notified for every event. Moreover, it handles hierarchies of classes. The concept of hierarchy (see Figure 2) has been derived from the Object Oriented inheritance technique. Since classes can be related in hierarchies, when a consumer subscribes to one class, it automatically subscribes to every upper class of the hierarchy.

The interface of the service exposes functions for subscribing and unsubscribing classes of events, notifying events, creating and handling hierarchies. Two hierarchies are used in the running scenario. The first hierarchy consists of three classes. Class MOBILITY contains the event NEW_LOCATION. Class PRESENCE contains the events NEW_DEVICE and DEVICE_HAS_LEFT. Finally, class LOCALIZATION groups all events. The second hierarchy consists of a single class, namely USER_PRESENCE, which contains events for logging in and out a user.

Topology Service

The topology service described in this paper relies on a location model that we have defined to provide a unique and uniform representation for location information, independently of the particular positioning system.

The model is based on the concepts of physical and semantic locations. A *physical* location specifies the position of a mobile entity and is characterized by different granularities and scopes, depending on the particular positioning system. Instead, a *semantic* location specifies the meaning of a location and usually groups

Figure 2. High level view of the event service

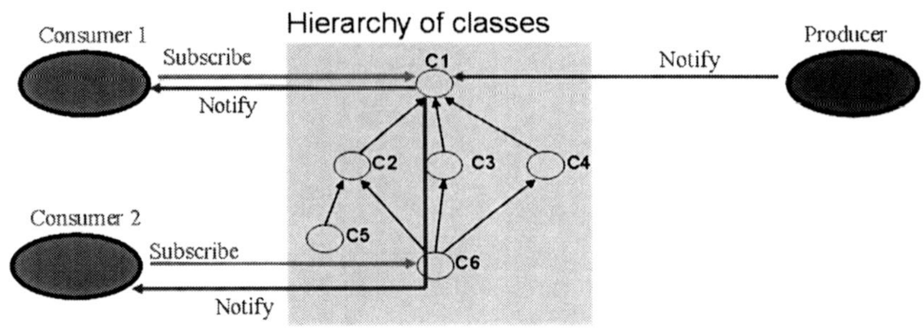

more physical locations. As an example, GPS coordinates represent physical locations, whereas a semantic location can be a building, an office inside a building, a meeting room, an area in front of a wall-monitor etc.

The proposed model describes physical locations as the proximity to well-known points. The technique of proximity is applicable when the environment is equipped with sensors to reveal the presence of mobile users, or with positioning systems to detect the position of mobile devices. In such cases, a sensor/positioning device, which covers a specific area, defines a physical location corresponding with the covered area. In the model, the covered area is called SensedArea.

We have adopted two specific positioning systems (Coronato, De Pietro, & Esposito, 2009). The former relies on the Wi-Fi technology to locate Wi-Fi enabled mobile devices. The latter uses RFID identification systems to locate RFID tagged mobile users.

Corresponding sensed areas are:

- *Wi-FiSensedArea*, which is identified by the physical area covered by a specific Wi-Fi AP, i.e. the region in which the AP is able to grant access to a Wi-Fi mobile device;
- *RFIDSensedArea*, which is identified by the physical area covered by a specific RFID reader; i.e., the region in which the RFID reader is able to detect an RFID tagged user.

In addition to these, a set of semantic locations, like Building, Floor, Room and Corridor, have been defined.

Finally, the concept of *AtomicLocation* is used to represent the linking element between physical and semantic locations. Its physical dimension corresponds with the one of the sensed areas of the finest positioning system in the environment. In the proposed example, an AtomicLocation corresponds with an RFIDSensedArea because an RFID reader covers a smaller area than the one covered by a Wi-Fi AP.

As shown in Figure 3.a, the concept of AtomicLocation is used to build a grid of locations in the physical environment (AtomicLocation Perspective). Therefore, some RFID readers are positioned in order to match with AtomicLocations. Not all the AtomicLocations are covered by an RFIDReader (RFIDSensed Perspective). Differently, each Wi-Fi AP spreads a signal over many AtomicLocations (Wi-FiSensedArea Perspective). Finally, semantic locations in turn group many AtomicLocations and correspond with well defined physical spaces (SemanticLocation Perspective).

As a result, relationships between SensedAreas and SemanticLocations are built by means of AtomicLocations. This makes the model able to adapt easily to changes like the introduction of

Figure 3. (a) Example of use of the location model (b) RFIDSensedArea Perspective (c) WiFiSensedArea Perspective (d) Semantic Location Perspective

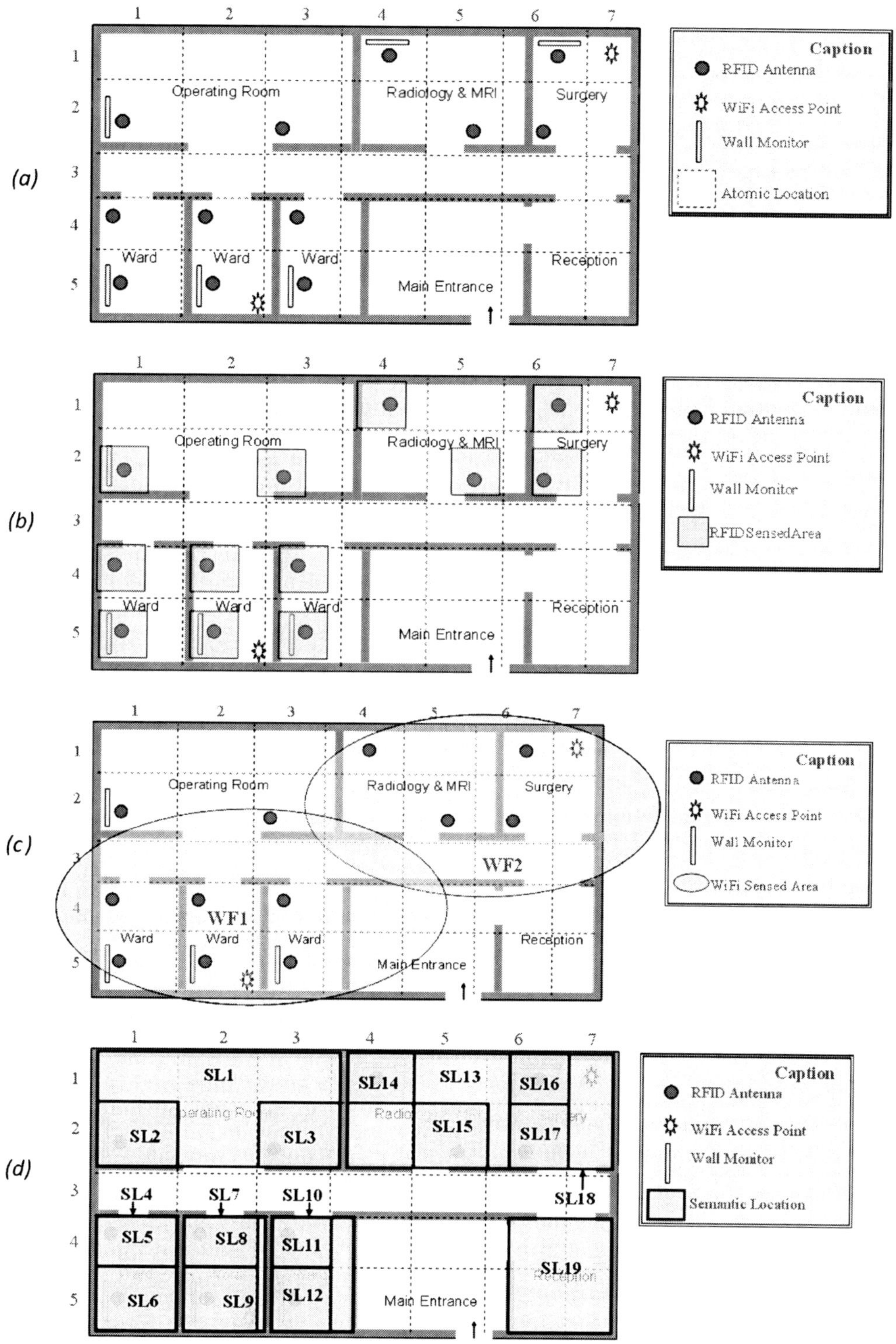

new positioning systems or the definition of new semantic locations. The introduction of a new positioning system obviously means that the physical dimension of an AtomicLocation has to be changed, but the location model still remains applicable.

In the following, some use cases, which need different localization capabilities, are reported:

- **Use Case 1:**whenever a patient is located within the Radiology, the system automatically retrieves X-Ray pictures and visualizes them through the wall monitor;
- **Use Case 2:** as a patient enters the surgery, the system automatically retrieves and shows his/her Electronic Health Record through the wall monitor;
- **Use Case 3:** when a doctor enters a ward (i.e., he/she is detected in the Ward entrance semantic location, say for example SL5 in Figure 3.d) and his/her tablet PC is connected to the Wi-FiSensedArea (see WF1 in Figure 3.c), the system automatically retrieves the patient Electronic Health Record and shows it on the doctor's device. After that, if the doctor approaches the wall monitor, the system automatically re-directs its output to the wall monitor for a better resolution;
- **Use Case 4:** when a doctor and a patient are both located in the surgery, the system automatically retrieves and shows the patient's Electronic Health Record either on the doctor's tablet PC or on the wall monitor depending on the doctor's position within the surgery, similarly to the use case 3. However, although the doctor is located in front of the wall monitor (SL16 in Figure 3.d), if another patient enters the surgery (i.e., he/she is detected at SL17), the system automatically re-directs the output onto the doctor's tablet PC for privacy reasons of privacy.

Use cases 1 and 2 require simple location functionalities. In contrast, Use Cases 3 and 4 require advanced location facilities and some reasoning capabilities. As a matter of fact, if we focus on Use Case 3, it is possible to conclude that the environment must be able to locate both RFID tagged users and Wi-Fi enabled devices. In addition to this, it must be able to reason on location information and to infer that in order to automatically show the Electronic Health Record on the tablet PC- the tablet PC is active in a RFID-SensedArea (the one at the entrance of the ward), which is also included in the Wi-FiSensedArea where it is located. The assumption is that the doctor does not leave his/her device active when he/she does not carry it with him/her.

Location Service

This service is able to locate active mobile objects like WiFi enabled devices and RFID tagged entities. It offers both locating and location functions; that is, the function *Locate_Object* returns the position of a specific object, whereas the function *Get_Objects* returns the list of objects that are active at a specific location. It notifies to the environment events of the class LOCALIZATION. In addition to location and locating functions, this service provides basic network facilities for connecting incoming mobile devices and detects leaving mobile objects.

The service architecture consists of two layers and the following components:

- **LocationComponent:** This component is in charge of handling global location states obtained by combining information coming from Locating components. When a mobile object changes its position the NEW_LOCATION event is notified. Moreover, when a mobile object is detected for the first time, the LocatingComponent notifies such an event (NEW_DEVICE) to the *Resource Service* that updates its registers.

- **WiFiLocatingComponent:** This component is in charge of locating WiFi enabled mobile devices. In particular, a WiFi location is identified by the area covered by a specific wireless Access Point (AP), that is, as the WiFiSendedArea of the location model. In the environment, one WiFiLocatingComponent is deployed per every wireless AP. Current implementation uses 3Com Office Connect Wireless 11g Access Points. Whenever a mobile device connects with the AP, the AP writes an event in its log file. The WiFiLocatingComponent periodically interrogates such a log file and communicates to the LocationComponent when a new device has connected. The WiFiLocatingComponent maintains information on devices locally connected to its AP.
- **RFIDLocatingComponent:** This component is in charge of locating RFID tagged objects. An RFID location is identified by the area covered by a specific RFID reader; that is, as the RFIDSensedArea of the location model. Current implementation uses the passive, short-range (30 cm), Feig Electronic RFID, model ISC. MR 100/101. When a tagged object enters the area covered by an antenna, the RFID reader generates an event that is caught by the RFIDLocatingComponent. Then, the RFIDLocatingComponent communicates to the LocationComponent such an event.
- **DHCPComponent:** This component implements a DHCP service. It provides network connectivity to incoming IP enabled devices as a standard DHCP, but it has also additional functionalities. In particular, it is able to release an IP address on demand. By this way, if a device has left the environment, the LocationComponent requires that the DHCPComponent free the IP address of that device.
- **EcoComponent:** This component sends ping messages towards mobile IP devices in order to detect leaving objects. When an implicit disconnection is detected, the component communicates such an event to the LocationComponent that notifies the DEVICE_HAS_LEFT event.

Resource Service

This service registers and monitors resources. For every resource, one can specify a description, if it is a mobile resource or not, several attributes like the IP address or MAC address.

User Service

It offers basic mechanisms for the registration of the users, specifically the monitored patients, and the resources (sensors) associated to them.

Utility Service

The architectural model of the Utility Service inspires to Hybrid Peer-to-Peer (P2P) networks. It relies on two logical entities: *Peer* – which is a hardware node that hosts the software platform and is able to execute tasks; and *Service Gateway* – which is a component that offers to users the service for submitting tasks to execute and is notified by Peers whenever they enter the community.

In greater detail, the software components are:

- **Service Gateway:** The Service Gateway represents the entry point for every Peer that wants to join the community. It is also the node that offers to users the service for submitting tasks. The Service Gateway is composed, as shown in Figure 4, by the following logic entities:
    - **Configuration Agent:** This agent receives connection requests from nodes that are willing to enter the community. In particular, a node com-

Figure 4. Service Gateway logical model

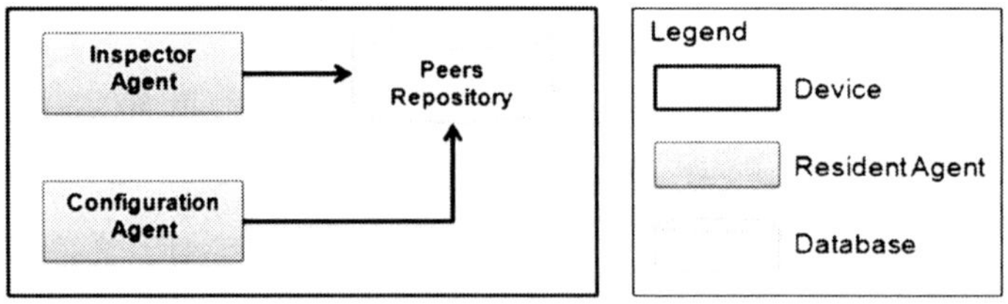

municates its IP and MAC addresses. Then, the Configuration Agent verifies its credentials and registers (into the Peers Repository) the new node as a Peer;

- ◦ **Peers Repository:** This is the repository that maintains information about all Peers and agents active in the community;
- ◦ **Inspector Agent:** This agent is in charge of monitoring Peers in order to verify their availability. Consequently, it updates the Peers' status in the Peers Repository.

- **Peer:** A Peer is a network node, either fixed or mobile, which has entered the community via the Service Gateway, and shares its computing power with all other Peers of the community. The logical architecture of a Peer is shown in Figure 5. It consists of the following components:
  - ◦ **Worker:** A Worker is a mobile agent that embeds a task in order to execute it. The mobility of this agent is a characteristic that the environment uses in order to redistribute the load in the platform.
  - ◦ **Worker Clone:** A Worker Clone is just a clone of a running task and is activated by the environment in case of failures of its related Worker. Obviously, in order to recover from node failures, a Peer maintains Worker Clones related to workers that are running on other Peers.
  - ◦ **Collector:** This agent is in charge of collecting elaboration results.

Figure 5. Peer logical model

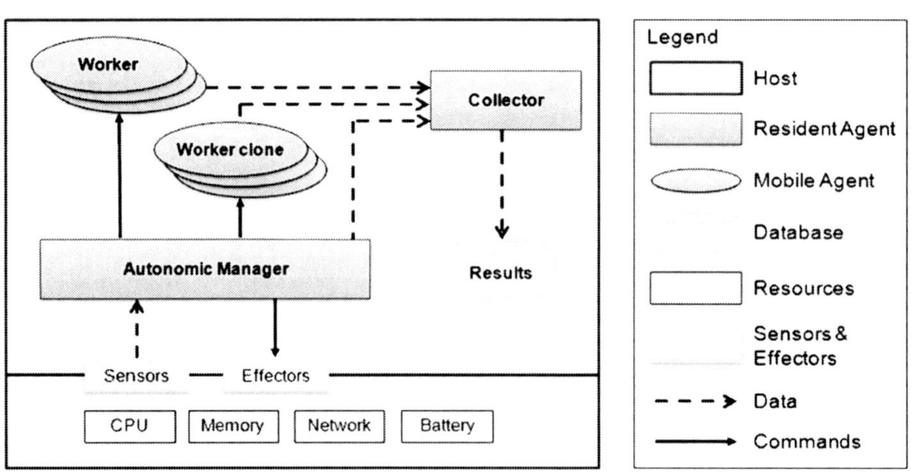

Figure 6. Volume ray casting results with a different number of rays per pixel

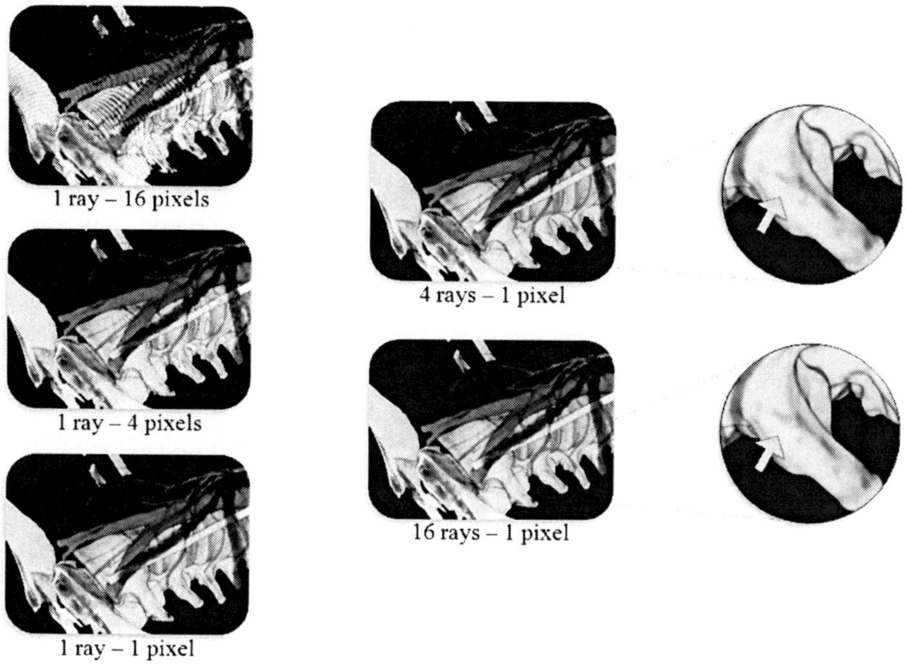

- **Autonomic Manager (AM):** This agent activates when the device enters in the community (i.e. it connects to the Service Gateway). From that moment on, it handles all activities that the Peer performs. In particular, it receives workers for execution, it can require workers to migrate, it can activate clones, and so on. This is achieved by executing the classic MAPE control loop for autonomic components (Kephart & Chess, 2003), which consists of four phases:
  - **Monitor phase:** The AM: monitors the state of its own device (i.e. the level of battery in the case of mobile devices, the memory occupancy, the processor load, the network connectivity, etc); periodically sends information about its state to all other peers of the community; collects information coming from other Peers;
  - **Analyze phase:** The AM models the state by using information gathered in the monitor stage;
  - **Plan phase:** The AM builds sequences of actions to execute in order to achieve specific goals;
  - **Execute phase:** The AM executes sequences of actions previously specified.

THE HIGH QUALITY 3D RENDERING SERVICE

Upon the middleware previously described, we developed a service for the distributed rendering of medical volume data via high quality volume ray casting with *supersampling* techniques.

Volume rendering via ray casting is an inherently parallelizable process. During image synthesis, the light propagation is computed by integrating light interaction effects along viewing rays based on the optical model. The corresponding integral is known as the volume rendering integral. Ray casting might be considered as the most direct numerical method for evaluating this integral. It is a process that, for each pixel in the image to render, casts a single ray from the eye through the pixel's center into the volume, and integrates the optical properties obtained from the encountered volume densities along the ray.

However, real-world objects have continuous, smooth curves and lines, whereas monitors can only display discrete points of light. This causes a problem known as aliasing. Supersampling is one of the ways of reducing the aliasing problem. Samples are taken at several instances inside the pixel (and not just at the center). In concrete terms, instead of sampling one ray per pixel, 4/8/16 rays are sampled per pixel.

In Figure 6, a comparison of the results of volume ray casting with supersampling on a CT male torso data set (361 16-bit grayscale slices with 1 mm thickness and 512 × 512 resolution) is reported. As we can see, supersampling (4 rays – 1 pixel and 16 rays – 1 pixel in Figure 5), greatly enhance the quality of the image. In particular, the stripes pattern which is also present when 4 rays per pixel are used, when 16 rays are used is not visible also when high zoom levels are used.

Recent advances in graphics hardware allow for the ray casting to be executed on a per-fragment level completely on the GPU leading to interactive frame rates, so making it possible to design more intuitive interface to manipulate medical data (Gallo, De Pietro, Coronato & Marra, 2008). Nonetheless, the rendering time considerably increases if supersampling techniques and high resolution displays are used. If the screen resolution is 800 × 600, there are "just" 480000 pixels to render, therefore 480000 rays to cast. On a display with a resolution of 2560 × 1600, there are 4096000 pixels, so the rendering load is almost decupled. In addition, when supersampling techniques are used to reduce aliasing artifacts, the computational load increases proportionally to the number of rays.

The high quality 3D rendering service we developed takes advantage of all the mechanisms the proposed middleware provides. Specifically, to distribute the rendering load across the platform, we used the Utility Service, which just requires to initialize each Worker with a portion of code and data. To partition large volume data sets among the Peers, we used a simple image-partition technique. Finally, the Collector agent was customized to build the final, high resolution image by adding all the rendering contributes. Once the image has been built, the Collector visualizes it on the most fitting video resource available, which is accessed by using the Topology Service.

CONCLUSION

In this paper, we have presented a software infrastructure for pervasive healthcare, which aims at supporting medical practitioners with pervasive access to medical data. The infrastructure is context-aware, since the modality to fruit data depends on the device used by the operator and on his physical position within the environment. Furthermore, the infrastructure realizes a P2P network that it is able to transparently handle the distribution of inherently parallelizable tasks in a lightweight grid of both fixed and mobile devices. We have also described a service which takes advantage of the P2P network to distribute the rendering of medical volume data over a dynamic community of both fixed and mobile devices in a way completely transparent to users.

REFERENCES

Anderson, D. P. (2004). BOINC: A System for Public-Resource Computing and Storage. In [Washington, DC: IEEE Computer Society.]. *Proceedings of GRID*, *04*, 4–10.

Chien, A., Calder, B., Elbert, S., & Bhatia, K. (2003). Entropia: architecture and performance of an enterprise desktop grid system. *Journal of Parallel and Distributed Computing*, *63*(5), 597–610. doi:10.1016/S0743-7315(03)00006-6

Cook, J., Augusto, J. C., & Jakkula, V. R. (2009). Ambient Intelligence: Technologies, applications, and opportunities. *Pervasive and Mobile Computing Journal*, *5*(4), 277–298. doi:10.1016/j.pmcj.2009.04.001

Cook, J., & Das, S. K. (2007). How smart are our environments? An updated look at the state of the art. *Pervasive and Mobile Computing Journal, 3*(2).

Coronato, A., & De Pietro, G. (2008). MiPeG: A Middleware Infrastructure for Pervasive Grids. *Journal of Future Generation Computer Systems*, *24*(1). doi:10.1016/j.future.2007.04.007

Coronato, A., & De Pietro, G. (in press). Formal Specification of Wireless and Pervasive Healthcare Applications. *ACM Transactions on Embedded Computing Systems.*

Coronato, A., De Pietro, G., & Esposito, M. (2009). A Multimodal Semantic Location Service for Intelligent Environments: An Application for Smart Hospitals. *Personal and Ubiquitous Computing Journal, 13*(7)

Coronato, A., De Pietro, G., & Gallo, L. (2007a). Automatic execution of tasks in MiPeG. In *GPC 2007* (LNCS 4459, pp. 702-709).

Coronato, A., De Pietro, G., & Gallo, L. (2007b). Dynamic Distribution and Execution of Tasks in Pervasive Grids. In *Proceedings of the 15th Euromicro international Conference on Parallel, Distributed and Network-Based Processing* (pp. 419-423). Washington, DC: IEEE Computer Society.

Coronato, A., De Pietro, G., & Gallo, L. (2008). An agent based platform for task distribution in virtual environments. *Journal of Systems Architecture*, *54*(9), 877–882. doi:10.1016/j.sysarc.2008.01.011

El-Khamra, Y., & Jha, S. (2009). Developing autonomic distributed scientific applications: a case study from history matching using ensemble kalman-filters. In *GMAC '09* (pp. 19-28). New York: ACM.

Fedak, G., Germain, C., Neri, V., & Cappello, F. (2001). XtremWeb: A Generic Global Computing System. In *Proceedings of the 1st International Symposium on Cluster Computing and the Grid.* Washington, DC: IEEE Computer Society.

Foster, I., & Kesselman, C. (1997). Globus: A metacomputing infrastructure toolkit. *The International Journal of Supercomputer Applications*, *11*(2), 115–128. doi:10.1177/109434209701100205

Gallo, L., De Pietro, G., Coronato, A., & Marra, I. (2008). Toward a natural interface to virtual medical imaging environments. In *Proceedings of the Working Conference on Advanced Visual Interfaces* (pp. 429-432). New York: ACM.

Gonzalez-Morcillo, C., Weiss, G., Jiménez, L., & Vallejo, D. (2007). A multi-agent approach to distributed rendering optimization. In. *Proceedings of AAAI*, *07*, 1775–1780.

Jara, A. J., Zamora, M. A., & Skarmeta, A. F. G. (2009). An Architecture for Ambient Assisted Living and Health Environments. In *Distributed Computing, Artificial Intelligence, Bioinformatics, Soft Computing, and Ambient Assisted Living* (LNCS 5518, pp. 882-889).

Kephart, J. O., & Chess, D. M. (2003). The Vision of Autonomic Computing. *Computer*, *36*(1), 41–50. doi:10.1109/MC.2003.1160055

Lee, R. G., Chen, K. C., Hsiao, C. C., & Tseng, C. L. (2007). A Mobile Care System with Alert Mechanism. *IEEE Transactions on Information Technology in Biomedicine*, *11*(5). doi:10.1109/TITB.2006.888701

Maibaum, N., & Mundt, T. (2002). JXTA: A Technology Facilitating Mobile Peer-To-Peer Networks. In *Proceedings of MobiWac '02* (p. 7). Washington, DC: IEEE Computer Society.
OASIS. (n.d.). *WSNotification*. Retrieved from http://www.oasis-open.org/committees/download.php/13485/wsn-ws-brokered_notification-1.3-spec-pr-01.pdf

Rangel-Kuoppa, R., Aviles-Cruz, C., & Mould, D. (2003). Distributed 3D rendering system in a multi-agent platform. In *Proceedings of ENC 2003* (pp. 168-175).

Sirvent, R., Merzky, A., Badia, R., & Kielmann, T. (2005). *Grid superscalar and SAGA: forming a high-level and platform-independent grid programming environment*. Paper presented at CoreGRID Integration WorkShop 2005.

Steg, H., et al. (2006). *Europe Is Facing a Demographic Challenge – Ambient Assisted Living Offers Solutions*. Paper presented at VDI/VDE/IT.

Tazari, M. R., Furfari, F., Ramos, J. P. L., & Ferro, E. (2009). The PERSONA Service Platform for AAL Spaces. In H. Nakashima, H. Aghajan, & J.C. Augusto (Eds.), *Handbook of Ambient Intelligence and Smart Environments (AISE)*. New York: Springer.

Thain, D., Tannenbaum, T., & Livny, M. (2003). *Grid Computing: Making the Global Infrastructure a Reality, chapter Condor and the grid*. New York: John Wiley & Sons.

Verbeke, J., Nadgir, N., Ruetsch, G., & Sharapov, I. (2002). Framework for peer-to-peer distributed computing in a heterogeneous, decentralized environment. In [London: Springer-Verlag.]. *Proceedings of GRID*, *02*, 1–12.

This work was previously published in International Journal of Healthcare Delivery Reform Initiatives, edited by Matthew W. Guah, pp. 68-61, copyright 2009 by IGI Publishing (an imprint of IGI Global).

Chapter 20
Seamless Access to Healthcare Folders with Strong Privacy Guarantees

Tristan Allard
University of Versailles & INRIA Rocquencourt, France

Nicolas Anciaux
INRIA Rocquencourt, France

Luc Bouganim
INRIA Rocquencourt, France

Philippe Pucheral
University of Versailles & INRIA Rocquencourt, France

Romuald Thion
INRIA Grenoble, France

ABSTRACT

During the past decade, many countries launched ambitious Electronic Health Record (EHR) programs with the objective to increase the quality of care while decreasing its cost. Pervasive healthcare aims itself at making healthcare information securely available anywhere and anytime, even in disconnected environments (e.g., at patient home). Current server-based EHR solutions badly tackle disconnected situations and fail in providing ultimate security guarantees for the patients. The solution proposed in this paper capitalizes on a new hardware device combining a secure microcontroller (similar to a smart card chip) with a large external Flash memory on a USB key form factor. Embedding the patient folder as well as a database system and a web server in such a device gives the opportunity to manage securely a healthcare folder in complete autonomy. This paper proposes also a new way of personalizing access control policies to meet patient's privacy concerns with minimal assistance of practitioners. While both proposals are orthogonal, their integration in the same infrastructure allows building trustworthy pervasive healthcare folders.

DOI: 10.4018/978-1-60960-183-6.ch020

1. INTRODUCTION

Driven by the need to improve the quality of care while decreasing costs, many countries around the world are setting up large scale Electronic Health Record (EHR) systems gathering the medical history of individuals. Interoperability among heterogeneous healthcare information systems and privacy preservation are two main challenges in this context. Pervasive healthcare on its side strive to remove location and time constraints to access patient's healthcare folders. Cares provided at home to elderly or disabled people illustrate well the need for pervasiveness. In this context healthcare data is often collected and consulted at home by practitioners having different privileges and acting at different time periods. Healthcare information must be safely exchanged among practitioners to improve care coordination but no connection to the Internet can be always guaranteed. Data can also be issued by institutions external to the care coordination (e.g., a medical lab) and join the patient's folder. The folder is sometimes accessed by practitioners outside patient's home (e.g., doctor's office, hospital). Finally, a large collection of folders can be targeted by epidemiological studies for a general health benefit. In this paper, we discuss how smart objects can provide a seamless access to healthcare folders without privacy breach in all these situations.

EHR systems aim at answering most of the requirements mentioned above. The objective of centralizing medical information in database systems is manifold[1]: completeness (i.e., to make the information complete and up to date), availability (to make it accessible through the internet 24h-7 days a week), usability (to organize the data and make it easily queryable and interpretable), consistency (to guarantee integrity constraints and enforce atomicity and isolation of updates) and durability (to protect the data against failure). A recent report identified more than 100 EHR running projects worldwide at the scale of a country or regions in 2007 (Door, 2008). Other reports suggest that about 25% of U.S. healthcare practices use EHR systems. Within Europe these figures vary greatly between countries, from 15% in Greece up to 90% in the Netherlands today.

Regarding pervasiveness, healthcare folders can be reached by allowing internet connections to the server(s) through mobile devices (e.g., laptop, PDA, tablet PC). This however requires that every point of the territory be connected through a secure, fast, reliable and cheap network, a situation uncommon in many countries and regions today.

In addition, and despite the unquestionable benefit of EHR systems in terms of quality of care, studies conducted in different countries show that patients are reluctant to use existing EHR systems arguing increasing threats on individual privacy (The Times, 2008; The International Council on Medical & Care Compunetics, 2009). This suspicion is fueled by computer security surveys pointing out the vulnerability of database servers against external and internal attacks (Gordon et al., 2006). Indeed, centralizing and organizing the information make it more valuable, thereby motivating attacks and facilitating abusive usages. Regardless of the legislation protecting the usage of medical data and of the security procedures put in place at the servers, the patient has the sense of losing control over her data.

Hence, implementing a trustworthy pervasive access to healthcare folders requires addressing accurately the following issues:

1. How to make patient's healthcare folder available in a disconnected mode?
2. How to make patient's healthcare folder seamlessly available in a connected area?
3. How to make the patient trust the EHR security?
4. How to get the patient consent about a pervasive use of her healthcare folder?

As discussed above, existing EHR systems answer well issue 2 but fail in answering issue 1 and issue 3. Therefore, EHR systems fail also in answering issue 4 precisely due to the lack of server trustworthiness.

This paper suggests a new way of organizing EHR to address issues 1 to 4 all at once. The solution proposed capitalizes on a new hardware device called Secure Portable Token (SPT) hereafter. Roughly speaking, a SPT combines a secure microcontroller (similar to a smart card chip) with a large external Flash memory (Gigabyte sized) on a USB key form factor (Eurosmart, 2008). A SPT can host on-board data and run on-board code with proven security properties. Embedding a database system and a web server in a SPT gives the opportunity to manage securely a healthcare folder in complete autonomy. Accessing the on-board folder at patient's home requires a simple rendering device (e.g., a netbook or PDA) equipped with an USB port and running a web browser. Then issue 1 is tackled by construction. The SPT security properties (tamper-resistant hardware, certified embedded software) answer issue 3 with a much higher confidence than any traditional server can provide.

Issue 2 becomes however more difficult to address. Indeed, the patient folder cannot be accessed without being physically in possession of the patient's SPT. We propose two complementary solutions to tackle situations where remote accesses to the folder are mandatory. The first solution is to reintroduce a server in the architecture so that a secure exchange of information can be organized between the patient and a trusted circle of persons (e.g., the family doctor expressing her opinion in an emergency situation without having the patient's folder on hand). The solution is such that patient's data is never stored in the clear on the server and encryption/decryption keys are known only by the SPT participating to the trusted circle of person defined by the patient. The second solution answers Privacy Preserving Data Publishing (PPDP) requirements (Fung, 2009), where patient's data must be made available to epidemiological studies. We propose a secure publishing mechanism such that a global anonymized view of data collected from different folders can be produced without disclosing any link to individuals. These two solutions together tackle issue 2 without compromising issue 3.

One may consider that answering issue 3 leads to answer issue 4 as well. This is unfortunately not true. Trusting the EHR security is a prerequisite for the patient to give her consent about a pervasive use of her medical folder but it is definitely not a sufficient condition. Expressing an enlightened consent means understanding and accepting an access control policy specifying who (individuals or roles) is granted access to which part of her folder. The high number of people interacting with the folder, the diversity of their roles, the complexity of the medical information and the intrinsic difficulty to determine which data (or data association) reveals a given pathology makes this objective highly difficult to reach. This paper proposes a new and pragmatic alternative to define access control policies manageable by a patient with minimal assistance of practitioners. This solution complements well the SPT-based EHR architecture by answering issue 4. This solution is however orthogonal to the SPT-based architecture and we believe it could apply to many healthcare information systems.

As a conclusion, the objective of this paper is twofold. First, it discusses to which extent existing EHR architectures can meet the four requirements introduced above (Section 2) and proposes an alternative based on the SPT hardware device (Sections 3 and 4). Second, it discusses whether existing access control policies and confidentiality mechanisms can capture the patient's consent (Section 5) and proposes a solution relying on a new access control model (Section 6). Section 7 relates an experimentation in the field of a pervasive EHR architecture combining both proposals, in the context of home care provided to elderly people.

2. BACKGROUND

An electronic health record system is a collection of electronic patient folders, each containing the complete medical history of an individual, managed and consulted by authorized health professionals across several organizations (Alliance, 2007). Building an EHR system requires interconnecting various heterogeneous health information systems of disparate organizations in order to aggregate the medical data they maintain separately (e.g., hospitals, practitioners and pharmacists data related to a same individual).

Hence, the first challenge tackled by EHR programs is providing interoperability between heterogeneous systems. As pointed out in the introduction, ensuring data availability even in disconnected environments and enforcing data security are two additional and mandatory challenges. The next subsections present a state of the art on these three challenges.

2.1. EHR Interoperability

Three main approaches can be distinguished according to the level of integration targeted between existing health information systems.

The first approach consists in interconnecting existing autonomous systems in a wider infrastructure with no data centralization and a minimal central control. The Danish Healthcare Data Network (Pedersen, 2006)[2] is representative of this category. It connects the already secure intranets of care organizations via VPNs over the Internet, progressively from organizations to counties, counties to regions, and regions to nation. The Danish EHR effort has mainly consisted in defining a common data model representing clinical data. The USA have adopted a federal approach to build the EHR. At the region scale, Regional Health Information Organizations (RHIOs) are multi-stakeholder organizations that enable the exchange of health information between local health organizations (e.g., CalRHIO for the Californian RHIO). At the nation scale, the Nationwide Health Information Network (NHIN) project, supervised by the Office of the National Coordinator for Health IT (ONC), aims at enabling secure health information exchange across the USA by using RHIOs as regional building blocks. The NHIN will be a "network of networks" built over the Internet.

The second approach strengthens the integration thanks to centralized indexes and/or data summaries. The National Health Society in the United Kingdom has launched the Care Record Service (CRS) project. First, CRS aims at linking together the existing Electronic Medical Record (EMR) of an individual, thus constituting a virtual unique health folder. Navigating between the EMRs of an individual and gathering detailed data will be easier; furthermore, by sharing data across EMRs, duplication of - e.g., administrative - data will be useless. Second, CRS aims at storing summaries of detailed data on the "Spine", an already existing central system currently in charge of delivering health related services (e.g., ePresciptions, eReservations). The Secondary Uses Service (SUS) of CRS will use summarized data to draw reports and analysis about collected care information. With its two-level functional architecture, the Diraya project from Andalusia is similar to the CRS UK project. First, detailed data in EMRs are kept where they are produced (e.g., hospitals) and the central Diraya system indexes them. Second, Diraya centralizes what is called the "main data", that is the data most frequently accessed. In the Netherlands, the National Healthcare Information Hub project (LSP in Dutch), lead by Nictiz is basically a central index storing the location of every individual's EMRs. The Austrian ELGA initiative (Husek, 2008) is similar to the LSP project. The Canadian national program Infoway-Inforoute funds provincial EHR projects, most of these focusing on interoperability between care organizations. For example, the Alberta Netcare EHR centralizes regionally the patients' summary data. The Yukon Telehealth project makes local EMRs accessible to remote specialist practitioners.

The most integrated approach seeks to gather all EMRs related to the same individual into a centralized healthcare folder. In the United States, some private organizations had already felt the need to aggregate all their patients' data in a single folder before the coming of RHIOs. For example, the Veteran Administration Medical Center developed the VistA system (Brown et al, 2003), a Health Information System (HIS) enabling health centers with VistA to share their patients' data. The French national program Dossier Medical Personnel (DMP) aims also at centralizing healthcare folders hosted by selected database service providers. In another spirit, systems like Google Health™ and Microsoft's HealthVault™ propose individuals to centralize their Personal Health Records (PHRs) on their own initiative. Both load medical data directly from the patient's health centers that do agree, offer practical tools for individuals (e.g., drug interactions, hospitals searches), and can provide a controlled access to the PHR to a selected set of persons. Both are free and the users are simply asked to trust their privacy policy.

2.2. EHR Availability

All EHR systems mentioned above provide a 24h/7day a week availability assuming the servers are active and an internet connection can be established to reach them. This is unfortunately not the case in every place and every situation, introducing the need for disconnected accesses to healthcare folders.

In the United Kingdom, the Health eCard is a private initiative that proposes to store encrypted copies of full EMRs in specifically designed smart cards, making patients' health data available in disconnected situations (e.g., emergency situations, home consultation).

The German organization Gematik leads the eGK, an ambitious project mixing a traditional infrastructure with smart cards in order to tackle connected and disconnected situations (Smart Card Alliance-b, 2006). Both patients and professionals are equipped with a smart card, patient smart cards storing EHRs while professional smart cards are being used for strong authentication, digital signature and encryption/decryption of documents. The infrastructure holds a centralized copy of the EHRs, accessible through the internet. This project is still at a preliminary stage.

In the USA, many private initiatives issued by care centers tackle the "disconnected access" requirement (Smart Card Alliance-a, 2006), e.g., the University of Pittsburgh Medical Center Health Passport Project (HPP), the Florida eLife-Card, Queens Health Network, Mount Sinai Medical Center Personal Health Card. All of them store a copy of critical health information encrypted on a smart card to make it available in case of emergency.

Taiwan has launched in 2001 a project to replace the traditional paper health cards by smart cards (Smart Card Alliance, 2005). Smart cards are used exactly as paper cards were used. They permanently store administrative personal and summary health data, and temporarily store the medical data related to the last six visits. Every six visits, the temporary medical data are uploaded into the Taiwanese health infrastructure. The smart card health project is seamlessly integrated with the previous health infrastructure, providing a strong patient authentication and a paperless data management.

While many initiatives tackle the disconnected access challenge, the low storage capacities of the smart cards used in the aforementioned projects (i.e., at best a few hundreds of kilobytes) severely limit the quantity of on-board data, and then the benefit of the approach.

2.3. EHR Security

Strong authentication is usually required to connect to EHR servers. Health professionals authenticate with a smart-card (e.g., the CRS in UK, the LSP in the Netherlands), as well as patients accessing to their medical folder (e.g., the Diraya initiative in Andalusia). In addition, communication channels can be protected by cryptographic techniques, based on protocols such as TLS (Internet Engineering Task Force, 2008), enabling entities to securely exchange messages (i.e., encryption, integrity protection, non repudiation of messages), and security measures are implemented on central servers. However, this is not sufficient to put trust in the system.

The suspicion is fueled by computer security surveys pointing out the vulnerability of database servers against external and internal attacks (Gordon et al., 2006). Database systems are identified as the primary target of computer criminality (Gordon et al., 2006), and even the most well defended servers, including those of Pentagon (The Financial Times, 2007; Liebert, 2008), FBI (The Washington Post, 2007) and NASA (Computer World, 2003), have been successfully attacked. In addition, nearly half of the attacks (Gordon et al, 2006) come from the inside (employees) of the companies or organizations. In addition, there are many examples where negligence leads to personal data leakages. To cite a few, thousands of Medicare and Medicaid patients in eight states have been lost in a HCA regional office (FierceHealthIT news, 2006) and Hospitals County published by accident medical records on the web (FierceHealthIT news, 2008; WFTV, 2008) including doctors' notes, diagnoses, medical procedures and possibly names and ages of patients. A recent study shows that 81% of US firms declare loosing employees laptops with sensitive data (Computer World, 2006). Data loss is so frequent that a research project called DataLossDB has been created to report such incidents.

In practice, EHRs are thus very difficult to protect. This legitimates the reserves expressed by both practitioners and patients about EHR programs (The Times, 2008; eHealth Insider, 2008). In the Netherlands, privacy and access concerns are major arguments for the postponement of the national EHR (The International Council on Medical & Care Compunetics, 2009). In particular, the lack of security measures limiting data access for service providers and the loss of control on their own data has been identified as a main reason for citizens to opt-out of the system.

Only EMRs stored in personal and secure hardware such as smart-cards (see Section 2.2) can benefit from true privacy enforcement. However, (1) the storage capacity of the smart-cards used by current projects (e.g., from KB to MB) is too low to store a complete EHR, limiting the data availability in disconnected situations, (2) their low connectivity makes the hosted data seldom available, and (3) their portable nature makes them subjects to losses or destruction. Moreover, to tackle availability, these projects rely on central servers unable to enforce the smart-cards security level (Eurosmart, 2008).

We believe that both data privacy and full availability can be achieved altogether. The solution we propose is centered on a personal smart-card based device storing (the most significant part of) the patient folder and extending the security sphere of its secure hardware to traditional central servers.

3. A SECURE, PORTABLE MEDICAL FOLDER

Researches conducted in the PlugDB[3] project led us to design a lightweight Database Management System (DBMS) embedded in a new form of tamper-resistant token, called hereafter Secure Portable Token (SPT). Roughly speaking, a SPT combines a secure microcontroller (similar to a smart card chip) with a large external Flash memory (Gigabyte sized) on a USB key form factor (Eurosmart, 2008). A SPT can host a large volume of on-board data and run on-board code with proven security properties thanks to its tamper-resistant hardware and a certified operating system (Eurosmart, 2008). The main target of the

PlugDB technology is the management of secure and portable personal folder. Healthcare folders are very good representative of large personal folders where security and portability are highly required.

Compared to smart cards used in other EHR projects (see Section 2), the storage capacity of a SPT is roughly four orders of magnitude higher. Henceforth, this makes sense to embed the whole patient folder in her SPT and make it available in disconnected mode. In addition to the data, a complete chain of software is embedded in the SPT microcontroller: (1) a Web server, (2) servlets implementing the application, (3) a JDBC bridge, (4) a DBMS engine managing the on-board database and enforcing access control. Hence, the SPT along with its embedded database and software can be seen as a full-fledged server accessible through any web browser running on any device equipped with a USB port (e.g., laptop, tablet-PC, PDA and even cell-phone). Compared to a regular server, the SPT server is personal, pluggable, does not require any network connection and provides unprecedented security guarantees.

The specific hardware architecture of the SPT introduces however many technical challenges. We detail below the most important ones.

3.1. SPT Hardware and Operating System

A SPT combines in the same hardware platform a secure chip and a mass storage NAND FLASH memory (several Gigabytes soon). The secure chip is of the smart card type, with a 32 bit RISC CPU clocked at about 50 MHz, memory modules composed of ROM, tens of KB of static RAM, a small quantity of internal stable storage (NOR FLASH) and security modules. The mass storage NAND FLASH memory is outside the secure chip, connected to it by a bus, and does not benefit from the chip hardware protection.

Gemalto, the smart card world leader has developed an experimental SPT platform. This platform includes a new multi-tasking operating system allowing the development of Web applications based on JAVA and Servlet technology, and thus offering a standardized means to integrate services or embedded Web applications to the SPT. The operating system supports natively: the USB 2.0 protocol and the internet protocol IP for communicating with the external world (Vandewalle, 2004); multi-threaded Java applications; cryptographic primitives (some of which implemented in hardware); memory management and garbage collection; Servlet management and Web server. For more technical details on the hardware platform and the operating system, we refer the reader to (http://www-smis.inria.fr/~DMSP).

3.2. Embedded Database System

DBMS designers have produced light versions of their systems for personal assistants (e.g. Oracle-lite, DB2 everyplace, SQLServer for Window CE) but they never addressed the more complex problem of embedding a DBMS in a chip. Initial attempts towards a smart card DBMS was ISOL's SQLJava Machine (Carrasco, 1999), the ISO standard SCQL (ISO/IEC, 1999) and the MasterCard Open Data Storage (MasterCard International, 2002). All these proposals concerned traditional smart cards with few resources and therefore proposed basic data management functionalities (close to sequential files). Managing embedded medical folders requires much more powerful storage, indexation, access control and query capabilities. PicoDBMS was the first full fledged relational DBMS embedded in a smart card (Pucheral et al, 2001) and was implemented on top of Gemalto's smart card prototypes (Anciaux et al., 2001). PicoDBMS has been designed for managing databases stored in a (Megabyte sized) EEPROM stable memory integrated in the secure chip and protected by the chip tamper-resistance.

The SPT framework introduces important new challenges (Anciaux et al., 2007):

Figure 1. Secure Portable Token

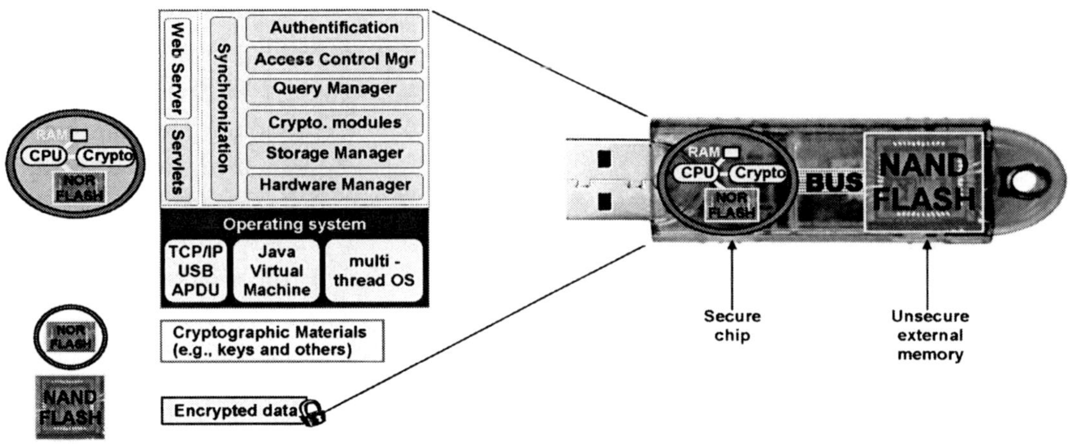

1. How to support complex queries over a large on-board database (Gigabyte sized) with very little RAM (a few kilobytes)?
2. How to organize the data storage and the indexes with an acceptable insert/update time considering the peculiarities of NAND Flash memory (fast reads, costly writes, block-erase-before-page-rewrite constraint)?
3. How to protect the on-board database against confidentiality and integrity attacks (the external Flash being not hardware protected) while keeping acceptable query performance?

The SPT architecture and the organization of the embedded software components are illustrated in Figure 1. The on-board code and sensitive data (e.g., cryptographic keys) reside in the secure chip; patient's data reside in the insecure external memory, previously encrypted by the secure execution environment. We detail below the components related to the technical challenges mentioned above.

The Query Manager is in charge of parsing the incoming database queries, building an optimal query execution plan and executing it. This module must consider peculiar execution strategies to answer complex SQL queries over a large quantity of data with little RAM (challenge 1). To tackle this challenge, we designed a massive indexing scheme presented in (Anciaux, Benzine, et al, 2007), which allows processing complex queries while consuming as little RAM as possible and still exhibiting acceptable performance. The idea is to combine in the same indexing model generalized join indices and multi-table selection indices in such a way that any combination of selection and join predicates can be evaluated by set operations over lists of sorted tuple identifiers. The operator library (algorithms for the operators of the relational algebra, e.g., select, project, join and aggregate) and the execution engine integrate those techniques.

The Storage Manager on which the query manager relies to access the database content (index and tables) is directly concerned with challenge 2. Indeed, the proposed massive indexation scheme causes a difficult problem in terms of Flash updates, due to the severe read/write constraints of NAND Flash (rewriting NAND Flash pages is a very costly operation). Therefore, we designed a structure which manages data and index keys sequentially so that the number of rewrites in Flash is minimized. The use of summarization structures based on bloom filters (Bloom, 1970) and vertical partitioning reduce the cost of index lookups (Yin et al, 2009). These additional structures are also managed in sequence. A first implementation of this principle has been patented jointly by INRIA and Gemalto (Pucheral & Yin, 2007) and is integrated in the current DBMS prototype.

The Hardware Manager embeds the methods for accessing the different memory modules of the SPT. It includes techniques associated with challenge 3 to protect the confidentiality and the integrity of the data, in an efficient way with respect to DBMS access patterns. Indeed, our massive indexation technique leads to numerous, random and fine grain accesses to raw data. We conducted preliminary studies (Anciaux et al., 2006), in which we combine encryption, hashing and timestamping techniques with query execution techniques in order to satisfy three conflicting objectives: efficiency, high security and compliance with the chip hardware resources.

The Access Control Manager is in charge of enforcing the access control policy defined to grant/deny access to pieces of the patient folder to the current user. Privileges can be associated to individual users or roles. To help collecting patients' consent, each patient should be given the chance to personalize a predefined access control policy. Hence, the Access Control Manager plays an important role in answering challenge 4 identified in the introduction. Access control is more deeply discussed in Section 6.

3.3. Data Availability and Security

Any terminal equipped with an USB port and a Web Browser can interact with the SPT and get the data he is granted access to. Hence, when no Internet connection is available (e.g., emergency situations, home intervention, remote server breakdown) SPTs guarantee patients' data availability, thereby achieving challenge 1 identified in the introduction. Furthermore, local connections to SPTs do not suffer from unpredictable performance due to overloaded remote servers or low quality connections: the embedded server is mono-user and USB-2 communication throughput is guaranteed.

In terms of security, patient's data resides in the external NAND Flash memory. As stated in section 3.2, this memory is not hardware protected so that its content must be encrypted to prevent confidentiality attacks and hashed to prevent integrity attacks. The cryptographic keys serving this purpose reside in the NOR Flash memory and are protected by the tamper-resistance of the secure chip. The encryption/decryption/hashing processes physically take place in the secure chip and are similarly hardware protected (i.e., see the red circle of Figure 1). More generally, the complete software chain (web server, servlets, DBMS) runs in the secure chip and benefits from its tamper-resistance. Hence, the authentication, access control, and query steps are all hardware protected. The security of the complete architecture thereby relies on the tamper-resistance of the secure chip. The security of our hardware platform and of the embedded code is under certification with the goal to reach the highest security level ($EAL4^+$), usually required for smart card chips used in the medical domain. This makes attacks highly improbable and extremely costly to conduct. Considering that the security of a system lies in the fact that the cost to conduct an attack outweighs its benefit, the security of our architecture is reinforced by the extreme cost of attacks and their small benefit (disclosure of a single patient's folder). Consequently, we argue that our architecture achieves convincingly challenge 4 identified in the introduction.

4. A SECURE, PERVASIVE MEDICAL FOLDER

Section 3 tackled challenges 1 and 3; this section focuses on challenge 2 that is making patient's healthcare folder seamlessly available in a connected area. Solving this challenge allows answering questions like: (1) how can the family doctor express her opinion about an emergency situation without the Patient's SPT on hand, or (2) how can survey institutes draw useful data analysis without having access to the patients' raw data? We introduce a central server in the architecture as a mean to obtain the required data availability.

This must be achieved without losing the benefits of the SPT in terms of security and control by its owner. This entails never revealing sensitive information to the central server. Two rules arise from this statement: (1) sensitive data must be stored encrypted on the server storage media, and (2) sensitive data must be encrypted and decrypted in a secure execution environment, i.e., a SPT.

To secure the communications, we use protocols such as TLS (Internet Engineering Task Force, 2008). TLS relies on a certificate authority to emit trusted certificates linking an identity to a public key. The Professionals, patients and central server safely communicate after having exchanged and checked their respective certificates. Certificates are inserted in the SPTs' secure internal memory at the beginning of their life cycle, before being delivered to its owner. The server is in charge of securing his own certificate. Note that SPTs are not durable: they may be lost or broken. Hence, to make certificates and pairs of (public key, private key) durable, they must be replicated in a Trusted Third Party (TTP). We do not detail those protocols further in this paper.

In this section, we first classify data according to their needs in terms of privacy and depict an SPT-centered architecture fulfilling these needs. Second, we focus on synchronization issues between the patient's SPT, the central server, and external entities (e.g., laboratories). Third, we present the Privacy Preserving Data Publishing protocol. Finally, we describe a comprehensive use case of the system.

4.1. A Data Classification Driven by Privacy Concerns

We call *Secret Data* (SD) the pieces of information the patient considers so sensitive (e.g., psychological analysis) that he cannot accept to delegate their storage to a remote server. Secret data remains confined to the patient's SPT. Hence SD durability is under the patient responsibility and SD availability requires the presence of the patient's SPT.

We call *Regular Data* (RD) the pieces of information the patient consents to replicate on a remote server in the clear. Such data is protected by the security policy enforced by the server and can be accessed on line by any practitioner having the required privileges. The access control policy enforced by the server and the SPT is assumed to be identical. However, the server does not benefit from the tamper-resistance of the SPT and RD can be accessed on the server without prior patient knowledge. What is actually considered as RD depends on the patient feeling, e.g., administrative data, non-sensitive medications (e.g., aspirin), non sensitive diagnosis (e.g., flue). Being replicated on the server, RD benefits from the server on-line availability and durability properties.

We call *Confined Data* (CD) the pieces of information which are too sensitive to be managed as RD but for which on-line availability and/or durability is mandatory for care practice (e.g., HIV diagnosis, chemotherapy medication, MRI image). CD is replicated encrypted on the server but the encryption keys are never present at the server. Hence CD is protected against server attacks. Encryption keys are stored and managed by SPT devices only. To ensure on-line availability, encryption keys can be shared by the SPTs of a selected set of persons, named hereafter *trusted circle* (e.g., the family doctor and some specialist physicians). Members of the trusted circle can access CD on the server and their SPT can decrypt them. Defining trusted circles is up to the patient. Durability is guaranteed by the server similarly to clear-text data. However, recovering CD entails recovering the related encryption keys. This can be achieved either by a pass phrase or by a TTP registering encryption keys. Note that Secret Data can be made durable by declaring them as confined, without sharing the encryption keys and assuming the patient trusts the cryptographic protocols.

Finally, we call *Anonymous Data* (AD) the pieces of information the patient agrees to externalize in order to contribute to a health survey (e.g., epidemiological study), provided these information will be properly anonymized. AD can be an extraction of – or a logical view built from – any data present in the folder (either SD, CD or RD). To preserve anonymity, AD can not be exported directly by the SPT hosting it but must go through a specific Privacy Preserving Data Publishing protocol.

Data classification is under patient responsibility, possibly with external help (e.g., his family doctor). The patient can change his mind afterwards (e.g., following the advice of his doctor) according to the following hierarchy: secret data → confined data → regular data → anonymous data. Any other change is uncertain, e.g., when changing from regular data to secret data, the clear regular data could have been queried or copied beforehand; the patient cannot be sure of its secrecy.

Figure 2 depicts the global architecture, showing where information resides and whether it is encrypted or not. Data located in dashed rectangles resides in a trusted storage (either the SPT's internal memory or the TTP) contrary to data located in solid rectangles. Data aside yellow locks is encrypted. This architecture provides stronger privacy preservation guarantees than any

Figure 2. Functional architecture

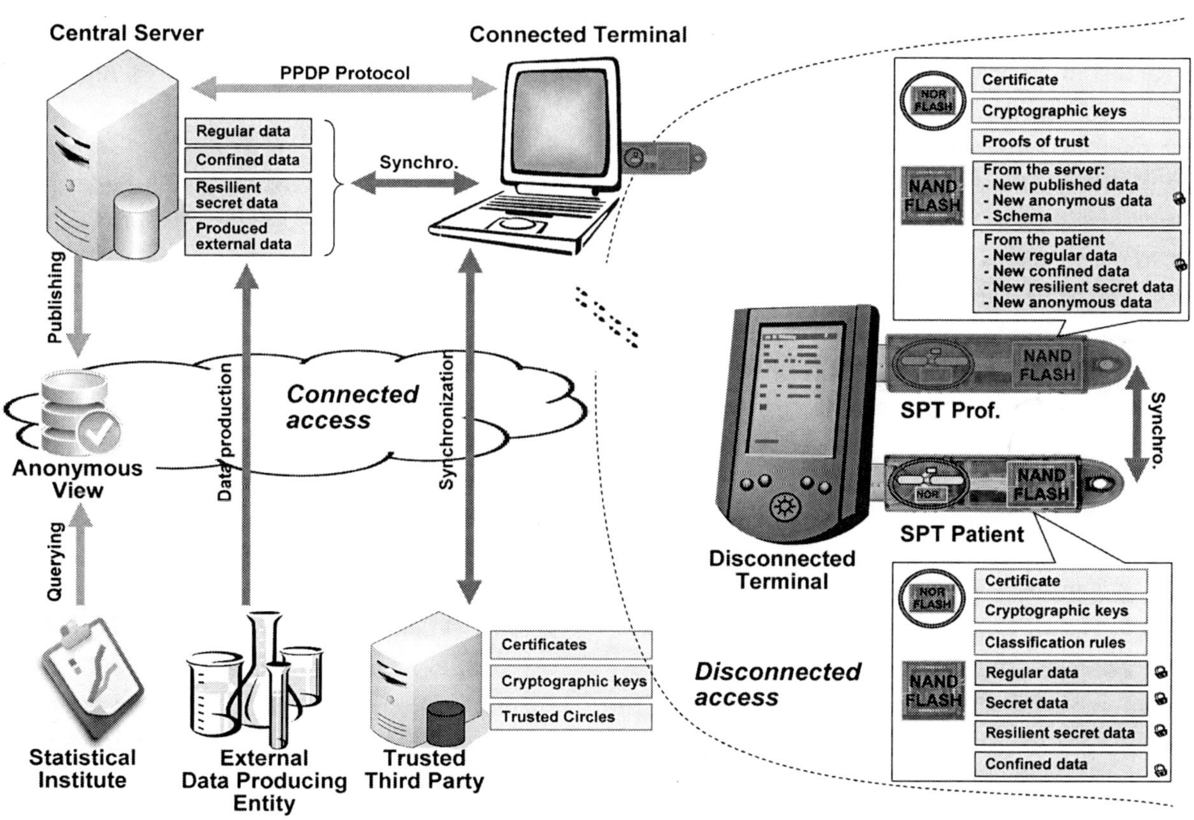

traditional EHR. Attacks conducted at the server (bypassing the traditional security measures) can only reveal regular data, secret data being absent from the server and confined data being encrypted with keys let under the control of the SPTs and the trusted third party. Attacks conducted over a patient's SPT are made highly difficult by its secure hardware.

4.2. Synchronization

Replicating data on the central server provides availability and durability, but raises a synchronization problem. When a server and a SPT are directly connected with each other, traditional synchronization methods apply. However, a SPT may never connect directly to the central server (e.g. a patient who never leaves home). In this case, SPTs of health professionals must behave as "proxies", carrying encrypted synchronization messages from patients' SPTs to the central server, and vice-versa.

Health professionals carry encrypted synchronization messages from patients' SPTs to the central server when they visit the patients. During the visit, the professional may insert new data in the patient's SPT. At the end of the visit, newly created regular and confined data (i.e., not present yet in the server) is copied into the professional's SPT. The central server is refreshed every time a professional connects to it. Conversely, the professional SPT carries encrypted data newly created at the server in order to refresh the patient's SPT replica. This situation occurs when external entities produce medical data directly on the central server, e.g., a laboratory producing examination results. However, data cannot be produced in the clear and the data is not yet classified by the patient. To circumvent this problem, external entities must encrypt data with the patient's public key before publishing them on the central server. At synchronization time, the patient will be able to decrypt this data, classify it, and store it according to its privacy class.

4.3. Privacy-Preserving Data Publishing of Data Stored in Spts

Hypothesis on the Anonymity Model

Among the various existing anonymity models, we consider in our context the most popular one, namely the *k*-anonymity model (Samarati & Sweeney, 1998). *k*-anonymity considers that a data row (also called a tuple) is made of three parts: <Identifier, {Quasi-Identifier}, {Sensitive Data}>. An Identifier (ID) identifies precisely an individual (e.g., SSN), Quasi-Identifier (QID) is a set of attributes which, combined with external knowledge, may identify an individual with a high probability (e.g., {age, zipcode}), and Sensitive Data is a set of attributes considered sensitive by the patient (e.g., {diagnosis}). To be *k*-anonymous, a tuple must not contain Identifier and have its Quasi-Identifier indistinguishable from the Quasi-Identifier of at least *k* other tuples. Generalization based algorithms (Sweeney, 1998; Samarati, 2001; Lefevre et al, 2006) aim at generalizing Quasi-Identifiers of an input set of tuples into equivalence classes such that each class contains at least *k* tuples. As an example, consider the schema <SSN, {age, zipcode}, {diagnosis}> and the tuples <1, {105, 75001}, Cancer>, <2, {31, 75002}, Cold>. 2-anonymizing these tuples would yield the following result: <{[31, 105], [75001, 75002]}, Cancer>, <{[31, 105], [75001, 75002]}, Cold>. Hence, an attacker would be unable to infer who has Cancer or Cold even with external knowledge.

The schema of Anonymous Data (i.e., Quasi-Identifiers, and Sensitive Data) depends on the statistical study. It is defined by data analysts, signed by the TTP (because AD specification is sensitive) and the patient must consent to externalize it. Note that for the sake of simplicity, the current version of the protocol does not cope with multiple anonymizations of overlapping Anonymous Data because it may lead to disclosures (Yao et al., 2005; Wang & Fung, 2006; Xiao &

Tao, 2007), nor with multiple tuples per individual (Nergiz et al., 2007).

Hypothesis on the PPDP Infrastructure

Computing the equivalence classes requires knowing the whole set of input quasi-identifiers. Due to their unpredictable connection patterns, it is difficult for SPTs to share their QIDs among them. Our PPDP protocol uses the central server to collect QIDs and compute the corresponding equivalence classes, taking care of never disclosing to the server the association between a given QID and a clear-text Sensitive Data. The PPDP protocol does the following assumptions on the infrastructure: (1) participating SPTs are considered seldom connected, powerful enough to perform simple tasks, and highly trustworthy; (2) the server is highly available (24h/7d) and highly powerful; (3) the server is untrusted and can adopt the following attack models:

- **Semi-Honest:** the server obeys the protocol it is participating in but tries to infer confidential data by exploiting in any possible way the result of each step of this protocol;
- **Weakly-Malicious:** the server may cheat the protocol to infer information, but does so only if SPTs can not detect the cheat and if the output remains correct (i.e., no deny of service attacks).

PPDP Protocols

Assuming the existence of an anonymous communication channel between SPTs and the server, a simple way to cope with the Semi-Honest attack model is to use the following three-phases protocol, called *Naive* hereafter:

1. **Collection Phase:** Each contributing SPT sends its QID to the server;
2. **Construction Phase:** When the server has gathered enough QIDs (this judgment can be based on any traditional data utility metric (Fung et al, 2010)), it computes the corresponding equivalence classes;
3. **Anonymization Phase:** The SPT that have contributed to the Collection Phase send their Sensitive Data to the server and tell him to which equivalence class they are associated.

The Naive protocol is secure but it incurs a high – and even unbounded latency – because each participating SPT must connect twice (in the Collection and the Anonymization phases).

By sharing a common encryption/decryption key among SPTs (e.g., inserted at initialization time), the set of SPTs participating to the Collection and the Anonymization phases can be different. Hence, the *Robust* protocol presented below overcomes the latency drawback of Naive:

1. **Collection Phase:** Each contributing SPT sends to the server its QID and its Sensitive Data encrypted with the common key. Note that in order to avoid inferences through encrypted patterns, Sensitive Data must be encrypted in such a way that two identical data do not yield the same encrypted value (e.g., by concatenating a random number to the Sensitive Data);
2. **Construction Phase:** When the server has gathered enough QIDs, it computes the corresponding equivalence classes;
3. **Anonymization Phase:** Every SPT which connects downloads an equivalence class, and returns the decrypted Sensitive Data in background. The time required by this task remains low since it depends on the size of a single equivalence class (i.e., between k and ($2k$-1) tuples, with k usually small).

The Weakly-Malicious attack model assumes that the server can cheat by producing two or more equivalence classes whose associated sets of QIDs overlap. By computing the differences between the *k*-anonymous overlapping results, the server is able to break the *k*-anonymity of tuples belonging to the overlapping classes. For example, let C1 and C2 be two overlapping classes, the QIDs belonging to C1 and not to C2 correspond to the tuples appearing in C1 anonymization and not in C2 anonymization, thereby decreasing the effective value of *k*. We call these cheats *Differential Attacks*. The *WM* protocol builds on the Robust protocol to forbid Differential Attacks. The respective Collection and Anonymization Phases are different in that more information is exchanged in order to allow the detection of attacks. The Construction Phase remains the same. We refer the interested reader to (Allard et al., 2010).

4.4. Use Case

Let us illustrate the behavior of the system through a scenario involving four participants: an elderly patient named Patrick, his family doctor David, a nurse Nora, and a spy Sandra. Patrick, David, and Nora have each their own SPT. Several medical examinations are prescribed to Patrick who classifies them as regular, confined, and secret data. Patrick recently went through blood exams into a medical laboratory. The medical lab performing the examination has published the encrypted results on the central server. Results were encrypted with Patrick's public key obtained from the trusted third party.

Nora frequently visits Patrick at home. Patrick has no internet connection and leaves home seldom. Thus, Nora acts as a synchronization means for Patrick's folder (as do any other person visiting Patrick and owning a SPT). Before the visit, Nora downloads from the central server the latest updates performed in Patrick's folder, encrypted with Patrick's public key. This includes the recent examination results. During the visit, Nora's and Patrick's SPTs synchronize: Nora's SPT send to Patrick's SPT the encrypted examination results, Patrick's SPT decrypts them with his private key, classifies and encrypts them accordingly to their classes – lab results are confined data – and sends them back to Nora's SPT which will refresh the central server the next time it connects to it. Nora's SPT also copies the latest updates performed in Patrick's local folder, if any. Nora cannot get access to this data, protected by the tamper resistance of the SPT.

During a previous visit, Patrick asked David to join his trusted circle. Patrick's SPT hashed and signed David's certificate and this proof of trust was uploaded onto the TTP. After Nora's visit, at his office, he can connect to the central server and view Patrick's up-to-date folder, including the results of the recent examinations (classified as confined data) and possible updates carried back by Nora (in the limit of David's access rights). When visiting Patrick at home, David gets the same information by accessing data directly through Patrick's SPT.

During another visit of David, Patrick's SPT warns Patrick that a nation-wide epidemiological study is being launched and discloses him the schema of the data required by the study. Following David advice, and because Patrick knows that his privacy is well protected, he agrees to contribute. Patrick's SPT forms Patrick's Anonymous data by following the desired schema and runs the collection phase of the PPDP protocol (either Robust or WM depending on the nation-wide policy). Once the construction phase has been completed by the server, every connected SPT can contribute to the anonymization phase of the protocol up to its completion, for the global benefit of all patients.

One day, Patrick's loses his SPT which is found by Sandra. Missing the PIN code, Sandra cannot authenticate to the SPT. She can open the SPT and snoop at the NAND FLASH memory content but data is encrypted. If she tries to tamper the secure chip to obtain the decryption key, security counter measures will destroy the embedded components. The only attack which could be successfully conducted is against the regular data on the central server. Any sensitive data is stored encrypted (the key being within SPTs or on the trusted third party). A few days after, Patrick receives a new SPT, containing both his keys and his data, and continues to receive visits at home from his health practitioners.

5. EXPRESSING PATIENT'S CONSENT

Trusting the EHR security is a prerequisite for the patient to give her consent about a pervasive use of her medical folder but it is definitely not a sufficient condition. Expressing an enlightened consent means understanding and accepting an access control policy specifying who (individuals or roles) is granted access to which part of her folder. This section details the notion of user's privacy and surveys the current models and mechanisms to achieve it.

5.1 Privacy Protection

Legal Approach

Roughly, privacy is the protection of Personally Identifiable Information (PII), by means of restricting access, transfer, storage, etc. of PII. The concept of "informed consent" is a cornerstone of most privacy regulations. The consent of use of personal data must be an enlightened, free, univocal and unilateral act. Protecting PII is a prime concern for the deployment of pervasive computing systems such as EHR (Langheinrich, 2005).

The European Union Directive 95/46/EC sets the protection of individuals with regard to the processing of personal data. Article 29 of this directive establishes a set of core principles of privacy, which are quite close to the ten founding principles of Hippocratic database systems (Agrawal et al., 2002):

1. The *purpose limitation principle*: data must be processed for a specific and declared purpose.
2. The *data quality and proportionality principle*: data must be accurate, adequate and relevant wrt the declared purpose.
3. The *transparency principle*: information must be provided as to the purpose of the processing, the identity of the data controller must be ensured.
4. The *security principle*: appropriate security measures must be taken.
5. The *rights of access, rectification and opposition*.
6. *Restrictions on onward transfers*.

As stated by the Article 29 Working party (Article 29 Data Protection Working Party, 2007), one of the essential principles concerning EHR is limiting access to a folder to only those healthcare professionals who are involved in the patient's treatment. Data protection could be enhanced by modular access rights: the patient should be given the chance to prevent access to his EHR data if he so chooses. This requires prior information about the possible consequences of not allowing access.

Privacy Preferences

A lot of attention has been dedicated to expression of privacy preferences, which are consent of use of PII expressed according to the above mentioned principles. The Platform for Privacy Preferences (P3P) defined by the W3C is a machine readable format of privacy preferences. The Platform for Enterprise Privacy Practices (E-P3P) (Karjoth et al., 2002) or EPAL (Ashley et al., 2003) define the enterprise privacy enforcement system for privacy policies internal to the enterprise. P3P is used to state an enterprise's privacy policy when collecting PII from the customers whereas E-P3P is used for internally enforcing the enterprise's policy to control accesses to the collected PII.

As coined by the title of (Massacci & Zannone, 2004) "Privacy Is Linking Permission to Purpose", the purpose (e.g. from P3P: marketing, surveys, payment etc.) is the intended use of the data queried and is the backbone of informed consent. Thus, integrating purpose (and obligations related to these purposes) into control is one of the main challenges and research directions investigated in privacy protection.

5.2. Control Mechanisms for Privacy

Traditional Access Control

An Access Control (AC) (or authorization) policy is a specialized form of security policy, dedicated to permission management. AC primarily aims at enforcing confidentiality (Samarati & Di Vimercati, 2001). Access control is one of the means to enhance privacy by restricting access to personal data. An AC policy is structured according to a model. The model formally describes the language in which policies are expressed and how to decide whether an access request should be granted or denied.

Traditional AC models are the Mandatory Access Control (MAC) and the Discretionary Access Control (DAC). MAC is a label-based (e.g. Unclassified, Confidential, Secret, Top Secret) AC mechanism. Each user and each data is associated to a unique label. Access on a data is allowed if the user is granted sufficient clearance level. DAC is a decentralized user-based mechanism where the creator of a data defines the set of authorizations.

Intermediate concepts between data and users have been introduced to simplify administration of AC policies. In the Role-Based Access Control (RBAC) models family, roles are assigned to users and permissions are assigned to those roles (Ferraiolo et al., 2003). Thus, an RBAC policy is a set of assignments between users and roles and between roles and permissions. The core rule of RBAC states that an access request is granted iff the issuer endorses a role with this privilege.

From the RBAC initiative, several models have been studied in the literature. These models may either extend RBAC (e.g. with temporal or geographical constraints), or organize policies by mean of additional concepts (e.g. team, task, organization) to enhance their expressive power and flexibility. First-order logic has been advocated as a general framework suitable to formalize AC models and policies (Halpern & Weissman, 2008).

Access Control for Privacy

Traditional AC models such as RBAC are commonly used to organize access rights. However, they are not adequate to express finer control on data usage. Usage CONtrol model (UCON) is a foundation for next-generation access control models. In this model, a usage control decision is determined by combining authorizations, obligations, and conditions (Zhang et al., 2005). Usage control is a way to implement digital rights management, for instance by providing guarantees of restriction on onward transfers.

In order to guarantee the purpose limitation principle, the notion of purpose should be used for access control. A policy should ensure that data can only be used for its intended purpose, and the access purpose should be compliant with the data's intended purpose. The authors (Yang et al., 2007) have proposed a purpose-based AC model on this basis. (Ni et al., 2007) have bound purposes to RBAC in an integrated model Privacy-Aware RBAC (P-RBAC). This model has been refined to include the definition of conditional obligations. The integration of purpose control and RBAC for privacy protection of relational data has been investigated too (Byun & Li, 2008).

Specialized Access Control Models for Health Record

Several models have been defined to organize rights on medical data. Alhaqbani and Fidge propose a cascaded AC architecture made of three AC layers (2007). First layer is based on DAC, second one on RBAC and last one on MAC. When all the three policies agree, access is granted. The authors of (Røstad & Nytrø, 2008) have more tightly combined DAC and RBAC into the Personally Controlled Health Record (PCHR) AC system. In their approach, two policies are defined: a common one and personalized one. Only the personalized one is defined by EHR's owner. A conflict resolution rule (e.g. deny overrides, permit overrides) is defined, it is used whenever the two policies disagree on the access decision.

Alhaqbani and Fidge (2007) and Røstad and Nytrø (2008) concentrate on policies defined by the owner of the EHR, data being centralized and held in a single device. Becker and Sewell focus on high level regulations expressed at national level (Becker & Sewell, 2004). They propose a logical language called Cassandra. This language is based on Datalog with constraints, a fragment of first-order logic studied by the databases community which enjoys good decidability properties.

5.3. Toward a Health Record Masking Model

Researches on usage control, purpose-based AC, privacy preferences and practices provide many valuable results to deal with privacy protection and consent expression. Current researches address a broad scope of privacy issues (e.g., enterprise-wide privacy practices or preference language) able to deal with complex rules (e.g., conditional obligations, time restricted usage, logic rules and constraints). However, access control policies usually defined to regulate accesses to EHR systems are far too complex to expect collecting an enlightened consent of the patients on them, as required by the law. This is due to two main characteristics of these policies:

C1. Huge number of AC rules, due to a high number of people interacting with a folder, combined with a large diversity of roles and privileges.

C2. Complexity of the data to be protected, usually described with a highly specialized terminology, and combined with an intrinsic difficulty to determine which data (or data association) reveals a given pathology.

The default access control policy defined for the future French DMP (Personal Medical Folder) illustrates this complexity quite well. As pictured in Figure 3, this RBAC-based policy is expressed as a matrix Document × Role, where elements of Document are the classes of documents constituting a healthcare folder, elements of Role are the roles which can be played by practitioners and each entry gives the corresponding Read and Write privileges. In its current form, this matrix already contains more than 400 entries while classes of documents are very coarse grain to implement an effective control (e.g., radiographies may reveal very different pathologies depending on the organ). What is finally revealed remains obscure to the patient.

In the light of this example, default access control policy must be considered as the expression of the need-to-know principle (i.e., a user should be granted access to the information strictly required to accomplish the tasks related to his role) rather than a tool which can be configured by the patient to better protect his own privacy. The right to hide part of his medical history has however been recognized by the law to the patients, with a prior information about the possible consequences of this action. We believe that collecting the enlightened consent of the patient requires providing them with effective and comprehensive tools to mask the undesirable information in his folder. To this end, we devised a masking model which consists in defining additional rules, semantically meaningful for each patient (based on self defined terms) and which takes priority over the default access control policy the patient cannot master.

Figure 3. Default matrix of the French DMP (Personal Medical Folder) http://www.d-m-p.org/docs/TabCxPS.pdf

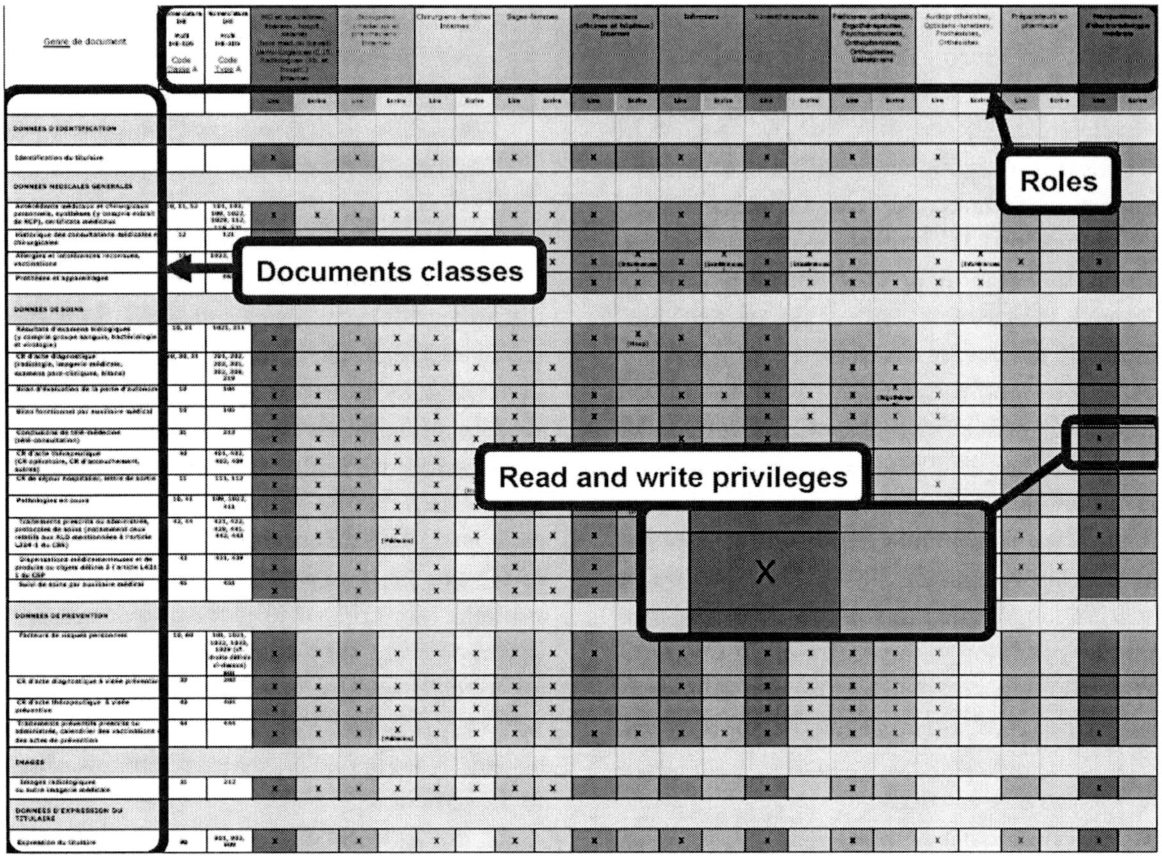

6. EBAC: AN EVENT-BASED ACCESS CONTROL MODEL

The Event-Based Access Control model (EBAC) has been designed to help the patient in masking sensitive healthcare records in his folder. Design rational of EBAC is simplicity and accuracy. The model is organized according to the main concepts of events, episodes and relation of confidence.

- **Event:** any document added to a medical folder is associated to an event. Events are endowed with properties, among which the *author* of the document (i.e., a practitioner) and the medical *episode* it belongs to.
- **Episode:** an *episode* is a set of events semantically linked and for which the patients wants to define a common masking policy. For example, the patient may define episodes "MyAbortion2008", "MySecondDepression" and associate incoming events to them, potentially with the help of his family doctor. The patient defines his masking policy on an episode basis by defining who (role or identified users) is granted to participate to this episode.
- **Relation of confidence:** the participation of a practitioner P to an episode is regulated by a relation of confidence with the patient stating (1) which event P can see in this episode and (2) who can see the events

produced by P himself in this episode (e.g., Dr Guru can see only the events he produces and nobody else than Guru and the patient can see these same events). In other words, the participants of an episode constitute a trusted circle as defined in Section 4.1 and the relation of confidence defines the scope of their respective actions in this episode. To make the model simple and intuitive, we introduce two scopes for the read the write actions termed *shared* (denoted by S) and *exclusive* (denoted by X). Combining these scopes leads to four possible relations of confidence:

SS: practitioner P can read the shared events in the episode, and produces himself shared events for the episode;

SX: practitioner P can read the shared events in the episode, and produces exclusive events for the episode;

XS: practitioner P can read the exclusive events produced by him in the episode, and produces shared events for the episode;

XX: practitioner P can read the exclusive events produced by him in the episode, and produces exclusive events for the episode;

The main ideas of the model are therefore:

- There exists a default (role-based) AC matrix which is defined at the regulation level and that cannot be modified by the owner of the EHR,
- Each healthcare record is associated to an event, itself related to (at most) one episode and the owner defines his masking policy at the episode level,
- Access decision is taken according to the identity of the querier, the author of the event and the episode the event belongs to, with priority given to the masking rule in case of conflict with the AC matrix,
- Only read permission is considered: the aim on the EBAC model is only to prevent from privacy disclosure, other actions are controlled at the regulation level.

The next section formalizes the EBAC model with sets and functions. Note that we do restrict ourselves to information related to AC decision. In a real implementation, basic types would be refined into more complex types. In the definitions, ∇ denotes the absence of value, $A \times B$ is the Cartesian products of sets A and B, and $\wp(U)$ denotes the set of all subsets of a set U.

6.1. Formal Definitions

Let's introduce basic types:

- **Identifiers:** the set of events' identifiers.
- **Users:** the set of users' identifiers.
- **Form:** the set of documents (or forms) constituting the medical folder.
- **Episodes:** the set of episodes.
- **SS, SX, XS and XX:** four functions that maps each episode to a set of users ($Episodes \rightarrow \wp(Users)$. Moreover $SS(e) \cap SX(e) \cap XS(e) \cap XX(e) = \varnothing$.
- **Events:** the set of events.
- $id : Events \rightarrow Identifiers$, $form : Events \rightarrow Forms$, $author : Events \rightarrow Users$ and $episode : Events \rightarrow Episodes \cup \{\nabla\}$:four functions that maps an event to (respectively) an identifier, a form, an author and an episode (if any).

Note that the sets S_{ep} and S_{∇} defined respectively as $S_{ep} = \{e \in Events | episode(e) = ep\}$ and $S_{\nabla} = \{e \in Events | episode(e) = \nabla\}$ define a partition of events according to the (unique) episode they belong: $\bigcup_{ep \in Episodes} S_{ep} \cup S_{\nabla} = Events$

Now we introduce two relations for the default access control matrix. Actually, it is role-based, but on more generic treatment it could be any access control model provided that a function exists. The definitions we propose are related to the flat RBAC model but may be easily extended by role hierarchy. Following definitions are from [Ferraiolo et al. 2003]:

- **Roles:** the set of roles
- $URA \subseteq Users \times Roles$: a relation for "user-role assignment"
- $PRA \subseteq Roles \times Forms$: a relation for "permission-role assignment"
- $DefaultMatrix \subseteq Users \times Forms = \{(u,f) \in Users \times Forms \mid \exists r \in Roles \wedge (u,r) \in URA \wedge (r,f) \in PRA\}$ the relation defined as the join on roles of *URA* and *PRA* relations.
- $defaultAccess :: Users \times Event \rightarrow \{true, false\}$ a function that determine whether a user's access query on an event is granted. The function is defined as:
  - $defaultAccess(u,e) = true$, iff *form(e)=f* and *(u,f)* $\in DefaultMatrix$

Now, we define the semantic of the sets of users SS, SX, XS and XX of a given episode e. The idea is to use these sets to define rights based on the identity of the user who try to access and the identity of the user who wrote the event. A user is always able to access an event he wrote himself.

- $perceive : Episodes \rightarrow \wp(Users), perceive(e) = SX(e) \cup SS(e)$ is the set of users who may read events related to the episode.
- $hidden : Episodes \rightarrow \wp(Users), hidden(e) = XX(e) \cup SX(e)$ is the set of users whose events are hidden to others.
- $access' : Episodes \times Users \times Users \rightarrow \{true, false\}$: the function that tell whether access to an episode *e* by a user *u*, on a event written by user *a* is granted. The function is defined as:
  - $access'(e,u,a) = true$ if $(a = u) \vee (u \in perceive(e) \wedge a \notin hidden(e))$
- $access : Users \times Events \rightarrow \{true, false\}$: the function that tell whether an access by a user *u* on an event *e* is granted or not. If the event is not related to any episode (∇), access is granted, else, we rely on function *access'*. The function *access* is defined as:
  - $access(u,e) = true$ if $episode(e) = \nabla$,
  - $access(u,e) = true$ if $episode(e) \neq \nabla$ and $access'(episode(e), u, author(e)) = true$,
  - $access(u,e) = false$ otherwise.

Finally, we combine the access decision based on the default access control model, which express the need to know based on role assignment, and on the episode related to the event. Access is granted if both access control decisions agree.

- $granted : Users \times Events \rightarrow \{true, false\}$: the function that combines *defaultAccess* and *access*, it is defined as:
  - $granted(u,e) = true$ iff $defaultAccess(u,e) \wedge access(u,e)$

6.2. Sample Policy

To illustrate the approach, we define a sample EBAC policy. Four professionals named Guru (an adept of alternative medicine), MyPhysician, MyNurse, and AnotherPhysician are acting with the system. The patient we consider has defined

Table 1.

	∇	E1	E2				
	e1	*e2*	*e3*	*e4*	*e5*	*e6*	*e7*
Guru	T	T	F	T	F	F	F
MyPhysician	T	T	T	F	T	T	F
MyNurse	T	F	T	F	F	F	F
AnotherPhys.	T	T	F	F	F	F	T

two episodes, one for a cancer and another one for an abortion, with the following rules:

- *E1*, "Cancer": *XX(E1)={Guru}, SS(E1)={ MyPhysician, MyNurse }*. This rule states that Guru, MyPhysician and MyNurse constitute the trusted circle for episode E1, in addition to the patient himself. No other user can read events in this episode whatever the default access control policy. MyPhysician and MyNurse share the documents produced in this episode, except those produced by Guru, because the patients wants to hide that he consults Guru for his cancer.
- *E2, "Abortion": SX(E2)={ MyPhysician, AnotherPhysician }, SS(E2)={ MyNurse }* MyPhysician, AnotherPhysician and MyNurse constitute the trusted circle of episode E2. MyNurse, who did practice the abortion, produces shared events. MyPhysician and AnotherPhysician share these events but what they produce themselves is kept invisible to each other. Such a rule may be defined by the patient after consulting MyPhysican about a problem following the abortion, and before consulting AnotherPhysician for a second opinion, whether the patient does not fully trust MyPhysician diagnosis.

Let us define a sample flat RBAC:

- $(Guru, Physician) \in URA$, $(MyPhysician, Physician) \in URA$, $(MyNurse, Nurse) \in URA$
- $(Physician, General) \in PRA$, $(Physician, Treatment) \in PRA$, $(Nurse, General) \in PRA$

The health record is composed of 7 events:

1. $e1 = (General, MyNurse, \nabla)$
2. $e2 = (Treatment, MyPhysician, \nabla)$
3. $e3 = (General, MyPhysician, E1)$
4. $e4 = (Treatment, Guru, E1)$
5. $e5 = (Treatment, MyPhysician, E2)$
6. $e6 = (General, MyPhysician, E2)$
7. $e7 = (General, AnotherPhysician, E2)$

Using function *granted* the following AC matrix can be computed, where T denotes true and F denotes false (see Table 1):

A proof of concept of the EBAC model has been developed in the Haskell (http://www.haskell.org) functional programming language.

6.3. Implementation Issues

This section sketches how the EBAC model is implemented in the embedded DBMS (see Section 3.2) and how it is used by patients.

A patient can incrementally define episodes (e.g., "Cancer", "Abortion") for his folder. Then, for each event, he chooses:

1. the set of practitioners constituting the trusted circle for this episode;
2. the relation of confidence attached to each.

To implement those access policies in the SPT using the relational model (Codd, 1970), the following relations are added to the database (the view below is simplified for the sake of simplicity):

Event (**Event_id**, *Episode_id*, *User_id*, Write_scope, …)
Episode (**Episode_id**, Label, …)
User (**User_id**, User_name, …)
Privilege (**Privilege_id**, *Episode_id*, *User_id*, read_scope, write_scope, …)
Notations: attributes in bold are primary keys; attributes in italic are foreign keys.

Relation Event logs the events occurring on the medical folder (e.g., insertion of a document), and refers to relations User and Episode. Relation User stores the set of practitioners interacting with the medical folder, and relation Episode stores the set of episodes defined by the patient. The relations of confidence are stored in the relation Privilege with references to relations Episode and User.

At the time of creation of each event, the reference to the user (User_id) originating the event is specified. The reference to the corresponding episode (Episode_id) is created on demand, i.e., at the time of the insertion or later, and the corresponding write scope (write_scope is set to S or X) is filled at that time by querying the relation Privilege.

For example, at creation of event $e3 = (General, MyPhysician, E1)$ of the previous example, event e3 in relation Event refers to the practitioner MyPhysician in relation User and is linked to the episode Cancer. Since the write scope of MyPhysician for episode Cancer is S, the attribute value write_scope in Event is set to S.

At execution time, a query Q issued by a practitioner P on the folder is rewritten to integrate access control. Our implementation requires joining each result of Q with relation Event, and projecting the event tuples on attributes Event.write_scope, Event.user_id and Event.episode_id. Before delivering the tuples to P, access control is checked by applying the following filtering condition:

Event.user_id = current_user OR (Event.write_scope = S AND Event.episode_id IN CC), where CC denotes the set of episodes the current user participates in (i.e., is member of the related trusted circle). This condition is checked by a system query on relation Privileges executed and stored at the time of the connection of the practitioner to the SPT.

Each result tuple qualified on this condition satisfies the access control policy defined by the user. Finally, attributes Event.write_scope, Event.user_id and Event.episode_id are removed before delivering the result tuple to P.

7. FUTURE WORK

The SPT hardware platform is today operational and the main software components described in the preceding sections have been developed and integrated: central server, embedded web server, embedded DBMS and synchronization protocol. The application itself is being developed and will be experimented in the field by the end of 2009 on a population of about 100 elderly patients and 25 practitioners. The ageing of population makes the health monitoring of elderly people at home crucial. In this context, sensitive data has to be shared between all participants of medical-social networks (doctors, nurses, social workers, home help and family circle) with different access rights. The data must be available at the patient's bedside for a better monitoring of their health cares. For this purpose, the Yvelines District in France has decided to carry out an experimental project of

Shared Medical-Social Folder (DMSP in French). In the first step, this project targets elderly people from two gerontology networks. At mid-term, it could be extended to other vulnerable people in unstable or handicapped situation.

ALDS (a home care association) has already carried out a "Common Medical Folder" in paper format, which enables professionals and participants from medical-social sectors to write down crucial facts related to the monitoring of elderly people. While the day-to-day use of this paper folder has proved its efficiency, two burning issues were still unresolved:

- **No privacy:** all participants (practitioners but also social workers, home help and family circle) can read all records in the patient's folder while some patients are facing complex human situations (diagnosis of terminal illness, addictions, financial difficulties, etc).
- **No remote access to the folder:** consequently, the folder is not updated consistently and timely, leading to a lesser accurate monitoring.

The objective of this experiment in the field is precisely to demonstrate the accuracy of the proposed technology to tackle these two issues. This project involves INRIA (the French National Research Institute in Computer Sciences), University of Versailles, SANTEOS (a French EHR provider), Gemalto (the smart card world leader), ALDS (a home care association) and COGITEY (a clinic for elderly people).

8. CONCLUSION

EHR projects are being launched in most developed countries. The benefits provided by centralizing the healthcare information in database servers in terms of information quality, availability and protection against failure are unquestionable. Yet, patients are reluctant to abandon the control over highly sensitive data (e.g., data revealing a severe or shameful disease) to a distant server. In addition, the access to the folder is conditioned by the existence of a high speed and secure internet connection at any place and any time.

This paper capitalizes on a new hardware portable device, associating the security of a smart card to the storage capacity of a USB key, to give the control back to the patient over his medical history. We have shown how this device can complement a traditional EHR server (1) to protect and share highly sensitive data among trusted parties and (2) to provide a seamless access to the data even in disconnected mode. From the architectural point of view, the key point is the embedding in a secure chip of the complete software chain usually running on traditional servers: web server, servlets, DBMS and finally the database itself. From the usage point of view, the key point is a new way of personalizing access control policies with minimal assistance of practitioners. While both contributions are orthogonal, their integration in the same infrastructure allows building trustworthy pervasive healthcare folders.

The solution proposed will be experimented in the context of a medical-social network providing medical care and social services at home for elderly people. The expected outcome of this experiment is to demonstrate the effectiveness of the proposed technology with a positive impact on the coordination of medical and social workers and on the acceptance of patients of an electronic usage of their medical history.

ACKNOWLEDGMENT

This work is partially funded by the Yvelines District Council through the DMSP project and by ANR (the French National Agency for Research) through the PlugDB project. The authors wish to thank Laurent Braconnier and Jean-François Navarre (Yvelines District Council),

Philippe Kesmarszky (ALDS), Sophie Lartigue (COGITEY), Morgane Berthelot (SANTEOS), Jean-Jacques Vandewalle (Gemalto) and Karine Zeitouni (University of Versailles) for their active participation in these two projects. Special thanks are also due to Benjamin Nguyen who participated to the definition of the Privacy Preserving Data Publishing protocol.

REFERENCES

Agrawal, R., Kiernan, J., Srikant, R., & Xu, Y. (2002). Hippocratic Databases. In. *Proceedings of VLDB*, *02*, 143–154.

Alhaqbani, B., & Fidge, C. J. (2007). Access Control Requirements for Processing Electronic Health Records Business. In *Proceedings of the Process Management Workshops* (pp. 371-382).

Allard, T., Nguyen, B., & Pucheral, P. (in press). *Safe Anonymization with Smart Tokens*. Retrieved from http://www-smis.inria.fr/Epublications.html

Alliance. (2008, April 28). *The National Alliance for Health Information Technology, on Defining Key Health Information Technology Term*. Retrieved February 17, 2009, from http://www.hhs.gov/healthit/documents/m20080603/10_2_hit_terms.pdf

Anciaux, N., Benzine, M., Bouganim, L., Pucheral, P., & Shasha, D. (2007). GhostDB: Querying visible and hidden data without leaks. In *Proceedings of the ACM SIGMOD Conference* (pp. 677-688).

Anciaux, N., Bobineau, C., Bouganim, L., Pucheral, P., & Valduriez, P. (2001). PicoDBMS: Validation and Experience. In *Proceedings of the International Conference on Very Large Data Bases (VLDB)* (pp. 709-710).

Anciaux, N., Bouganim, L., & Pucheral, P. (2006). Data Confidentiality: to which extent cryptography and secured hardware can help. *Annales des Télécommunications*, *61*(3-4), 267–283.

Anciaux, N., Bouganim, L., & Pucheral, P. (2007). Future Trends in Secure Chip Data Management. *A Quarterly Bulletin of the Computer Society of the IEEE Technical Committee on Data Engineering*, *30*(3), 49–57.

Article 29 Data Protection Working Party. (2007). *Working Document on the processing of personal data relating to health in electronic health records (EHR)* (Tech. Rep. 00323/07/EN WP 131). Brussels, Belgium: European Commission.

Ashley, P., Hada, S., Karjoth, G., Powers, C., & Schunter, M. (2003). *Enterprise Privacy Authorization Language (EPAL 1.2)*. IBM Tivoli Software, IBM Research.

Becker, M. Y., & Sewell, P. (2004). Cassandra: Flexible Trust Management, Applied to Electronic Health Records. *Computer Security Foundations Workshop* (pp. 139-154).

Bloom, B. (1970). Space/time tradeoffs in hash coding with allowable errors. *Communications of the ACM*, *13*(7), 422–426. doi:10.1145/362686.362692

Brown, S. H., Lincoln, M. J., Groen, P. J., & Kolodner, R. M. (2003). VistA, U.S. Department of Veterans Affairs national scale HIS. *International Journal of Medical Informatics*, *69*, 135–156. doi:10.1016/S1386-5056(02)00131-4

Byun, J., & Li, N. (2008). Purpose based access control for privacy protection in relational database systems. *The VLDB Journal*, *17*, 603–619. doi:10.1007/s00778-006-0023-0

Carrasco, L. C. (1999). *RDBMS's for Java Cards? What a Senseless Idea!* ISOL Corp.

Codd, E. F. (1970). A Relational Model of Data for Large Shared Data Banks. *Communications of the ACM*, *13*(6), 377–387. doi:10.1145/362384.362685

Computer World. (2003, December). *NASA Sites Hacked*. Retrieved February 17, 2009, from http://www.computerworld.com/securitytopics/security/cybercrime/story/0,10801,88348,00.html

Computer World. (2006, August). *Survey: 81% of U.S. firms lost laptops with sensitive data in the past year*. Retrieved February 17, 2009, from http://www.computerworld.com/action/article.do?command=viewArticleBasic&articleId=9002493&source=NLT_PM&nlid=8

Dahl, M. R. (2006). *Status and perspective of personal health informatics in Denmark*. Aarhus, Denmark: University of Aarhus, Section for Health Informatics, Institute of Public Health. Retrieved February 17, 2009, from http://www.ieee2407.org/files/ws01_mads01.pps

Door, J.-P. (2008). *Le dossier médical personnel* (Information Rep. No. 659). Paris: Assemblée Nationale. eHealth Insider. (2008, January 16). *German doctors say no to centrally stored patient records*. Retrieved February 17, 2009, from http://www.e-health-insider.com/news/3384/.

Eurosmart. (2008, April). *Smart USB Token*. Retrieved February 17, 2009, from http://www.eurosmart.com/images/doc/WorkingGroups/NewFF/Papers/eurosmart_smart_usb_token_wp_april08.pdf

Ferraiolo, D. F., Kuhn, R. D., & Chandramouli, R. (2003). *Role-Based Access Control*. Norwood, MA: Artech House Publishers.

FierceHealthIT news. (2006, August 20). *Massive data loss at HCA*. Retrieved February 17, 2009, from http://www.fiercehealthit.com/story/massive-data-loss-at-hca/2006-08-21

FierceHealthIT news. (2008, September). *GA hospital health data breach due to outsourcing error.* Retrieved February 17, 2009, from http://www.fiercehealthit.com/story/ga-hospital-health-data-breach-due-outsourcing-error/2008-09-28

Fung, B. C. M., Wang, K., Chen, R., & Yu, P. S. (in press). Privacy-preserving data publishing: A survey on recent developments. *ACM Computing Surveys*.

Gordon, L. A., Loeb, M. P., Lucyshin, W., & Richardson, R. (2006). *2006 CSI/FBI Computer Crime and Security Survey*. Retrieved February 17, 2009, from http://i.cmpnet.com/gocsi/db_area/pdfs/fbi/FBI2006.pdf

Halpern, J. Y., & Weissman, V. (2008). Using First-Order Logic to Reason about Policies. *ACM Transactions on Information and System Security*, *11*, 1–41. doi:10.1145/1380564.1380569

Husek, C. (2008, August). *ELGA: The Electronic Health Record in Austria*. Paper presented at the International Conference of Society for Medical Innovation and Technology, Vienna, Austria.

Internet Engineering Task Force. (2008). *The Transport Layer Security (TLS) Protocol Version 1.2*. Retrieved February 17, 2009, from http://tools.ietf.org/html/rfc5246

ISO/IEC. (1999). Integrated Circuit(s) Cards with Contacts – Part 7: Interindustry Commands for Structured Card Query Language (SCQL). Standard ISO/IEC 7816-7.

Karjoth, G., Schunter, M., & Waidner, M. (2002). Platform for Enterprise Privacy Practices: Privacy-Enabled Management of Customer Data. In *Privacy Enhancing Technologies* (pp. 69-84).

Langheinrich, M. (2005). *Personal Privacy in Ubiquitous Computing*. Unpublished doctoral dissertation, ETH Zurich.

LeFevre, K., DeWitt, D. J., & Ramakrishnan, R. (2006). Mondrian multidimensional k-anonymity. In *Proceedings of the 22nd IEEE International Conference on Data Engineering (ICDE)*, Atlanta, GA.

Liebert, T. (2008, March). Ongoing concern over Pentagon network attack. *IT News Digest*. Retrieved February 17, 2009, from http://blogs.techrepublic.com.com/tech-news/?p=2098

Massacci, F., & Zannone, N. (2004). Privacy Is Linking Permission to Purpose. In *Proceedings of the Security Protocols Workshop* (pp. 179-191).

MasterCard International. (2002). *MasterCard Open Data Storage Version 2.0. Technical Specifications*. Purchase, NY: Author.

Nergiz, M. E., Atzori, M., & Clifton, C. W. (2007). Hiding the presence of individuals from shared databases. In *Proceedings of ACM SIGMOD*, Vancouver, BC, Canada (pp. 665-676).

Ni, Q., Trombetta, A., Bertino, E., & Lobo, J. (2007). Privacy-aware role based access. In *Proceedings of the 12th ACM Symposium on Access Control Models and Technologies* (pp. 41-50).

Pedersen, C. D. (2006, September 8). *MedCom - the Danish Healthcare Data Network*. Paper presented at the Meeting of the AGFA.

Pucheral, P., Bouganim, L., Valduriez, P., & Bobineau, C. (2001). PicoDBMS: Scaling down database techniques for the smartcard. [VLDBJ]. *Very Large Data Bases Journal, 10*(2-3), 120–132.

Pucheral, P., & Yin, S. (2007). *System and Method of Managing Indexation of Flash Memory* (Patent by Gemalto and INRIA No. 07290567.2).

Røstad, L., & Nytrø, O. (2008). Personalized access control for a personally controlled health record. *Proceedings of the 2nd ACM workshop on Computer security architectures* (pp. 9-16).

Samarati, P. (2001). Protecting respondents' identities in microdata release. [TKDE]. *IEEE Transactions on Knowledge and Data Engineering, 13*(6), 1010–1027. doi:10.1109/69.971193

Samarati, P., & di Vimercati, S. D. C. (2000). Access Control: Policies, Models, and Mechanisms. In *Proceedings of the Foundations of Security Analysis and Design on Foundations of Security Analysis and Design 2000 Conference* (pp. 137-196).

Samarati, P., & Sweeney, L. (1998). Generalizing data to provide anonymity when disclosing information. In *Proceedings of the 17th ACM SIGACT-SIGMOD-SIGART PODS*, Seattle, WA (p. 188).

Smart Card Alliance. (2005). *The Taiwan Health Care Smart Card Project*. Retrieved February 17, 2009, from http://www.smartcardalliance.org/resources/pdf/Taiwan_Health_Card_Profile.pdf

Smart Card Alliance. (2006a). *Smart Card Applications in the U.S. Healthcare Industry* (White Paper No. HC-06001). Retrieved February 17, 2009, from http://www.smartcardalliance.org/resources/hc/Smart_Card_Healthcare_Applications_FINAL.pdf

Smart Card Alliance. (2006b). *German Health Card*. Retrieved February 17, 2009, from http://www.smartcardalliance.org/resources/pdf/German_Health_Card.pdf

Sweeney, L. (1998). Datafly: A system for providing anonymity in medical data. In *Proceedings of the IFIP TC11 WG11.3 11th International Conference on Database Security XI: Status and Prospects* (pp. 356-381).

The Financial Times. (2007, September). *Chinese military hacked into Pentagon*. Retrieved February 17, 2009, from http://www.ft.com/cms/s/0/9dba9ba2-5a3b-11dc-9bcd-0000779fd2ac.html

The International Council on Medical & Care Compunetics. (2009, January 23). *Dutch nationwide EHR postponed. Are they in good company?* Retrieved February 17, 2009, from http://articles.icmcc.org/2009/01/23/dutch-ehr-postponed-are-they-in-good-company

The Times. (2008, December 26). *Patients avoid NHS database blunders by keeping cards close to their chest.* Retrieved February 17, 2009, from http://www.timesonline.co.uk/tol/life_and_style/health/article5397883.ece

The Washington Post. (2007, July). *Consultant Breached FBI's Computers.* Retrieved February 17, 2009, from http://www.washington-post.com/wp-dyn/content/article/2006/07/05/AR2006070501489_pf.html

Vandewalle, J-J. (2004). Smart Card Research Perspectives. *LNCS Construction and Analysis of Safe, Secure and Interoperable Smart devices.*

Wang, K., & Fung, B. C. M. (2006). Anonymizing sequential releases. In *Proceedings of the 12th ACM SIGKDD Conference*, Philadelphia.

WFTV. (2008, August 14). *Medical Center Patient Records Posted On Internet.* Retrieved February 17, 2009, from http://www.wftv.com/news/17188045/detail.html?taf=orlc

Xiao, X., & Tao, Y. (2007). m-invariance: Towards privacy preserving re-publication of dynamic datasets. In *Proceedings of the ACM SIGMOD Conference,* Beijing, China.

Yang, N., Barringer, H., & Zhang, N. (2007). A Purpose-Based Access Control Model. In *Proceedings of the Symposium in Information Assurance and Security* (pp. 143-148).

Yao, C., Wang, X. S., & Jajodia, S. (2005). Checking for k-anonymity violation by views. In *Proceedings of the 31st Very Large Data Bases (VLDB) Conference,* Trondheim, Norway (pp. 910-921).

Yin, S., Pucheral, P., & Meng, X. (2009). *A Sequential Indexing Scheme for Flash-Based Embedded Systems.* Paper presented at the International Conference on Extending Database Technology (EDBT).

Zhang, X., Parisi-Presicce, F., Sandhu, R., & Park, J. (2005). Formal model and policy specification of usage control. *ACM Transactions on Information and System Security, 8,* 351–387. doi:10.1145/1108906.1108908

ENDNOTES

1 The term centralization refers to the fact that the data is stored, organized, made available and controlled by database servers, whatever the computer system infrastructure is (either centralized or distributed).

2 The Danish health minister stopped the EHR effort in 2006 to make the EHR centrally controllable (Dahl, 2006).

3 PlugDB is a project funded by ANR, the French National Research Agency: http://www-smis.inria.fr/~DMSP

This work was previously published in International Journal of Healthcare Delivery Reform Initiatives, edited by Matthew W. Guah, pp. 82-107, copyright 2009 by IGI Publishing (an imprint of IGI Global).

Compilation of References

Aanestad, M., *et al.* (2005) "Strategies for Development and Integration of Health Information Systems: Coping with Historicity and Heterogeneity", *Information Systems Group Working Article: University of Oslo,* 5.

Aaronson, J. W., Murphy-Cullen, C. L., Chop, W. M., & Frey, R. D. (2001). Electronic medical records: the family practice resident perspective. *Family Medicine*, *33*(2), 128–132.

AbouZahr, C., & Boerma, T. (2005). Health Information Systems: The Foundations of Public Health. *Bulletin of the World Health Organization*, *83*(8), 578–583.

ABS. (2003). *Population Projections, Australia, 2002-2011, Cat. No. 3222.0*. Canberra: Australian Bureau of Statistics.

Adamodt, K. (2006). [Location Engine]. *Application Note*, *AN042*, CC2431.

Adams, C. P., & Brantner, V. V. (2006). Estimating the cost of new drug development: Is it really $802 million? *Health Affairs*, *25*(2), 420–428. doi:10.1377/hlthaff.25.2.420

Adams, M. R. (2007). Databases and the future of clinical trials in bladder cancer. *Urologic Oncology: Seminars and Original Investigations*, *25*, 330–332. doi:10.1016/j.urolonc.2007.05.003

Adams, J., Archbold, B., Mounib, E. L., & New, D. (2007). *Healthcare 2015 and U.S. health plans. New roles, new competencies. IBM Institute for Business Value*. IBM Corporation.

Adams, J., Mounib, E., Pai, A., Stuart, N., Thomas, R., & Tomaszewicz, P. (2006). [Win-win or lose-lose? *A portrait and a path to successful transformation*. IBM Institute for Business Value, IBM Corporation.]. *Health Care*, 2015.

Adams, J. S. (1965). Inequity in social exchange. In Berkowitz, L. (Ed.), *Advances in experimental social psychology*. New York: Academic Press.

Adeyemo, A. (2005). Local Government and Health Care Delivery in Nigeria: A Case Study. *Journal of Human Ecology (Delhi, India)*, *18*(2), 149–160.

Adler, R. (2007). *Health Care Unplugged: The Evolving Role of Wireless Technology*. Oakland, CA: California HealthCare Foundation.

Agency, U. S. A. a. R. E. P. (1991). Indoor Air Facts No. 4 (revised) Sick Building Syndrome. [Government publication].

Agrawal, R., Kiernan, J., Srikant, R., & Xu, Y. (2002). Hippocratic Databases. In. *Proceedings of VLDB*, *02*, 143–154.

Agresti, A. (2002). *Categorical Data Analysis* (2nd ed.). Canada: John Wiley & Sons. doi:10.1002/0471249688

Aichholzer, G. (2003). Scenarios of e-Government in 2010 and implications for strategy design. *Electronic Journal of E-government*. Available at http://www.ejeg.com

AIHW. (2007). *National Indicators for Monitoring Diabetes: Report of the Diabetes Indicators Review Subcommittee of the National Diabetes Data Working Group: AIHW cat. no. CVD 38*. Canberra: AIHW.

AIHW. (2008). *Diabetes: Australian Facts 2008*. Canberra: Australian Institute of Health and Welfare.

Ajzen, I. (1991). The theory of planned behaviour. *Organizational Behavior and Human Decision Processes*, *50*, 179–211. doi:10.1016/0749-5978(91)90020-T

Ajzen, I., & Fishbein, M. (1980). *Understanding Attitudes and Predicting Social Behaviour*. Eaglewood Cliffs, NJ: Prentice-Hall.

Al-adawi, Z., Yousafzai, S., & Pallister, J. (2005). Conceptual Model of Citizen Adoption of E-government. *The Second International Conference on Innovations in Information Technology (IIT'05).*

Alasaarela, E. (2008). *Wirhe – Wireless Solutions in Healthcare. International strategy and roadmap towards 2014*. Helsinki: Tekes.

Alasaarela, E. (2009). Finnish Perspectives of Wireless in Healthcare. *International Journal of Electronic Healthcare*, *5*, 177–192. doi:10.1504/IJEH.2009.029224

Alasaarela, E., DeMello, S., & Nemana, R. (2009). Comparative National Perspectives on the Future of Wireless in Health Care: Finland and the United States. *Journal of Management and Marketing in Healthcare*, *2*(4), 1–18.

Alasaarela, E., Nemana, R., DeMello, S., Oliver, N. S., & Miyazaki, M. (2009, April-June). Wireless for Managing Healthcare – the Wirhe Framework. *International Journal of Healthcare Delivery Reform Initiatives*, *1*(2), 52–73.

Alasaarela, E., & Oliver, N. S. (2009). Wireless solutions for managing diabetes. *International Journal of Technology and Health Care*, *17*, 353–367.

Alasaarela, E., Nemana, R., & DeMello, R. (2009, February), Drivers and challenges of wireless solutions in future healthcare. *International Conference on eHealth, Telemedicine, and Social Medicine, eTelemed'09*. Cancun, Mexico 1-7.2.2009. Available in IEEEXplore.

Alexander, G. L. (2008). A Descriptive Analysis of a Nursing Home Clinical Information System with Decision Support. *Perspectives in Health Information Management / AHIMA, American Health Information Management Association, 5*(12).

Alhaqbani, B., & Fidge, C. J. (2007). Access Control Requirements for Processing Electronic Health Records Business. In *Proceedings of the Process Management Workshops* (pp. 371-382).

Allard, T., Nguyen, B., & Pucheral, P. (in press). *Safe Anonymization with Smart Tokens*. Retrieved from http://www-smis.inria.fr/Epublications.html

Alliance. (2008, April 28). *The National Alliance for Health Information Technology, on Defining Key Health Information Technology Term*. Retrieved February 17, 2009, from http://www.hhs.gov/healthit/documents/m20080603/10_2_hit_terms.pdf

Allyn, W. (n.d.). *Welch Allyn Micropaq Monitor model Micropaq 404 Monitor (ECG/SpO$_2$) Directions for use*. Retrieved February 13, 2009, from http://www.welchallyn.com/documents/Patient%20Monitoring/Continuous%20Monitoring/Micropaq/usermanual_20070615_402_404_micropaq.pdf

Alschuler, L., Kush, R., & Bain, L. (2004). Improving Data Collection for Patient Care and Clinical Trials. *Science*, (March): 26.

Alter, C., & Hage, J. (1993). *Organisations working together*. Newbury Park, CA: Sage Publications.

Alvarez, A. J. S. (2003). Towards an Interpretative Integrative Framework to Conceptualise Social Processes in Large Information Systems Implementations. *Information Technology for Development*, *10*, 233–247. doi:10.1002/itdj.1590100403

Alvarez, R.C. (2003). The promise of e-health: a Canadian perspective. *e-Health International, 1*(1), 4.

American Association of Homes and Services for the Aging. (2007). *Staff Turnover and Retention*. Washington, DC: Author.

American Health Information Management Association. (2005). *A road map for health IT in long-term care.* Chicago: Author.

Ammenwerth, E., & Shaw, N. T. (2005). Bad Health informatics can kill--is evaluation the answer? *Methods of Information in Medicine*, *44*(3), 215–231.

Anciaux, N., Bouganim, L., & Pucheral, P. (2006). Data Confidentiality: to which extent cryptography and secured hardware can help. *Annales des Télécommunications*, *61*(3-4), 267–283.

Anciaux, N., Bouganim, L., & Pucheral, P. (2007). Future Trends in Secure Chip Data Management. *A Quarterly Bulletin of the Computer Society of the IEEE Technical Committee on Data Engineering*, *30*(3), 49–57.

Anciaux, N., Benzine, M., Bouganim, L., Pucheral, P., & Shasha, D. (2007). GhostDB: Querying visible and hidden data without leaks. In *Proceedings of the ACM SIGMOD Conference* (pp. 677-688).

Anciaux, N., Bobineau, C., Bouganim, L., Pucheral, P., & Valduriez, P. (2001). PicoDBMS: Validation and Experience. In *Proceedings of the International Conference on Very Large Data Bases (VLDB)* (pp. 709-710).

Andersen, J. G. (1997). Clearing the way for physicians' use of clinical information systems. *Communications of the ACM*, *40*(8), 83–90. doi:10.1145/257874.257895

Anderson, D. M., Asher, L. M., & Wilson, E. A. (2007). Physician computer skills: A prerequisite to the future in healthcare services. *The Journal of the Kentucky Medical Association*, *105*(2), 67–71.

Anderson, R., Issel, L. M., & McDaniel, R. R. (2003). Nursing homes as complex adaptive systems: relationship between management practice and resident outcomes. *Nursing Research*, *52*(1), 12–21. doi:10.1097/00006199-200301000-00003

Anderson, S., & Wittwer, W. (2004). Using bar-code point-of-care technology for patient safety. *Journal for Healthcare Quality*, *26*(6), 5–11.

Anderson, D. P. (2004). BOINC: A System for Public-Resource Computing and Storage. In [Washington, DC: IEEE Computer Society.]. *Proceedings of GRID*, *04*, 4–10.

Anderson, G. (2004). Chronic Conditions: Making the Case for Ongoing Care. *Partnership for Solutions*, Sept. 2004. Available at http://www.partnershipforsolutions.org/DMS/files/chronicbook2004.pdf, last accessed on 13 August 2010.

Andrews, D. C. (2002). Audience-specific online community design. *Communications of the ACM*, *45*(4), 64–68. doi:10.1145/505248.505275

Andrews, J. E., Pearce, K. A., Sydney, C., Ireson, C., & Love, M. (2004). Current state of information technology use in a US primary care practice-based research network. *Informatics in Primary Care*, *12*(1), 11–18.

Andrews, J. (2009). Keeping record: long-term care may not deserve its reputation as a tech laggard. But more could be done to prepare for the electronic health record. *McKnight's Long-Term Care News*, *30*(1), 42–43.

Anon. (2007). Khomas region. Wikipedia. http://en.wikipedia.org/wiki/Khomas [date accessed: 28 May 2007].

Anonymous. (2007). TrialCheck(R) Cancer Clinical Trial Matching Interface to Debut on American Cancer Society Web Site, Retrieved on February 27, 2008 from *PR Newswire*, http://proquest.umi.com

Aoki, M. (1988). *Information, incentives and bargaining in the Japanese economy*. Cambridge, UK: Cambridge University Press. doi:10.1017/CBO9780511571701

Arisoylu, M., Mishra, R., Rao, R., & Lenert, L. A. (2005). 802.11 wireless infrastructure to enhance medical response to disasters. In *Proceedings of the AMIA Annual Symposium* (pp. 1-5).

Armfield, N., Donovan, T., & Wootton, R. (2005). Real-time video in the neonatal intensive care nursery. *Journal of Telemedicine and Telecare*, *11*, 238–245.

Article 29 Data Protection Working Party. (2007). *Working Document on the processing of personal data relating to health in electronic health records (EHR)* (Tech. Rep. 00323/07/EN WP 131). Brussels, Belgium: European Commission.

Asheim, B. T. (2002). Temporary Organisations and Spatial Embeddedness of Learning and Knowledge Creation. *Geografiska Annaler. Series B, Human Geography*, *84*(2), 111–124. doi:10.1111/j.0435-3684.2002.00117.x

Ashley, P., Hada, S., Karjoth, G., Powers, C., & Schunter, M. (2003). *Enterprise Privacy Authorization Language (EPAL 1.2)*. IBM Tivoli Software, IBM Research.

Athey, S., & Stern, S. (2002). The impact of information technology on emergency health care outcomes. *The Rand Journal of Economics*, *33*(3), 399–388. doi:10.2307/3087465

Athey, S., & Stern, S. (2002). The impact of information technology on emergency health care outcomes. *The Rand Journal of Economics*, *33*, 399–388. doi:10.2307/3087465

Atkinson, S. (1995). Restructuring Health Care: Tracking the Decentralization Debate. *Progress in Human Geography*, *19*(4), 486–503. doi:10.1177/030913259501900403

Atkinson, S., Fernandes, L., Caprara, S., & Gideon, J. (2005). Prevention and Promotion in Decentralized Rural Health Systems: A Comparative Study from Northeast Brazil. *Health Policy and Planning*, *20*(2), 69–79. doi:10.1093/heapol/czi009

Atkinson, S., Medeiros, R., Oliveira, P., & Dias de Almeida, R. (2000). Going Down to the Local: Incorporating Social Organisation and Political Culture into Assessments of Decentralised Health Care. *Social Science & Medicine*, *51*, 619–636. doi:10.1016/S0277-9536(00)00005-8

Atreja, A., Mehta, N., Miller, D., Moore, S., Nichols, K., Miller, H., et al. (2005). One size does not fit all: using qualitative methods to inform the development of an Internet portal for multiple sclerosis patients. Paper presented at the AMIA Annual Symposium, Cleveland, OH.

Audet, A., Doty, M., Peugh, J., Shamasdin, J., Zapert, K., & Schoenbaum, S. (2004). Information technologies: When will they make it into physicians' black bags? *Medscape General Medicine*, *6*(4), 843–853.

Australian Bureau of Statistics. (2006). *4102.0 - Australian Social Trends, 2006*. Retrieved from http://www.abs.gov.au/ausstats/abs@.nsf/Latestproducts/6F443192D27B9360CA2571B00013D954?opendocument

Australian Bureau of Statistics. (2008). *3222.0 - Population Projections, Australia, 2006 to 2101*. Retrieved from http://www.abs.gov.au/ausstats/abs@.nsf/mf/3222.0

Australian Government. (2007a). *Clinical IT in Aged Care Product Trial - Trial of a Medication Management System - Report*. Retrieved from http://www.health.gov.au/internet/main/publishing.nsf/Content/ageing-rescare-econnect-med-mgt-trial.htm

Australian Government. (2007b). *Clinical IT in Aged Care Product Trial - Trial of a System for Monitoring Clinical Well-Being - Report*. Retrieved from http://www.health.gov.au/internet/main/publishing.nsf/Content/1E896B258E583DF8CA2573B5007C788D/$File/Clinical%20Monitoring.pdf

Australian Institute of Health and Welfare. (2008). *Australia's health 2008*. Retrieved from http://www.aihw.gov.au/publications/index.cfm/title/10585

Ax, R. K., Fagan, T. J., Magaletta, P. R., Morgan, R. D., Nussbaum, D., & White, T. W. (2007). Innovations in correctional assessment and treatment [Special issue]. *Criminal Justice and Behavior*, *34*, 893–905. doi:10.1177/0093854807301555

Aziz, O., Lo, B., Pansiot, J., Atallah, L., Yang, G.-Z., & Darzi, A. (2008, Oct). From computers to ubiquitous computing by 2010: Health Care. *Philosophical Transactions of the Royal Society A*, *366*(1881), 3805-3811.

Bagozzi, R. P., Davis, F. D., & Warshaw, P. R. (1992). Development and test of a theory of technological learning and usage. *Human Relations*, *45*(7), 659–686. doi:10.1177/001872679204500702

Baldwin, L. P., Clarke, M., Eldabi, T., & Jones, R. W. (2002). Telemedicine and its role in improving communication in healthcare. [October.]. *Logistics Information Management*, *15*(4), 309–319. doi:10.1108/09576050210436147

Ball, C., & Puffet, A. (1998). The assessment f cognitive functioning in the elderly using videoconferencing. *Journal of Telemedicine and Telecare*, *4*, 36–38. doi:10.1258/1357633981931362

Ballantine, J. A., Galliers, R. D., & Stray, S. J. (1999). Information Systems Technology Evaluation Practices: Evidence from UK Organizations. In Willcocks, L. P., & Lester, S. (Eds.), *Beyond the IT Productivity Paradox* (pp. 123–149). Chichester, England: John Wiley & Sons.

Ballou, D., & Pazer, H. (1985). Modeling data and process quality in multi-input multi-output information systems. *Management Science*, *31*(2), 150–162. doi:10.1287/mnsc.31.2.150

Ballou, D., & Pazer, H. (2003). Modeling completeness versus consistency tradeoffs in information decision contexts. *IEEE Transactions on Knowledge and Data Engineering*, *15*(1), 240–243. doi:10.1109/TKDE.2003.1161595

Ballou, D., Wang, R., Pazer, H., & Tayi, G. K. (1998). Modeling Information Manufacturing Systems to Determine Information Product Quality. *Management Science*, *44*(4), 462–484. doi:10.1287/mnsc.44.4.462

Ballou, D. P., & Pazer, H. L. (1995). Designing information systems to optimize the accuracy-timeliness tradeoff. Information Systems Research: ISR: A Journal of the Institute of Management Sciences, 6(1), 51-72.

Bardram, J. E., & Christensen, H. B. (2007). Pervasive computing support for hospitals: An overview of the activity-based computing project. *IEEE Pervasive Computing / IEEE Computer Society [and] IEEE Communications Society*, *6*(1), 44–51. doi:10.1109/MPRV.2007.19

Barlow, I., Liu, L., & Sekulic, A. (2009). Wheelchair Seating Assessment and Intervention: A Comparison Between Telerehabilitation and Face-to-Face Service. International. *Journal of Telerehabilitation*, *1*(1).

Baron, R. J., Fabens, E. L., Schiffman, M., & Wolf, E. (2005). Electronic health records: Just around the corner? Or over the cliff? *Annals of Internal Medicine*, *143*(3), 222–226.

Barrick, A., & Rader, J. (2008). *Bathing without a battle: Person-directed care of individuals with dementia.* New York: Springer.

Bates, D. W., Cohen, M., Leape, L. L., Overhage, J. M., Shabot, M. M., & Sheridan, T. (2001). Reducing the frequency of errors in medicine using information technology. *Journal of the American Medical Informatics Association*, *8*(4), 299–308.

Bates, D. W., Leape, L. L., Cullen, D. J., Laird, N., Petersen, L. A., & Teich, J. M. (1998). Effect of computerized physician order entry and a team intervention on prevention of serious medication errors. *Journal of the American Medical Association*, *280*(15), 1311–1316. doi:10.1001/jama.280.15.1311

Bates, D. W., Teich, J. M., Lee, J., Seger, D., & Kuperman, G. J., Ma'Luf, N., et al. (1999). The impact of computerized physician order entry on medication error prevention. *Journal of the American Medical Informatics Association*, *6*(4), 313–321.

Battlefield Medical Information System Tactical - Joint. (n.d.). *BMIST-J home page*. Retrieved February 13, 2009, from http://www.mc4.army.mil/AHLTA-Mobile_CBT.asp#

Becker, M. Y., & Sewell, P. (2004). Cassandra: Flexible Trust Management, Applied to Electronic Health Records. *Computer Security Foundations Workshop* (pp. 139-154).

Benowitz, S. (2005). Clinical Trial Transparency: Registries, Databases Raise Questions, Stir Debate. *Journal of the National Cancer Institute*, *97*(22), 1640–1641. doi:10.1093/jnci/dji421

Berg, M. (2001). Implementing Information Systems in Health Care Organizations: Myths and Challenges. *International Journal of Medical Informatics*, *64*, 143–146. doi:10.1016/S1386-5056(01)00200-3

Berger, L. (2006, January 13). Information technology feature: The IT payback. *McKnight's Long-Term Care News*, 34-37.

Bergeron, B. P. (2006). I have an EMR system – now what? *The Journal of Medical Practice Management*, *22*(3), 131–132.

Bergqvist, J., Dahlberg, P., & Ljungberg, F. (2006) *Scalability through Cultivation. Designing It Support for Co-Ordination Work* Last accessed: 6 February 2007 Last updated: Address: http://citeseer.ist.psu.edu/cache/articles/cs/23947/http:zSzzSzwww.dahlberg.sezSzpubzSzmaster.pdf/scalability-through-cultivation-designing.pdf.

Berkowitz, L. L. (2002). Clinical informatics tools in physician practice. *Healthcare Informatics*, *19*(4), 41–44.

Berman, P. (Ed.). (1995). *Health Sector Reform: Making Health Development Sustainable*. Boston: Harvard University Press.

Berman, P., & Bossert, T. (2000). *Appraising a Decade of Health Sector Reform in Developing Countries*. Washington, DC: Havard School of Public Health.

Bernstam, E. V., Shelton, S. M., Walji, M., & Meric-Bernstam, F. (2005). Instruments to assess the quality of Health Information on the World Wide Web: What can our Patients Actually Use? *International Journal of Medical Informatics*, *74*, 13–19. doi:10.1016/j.ijmedinf.2004.10.001

Bevan, N., & Macleod, M. (1993). Usability assessment and measurement. In Kelly, M. (Ed.), *The management and measurement of software quality*. Ashgate Technical/Gower Press.

Bevan, N., Petrie, H., & Claridge, N. (2007). Strategies for Providing Guidance on Usability and Accessibility. In *Proceedings HCI International 2007*. Springer.

Beynon-Davies, P. (2005). Constructing Electronic Government: the case of the UK Inland Revenue. *International Journal of Information Management*, *25*(1), 3–20. doi:10.1016/j.ijinfomgt.2004.08.002

Bharati, P. (2002/2003). People and information matter: Task support satisfaction from the other side. *Journal of Computer Information Systems*, *43*(2), 93–102.

Bhasker, R. (1998). Philosophy and Scientific Realism. In Archer, M., Bhasker, R., Collier, A., Lawson, T., & Norrie, A. (Eds.), *Critical Realism: Essential Readings* (pp. 16–48). London: Routledge.

Bischoff, R. J., Hollist, C. S., Smith, C. W., & Frank, P. (2004). Addressing the mental health needs of the rural underserved: Findings from a multiple case study of a behavioral telehealth project. *Contemporary Family Therapy*, 26.

Blaauw, D., Gilson, L., Penn-Kekana, L., & Schneider, H. (2003). *"Organisational Relationships and the 'Software' of Health Sector Reform. Background Article Disease Control Priorities Project (Dcpp) Capacity Strengthening and Management Reform" Centre for Health Policy, Schoolff Public Health*. University ofThe Witwatersrand.

Black, P. C., & Penson, D. F. (2006). Prostrate Cancer on the Internet--information or misinformation? *The Journal of Urology*, *175*(5), 1836–1842. doi:10.1016/S0022-5347(05)00996-1

Blackler, F. (1995). Knowledge, knowledge work and organizations: an overview and interpretation. *Organization Studies*, *16*(6), 1021–1046. doi:10.1177/017084069501600605

Blackmon, L. A., Kaak, H. O., & Ranseen, J. (1997). Consumer satisfaction with telemedicine child psychiatry consultation in rural Kentucky. *Psychiatric Services (Washington, D.C.)*, *48*, 1464–1466.

Bleicher, P. (2003). Clinical trial technology: at the inflection point. *BIOSILICO*, *1*(15), 163–168. doi:10.1016/S1478-5382(03)02373-4

Bloom, B. (1970). Space/time tradeoffs in hash coding with allowable errors. *Communications of the ACM*, *13*(7), 422–426. doi:10.1145/362686.362692

Bof, F., & Previtali, P. (2007). Organisational Pre-Conditions for e-Procurement in Governments: the Italian Experience in the Public Health Care Sector. *The Electronic. Journal of E-Government*, *5*(1), 1–10.

Booysen, C. (2006). *The application of discriminant analysis and logistical regression as methods of compilation in the research function in youth rugby*. Pretoria: University of Pretoria.

Bossert, T. (1979). Health Policies in Africa and Latin America: Adopting the Primary Care Approach. *Social Science & Medicine*, *13*(C), 65.

Bossert, T. (1998). Analyzing the Decentralization of Health Systems in Developing Countries: Decision Space, Innovation and Performance. *Social Science & Medicine*, *47*(10), 1513–1527. doi:10.1016/S0277-9536(98)00234-2

Boumans, N., Berkhout, A., & Landeweerd, A. (2005). Efforts of resident-oriented care on quality of care, well-being and satisfaction with care. *Scandinavian Journal of Caring Sciences*, *19*(3), 11–15. doi:10.1111/j.1471-6712.2005.00351.x

Bower, A. G. (2005). *The diffusion and value of healthcare information technology*. Santa-Monica, CA: Rand Publishing.

Bowker, G., & Star, S. (1999). *Sorting Things Out: Classification and Its Consequences*. Cambridge, MA: The MIT Press.

Braa, J., Monteiro, E., & Sahay, S. (2004). Networks of Action: Sustainable Health Information Systems across Developing Countries. *MIS Quarterly: Management Information Systems*, *28*(3), 337–362.

Braa, J. (2000) "Developing District-Based Health Care Information Systems: The South African Experience". in *Proceedings of IRIS 23. Laboratorium for Interaction Technology,* University of Trollhättan Uddevalla, Braa, J., *et al.* (2001) "A Study of the Actual and Potential Usage of Information and Communication Technology at District and Provincial Levels in Mozambique with a Focus on the Health Sector", *EJISDC,* 5 (2), pp. 1-29.

Breen, G., & Zhang, N. (2008). Theoretical Analysis of Improving Resident Care. *Journal of Medical Systems*, *32*(2), 18–23. doi:10.1007/s10916-007-9121-9

Breen, G. M., & Matusitz, J. (2007). An interpersonal examination of telemedicine: Applying relevant communication theories. *E-health. International Journal (Toronto, Ont.)*, *3*(1), 187–192.

Brender, J. (2006). *Handbook of Evaluation Methods for Health Informatics*. Elsevier Academic Press Publications.

Britt, H., Miller, G. C., Charles, J., Pan, Y., Valenti, L., & Henderson, J. (2007). *General Practice Activity in Australia 2005-06, Cat. no. GEP 16*. Canberra: AIHW.

Brown, S. H., Lincoln, M. J., Groen, P. J., & Kolodner, R. M. (2003). VistA, U.S. Department of Veterans Affairs national scale HIS. *International Journal of Medical Informatics*, *69*, 135–156. doi:10.1016/S1386-5056(02)00131-4

Burgess, L. (2004, October 13-15). A Conceptual Framework for Understanding and Measuring Perceived Service Quality in Net-based Customer Support Systems. *CollECTeR LatAm Conference*, Santiago, Chile.

Burland, E. M. J. (2008). An Evaluation of a Fall Management Program in a Personal Care Home Population. *Healthcare Quaterly*, *11*(3), 137–140.

Burt, C. W., Hing, E., & Woodwell, D. (2005). Electronic medical record use by office-based physicians: National Center for Health Statistics. Retrieved February 4, 2008 from http://www.cdc.gov/nchs/products/pubs/pubd/hestats/electronic/electronic.htm

Buse, K., & Watt, G. (1996). Aid Coordination for Health Sector Reform: A Conceptual Framework for Analysis and Assessment. *Health Policy (Amsterdam)*, *38*, 173–187. doi:10.1016/0168-8510(96)00855-X

Byun, J., & Li, N. (2008). Purpose based access control for privacy protection in relational database systems. *The VLDB Journal*, *17*, 603–619. doi:10.1007/s00778-006-0023-0

CaBig. (2007). Retrieved on November 26, 2007, from http://cabig.cancer.gov/connection/principles.asp

Caldwell, B., Cooper, M., Reid, L., & Vanderheiden, G. (2007, December). *Web Content Accessibility Guidelines 2.0.*

Carrasco, L. C. (1999). *RDBMS's for Java Cards? What a Senseless Idea!* ISOL Corp.

Carrillo, H., & Harrington, C. (2006). *Cross the States 2006: Profiles of Long-Term Care and Independent Living.* Washington, DC: AARP.

Carroll, R., Cnossen, R., Schnell, M., & Simons, D. (2007). Continua: An Interoperable Personal Healthcare Ecosystem. *IEEE Pervasive Computing / IEEE Computer Society [and] IEEE Communications Society*, *6*(4). doi:10.1109/MPRV.2007.72

Carter, L., & Belanger, F. (2004). Citizen Adoption of Electronic Government Initiatives. In *Proceedings of 37th Annual Hawaii International Conference on System Sciences*, Big Island, Hawaii.

Casa, A., Troosters, T., & Garcia-Aymerich, J. (2006). Integrated care prevents hospitalisations for exacerbations in COPD patients. *The European Respiratory Journal*, *28*, 1–8.

Casper, E. S. (2004). A formative evaluation of a rent subsidy program for homeless substance abusers. *Journal of Service Research*, *31*(2), 25–39.

Casper, V. (2004). Beyond feeders and growers: Changing conceptions of care in the Western Cape. *Journal of Child and Adolescent Mental Health*, *16*(1), 55–59.

Casper, L.M., & King, Rosalind, K.B. (2004). Changing families, shifting economic fortunes, and meeting basic needs [Comment/Reply]. *Work Family Challenges for Low-Income Parents and Their Children, 55-79.*

Castle, N. G. (2008). Nursing Home Evacuation Plans. *American Journal of Public Health*, *98*(7), 1235–1241. doi:10.2105/AJPH.2006.107532

CDISC. (2007). Retrieved on November 23, 2007 from http://www.cdisc.org/about/index.html

Celler, B. G., Earnshaw, W., Ilsar, E. D., Betbeder-Matibet, L., Harris, M., & Clark, R. (1995). Remote monitoring of the elderly at home. A multidisciplinary project on aging at the University of New South Wales. *International Journal of Bio-Medical Computing*, *40*, 147–155. doi:10.1016/0020-7101(95)01139-6

Celler, B. G., Basilakis, J., Budge, M., & Lovell, N. H. (2006). A Clinical Monitoring and Management System for Residential Aged Care Facilities. In *Proceedings of the 28th IEEE EMBS Annual International Conference* (pp. 3301).

CHA. (2009). The Next Generation of Personal Telehealth is Here. Continua Overview Presentation. *Continua Health Alliance*. Available at http://www.continuaalliance.org/about-the-alliance.html, last accessed on 13 August 2010.

Chan, L. L., Zhang, J. Z., Narayanan, M. R., Celler, B. G., & Lovell, N. H. (2008, February 13-15). *A Health Monitoring and Evaluation System for Assessing Care Needs of Residents in Aged-Care Facilities.* Paper presented at the IASTED Biomed. Eng., Innsbruck, Austria.

Chandrasekhar, C. P., & Ghosh, J. (2001). Information and communication technologies and health in low income countries: the potential and the constraints. *Bulletin of the World Health Organization*, *79*(9), 850–855.

Chao, C.C., Jen, W.Y., Hung, M.C., Li, Y.C. & Y.P. Chi. (2006). An innovative mobile approach for patient safety services: The case of a Taiwan health care provider.

Charatan, F. (2000). US launches new clinical trials database. *BMJ (Clinical Research Ed.)*, *320*(7236), 668. doi:10.1136/bmj.320.7236.668

Charnock, D., & Sheppard, S. (2004). Learning to DISCERN online: applying an appraisal tool to health websites in a workshop setting. *Health Education Research*, *19*(4), 440–446. doi:10.1093/her/cyg046

Chatora, R., & Tumusime, P. (2004). Primary Health Care: A Review of Its Implementation in Sub-Saharan Africa. *Primary Health Care Research and Development*, *5*, 296–306. doi:10.1191/1463423604pc220oa

Chau, P. Y. K., & Hu, P. J.-H. (2002). Investigating healthcare professionals' decision to accept telemedicine technology: An empirical test of competing theories. *Information & Management*, *39*, 297–311. doi:10.1016/S0378-7206(01)00098-2

Chau, S., & Turner, P. (2006). Utilization of mobile handheld devices for care management at an Australian aged care facility. [Winter.]. *Electronic Commerce Research and Applications*, *5*(4), 305–312. doi:10.1016/j.elerap.2006.04.005

Chau, P., & Hu, P. (2001). Information Technology Acceptance by Individual Professionals: A Model Comparison Approach. *Decision Sciences*, *32*(4). doi:10.1111/j.1540-5915.2001.tb00978.x

Chau, P. Y. K., & Hu, P. J. (2002). Examining a model of information technology acceptance by individual professionals: An exploratory study. *Management Information Systems*, *18*(4), 191–229.

Chestnutt, I. G., & Reynolds, K. (2003). Perceptions of how the Internet has impacted Dentistry. *British Dental Journal*, *11*(2), 161–165.

Chetty, K. S. (2007). *Equity Promoting Health Care Policies in South Africa.* Report to the Health Systems Knowledge Network. Retrieved Jan 10, 2008 from: http://www.wits.ac.za/chp/kn/Chetty%202007%20Equity.pdf

Cheung, B. K., Morze, C. J., Jones, M. A., & Venkatesh, B. (2006). Information on the Internet about head injury pertaining to intensive care: less quantity and more quality is needed. *Critical Care and Resuscitation, 8*(2), 100–106.

Chiasson, M., Davidson, E., Kaplan, B., Lau, F., & Reddy, M. (2004, September). *Interdisciplinary windows for studying information systems in healthcare: Challenges and opportunities.* Paper presented at IT in healthcare: Socio-technical Approaches Second International Conference, Oregon, USA.

Chien, A., Calder, B., Elbert, S., & Bhatia, K. (2003). Entropia: architecture and performance of an enterprise desktop grid system. *Journal of Parallel and Distributed Computing, 63*(5), 597–610. doi:10.1016/S0743-7315(03)00006-6

Childs, S. (2004). Developing Health Website Quality Assessment Guidelines for the Voluntary Sector: Outcomes from the Judge Report. *Health Information and Libraries Journal, 21*(2), 14–26. doi:10.1111/j.1740-3324.2004.00520.x

Chilundo, B., & Aanestad, M. (2003) "Vertical of Integrated Health Programmes? The Consequence for the Laboratory Information Systems in Mozambique". in *Electronic Proceedings of the IFIP TC8 & TC9. WG8.2 + 9.4 Working Conference on Information Systems Perspectives and Challenges in the Context of Globalization,* Athens, Greece, Chilundo, B. and M. Aanestad (2004) "Negotiating Multiple Rationalities in the Process of Integrating the Information Systems of Disease-Specific Health Programmes", *EJISDC,* 20 (2), pp. 1-28.

Chilvers, R. & Macdonald, G. & Hayes A (2003). Supported housing for people with severe mental disorders. Cochrane Library.

Chismar, W. R., & Wiley-Patton, S. (2006). Predicting Internet Use: Applying teh Extended Technology Acceptance Model to the Healthcare Environment. In Spil, T. A. M., & Schuring, R. W. (Eds.), *E-Health Systems Diffusion and USe: The Innovation, the USer and the USE IT Model.* Hershey, PA: Idea Group Publishing.

Chismar, W. G., & Patton, S. W. (2003). Does the extended technology acceptance model apply to physicians? *36th Hawaii International Conference on System Sciences,* Hawaii.

Christopher, J., Hardwick, R., & McKenzie, F. M. (2003). Information contained in miscarriage-related websites and the predictive value of website scoring systems. *European Journal of Obstetrics and Gynecology, 106,* 60–63. doi:10.1016/S0301-2115(02)00357-3

Ciborra, C. (Ed.). (2000). *From Control to Drift. The Dynamics of Corporate Information Infrastructures.* Oxford: Oxford University Press.

Ciborra, C. (2002). *The Labyrinths of Information: Challenging the Wisdom of Systems.* Oxford: Oxford University Press.

Cicchetti, A. (2004). *La progettazione organizzativa.* Milano: FrancoAngeli.

CleveMed. (n.d.). *Home page.* Retrieved February 13, 2009, from http://www.clevemed.com/

Cline, R. J., & Haynes, K. M. (2001). Consumer Health Information Seeking on the Internet: The State of the Art. *Health Education Research, 16,* 671–692. doi:10.1093/her/16.6.671

Codd, E. F. (1970). A Relational Model of Data for Large Shared Data Banks. *Communications of the ACM, 13*(6), 377–387. doi:10.1145/362384.362685

Colagiuri, S., Colagiuri, R., & Ward, J. (1998). *National Diabetes Strategy and Implementation Plan.* Canberra: Diabetes Australia.

Colfer, C. J. P., Woelfel, J., Wadley, R. L., & Harwell, E. (2001). Assessing people's perceptions of forests: Research in West Kalimantan, Indonesia. In Colfer, C. J. P., & Byron, Y. (Eds.), *People Managing Forests: The Links between Human Well-Being and Sustainability* (pp. 135–154). Washington, D.C.: Resources for the Future.

Collins, H. M. (1993). The structure of knowledge. *Social Research*, *60*(1), 95–116.

Collins, C., & Green, A. (1994). Decentralization and Primary Health Care: Some Negative Implications in Developing Countries. *International Journal of Health Services*, *24*(3), 459–475.

Computer World. (2003, December). *NASA Sites Hacked.* Retrieved February 17, 2009, from http://www.computerworld.com/securitytopics/security/cybercrime/story/0,10801,88348,00.html

Computer World. (2006, August). *Survey: 81% of U.S. firms lost laptops with sensitive data in the past year.* Retrieved February 17, 2009, from http://www.computerworld.com/action/article. do?command=viewArticleBasic&articleId=9002493&source=NLT_PM&nlid=8

Connell, N., & Young, T. (2007, June). Evaluating healthcare information systems through an "enterprise" perspective. *Information & Management*, *44*(4), 433–440. doi:10.1016/j.im.2007.04.002

Connolly, C. (2005, March, 21). Cedars-Sinai Doctors Cling to Pen and Paper. The Washington Post, p. A01. Retrieved February 4, 2008 from http://www.washingtonpost.com/wp-dyn/articles/A52384-2005Mar20.html

CONSIP. (2003). *Il Programma di razionalizzazione della spesa per beni e servizi della Pubblica Amministrazione.* CONSIP Annual Report (*house journal*), Rome.

Cook, J., Augusto, J. C., & Jakkula, V. R. (2009). Ambient Intelligence: Technologies, applications, and opportunities. *Pervasive and Mobile Computing Journal*, *5*(4), 277–298. doi:10.1016/j.pmcj.2009.04.001

Cook, J., & Das, S. K. (2007). How smart are our environments? An updated look at the state of the art. *Pervasive and Mobile Computing Journal, 3*(2).

Corey, C., & Grossman, J. M. (2007). Clinical information technology adoption varies across physician specialties. Center for Studying Health System Change. Data Bulletin, Number 34. Retrieved February 4, 2008 from http://www.hschange.com/CONTENT/945/

Cornia, G. A. (2001). Globalization and Health: Results and Options. *Bulletin of the World Health Organization*, *79*, 834–841.

Cornwall, A., Lucas, H., & Pasteur, K. (2000). Introduction: Accountability through Participation:Developing Workable Partnership Models in the Health Sector. *IDS Bulletin*, *31*(1), 1–13. doi:10.1111/j.1759-5436.2000.mp31001001.x

Coronato, A., & De Pietro, G. (2008). MiPeG: A Middleware Infrastructure for Pervasive Grids. *Journal of Future Generation Computer Systems*, *24*(1). doi:10.1016/j.future.2007.04.007

Coronato, A., & De Pietro, G. (in press). Formal Specification of Wireless and Pervasive Healthcare Applications. *ACM Transactions on Embedded Computing Systems.*

Coronato, A., De Pietro, G., & Gallo, L. (2008). An agent based platform for task distribution in virtual environments. *Journal of Systems Architecture*, *54*(9), 877–882. doi:10.1016/j.sysarc.2008.01.011

Coronato, A., & Esposito, M. (2008). Towards an implementation of smart hospital: A localization system for mobile users and devices. In *Proceedings of the Sixth Annual IEEE International Conference on Pervasive Computing and Communications PERCOM 2008* (pp. 715-719).

Coronato, A., De Pietro, G., & Esposito, M. (2009). A Multimodal Semantic Location Service for Intelligent Environments: An Application for Smart Hospitals. *Personal and Ubiquitous Computing Journal, 13*(7)

Coronato, A., De Pietro, G., & Gallo, L. (2007a). Automatic execution of tasks in MiPeG. In *GPC 2007* (LNCS 4459, pp. 702-709).

Coronato, A., De Pietro, G., & Gallo, L. (2007b). Dynamic Distribution and Execution of Tasks in Pervasive Grids. In *Proceedings of the 15th Euromicro international Conference on Parallel, Distributed and Network-Based Processing* (pp. 419-423). Washington, DC: IEEE Computer Society.

CosmoCom. (2009). *CosmoCom Showcases Telehealth at World Health Care Congress*. Melville, NY: Author.

Crane, J., & Crane, F. G. (2006). Preventing medication errors in hospitals through a systems approach and technological innovation: A prescription for 2010. *Hospital Topics*, *84*(4), 3–8. doi:10.3200/HTPS.84.4.3-8

Crede, A., & Masell, R. (1998). *Knowledge societies... in a nutshell: Information technology for sustainable Development*. Canada: IDRC Books.

Creswell, J. W. (2003). *Research Design. Qualitative, Quantitative, and Mixed Methods Approaches*. Thousand Oaks, CA, USA: Sage.

Crocco, A. G., Villasis-Keever, M., & Jadad, A. R. (2002). Two Wrongs Don't Make a Right: Harm Aggravated by Inaccurate Information on the Internet. *Pediatrics*, *109*(3), 522–523. doi:10.1542/peds.109.3.522

Cronholm, S., & Goldkuhl, G. (2003, September 25-26). Six Generic Types of Information Systems Evaluation. *The 10th European Conference on Information Technology Evaluation (ECITE-2003)*, Madrid.

Crossbow. (n.d.). *Home page*. Retrieved February 13, 2009, from http://www.xbow.com

Cueto, M. (2004). The Origins of Primary Health Care and Selective Primary Health Care. *American Journal of Public Health*, *94*(11), 1864–1874. doi:10.2105/AJPH.94.11.1864

Culver, M., & Chadwick, A. (2005). Internet Information on Rheumatoid Arthritis: An Evaluation. *Musculoskeletal Care*, *3*(1), 33–43. doi:10.1002/msc.24

Curtis, D. W., Pino, E. J., Bailey, J. M., Shih, E. I., Waterman, J., & Vinterbo, S. A. (2008). SMART - An Integrated Wireless System for Monitoring Unattended Patients. *Journal of the American Medical Informatics Association*, *15*(1), 44–53. doi:10.1197/jamia.M2016

Daft, R. L. (2003). *Organization Theory and Design*. Chula Vista, CA: South-Western College Pub.

Dahl, M. R. (2006). *Status and perspective of personal health informatics in Denmark*. Aarhus, Denmark: University of Aarhus, Section for Health Informatics, Institute of Public Health. Retrieved February 17, 2009, from http://www.ieee2407.org/files/ws01_mads01.pps

Darr, A., Harrison, M. I., Shakked, L., & Shalom, N. (2003). Physicians' and nurses' reaction to electronic medical records. *Journal of Health Organization and Management*, *17*(5), 349–359. doi:10.1108/14777260310505129

David, P. (1994). *A revolution in seating - Nursing Home Technology*. Retrieved November 3, 2008, from http://findarticles.com/p/articles/mi_m3830/is_n9_v43/ai_16539882/

Davies, F. D., Bagozzi, R. P., & Warshaw, P. R. (1989). User acceptance of computer technology: A comparison of two theoretical models. *Communications of the ACM*, *35*(8), 982–1003.

Davis, R. (2002). Pursue front end solutions to revenue problems. *Healthcare Financial Management*, *56*(8), 30–36.

Davis, F. (1989). Perceived Usefulness, Perceived Ease of Use and User Acceptance of Information Technology. *Management Information Systems Quarterly*, *13*(3), 319–340. doi:10.2307/249008

Davis, L., Domm, J., Konikoff, M., & Miller, R. (1999, Jan–Feb). Attitudes of First-year Medical Students toward the Confidentiality of Computerized Patient Records. *Journal of the American Medical Informatics Association*, *6*(1).

Davis, R. (2002). Pursue front end solutions to revenue problems. *Healthcare Financial Management*, *56*, 30–36.

Deaton, A. (2003). Health, Inequality, and Economic Development. *Journal of Economic Literature*, *XLI*, 113–158. doi:10.1257/002205103321544710

Debra, O., & Brain, H. (2006). A promising Technology to Reduce Social Isolation of Nursing Home Residents. *Journal of Nursing Care Quality*, *21*(4), 302–306.

Delanyo, D. (2001). Namibia country briefing paper. Department for international Development Health systems resource centre for the UK DFID. http://www.dfidhealthrc.org/shared/publications/Country_health/Namibia.pdf [date accessed: 10 March 2006].

DeLeon, P. H., Crimmins, D. B., & Wolf, A. W. (2003). Afterword-the 21st century has arrived. *Psychotherapy (Chicago, Ill.)*, *40*(1-2), 164–169. doi:10.1037/0033-3204.40.1-2.164

Demiris, G., Speedie, S. M., & Finkelstein, S. (2001). Change of patients' perceptions of Tele-HomeCare. *Telemedicine & E-Health*, *7*(3), 241–249. doi:10.1089/153056201316970948

Department of Health. (2004). *National HIV and Syphillis Antenatal Seroprevalence Survey in South Africa 2003*. Retrieved January 10, 2008, from http://www.doh.gov.za/docs/2003hiv-f.html.

Devadoss, P. R., Pan, S. L., & Huang, J. C. (2002). Structurational Analysis of e-Government initiatives: a case study of SCO. *Decision Support Systems*, *34*, 253–269. doi:10.1016/S0167-9236(02)00120-3

DiabetesAustralia. (2008). *Diabetes in Australia*. Retrieved from http://www.diabetesaustralia.com.au/Understanding-Diabetes/Diabetes-in-Australia/

District of Columbia Department of Human Services. (n.d.). *Home Care and Nursing Home Services*. Retrieved December 12, 2008, from http://dhs.dc.gov/dhs/cwp/view,a,3,Q,613301.asp

Dixon, T., & Webbie, K. (2006). *The National System for Monitoring Diabetes in Australia (AIHW Cat. No. CVD 32). Canberra: Australian Institute of Health and Wealfare.* eHealthImpact. (2006). *Study on Economic Impact of eHealth: Developing an evidence-based context-adaptive method of evaluation for eHealth*. Bonn: Information Society and Media.

Dobrow, M., Goel, V., & Upshur, R. (2004). Evidence-Based Health Policy: Context and Utilisation. *Social Science & Medicine*, *58*, 207–217. doi:10.1016/S0277-9536(03)00166-7

Doerfel, M. L., & Barnett, G. A. (1999). A Semantic Network Analysis of the International Communication Association. *Human Communication Research*, *25*(4), 589–603. doi:10.1111/j.1468-2958.1999.tb00463.x

Door, J.-P. (2008). *Le dossier médical personnel* (Information Rep. No. 659). Paris: Assemblée Nationale. eHealth Insider. (2008, January 16). *German doctors say no to centrally stored patient records*. Retrieved February 17, 2009, from http://www.e-health-insider.com/news/3384/.

Dyer, O. (2003). Patients will be reminded of appointments by text messages. *British Medical Journal*, *326*(402), 281. doi:10.1136/bmj.326.7402.1281-a

Egan, G. F., & Liu, Z. (1995). Computers and networks in medical and Healthcare systems. [May.]. *Computers in Biology and Medicine*, *25*(3), 355–365. doi:10.1016/0010-4825(95)00016-W

Eisenhardt, K. (1989). Building Theories from Case Study Research. *Academy of Management Review*, *14*(4), 532–550. doi:10.2307/258557

Ekman, A., Hall, P., & Litton, J.-E. (2005). Can we Trust Cancer Information on the Internet? - A Comparison of interactive cancer Risk Sites. *Cancer Causes & Control*, *16*(6), 765–772. doi:10.1007/s10552-005-1722-3

Eley, R., Fallon, T., Soar, J., Buikstra, E., & Hegney, D. (2008). The status of training and education in information and computer technology of Australian nurses: a national survey. *Journal of Clinical Nursing*, *17*, 2758–2767. doi:10.1111/j.1365-2702.2008.02285.x

Elite Care. (2008). *Elite Care*. Retrieved from http://www.elitecare.com/

ELJAY. LCC. (2006). *A Report on Shortfalls in Medicaid Funding for Nursing Home Care*. Washington, DC: American Health Care Association.

El-Khamra, Y., & Jha, S. (2009). Developing autonomic distributed scientific applications: a case study from history matching using ensemble kalman-filters. In *GMAC '09* (pp. 19-28). New York: ACM.

Eng, T. R. (2001). *The e-health landscape: A terrain map of emerging information and communication technologies in health and health care*. Princeton, NJ: The Robert Wood Johnson Foundation.

Eng, T. R. (2002). E-health research and evaluation: challenges and opportunities. *Journal of Health Communication*, *7*(4), 267–272. doi:10.1080/10810730290001747

Equity Network for Southern Africa (EQUINET). (2005). Equity in health Care in Namibia Towards needs-based allocation formula. MOHSS World Health Organization. EQUINET policy paper number 26, Windhoek, Namibia. http://www.healthnet.org.na [date accessed: 12 May 2006].

Eurosmart. (2008, April). *Smart USB Token*. Retrieved February 17, 2009, from http://www.eurosmart.com/images/doc/WorkingGroups/NewFF/Papers/eurosmart_smart_usb_token_wp_april08.pdf

Eurostat/US Bureau of the Census. (2008). *People by age classes*. Retrieved January 28, 2009, from http://epp.eurostat.ec.europa.eu/portal/page?_pageid=1996,39140985&_dad=portal&_schema=PORTAL&screen=detailref&language=en&product=REF_TB_population&root=REF_TB_population/t_popula/t_pop/t_demo_pop/tps00010

Farbey, B., Land, F., & Targett, D. (1995). A Taxonomy of information systems applications: the benefits evaluation Ladder. *European Journal of Information Systems*, *4*, 41–50. doi:10.1057/ejis.1995.5

Farbey, B., Land, F., & Targett, D. (1999). Evaluating Investments in IT: Findings and a Framework. In Willcocks, L. P., & Lester, S. (Eds.), *Beyond the IT Productivity Paradox* (pp. 183–215). Chichester, England, UK: John Wiley & Sons.

FDA. (1997). 21 CFR Part 11: Electronic records; electronic signatures. Retrieved on November 20, 2007 from http://www.accessdata.fda.gov/scripts/cdrh/cfdocs/ cfcfr/CFRSearch.cfm?CFRPart=11

FDA. (2007). Guidance for Industry Computerized System Used in Clinical Investigations. Retrieved on November 20, 2007 from www.fda.gov/OHRMS/DOCKETS/98fr/04d-0440-gdl0002.pdf

Fedak, G., Germain, C., Neri, V., & Cappello, F. (2001). XtremWeb: A Generic Global Computing System. In *Proceedings of the 1st International Symposium on Cluster Computing and the Grid*. Washington, DC: IEEE Computer Society.

Federici, T. (2009). Introducing e-Procurement in a Local Healthcare Agency. In Scupola, A. (Ed.), *Cases on Managing E-services*. Hershey, PA, USA: Roskilde University, Denmark. Information Science Reference. doi:10.4018/978-1-60566-064-6.ch015

Federici, T. (2005). An Integrated Approach in Healthcare e-procurement: The Case-Study of the ASL of Viterbo. In Böhlen, M. et al. (eds.) *Proceedings of E-Government: Towards Electronic Democracy, TCGOV 2005* (LNAI 3416, p. 298). Berlin:Springer.

Federici, T. (2006). Public Healthcare: changes introduced when implementing e-procurement. In *Proceedings of the: Mediterranean Conference on Information Systems, MCIS 2006*. Venice, Italy, October 2006.

Federici, T., & Resca, A. (2007), Managing a widespread e-Procurement implementation in Public Healthcare. Proceedings of the *"Mediterranean Conference on Information Systems, MCIS 2007"*, Venice, Italy, 4-8 October.

Ferraiolo, D. F., Kuhn, R. D., & Chandramouli, R. (2003). *Role-Based Access Control*. Norwood, MA: Artech House Publishers.

Field, T. S., Rochon, P., Lee, M., Gavendo, L., Subramanian, S., & Hoover, S. (2008). Costs associated with developing and implementing a computerized clinical decision support system for medication dosing for patients with renal insufficiency in the long-term care setting. *Journal of the American Medical Informatics Association*, *15*(4), 466–472. doi:10.1197/jamia.M2589

FierceHealthIT news. (2006, August 20). *Massive data loss at HCA*. Retrieved February 17, 2009, from http://www.fiercehealthit.com/story/massive-data-loss-at-hca/2006-08-21

FierceHealthIT news. (2008, September). *GA hospital health data breach due to outsourcing error.* Retrieved February 17, 2009, from http://www.fiercehealthit.com/story/ga-hospital-health-data-breach-due-outsourcing-error/2008-09-28

Filmer, D., Pritchett, L., & Hammer, J. (1998). *Health Policy in Poor Countries: Weak Links in the Chain?* Washington, D.C.: World Bank, Development Research Group, Poverty and Human Resources.

Finnema, E., de Lange, J., Droes, R. M., Ribbe, M., & Tilburg, W. (2001). The quality of nursing home care: Do the opinions of family members change after implementation of emotion-oriented care? *Journal of Advanced Nursing*, *35*(5), 728–732. doi:10.1046/j.1365-2648.2001.01905.x

Fitzgerald, B., & Howcroft, D. (1998, December). Competing dichotomies in IS research and possible strategies for resolution. *AIS International Conference on Information Systems*, Helsinki, Finland.

Fitzmaurice, J. M., Adams, K., & Eisenberg, J. M. (2002). Three decades of research on computer applications in health care: Medical informatics support at the agency for healthcare research and quality. *Journal of the American Medical Informatics Association*, *9*(2), 144–160. doi:10.1197/jamia.M0867

Fonkych, K., & Taylor, R. (2005). The state and pattern of health information technology adoption. The Rand Corporation Monograph. Retrieved February 4, 2008 from http://www.rand.org/pubs/monographs/MG409/

Foster, I., & Kesselman, C. (1997). Globus: A metacomputing infrastructure toolkit. *The International Journal of Supercomputer Applications*, *11*(2), 115–128. doi:10.1177/109434209701100205

Fourty, N., Val, T., Fraisse, P., & Mercier, J.-J. (2005). Comparative analysis of new high data rate wireless communication technologies "from Wi-Fi to WiMAX". In. *Proceedings of the Joint International Conference on Autonomic and Autonomous Systems and International Conference on Networking and Services, ICAS-ICNS, 2005*, 66–71. doi:10.1109/ICAS-ICNS.2005.34

Fox, C., Levitin, A., & Redman, T. C. (1994). The notion of data and its quality dimensions. *Information Processing & Management*, *30*(1), 9–19. doi:10.1016/0306-4573(94)90020-5

Francis, C. F., Feyer, A.-M., & Smith, B. J. (2007). Implementing chronic disease self-management in community settings: lessons from Australian demonstration projects. *Australian Health Review*, *31*(4), 499–509. doi:10.1071/AH070499

Freeman, R. E. (1984). *Strategic Management: A stakeholder Approach.* Cambridge: Ballinger Publishing Co.

Friedman, C., & Wyatt, J. (2000). *Evaluation methods in medical informatics*. New York: Springer-Verlag.

From clipboards to keyboard (2007, May 19). The Economist, pp. 68-69.

Frost, & Sullivan. (2004). Frost and Sullivan Country Industry Forecast - European Union Healthcare Industry, May 11, 2004. http://www.news-mdical.net/print_article.asp? id=1405.

Fruhling, A., & Lee, S. (2004, September). Designing Trustworthy e-Health Services for Rural Consumers. *MedInfo. American Medical Informatics Association Proceedings.*

Fung, B. C. M., Wang, K., Chen, R., & Yu, P. S. (in press). Privacy-preserving data publishing: A survey on recent developments. *ACM Computing Surveys.*

Gagliardi, A., & Jadad, A. R. (2002). Examination of instruments used to rate quality of health information on the Internet: chronicle of a voyage with an unclear destination. *BMJ (Clinical Research Ed.)*, *9*, 569–576. doi:10.1136/bmj.324.7337.569

Gagnon, M., Lamothe, L., Fortin, J., Cloutier, A., Godin, G., Gagne, C., & Reinharz, D. (2005). Teleadoption in hospitals: an organizational perspective. *Journal of Health Organization and Management*, *19*(1), 32–56. doi:10.1108/14777260510592121

Gallego, G., Fowler, S., & van Gool, K. (2008). Decision makers' perceptions of health technology decision making and priority setting at the institutional level. *Australian Health Review*, *32*(3), 520–526. doi:10.1071/AH080520

Gallo, L., De Pietro, G., Coronato, A., & Marra, I. (2008). Toward a natural interface to virtual medical imaging environments. In *Proceedings of the Working Conference on Advanced Visual Interfaces* (pp. 429-432). New York: ACM.

Galloway, L., & Mochrie, R. (2005). The use of ICT in rural firms: a policy-oriented literature review. *Info*, *7*(3), 33–46. doi:10.1108/14636690510596784

Gallup, J. L. and J. D. Sachs (2001) "The Economic Burden of Malaria", *The American Society of Tropical Medicine and Hygiene,* 64 (1,2), pp. 85-96.

Gao, T., Massey, T., Selavo, L., Crawford, D., Chen, B., & Lorincz, K. (2007). The advanced health and disaster aid network: A light-weight wireless medical system for triage. *IEEE Transactions on Biomedical Circuits and Systems*, *1*(3), 203–216. doi:10.1109/TBCAS.2007.910901

Gao, T., Kim, M. I., White, D., & Alm, A. M. (2006). Iterative user-centered design of a next generation patient monitoring system for emergency medical response. In *Proceedings of the AMIA Annual Symposium* (pp. 284-288).

Gao, T., Pesto, C., Selavo, L., Chen, Y., Ko, J. G., Lim, J. H., et al. (2008) Wireless Medical Sensor Networks in Emergency Response: Implementation and Pilot Results. In *Proceedings of the 2008 IEEE Conference on Technologies for Homeland Security* (pp. 187-192).

Garcia-Aymerich, J. & Hernandez, C. & Alonso A. (2007). Effects of an integrated care intervention on risk factors of COPD readmission. *Respiratory Medicine*, 10.1016.

Garrett, L. (2007) *The Challenge of Global Health* Foreign Affairs Last accessed: 1 March 2007 Last updated: Address: http://www.foreignaffairs.org/20070101faessay86103/laurie-garrett/the-challenge-of-global-health.html.

Garritty, C., & Emam, K. E. (2006). Who's Using PDAs? Estimates of PDA Use by Health Care Providers: A Systematic Review of Surveys. *Journal of Medical Internet Research*, *8*(2), e7. doi:10.2196/jmir.8.2.e7

Garson, G. D. (1998). Statnotes: Logistic regression. Raleigh, North Carolina: Carolina State University. http://www2.chass.ncsu.edu/garson/pa765/logistic.htm) [date accessed: 2 April 2006].

Gearing, P., Olney, C. M., Davis, K., Lozano, D., Smith, L. B., & Friedman, B. (2006). Enhancing patient safety through electronic medical record documentation of vital signs. *Journal of Healthcare Information Management*, *20*(4), 40–45.

Geertz, C. (1973). *The Interpretation of Cultures*. New York: Basic Books.

Geldenhuys, E., Herbst, D., & Dixon, B. J. Schnetler, J. (ed) & Stoker, D., J. (1989). Survey methods and practice. Revised Ed. Pretoria: Opinion Survey Centre. HSRC.

Ghosh, G. J., McLaren, P. M., & Watson, J. P. (1997). Evaluating the alliance in video-link teletherapy. *Journal of Telehealth*, *3*(suppl. 1), 33–35.

Gill, T. M., Allore, H. G., & Han, L. (2006). Bathing disability and the risk of long-term admission to a nursing home. *Journal of Gerontology*, *61*(8), 821–825.

Glasgow, R. E. (2007). E-health evaluation and dissemination research. *American Journal of Preventive Medicine*, *32*(5Suppl), S119–S126. doi:10.1016/j.amepre.2007.01.023

Glasser, B. G., & Strauss, A. L. (1967). *The discovery of grounded theory*. New York: Aldine.

Godlee, F. (2004). Can We Achieve Health Information for All by 2015. *Lancet*, *364*, 295–300. doi:10.1016/S0140-6736(04)16681-6

Golant, S. M. (2008). The Future of Assisted Living Residences. In S. M. Golant & J. Hyde (Eds.), *The Assisted Living Residence* (pp. 3-45). Baltimore, MD: John Hopkins University Press.

Goldberg, S. a. (2002a). *Building the Evidence for a standardized Mobile Internet (wireless) Environment in Ontario, Canada, January Update, Internal INET Documentation*. Ontario, Canada: INET.

Goldberg, S. a. (2002b). *HTA Presentational Selection and Aggregation Component Summary. Internal INET Documentation*. Ontario, Canada: INET.

Goldberg, S. a. (2002c). *Wireless POC Device Component Summary, Internal INET documentation*. Ontario, Canada: INET.

Goldberg, S. a. (2002d). *HTA Presentation Rendering Component Summary, Internal INET documentation*. Ontario, Canada: INET.

Goldberg, S. a. (2002e). *HTA Quality Assurance Component Summary, Internal INET documentation*. Ontario, Canada: INET.

Golden Living Centers. (2008). *Fun Times*. Retrieved October 20, 2008, from http://www.goldenlivingcenters.com/GGNSC

Goldsborough, R. (2001). Mastering Computers: Can the Internet be trusted? *Tech Directions*, *61*(4), 13–14.

Gonzalez, C. M., & Puri, L. (2008). Productivity and cost implications of implementing electronic medical records into an ambulatory surgical subspecialty clinic. *Urology*, *71*(2), 173–177. doi:10.1016/j.urology.2007.09.024

González, M. E., Quesada, G., Urrutia, I., & Gavidia, V. (2006). Conceptual design of an e-health strategy for the Spanish health care system. *International Journal of Health Care Quality Assurance*, *19*(2), 146–157. doi:10.1108/09526860610651681

Gonzalez-Morcillo, C., Weiss, G., Jiménez, L., & Vallejo, D. (2007). A multi-agent approach to distributed rendering optimization. In. *Proceedings of AAAI*, *07*, 1775–1780.

Goodman, N. (1978). *Ways of Worldmaking*. Indianapolis: Hackett.

Gordon, L. A., Loeb, M. P., Lucyshin, W., & Richardson, R. (2006). *2006 CSI/FBI Computer Crime and Security Survey*. Retrieved February 17, 2009, from http://i.cmpnet.com/gocsi/db_area/pdfs/fbi/FBI2006.pdf

Green, A. (1999). *An Introduction to Health Planning in Developing Countries* (2nd ed.). Oxford: Oxford University Press.

Greenfield, T. (Ed.). (2002). *Research methods for postgraduates* (2nd ed.). London: Arnold.

Greenly, M., & Gugerty, B. (2002). How bar coding reduces medication errors. *Nursing*, *32*(5), 70.

Griffith, J. A. G. (1966) Central Departments and Local Authorities. University of Toronto Press, Toronto, Ont.

Gröne, O., & Garcia-Barbero, M. (2002). Trends in Integrated Care – Reflections on Conceptual Issues. WHO, Copenhagen, EUR/02/5037864.

Grover, V., Jeong, S. R., & Segars, A. H. (1996). Information Systems Effectiveness: The Construct Space and Patterns of Applications. *Information & Management*, *31*(4). doi:10.1016/S0378-7206(96)01079-8

Groves, R. M., Fowler, F. J., Couper, M. P., Lepkowski, J. M., Singer, E., & Tourangeau, R. (Eds.). (2004). *Survey Methodology*. New Jersey: John Wiley & Sons.

Guevara, J. P., Wolf, F. M., & Grum, C. M. (2003). Effects of educational Interventions for self management of asthma in children and adolescents: systematic review and meta-analysis. *BMJ (Clinical Research Ed.)*, *326*, doi:10.1136/bmj.326.7402.1308

Gupta, M., Gauri, V., & Khemani, S. (2003). *"Decentralized Delivery of Primary Health Services in Nigeria. Survey Evidence from the States of Lagos and Kogi" The world Bank*. Africa Region.

Gururajan, R., & Murugesan, S. (2005). *Wireless solutions developed for the Australian healthcare: A review.* Paper presented at the 4th International Conference on Mobile Business, Sydney, Australia.

Gururajan, R., Hafeez-Baig, A., & Gururjan, V. (2008). Clinical Factors And Technological Barriers As Determinants For The Intention To Use Wireless Handheld Technology In Healthcare Environment: An Indian Case Study. In *16th European Conference on Information Systems*, National University of Ireland, Galway.

Gururajan, R., Moloney, C., & Kerr, D. (2005). Drivers for wireless handheld technology: Views from Queensland nurses. In *Australian Business & Behavioural Sciences Association (ABBSA) Conference,* Cairns, Australia, James Cook University (pp. 258-267).

Gururajan, R., Quaddus, M., Fink, D., Vuori, T., & Soar, J. (2005). *Drivers and Barriers to adoption of wireless handheld system in WA healthcare: Selected views.* Paper presented at the HIC 2005, Melbourne.

Gururajan, R., Toleman, M., & Soar, J. (2004, 25-27 July). *Necessity for a new technology acceptance model to predict adoption of wireless technology in healthcare.* Paper presented at the Let's Make a Difference with Health ICT, HIC Conference.

Gustafson, D., Hawkins, R., Pingree, S., McTavish, F., Arora, N., & Salner, J. (2001). Effect of computer support on younger women with breast cancer. *Journal of General Internal Medicine*, *16*, 435–445. doi:10.1046/j.1525-1497.2001.016007435.x

Gustafson, D., & Wyatt, J. (2004). Evaluation of e-health systems and services. *British Medical Journal*, *328*, 1150. .doi:10.1136/bmj.328.7449.1150

Gwatkin, D. (2000). Critical Reflection: Health Inequalities and the Health of the Poor. What Do We Know? What Can We Do? *Bulletin of the World Health Organization*, *78*(1), 3–18.

Haag, S., Baltzan, P., & Phillips, A. (2006). *Business Driven Technology* (2nd ed.). McGraw-Hill.

Hafeez-Baig, A. (2007). *Technology Management, Data management, Improved outcomes, Efficiency and Software limitation influencing the use of wireless technology for healthcare in Pakistan* Paper presented at the 6th IEEE/ACIS International Conference on Computer and Information Science (ICIS 2007) Melbourne.

Hair, J. F., Anderson, R. E., Tatham, R. L., & Black, W. C. (1995). *Multivariate Data Analysis with Readings* (4th ed.). London: Prentice-Hall.

Hall, J. J., & Taylor, R. (2003). Health for All Beyond 2000: The Demise of the Alma-Ata Declaration and Primary Health Care in Developing Countries. *The Medical Journal of Australia*, *178*(1), 17–20.

Halpern, J. Y., & Weissman, V. (2008). Using First-Order Logic to Reason about Policies. *ACM Transactions on Information and System Security*, *11*, 1–41. doi:10.1145/1380564.1380569

Hameed, K. (2003). The application of mobile computing and technology to health care services. [May.]. *Telematics and Informatics*, *20*(2), 99–106. doi:10.1016/S0736-5853(02)00018-7

Hamilton, B. (2006). *Evaluation design of the business case of health information technology in long-term care (Final report).* Baltimore: Centers for Medicare and Medicaid Services. Harding Nursing Home. (n.d.) *Activities.* Retrieved October 20, 2008, from http://www.hardingnh.com/

Hammersley, M., & Atkinson, P. (1983). *Ethnography: Principles in Practice.* London: Tavistock.

Handy, J., Whiddett, R., & Hunter, I. (2001). A technology acceptance model for inter-organizational electronic medical records systems. *AJIS*, *9*(1), 39–50.

Hans, O., Rizo, C., Enkin, M., & Jadad, A. (2005, February 24). What is e-health? *A Systematic Review of Published Definitions. Journal of Medical Internet Research.* doi:. doi:10.2196/jmir.7.1.e1

Haoses-Gorases, L. (2005). Utilization of Health Information System (HIS) in Namibia: Challenges and opportunities faced by the health care delivery system. Paper presented at the international workshop on Strategies for Permanent Access to Scientific Information in Southern Africa: Focus on Health and Environmental Information for Sustainable Development, Pretoria, 5-7. September 2005.

Hardy, C., & Williams, S. P. (2005). Public eProcurement in Action: Policies, Practice and Technologies. In Böhlen, M. et al. (eds.) Proceedings of E-Government: Towards Electronic Democracy, TCGOV 2005 (LNAI 3416, p.286). Berlin: Springer.

Harkke, V. (2005). Physicians' usage experiences of a mobile information system. *38th Hawaii International Conference on System Sciences*, Hawaii.

Harris, Y., & Clauser, S. B. (2002). Achieving improvement through nursing home quality measurement. *Health Care Financing Review*, *23*(4), 13.

Harrison, S. (2002). Telehealth skills hailed as answer to discharge delays: Costs of high-tech monitoring systems compare favourably with long-term care. *Nursing Standard*, *17*(12), 7.

Harvey, P. W., Petkov, J. N., Misan, G., Fuller, J., Battersby, M. W., & Cayetano, T. N. (2008). Self-management support and training for patients with chronic and complex conditions improves health-related behaviour and health outcomes. *Australian Health Review*, *32*(2), 330–338. doi:10.1071/AH080330

Health IT Strategic Framework. (2004), Office for the National Coordinator for Health Information Technology. United States Department of Health and Human Services. Retrieved February 4, 2008 from http://www.hhs.gov/healthit/preface.html

Heeks, R. (2006). Health Information Systems: Failure, Success and Improvisation. *International Journal of Medical Informatics*, *75*, 125–137. doi:10.1016/j.ijmedinf.2005.07.024

Helene, B., & Ford, P. (2000). Mind-body Innovations, an Integrative Care Approach. *Psych Quart*, *71*(1), 47–58. doi:10.1023/A:1004614717641

Henriksen, H. Z., & Mahnke, V. (2005). E-Procurement Adoption in the Danish Public Sector. *Scandinavian Journal of Information Systems*, *17*(2), 85–106.

Herper, M. (2005). *The most expensive diseases*. Forbes. Available at http://www.forbes.com/2005/04/14/cx_mh_0414healthcosts.html, last accessed on 13 August 2010.

Hess, H. M. (2005). Aligning technology and business: Applying patterns for legacy transformation. *IBM Systems Journal*, *44*(1), 25–45. doi:10.1147/sj.441.0025

Hesselmark, O., & Miller, J. (2002). A country ICT survey for Namibia. http://www.cyberzoo.co.za/download/milless/newdocs/Namrep%20v5.pdf [Date accessed: 10 March 2006].

Hesterly, W. S., Liebeskind, J., & Zenger, T. R. (1990). Organizational economics: an impeding revolution in organizational theory. *Academy of Management Review*, *15*(3), 402–420. doi:10.2307/258016

Hesterly, W. S., & Zenger, T. R. (1993). The myth of a monolithic economics: Fundamental assumptions and the use of economic models in policy and strategy research. *Organization Science*, *4*, 496–510. doi:10.1287/orsc.4.3.496

Hillestad, R., Bigelow, J., Bower, A., Girosi, F., Meili, R., Scoville, R., & Taylor, R. (2005). Can electronic medical record systems transform health care? Potential health benefits, savings, and costs. *Health Affairs*, *24*(5), 1103–1117. doi:10.1377/hlthaff.24.5.1103

Hoban, S. (2003). Activities plus at Montgomery Place: The "new" active senior wants to be entertained, enlightened, and engaged--and will let you know how. *Nursing Homes*, *52*(6), 52–56.

Hobart, J. C., Lamping, D. L., & Freeman, J. A. (2001). Evidence-based measurement. Which disability scale for neurologic rehabilitation? *Neurology*, *2001*, 57.

Hoffman-Goetz, L., & Clarke, J. N. (2000). Quality of Breast cancer sites on the World Wide Web. *Canadian Journal of Public Health*, *91*(4), 281–284.

Hogan, W. (2007). *The Organisation of Residential Aged Care for an Ageing Population.* St. Leonards, NSW, Australia: The Centre of Independent Studies.

Holliday, I., & Tam, W. (2004). E-health in the East Asian tigers. *International Journal of Medical Informatics*, *73*(11-12), 759–769. doi:10.1016/j.ijmedinf.2004.08.001

Holman, H. (2004). Chronic disease – the need for a new clinical education. *Journal of the American Medical Association*, *292*, 1057–1059. doi:10.1001/jama.292.9.1057

Holmes, D. (2007). An evaluation of a monitoring system intervention: falls, injuries, and affect in nursing homes. *Clinical Nursing Research*, *16*(4), 317–335. doi:10.1177/1054773807307870

Holmes-Smith, P. (2000). *Introduction to Structural Equation Modeling Using AMOS 4.0.* Melbourne: SREAMS.

Hopkinson, G. C., & Pujari, D. (1999). A factor analytic study in hedonic consumption. [April.]. *European Journal of Marketing*, *33*(3/4), 273–290. doi:10.1108/03090569910253053

Horan, T. A., Tule, B., & Hilton, B. N. (2006). Understanding physician use of online systems: An empirical assessment of an electronic disability evaluation system. In Spil, T. A. M., & Schuring, W. R. (Eds.), *E-Health Systems Diffusion and Use: The Innovation, the User and the USE IT Model.* Hershey, PA, USA: IGI Global.

Horan, T. A., Tulu, B., Hilton, B., & Burton, J. (2004). Use of online systems in clinical medical assessments: An analysis of physician acceptance of online disability evaluation systems. *37th Hawaii International Conference on System Sciences*, Hawaii.

Horan, T., Abhichandani, T., & Rayalu, R. (2006). Assessing User Satisfaction of E-Government Services: Development and Testing of Quality-in-Use Satisfaction with Advanced Traveler Information Systems (ATIS). *Proceedings of the 39th Hawaii International Conference on System Sciences.*

Houlton, S. (2004). Time for Transparency. *Pharmaceutical Executive*, *24*(11), 40.

Howard, A., Gururajan, R., Hafeez-Baig, A., et al. (2006). Clinical Usefulness of Wireless Technology in Healthcare: An Indian Study. In *The Australasian Conference on Information Systems*, University of South Australia.

Hsu, L. L., Li, H., & Zhi, Z. (2004). Establishing evaluation indicators in health and medical websites. *Hu Li Za Zhi*, *51*(3), 47–52.

Hsu, J., Huang, J., Fung, V., Robertson, N., & Jimison, H. (2005). Health information technology and physician-patient interactions: Impact of computers on communication during outpatient visits. *Journal of the American Medical Informatics Association*, *12*, 474–480. doi:10.1197/jamia.M1741

Hu, P. J., Chau, P. Y. K., & Liu Sheng, O. R. (2002). Adoption of telemedicine technology by health care organisations: An exploratory study. *Journal of Organizational Computing and Electronic Commerce*, *12*(3), 197–222. doi:10.1207/S15327744JOCE1203_01

Hu, P., Chau, P., & Tam, K. (1999). Examining the technology acceptance model using physician acceptance of telemedicine technology. *Journal of Management Information Systems*, *16*(2), 91–112.

Hufnagel, E. M., & Conca, C. (1994). Use Response Data: The Potential for Errors and Biases. *Information Systems Research*, *5*, 48–73. doi:10.1287/isre.5.1.48

Hundie, K. (2002). free medical journals Website: an exemplary service. *Campus-Wide Information Systems*, *19*(3), 113–116.

Hunt, D. (2007). *Urgent health system reform needed to tackle disease epidemic, says head of new University of Melbourne centre.* Retrieved 25 November, 2008, from http://uninews.unimelb.edu.au/view.php?articleID=4615

Husek, C. (2008, August). *ELGA: The Electronic Health Record in Austria.* Paper presented at the International Conference of Society for Medical Innovation and Technology, Vienna, Austria.

Hutton, P., Trueman, P., & Henshall, C. (2007). Coverage with Evidence Development. *International Journal of Technology Assessment in Health Care, 23*(4), 425–435.

Hyde, J., Perez, R., & Reed, P. S. (2008). The Old Road Is Rapidly Aging. In S. M. Golant & J. Hyde (Eds.), *The Assisted Living Residence* (pp. 46-85). Baltimore, MD: Johns Hopkins University Press.

ICIC. (2008). *Improving Chronic Illness Care: The Chronic Care Model.* Retrieved from http://www.improvingchroniccare.org/indix.php?p=The_Chronic_Care_Model&s=2

Ikemba, C. M., Kozinetz, C. A., Feltes, T. F., Fraser, C. D., McKenzie, D., & Shah, N. (2002). Internet Use in Families with Children requiring Cardiac Surgery for Congenital Heart Disease. *Pediatrics, 109*(3), 419–422. doi:10.1542/peds.109.3.419

Ilie, V., Courtney, J. F., & Slyke, C. V. (2007). Paper versus electronic: Challenges associated with physicians' usage of electronic medical records. Proceedings of the 40th Hawaii International Conference on Systems Science.

Informa. (2005a). *Mobile Content and Services: Worldwide Market Analysis & Strategic Outlook.* London: Informa Telecoms & Media.

Informa. (2005b). *Global Mobile Forecasts to 2010: Worldwide Market Analysis & Strategic Outlook 2005-2010* (5th ed.). London: Informa Telecoms & Media.

Informa. (2006a). *Global Mobile: The International Business Newsletter of Mobile Communications Markets. 13*(6).

Initiatives, F. D. A. (2007). FDA and Duke Launch Public-Private Partnership to Modernize Clinical Trials. Retrieved on March 31, 2008 from http://www.fda.gov/oc/initiatives/criticalpath/partnership.html

Institute of Medicine. (2001). *Crossing the quality chasm: A new health system for 21st century.* Washington, DC: National Academy Press.

Intel Health. (2007). Reconceiving Disease Management: A Technology Perspective. *Whitepaper of Intel Health.* Available at http://www.intel.com/pressroom/kits/healthcare/DiseaseMgmt_whitepaper.pdf, last accessed on 13 August 2010.

Internet Engineering Task Force. (2008). *The Transport Layer Security (TLS) Protocol Version 1.2.* Retrieved February 17, 2009, from http://tools.ietf.org/html/rfc5246

Intille, S. S. (2002). Designing a Home of the Future. *IEEE Pervasive Computing / IEEE Computer Society [and] IEEE Communications Society, 1*(2), 76–82. doi:10.1109/MPRV.2002.1012340

ISO/IEC. (1999). Integrated Circuit(s) Cards with Contacts – Part 7: Interindustry Commands for Structured Card Query Language (SCQL). Standard ISO/IEC 7816-7.

Istepanian, R. S. H., Jovanov, E., & Zhang, Y. T. (2004). Guest Editorial: Introduction to the special section on m-health: beyond seamless mobility and global wireless healthcare connectivity. *IEEE Transactions on Information Technology in Biomedicine, 8*(4), 405–414. doi:10.1109/TITB.2004.840019

Istepanian, R. S. H., & Lacal, J. C. (2003). *Emerging mobile communication technologies for health: some imperative notes on m-health.* Paper presented at the 25th Annual International Conference of the IEEE EMBS, New York.

Ivanitskaya, L., O'Bole, I., & Casey, A. M. (2006). Health Information Literacy and Compentencies of Information Age Students: Results from Interactive Online Research readiness Self-Assessment (RRSA). *Journal of Medical Internet Research, 8*(2), 1–15. doi:10.2196/jmir.8.2.e6

Ivers, B., & Gururajan, R. (2006). Management issues in telecommunications: videoconferencing & telehealth. In *International Conference on Recent Trends in Information Systems Proceedings* (pp. 796-806), India: Allied Publishers Pvt Ltd.

Jaarsma, T., Strömberg, A., & De Geest, S. (2006). Heart failure management programmes in Europe. *European Journal of Cardiovascular Nursing, 5*, 197–205. doi:10.1016/j.ejcnurse.2006.04.002

Jamison, D., & Mosley, W. (1991). Disease Control Priorities in Developing Countries: Health Policy Responses to Epidemiological Change. *American Journal of Public Health, 81*(1), 15–22. doi:10.2105/AJPH.81.1.15

Japan Statistics Bureau & Statistics Center. (2008, April 15). *Population by Age (Single Year), Sex and Sex ratio - Total population, Japanese population.* Retrieved January 28, 2009, from http://www.e-stat.go.jp/SG1/estat/ListE.do?lid=000001026128

Jara, A. J., Zamora, M. A., & Skarmeta, A. F. G. (2009). An Architecture for Ambient Assisted Living and Health Environments. In *Distributed Computing, Artificial Intelligence, Bioinformatics, Soft Computing, and Ambient Assisted Living* (LNCS 5518, pp. 882-889).

Jarvinen, O. (2005). *Privacy Management of E-health, Content Analysis of 39 US Health Providers' Privacy Policies.* Publication of Turku School of Economics and Business Administration. *Series, A-3,* 2005.

Jayasuriya, R. (1998). Determinants of microcomputer technology use: Implications for education and training of health staff. *International Journal of Medical Informatics, 50,* 187–194. doi:10.1016/S1386-5056(98)00067-7

Jeppsson, A., & Okuonzi, S. A. (2000). Vertical or Holistic Decentralization of the Health Sector? Experiences from Zambia and Uganda. *The International Journal of Health Planning and Management, 15*(4), 273–289. doi:10.1002/hpm.597

John, A. K. (2006). A Critical Appraisal of Internet Resources on Colorectal Cancer. *Colorectal Disease, 8*(3), 217–223. doi:10.1111/j.1463-1318.2005.00882.x

Johnson, B., Wheeler, L., Dueser, J., & Sousa, K. (2000). Outcomes of the Kaiser Permanente Tele-Home Health Research Project. *Archives of Family Medicine, 9*(4), 40–45. doi:10.1001/archfami.9.1.40

Johnson, A. M. (2005). The technology acceptance model and the decision to invest in Information security. Southern Association of Information systems conference. Savannah, Georgia, USA, 25-26, 2005.

Joint Report by the Commission and the Council on supporting national strategies for the future health care and care for the elderly. EU 7166/03 SOC 116 ECOFIN 77 SAN 41.

Jones, S., & Hughes, J. (2001). Understanding IS Evaluation as a Complex Social Process: A Case Study of a United Kingdom Local Authority. *European Journal of Information Systems, 10*(1).

Jones, C., Hesterly, W. S., & Borgatti, S. P. (1997). A general theory of network governance: exchange conditions and social mechanisms. *Academy of Management Review, 22*(4), 911–945. doi:10.2307/259249

Joos, D., Chen, Q., Jirjis, J., & Johnson, K. B. (2006). An electronic medical record in primary care: Impact on satisfaction, work efficiency, and clinical processes. AMIA Symposium Proceedings, 394-398.

Joy, S., & Benrubi, G. (2004). Personal digital assistant use in Florida in obstetrics and gynaecology residency programs. *Southern Medical Journal, 97*(5), 430–433. doi:10.1097/00007611-200405000-00002

Kahn, B. K., Strong, D. M., & Wang, R. Y. (2002). Information quality benchmarks: product and service performance. *Communications of the ACM, 45*(4), 184–193. doi:10.1145/505248.506007

Kallinikos, J. (2006). *The Consequences of Infformation. Institutional Implications of Technological Change.* Cheltenham: Edward Elgar.

Kalorama (2007). *Wireless Opportunities in Healthcare.* Rockville, MD:Kalorama Information.

Kang, S. W., Yoo, J. S., & Ko, I. S. (2006). Development of a-health information website: evaluation categories with items for diabetes mellitus. *Studies in Health Technology and Informatics, 122,* 777.

Karantonis, D. M., Narayanan, M. R., Mathie, M., Lovell, N. H., & Celler, B. G. (2006). Implementation of a Real-Time Human Movement Classifier Using a Triaxial Accelerometer for Ambulatory Monitoring. *IEEE Transactions on Information Technology in Biomedicine, 10*(1), 156–167. doi:10.1109/TITB.2005.856864

Karjoth, G., Schunter, M., & Waidner, M. (2002). Platform for Enterprise Privacy Practices: Privacy-Enabled Management of Customer Data. In *Privacy Enhancing Technologies* (pp. 69-84).

Kassim, E. S., & Hussin, H. (2010). *Public E-procurement: A Research Synthesis, e-Education, e-Business, e-Management and e-Learning*. International Conference on, 150-154, 2010 International Conference on e-Education, e-Business, e-Management, IEEE.

Kavanagh, S., & Yellowlees, P. (1995). Telemedicine: Clinical applications in mental health. *Australian Family Physician*, *24*, 1242–1246.

Kavas, A. (2007). Comparative analysis of WLAN, WiMAX and UMTS Technologies. In *Proceedings of the Progress In Electromagnetics Research Symposium 2007*, Prague, Czech Republic (pp. 140-144).

Kemper, P., Komisar, H. L., & Alecixh, L. (2005). Long-Term Care over what can Current Retirees Expect? *Inquiry*, *42*, 15.

Kenny, C. (2002). Information and communication technologies for direct poverty alleviation: costs and benefits. *Development Policy*, *20*(2), 141–157. doi:10.1111/1467-7679.00162

Kephart, J. O., & Chess, D. M. (2003). The Vision of Autonomic Computing. *Computer*, *36*(1), 41–50. doi:10.1109/MC.2003.1160055

Khambati, A., Warren, J., Grundy, J., & Hosking, J. (2008). *A model driven approach to care planning systems for consumer engagement in chronic disease management*. Paper presented at the HIC 2008 Australia's Health Informatics Conference, Health Informatics Society of Australia Ltd (HISA).

Khoumbati, K., & Themistocleous, M. (2006). Integrating the IT Infrastructures in Healthcare Organisations: a Proposition of Influential Factors. *The Electronic. Journal of E-Government*, *4*(1), 27–36.

Kidd, C. D., Orr, R., Abowd, G. D., Atkeson, C. G., Essa, I. A., MacIntyre, B., et al. (1999). *The Aware Home: A Living Laboratory for Ubiquitous Computing Research*. Paper presented at the Second International Workshop on Cooperative Buildings, Integrating Information, Organization, and Architecture.

Killeen, J. P., Chan, T. C., Buono, C., Griswold, W. G., & Lenert, L. A. (2006). A wireless first responder handheld device for rapid triage, patient assessment and documentation during mass casualty incidents. In *Proceedings of the AMIA Annual Symposium* (pp. 429-433).

Kim, J., & Shunk, D. L. (2004). Matching indirect procurement process with different B2B e-procurement systems. *Computers in Industry*, *53*, 153–164. doi:10.1016/j.compind.2003.07.002

Kimaro, H., & Nhampossa, J. (2005). Analysing the Problem of Unsustainable Health Information Systems in Less-Developed Economies: Case Studies from Tanzania and Mozambique. *Information Technology for Development*, *11*(3), 273–298. doi:10.1002/itdj.20016

King, W. R., & He, J. (2006). A meta-analysis of the technology acceptance model. *Information & Management*, *43*(6), 740–755. doi:10.1016/j.im.2006.05.003

Kirshner, M., Salomon, H., & Chin, H. (2004). An evaluation of one-on-one advanced proficiency training in clinicians' use of computer information systems. *International Journal of Medical Informatics*, *73*(4), 341–348.

Kleeman, E. (2006). Clinical trials face shortage of candidates. *Knight Ridder Tribune Business News, 1, October 2nd, RetrievedMarch5, 2008, from ABI/INFORM Dateline database. (Document ID: 1139651541).*

Klein, H., & Myers, M. (1999). A Set of Principles for Conducting and Evaluating Interpretive Field Studies. *Management Information Systems Quarterly*, *23*(1), 67–93. doi:10.2307/249410

Klein, B. D. (2001). User perceptions of data quality: Internet and traditional text sources. *Journal of Computer Information Systems*, *41*(4), 9–15.

Klein, H. K., & Myers, M. D. (1999). A set of principles for conducting and evaluating interpretive field studies in information systems. *Management Information Systems Quarterly*, *23*(1), 67–94. doi:10.2307/249410

Knuiman, M. W., Welborn, T. A., & Bartholomew, H. C. (1996). Self-reported health and use of health services: a comparison of diabetic and nondiabetic persons from a national sample. *Australian and New Zealand Journal of Public Health*, *20*(3), 241–247. doi:10.1111/j.1467-842X.1996.tb01023.x

Ko, Y., Brown, M., Frost, R., & Woosley, R. L. (2006). Brief Report: Development of a Prescription Mediation Information Webliography for Consumers. *Journal of General Internal Medicine*, *21*(12), 1313–1316. doi:10.1111/j.1525-1497.2006.00620.x

Kohn, L. T., Corrigan, J. M., & Donaldson, M. S. (1999). *To err is human: Building a safer human system.* Washington, DC: National Academy Press.

Korhonen, I., & Bardram, J. E. (2004). Guest editorial introduction to the special section on pervasive healthcare. *IEEE Transactions on Information Technology in Biomedicine*, *8*(3), 229–234. doi:10.1109/TITB.2004.835337

Kramer, A., Bennett, R., Fish, R., Lin, C. T., Floersch, N., Conway, K., et al. (2004). *Case studies of electronic health records in post-acute and long-term care*. Washington, DC: U.S. Department of Health and Human Services.

Kreuter, M. W., Strecher, V. J., & Glassman, B. (1999). One size does not fit all: The case for tailoring print materials. *Annals of Behavioral Medicine*, *21*(4), 276–283. doi:10.1007/BF02895958

Kulkarni, R., & Nathanson, L. A. (2005). *Medicine Informatics in Medicine. Available:*http://www.emedicine.com/emerg/topic879.htm.

Kutzik, D. M., Glascock, A. P., Lundberg, L., & York, J. (2008). Technological Tools of the Future. In S. M. Golant & J. Hyde (Eds.), *The Assisted Living Residence*. Baltimore, MD: Johns Hopkins University Press.

Labiod, H., Afifi, H., & De Santis, C. (2007). *Wi-Fi Bluetooth Zigbee and WiMax*. Dordrecht, The Netherlands: Springer.

LaBrie, R. A., LaPlante, D. A., & Peller, A. J. (2007). The interdependence of behavioural and somatic health: implications for conceptualizing health and measuring treatment outcomes. [May.]. *International Journal of Integrated Care*, *7*, 16.

Lacroix, A. (1999). International concerted action on collaboration in telemedicine: G8sub-project 4. *Studies in Health Technology and Informatics*, *64*, 12–19.

Lam, A. (1997). Embedded Firms, Embedded Knowledge: Problems of Collaboration and Knowledge Transfer in Global Cooperative Ventures. *Organization Studies*, *18*(6), 973–996. doi:10.1177/017084069701800604

Lam, A. (2000). Tacit knowledge, organizational learning and societal institutions: an integrated framework. *Organization Studies*, *21*(3), 487–513. doi:10.1177/0170840600213001

Lam, A. (2002). Alternative societal models of learning and innovation in the knowledge economy. *International Social Science Journal*, *54*(171), 67–82. doi:10.1111/1468-2451.00360

Lampe, A. J., & Weiler, J., M. (1998). Data capture from the sponsors' and investigators' perspectives: Balancing quality, speed, and cost. *Drug Information Journal*, *32*(4), 871–886.

Langheinrich, M. (2005). *Personal Privacy in Ubiquitous Computing*. Unpublished doctoral dissertation, ETH Zurich.

Langhorne, P., & Taylor, G. (2005). Early supported discharge services for stroke patients: an individual patient data meta-analysis. *Lancet*, *365*, 501–506.

Langhorne, P., & Widén-Holmquist, L. (2007). Early Supported Discharge after Stroke. *Journal of Rehabilitation Medicine*, *39*, 103–108. doi:10.2340/16501977-0042

Lapointe, L., Lamothe, L., & Fortin, J. (2006). The dynamics of IT adoption in a major change process in healthcare delivery. In Spil, T. A. M., & Schuring, R. W. (Eds.), *E-Health Systems Diffusion and Use: The Innovation, the User and the USE IT Model*. Hershey, PA, USA: IGI Global.

Lapointe, L., Lamothe, L., & Fortin, J. P. (2002). The dynamics of IT adoption in a major change process in healthcare delivery. *Proceedings of the 35th HICSS conference,* Big Island, Hawaii.

Larsen, T. (2010). Neuroeconomics and Public Health. *Acta Systemica*, *X*(1).

Larsen, T., Olsen, T. S., & Sorensen, J. (2006). Early Home-supported Discharge of Stroke Patients: a Health Technology Assessment. *International Journal of Technology Assessment in Health Care*, *22*(3), 313–320. doi:10.1017/S0266462306051208

Lauer, T., Joshi, K., & Browdy, T. (2000, Jan–Feb). Use of the Equity Implementation Model to Review Clinical System Implementation Efforts. *Journal of the American Medical Informatics Association*, *7*(1),

Laurence, G. G., & Paul, R. Y. (eds). (2000). Reading and Understanding more multivariate statistics. American Psychological Association.

Lee, K. (1998). Shaping the Future of Global Health Cooperation: Where Can We Go from Here? *Lancet*, *351*, 899–902. doi:10.1016/S0140-6736(97)11455-6

Lee, E., Kwon, J., & Schumann, D. W. (2005). Segmenting the non-adopter category in the diffusion of Internet banking. *International Journal of Bank Marketing*, *23*(5), 414–437. doi:10.1108/02652320510612483

Lee, R. G., Chen, K. C., Hsiao, C. C., & Tseng, C. L. (2007). A Mobile Care System with Alert Mechanism. *IEEE Transactions on Information Technology in Biomedicine*, *11*(5). doi:10.1109/TITB.2006.888701

LeFevre, K., DeWitt, D. J., & Ramakrishnan, R. (2006). Mondrian multidimensional k-anonymity. In *Proceedings of the 22nd IEEE International Conference on Data Engineering (ICDE)*, Atlanta, GA.

Leff, J. (1997). *Care in the community: illusion or reality*. London: Wiley.

Leichsenring, K. (2004). Developing integrated health and social care services for older persons in Europe. *International Journal of Integrated Care*, 4.

Lemon, M., & Sahota, P. S. (2004). Organizational culture as a knowledge repository for increased innovative capacity. *Technovation*, *24*(6), 483–498. doi:10.1016/S0166-4972(02)00102-5

Lenert, L., Palmer, D., Chan, T., & Rao, R. (2005). An intelligent 802.11 triage tag for medical response to disasters. In *Proceedings of the AMIA Annual Symposium* (pp. 440-444).

Lenhart, A., Horrigan, J., Rainie, L., Allen, K., Boyce, A., & Madden, M. (2003). *The ever-shifting Internet population. A new look at Internet access and the digital divide*. Washington, DC: Pew Internet & American Life Project.

Lewiecki, E. M., Rudolph, L. A., Kiebzak, G. M., Chavez, J. R., & Thorpe, B. M. (2006). Assessment of Osteoporosis Quality. *Osteoporosis International*, *17*(5), 741–752. doi:10.1007/s00198-005-0042-5

Li, Y. C., Chang, I. C., Hung, W. F., & Fu, H. K. (2005). The critical factors affecting hospital adoption of mobile nursing technologies in Taiwan. *Proceedings of the 38th Hawaii International Conference on System Sciences*, Hawaii, USA.

Liebert, T. (2008, March). Ongoing concern over Pentagon network attack. *IT News Digest*. Retrieved February 17, 2009, from http://blogs.techrepublic.com.com/tech-news/?p=2098

Lilley, R., Lambden, P., & Gillies, A. (2006). *Medicines management for residential and nursing homes: A toolkit for best practice and accredited learning*. Seattle, WA: Radcliffe.

Lin, Y.-H., Jan, I.-C., Ko, P. C.-I., Chen, Y.-Y., Wong, J.-M., & Jan, G.-J. (2004). A wireless PDA-based physiological monitoring system for patient transport. *IEEE Transactions on Information Technology in Biomedicine*, *8*(4), 439–447. doi:10.1109/TITB.2004.837829

Lincoln, Y. S., & Cuba, E. G. (1985). *Naturalistic Inquiry*. Newbury Park: Sage.

Lind-Albrecht, G. (2006). Patientenschulung in der Rheumatologie: Ein Weg zum besseren Krankheitsmanagement durch Kompetenzsteigerung bei den Betroffenen. *Wiener Medizinische Wochenschrift*, *156*(21–22), 583–586. doi:10.1007/s10354-006-0350-1

Lindars, E. S., & Spickett, J. T. (2000). The content and efficacy of environmental public health journal homepages. *Asia-Pacific Journal of Public Health*, *12*(1), 32–36.

Linder, J. A., Bates, D. W., Middleton, B., & Stafford, R. S. (2007). Electronic health records use and the quality of ambulatory care in the United States. *Archives of Internal Medicine*, *167*(13), 1400–1405. doi:10.1001/archinte.167.13.1400

Littlejohns, P., Wyatt, J. C., & Garvican, L. (2003). Evaluating Computerised Health Information Systems: Hard Lessons Still to Be Learnt. *BMJ (Clinical Research Ed.)*, *326*, 860–863. doi:10.1136/bmj.326.7394.860

Liu, Y., & Liu, M. (2006). Osteosarcoma: Evaluation Information on the Internet. Telemedicine and e-Health, 12(5), 542-545.

Loewenson, R. (1993). Structural Adjustment and Health Policy in Africa. *International Journal of Health Services*, *23*(4), 717–730.

Löfstedt, U. (2007). E-Government Services in Local Governments – A study of Development in Swedish Municipalities. *Journal of Organisational Transformation and Social Change*, *4*(2), 157–167. doi:10.1386/jots.4.2.157_1

Loiacono, E. T., Watson, R. T., & Goodhue, D. L. (2002). Webqual: A Web Site Quality Instrument. In *Proceedings of the AMA Winter Marketing Educators' Conference*, Austin, TX, USA.

Lopez, F. R. P. (2004). An Evaluation of the contents and Quality of Menopause Information on the World Wide Web. *The European Menopause Journal*, *49*, 276–282.

Lovell, N. H., Celler, B. G., Basilakis, J., Magrabi, F., Huynh, K., & Mathie, M. (2002). *Managing chronic disease with home telecare: a system architecture and case study*. Paper presented at the Proceedings of the Second Joint EMBS/BMES Conference.

Lowery, D., & Evans, K. G. (2004). The iron cage of methodology. *Administration & Society*, *36*(3), 306–327. doi:10.1177/0095399704265298

Lu, J., Yu, C., Liu, C., & Yao, J. E. (2003). Technology acceptance model for wireless Internet. *Electronic Networking Applications and Policy*, *1*(3), 206–222. doi:10.1108/10662240310478222

Lu, Y. C., Xiao, Y., Sears, A., & Jacko, J. A. (2005). A review and a framework of handheld computer adoption in healthcare. *International Journal of Medical Informatics*, *74*(5), 409–422. doi:10.1016/j.ijmedinf.2005.03.001

Ma, Q., & Liu, L. (2004). The technology acceptance model: a meta-analysis of empirical finings. *Journal of Organizational and End User Computing*, *16*(1), 59–74.

Macfarlane, S., Racelis, M., & Muli-Musiime, F. (2000). Public Health in Developing Countries. *Lancet*, *356*, 841–846. doi:10.1016/S0140-6736(00)02664-7

Mackay, M. M., & Weidlich, O. (2007, March 2007). *Australian Mobile Phone Lifestyle Index, 3rd Edition, Australian Interactive Media Industry Association (AIMIA), Mobile Content Industry Development Group (MCIDG)*. Retrieved 8 April, 2007, from http://www.aimia.com.au/mobile

MacLaughlin, E. J. (2005). Assessing medication adherence in the elderly: which tools to use in clinical practice? *Drugs & Aging*, *22*(3), 55–231. doi:10.2165/00002512-200522030-00005

MacManus, S. A. (2002). Understanding the Incremental Nature of E-procurement. Implementation at the State and Local levels. *Journal Public Procurement*, *2*, 5–28.

Magnussen, L., Ehiri, J., & Jolly, P. (2004). Comprehensive Versus Selective Primary Health Care: Lessons for Global Health Policy. *Health Affairs*, *23*(3), 167–176. doi:10.1377/hlthaff.23.3.167

Mahue, M., Whitten, P., & Allen, A. (2001). *E-health, telehealth, and telemedicine: A practical guide to start-up and success*. San Francisco: Jossey-Bass.

Maibaum, N., & Mundt, T. (2002). JXTA: A Technology Facilitating Mobile Peer-To-Peer Networks. In *Proceedings of MobiWac '02* (p. 7). Washington, DC: IEEE Computer Society. OASIS. (n.d.). *WSNotification*. Retrieved from http://www.oasis-open.org/committees/download.php/13485/wsn-ws-brokered_notification-1.3-spec-pr-01.pdf

Malan, D., Fulford-Jones, T., Welsh, M., & Moulton, S. (2004). *Codeblue: An ad hoc sensor network infrastructure for emergency medical care*. Paper presented at the International Workshop on Wearable and Implantable Body Sensor Networks.

Mantzana, V., & Themistocleous, M. (2006). A Method for the Identification of Actors Involved in the Adoption of Innovations in Healthcare Organizations. In *Proceedings of the 39th Hawaii International Conference on System Sciences*.

Margalit, R. S., Roter, D., Dunevant, M. A., Larson, S., & Reis, S. (2006). Electronic medical record use and physician-patient communication: An observational study of Israeli primary are encounters. *Patient Education and Counseling*, *61*(1), 134–141. doi:10.1016/j.pec.2005.03.004

Markman, M., Petersen, J., & Montgomery, R. (2008). An examination of the influence of patient race and ethnicity on expressed interest in learning about cancer clinical trials. *Journal of Cancer Research and Clinical Oncology*, *134*(1), 115–118. doi:10.1007/s00432-007-0263-4

Marquie, J. C., Jourdan-Boddaert, L., & Huet, N. (2002). Do older adults underestimate their actual computer knowledge? *Behaviour & Information Technology*, *21*(4), 273–280. doi:10.1080/0144929021000020998

Marsden, D. (1986). *The end of economic man*. New York: St. Martin's Press.

Martin, S. (2003). More than half of MDs under age 35 now using PDAs. *Canadian Medical Association Journal*, *16*(2), 952–952.

Martins, E. N., & Morse, L. S. (2005). Evaluation of Internet Websites about Retinopathy of Prematurity Patient Education. *Journal of Ophthalmology*, *89*, 565–568.

Masaiganah, M. S. (2004). Primary Health Care for the People: Health Policy in Tanzania. *Development*, *47*(2), 136–139. doi:10.1057/palgrave.development.1100041

Massacci, F., & Zannone, N. (2004). Privacy Is Linking Permission to Purpose. In *Proceedings of the Security Protocols Workshop* (pp. 179-191).

Massachusetts Institute of Technology. (2003). *PlaceLab: A House_n + TIAX Initiative*. Cambridge, MA: Author. Retrieved from http://architecture.mit.edu/house_n/placelab.html

Massey, T., Gao, T., Welsh, M., Sharp, J. H., & Sarrafzadeh, M. (2006). The design of a decentralized electronic triage system. In *Proceedings of the AMIA Annual Symposium* (pp. 544-548).

MasterCard International. (2002). *MasterCard Open Data Storage Version 2.0. Technical Specifications*. Purchase, NY: Author.

Mathie, M. J., Coster, A. C., Lovell, N. H., & Celler, B. G. (2004). Accelerometry: Providing an integrated, practical method for long-term, ambulatory monitoring of human movement. *Physiological Measurement*, *25*(2), R1–R20. doi:10.1088/0967-3334/25/2/R01

Mathie, M. J., Coster, A. C., Lovell, N. H., Celler, B. G., Lord, S. R., & Tiedemann, A. (2004). A pilot study of long-term monitoring of human movements in the home using accelerometry. *Journal of Telemedicine and Telecare*, *10*(3), 144–151. doi:10.1258/135763304323070788

Mathieson, K. (1991). Predicting user intention: comparing the technology acceptance model with the theory of planned behavior. *Information Systems Research*, *2*(3), 173–191. doi:10.1287/isre.2.3.173

Matusitz, J., & Breen, G. M. (2007). Telemedicine: Its effects on health communication. *Health Communication, 21*(1), 10–21.

Maumbe, B. M., & Owei, V. (2007). e-Government policy development in South Africa: distributional issues and implementation hurdles. *Proceedings of the 2007 conference of the IST Africa*, Maputo, 9-11 May 2007: Ireland, IIMC International Information Management Corporation Ltd.

Maurice, M., Sellier, F., & Silvestre, J. J. (1986). *The social foundation of industrial power: a comparison of France and Germany*. Cambridge, MA: The MIT Press.

Mayer, R. C., Davis, J. H., & Schoorman, F. D. (1995). An integrative model of organizational trust. *Academy of Management Review, 20*(3), 709–734. doi:10.2307/258792

Mayo, E. (1949). *Hawthorne and the Western Electric Company, the Social Problems of an Industrial Civilization*. Routledge.

Mazzoleni, M. C., Baiardi, P., Giorgi, I., Franchi, G., & Cortesi, M. (1996). Assessing users' satisfaction through perception of usefulness and ease of use in the daily interaction with a hospital information system. Proceeding of the AMIA Annual Fall Symposium.

Mcconaghy, J. (2006). Evolving Medical Knowledge: Moving Toward Efficiently Answering Questions and Keeping Current. [Elsevier Inc.]. *Primary Care: Clinics in Office Practice, 33*(4), 831–837. doi:10.1016/j.pop.2006.10.002

McGowan, J. J., Passiment, M., & Hoffman, H. M. (2007). Educating medical students as competent users of health information technologies: The MSOP data. *Medinfo, 12*, 1414–1418.

McGrail, K., & Black, C. (2005). Access to Data in Health Information Systems. *Bulletin of the World Health Organization, 83*(8), 563.

McGrath, J. M., Arar, N. H., & Pugh, J. A. (2007). The influence of electronic medical record usage on nonverbal communication in the medical interview. *Health Informatics Journal, 13*(2), 105–118. doi:10.1177/1460458207076466

McGrath, S., Grigg, E., Wendelken, S., Blike, G., Rosa, M. D., Fiske, A., et al. (2003, November). *ARTEMIS: A vision for remote triage and emergency management information integration*. Hanover, NH: Dartmouth University.

McGraw, C. (2004). Multi-compartment medication devices and patient compliance. *British Journal of Community Nursing, 9*(7), 90–285.

McKnight's LTC News. (2005, July). 2005 software. *McKnight's Long-Term Care News*, 43.

McLaren, P., Blunden, J., Lipsedge, M., & Summerfield, A. (1996). Telepsychiatry in an innercity community psychiatric service. *Journal of Telemedicine and Telecare, 2*, 57–59. doi:10.1258/1357633961929178

McMichael, C., Waters, E., & Volmick, J. (2005). Evidence-Based Public Health: What Does It Offer Developing Countries? *Journal of Public Health, 27*(2), 215–221. doi:10.1093/pubmed/fdi024

McPake, B., & Banda, E. (1994). Contracting out of Health Services in Developing Countries. *Health Policy and Planning, 9*(1), 25–30. doi:10.1093/heapol/9.1.25

Mcwhirter, G. (2003). The potential for using hospital bedside TV services in England to provide patients with access to information. [December.]. *Aslib Proceedings, 55*(5/6), 339–345. doi:10.1108/00012530310498914

Meadows, B. J. (2003). Eliciting Remote Data Entry System Requirements for the Collection of Cancer Clinical Trial Data. *Computers, Informatics, Nursing, 21*(5), 234–240. doi:10.1097/00024665-200309000-00010

MedApps. (2010). *m-Health's Enabling Role in Healthcare Reform*. Whitepaper of MedApps Inc. Available at http://www.medapps.net/RefDocs/MedAppsRole_HealthReform_041010.pdf, last accessed on 13 August, 2010.

Melander-Wikman, A., Jansson, M., & Gard, G. (2005). The MobiHealth Usability Evaluation Questionnaire. *E-health International Journal*.

Melone, N. P. (1990). A Theoretical Assessment of the User Satisfaction Construct in Information Systems Research. *Management Science, 36*, 76–91. doi:10.1287/mnsc.36.1.76

Mengiste, S., & Nielsen, P. (2006) *Scaling Health Information Systems in Developing Countries: On the Essence of Being Installed Base Friendly* Last accessed: 6 February 2007 Last updated: Address: http://www.itu.dk/iris29/IRIS29/14-5.pdf.

Michael, S. J. C. (2000). Wireless clinical alerts for physiologic, laboratory and medication data. In *Proceedings of the AMIA 2000 Annual Symposium* (pp. 789-793).

Miles, M. B., & Huberman, A. M. (1994). *Qualitative Data Analysis: An Expanded Sourcebook.* Beverly Hills, CA: Sage.

Miller, R. H., & Sim, I. (2004). Physicians' use of electronic medical records: Barriers and solutions. *Health Affairs, 23*(2), 116–126. doi:10.1377/hlthaff.23.2.116

Miller, T. W. (1998). The psychologist with 20/20 vision. *Consulting Psychology Journal: Practice and Research, 50*(1), 25–35. doi:10.1037/1061-4087.50.1.25

Miller, T. W. (2006). Telehealth issues in consulting psychology practice. *Consulting Psychology Journal: Practice and Research, 58*(2), 82–90. doi:10.1037/1065-9293.58.2.82

Miller, T. W. (2007). (Accepted). Telehealth Issues in Consulting Psychology Practice. *Consulting Psychology Journal: Practice and Research.*

Miller, T. W., & Holcomb, T. F. (2007). Telehealth Applications for Counselors in the Schools. *Kentucky Counseling Association Journal, 26*(1), 6–13.

Miller, T. W., & Hutchins, S. A. (2008). (Accepted). 21st Century Teaching technology: Best Practices and Effectiveness in Teaching Psychology. *International Journal of Instructional Media.*

Miller, T. W., & Miller, J. (1999). Telemedicine: New directions for health care delivery in Kentucky schools. *The Journal of the Kentucky Medical Association, 97*(4), 163–166.

Miller, T. W., Miller, J. M., Burton, D., Sprang, R., & Adams, J. M. (2003). A Telehealth Model for Clinical Supervision In Allied Health. *Internet Journal of Allied Health, 2*(1), 1–10.

Miller, T. W., Miller, J. M., Kraus, O. F., & Sprang, R. (2003). Telehealth a clinical application model for rural consultation. *Consulting Psychology Journal, 55*(2), 119–127. doi:10.1037/1061-4087.55.2.119

Miller, T. W., & Wader, B. (2002). Best Practices for Psychologist using 21st Century Technology. Annual Convention Connecticut Psychological Association, November 1-2, 2002. Westbrook, CT.

Miller, TW, DeLeon, P., Morgan, R., Penk, W. Magaletta, P. (2006) The Public Sector Psychologist with 2020 vision. *Professional Psychology: Research and Practice. 37-2*, 531-538.

Milliken, F. J. (1987). Three types of perceived uncertainty about the environment: state, effect, and response uncertainty. *Academy of Management Review, 12*(1), 133–143. doi:10.2307/257999

Mills, A. (2004). The Performance of Different Models of Primary Care Provision in Southern Africa. *Social Science & Medicine, 59*(5), 931–943. doi:10.1016/j.socscimed.2003.12.015

Mingers, J. (2001). Combining IS research methods: Towards a pluralist methodology. *Information Systems Research, 12*(3), 240–259. doi:10.1287/isre.12.3.240.9709

Mingers, J., & Stowell, F. (1997). *Information Systems: An Emerging Discipline? Information Systems Series* (pp. 239–266). London: McGraw-Hill.

Mingers, J. (2001). Combining IS research methods: Towards a pluralist methodology. *Information Systems Research, 12*, 240–259. doi:10.1287/isre.12.3.240.9709

Mintzberg, H. (1979). *The structure of organizations.* Englewood Cliffs, NJ: Prentice Hall.

Mirza, F., Norris, T., & Stockdale, R. (2008). Mobile technologies and the holistic management of chronic diseases. *Health Informatics Journal, 14*(4), 309–321. doi:10.1177/1460458208096559

Mitchell, J. A., Fomous, C., & Fun, J. (2006). Challenges and Strategies of the Genetics Home Reference. *Journal of the Medical Library Association, 94*(3), 336–342.

Mitka, M. (2003). Telemedicine eyed for mental health services. Approach could widen access for older patients. *Journal of the American Medical Association, 290*(14), 22–25.

Miyazaki, M., Rowe, M., Ohyanagi, T., Liu, L., Clark, C., Cook, A., & Duguay, R. (2008, April). Bidirectional wireless physiological monitoring of homecare clients. Presented in13th *Annual International Meeting of the American Telemedicine Association*.Seattle, Washington.

Moller, J., & Renegar, C. (2003). Bathing as a wellness experience. *Nursing Homes Long Term Care Management, 52*(10), 108.

Monagan, B. (2010) *Telehealth Tools Seen as Key to VA's Rural Health Care Strategy*. Healthcare IT News June 28, 2010. Web Based retrieval at: http://www.ihealthbeat.org/articles/2010/6/24/telehealth-tools-seen-as-key-to-vas-rural-health-care-strategy.aspx

Mont, D. (2007). *Measuring Disability Prevalence* (SP Discussion Paper NO. 0706). Available at: http://siteresources.worldbank.org/DISABILITY/Resources/Data/MontPrevalence.pdf.

Moor, J. H. (1997). Towards a Theory of Privacy in the Information Age. *Computers & Society, 27*(3), 27–32. doi:10.1145/270858.270866

Mor, V., Berg, K., Angelelli, J., Gifford, D., Morris, J., & Moore, T. (2003). The quality of quality measurement in U.S. nursing homes. *The Gerontologist, 43*(2), 37–46.

Morey, R. C. (1982). Estimating and improving the quality of information in the MIS. *Communications of the ACM, 25*(5), 337–342. doi:10.1145/358506.358520

Morgan, R. D., Patrick, A. R., & Magaletta, P. R. (2008). Does the use of telemental health alter the treatment experience?: Inmates' perceptions of telemental health vs. face-to-face treatment modalities. *Journal of Consulting and Clinical Psychology, 76*, 158–162. doi:10.1037/0022-006X.76.1.158

Mori, T., Noguchi, H., Takada, A., & Sato, T. (2004). Sensing Room: Distributed Sensor Environment for Measurement of Human Daily Behavior. In *Proceedings of the First International Workshop on Networked Sensing Systems (INSS2004)* (pp. 40-43).

Mukamel, B. D., & Spector, D. W. (2000). Nursing home Costs and Risk-Adjusted Outcome Measures of Quality. *Medical Care, 38*(1), 32–35. doi:10.1097/00005650-200001000-00009

Mullen, D. R., Fontaine, M. A., & Muller, M. J. (2002). Understanding the Benefit and Costs of Communities of Practice. *Communications of the ACM, 45*(4), 64–68.

Mullen, R., & Donnelly, J. T. (2006). Keeping it real--building an ROI model for an ambulatory EMR initiative that the physician practices espouse. *Journal of Healthcare Information Management, 20*(1), 42–52.

Munukka.K. (2005). Bridging the digital divide? Development of information society in Namibia- Conceptions of the local actors. University of Tempere.

Murray, C., & Frenk, J. (2001). World Health Report 2000: A Step Towards Evidence-Based Health Policy. *Lancet, 357*, 1698–1700. doi:10.1016/S0140-6736(00)04826-1

My Health. *e*Vet. (n.d.). Retrieved June 2, 2006, from https://www.myhealth.va.gov/mhvPortal/anonymous.portal?_nfpb=true&_nfto=false&_pageLabel=mhvHome

Myers, M. (1997). Qualitative Research in Information Systems. *MISQ Quarterly, 21*(2), 241–242. doi:10.2307/249422

Myers, M. D., & Newman, M. (2007). The Qualitative Interview in Is Research: Examining the Craft. *Information and Organization, X*(x).

Myers, M. D., & Avison, D. (2002). *Qualitative Research in Information Systems*. London: Sage Publications.

Namibia, M. O. H. S. S. (2004b). The technical efficiency of District Hospitals in Namibia. Windhoek: Directorate: Policy, Planning and Human Resources Development. Mcwhirter, G. (2003). The potential for using hospital bedside TV services in England to provide patients with access to information. [December]. *Aslib Proceedings, 55*(5/6), 339–345.

Namibia. (2004)c. Namibia Vision 2030: Policy Framework for Long-Term National Development. Windhoek: National Planning Commission Secretariat.

Namibia. Ministry of Foreign Affairs, Information and Broadcasting. (2002a). Information and communication technology policy for the Republic of Namibia. http://www.uneca.org/aisi/nici/Documents/ICT%20Policy%20Document%20Ver%208.2.pdf [date accessed: 8 March 2006].

Namibia. Ministry of Health and Social Services. (2005). Follow-up to the declaration of commitment on HIV/AIDS (UNGASS): Namibia Country Report. Windhoek: Directorate: Special Programmes (HIV/AIDS, TB & Malaria).

Namibia. Ministry of Health and Social Services.2006. Health Facilities. http://www.healthnet.com.na [date accessed: 20 April 2006].

Namibia. MOHSS. (2003). Namibia National Health Accounts November 2003.Windhoek: Directorate: Policy, Planning and Human Resources Development.

Namibia. MOHSS. (2004a). Annual Report of Oshana region: 2003-2004.Windhoek: Ministry of Health and Social Services.

Namibia.MOHSS.(1998).The referral system. Performance audit report of the Auditor General. Windhoek.

National Advisory Committee on Rural Health and Human Services. (2004).*The 2004 Report to the Secretary: Rural Health and Human Services*. Available at: ftp://ftp.hrsa.gov/ruralhealth/NAC04web.pdf

NCI and FDA. (2007). Memorandum of Understanding on Janus Study Data Repository. Retrieved on November 21, 2007, from http://www.fda.gov/OHRMS/DOCKETS/98fr/FDA-225-07-4301-mou0001.PDF

Nergiz, M. E., Atzori, M., & Clifton, C. W. (2007). Hiding the presence of individuals from shared databases. In *Proceedings of ACM SIGMOD*, Vancouver, BC, Canada (pp. 665-676).

Netsize. (2009). *Netsize Guide 2009 Edition: Mobile Society and Me: When worlds combine*. Levallois-Perret: Netsize.

Neville, G., Greene, A., McLeod, J., & Tracy, A. (2002). Mobile phone text messaging can help young people with asthma. *British Medical Journal*, *325*, 600. doi:10.1136/bmj.325.7364.600/a

Newell, K. (1989). The Way Ahead for District Health Systems. *World Health Forum*, *10*(1), 80–87.

Ni, Q., Trombetta, A., Bertino, E., & Lobo, J. (2007). Privacy-aware role based access. In *Proceedings of the 12th ACM Symposium on Access Control Models and Technologies* (pp. 41-50).

Nicholson, B & Sundeep Sahay. (2004). Embedded knowledge and offshore software development. *Information and Organization*, *14*(4), 329–365. doi:10.1016/j.infoandorg.2004.05.001

Nickelson, D. (1996). Behavioral telehealth: Emerging practice, research, and policy opportunities. *Behavioral Sciences & the Law*, *14*, 443–457. doi:10.1002/(SICI)1099-0798(199623)14:4<443::AID-BSL256>3.0.CO;2-G

Nickelson, D. W. (1998). Telehealth and the evolving health care system: Strategic opportunities for professional psychology. *Professional Psychology, Research and Practice*, *29*, 527–534. doi:10.1037/0735-7028.29.6.527

Nielsen, J. (1993). *Usability engineering (Interactive Technologies)*. New York: Academic Press.

Niessen, L., Grijseels, E., & Rutten, F. (2000). The Evidenced-Based Approach in Health Policy and Health Care Delivery. *Social Science & Medicine*, *51*, 859–869. doi:10.1016/S0277-9536(00)00066-6

NNHS. (2004). *Analysis of the National Nursing Home Survey*. Washington, DC: AARP Public Policy Institute.

Norman, S. (2006). The use of telemedicine in psychiatry. *Journal of Psychiatric and Mental Health Nursing*, *13*, 771–777. doi:10.1111/j.1365-2850.2006.01033.x

Norris, A. C. (2002). *Essentials of Telemedicine and Telecare*. Chichester, UK: Wiley.

O'Connor, J. (2008). Nursing homes up on technology. *McKnight's Long-Term Care News*, *29*(12), 3.

O'Connor, J. (2005). Feds provide info on LTC tech products on market. *McKnight's Long-Term Care News, 14*(11).

O'Doherty, K., Rao Hill, S., Mackay, M. M., & McPherson, J. (2010). Mobile Data Service usage and preference: an investigation of Australian consumers. *International Journal of Mobile Communications, 8*(1), 106–127. doi:10.1504/IJMC.2010.030523

Office of Rural Health Policy, Health Resources and Services Administration. (1994). *Reaching: Rural health travel in the telecommunications highway*. Rockville, MD: Federal Office of Rural Health Policy.

Oh, S., Yang, S., Kurnia, S., Lee, H., Mackay, M. M., & O'Doherty, K. (2008). The characteristics of mobile data users in Australia. *International Journal of Mobile Communications, 8*(2), 217–230. doi:10.1504/IJMC.2008.016578

Ohta, S., Nakamoto, H., Shinagawa, Y., & Tanikawa, T. (2002). A health monitoring system for elderly people living alone. *Journal of Telemedicine and Telecare, 8*(3), 151–156. doi:10.1258/135763302320118997

Okuonzi, S. A., & Macrae, J. (1995). Whose Policy Is It Anyway? International and National Influences on Health Policy Development in Uganda. *Health Policy and Planning, 10*(2), 122–132. doi:10.1093/heapol/10.2.122

Opie, A. (1998). Nobody's asked me for my view: users' empowerment by multidisciplinary health teams. *Qualitative Health Research, 18*, 188–206. doi:10.1177/104973239800800204

Oracle (2007). Retrieved on November 20, 2007, from http://www.oracle.com/industries/life_sciences/pharma.html.

Orwat, C., Graefe, A., & Faulwasser, T. (2008). Towards pervasive computing in health care - a literature review. *BMC Medical Informatics and Decision Making, 8*, 26. doi:10.1186/1472-6947-8-26

Otis, P. (1997). Don't worry, The Carpet is Keep Watching. *Business Week*, 1.

Ouwens, M., Wollersheim, H., & Hermens, R. (2005). Integrated care programmes for chronically ill patients: a review of systematic reviews. *International Journal for Quality in Health Care, 17*(2). doi:10.1093/intqhc/mzi016

Ovretveit, J., Scott, T., Rundall, T. G., Shortell, S. M., & Brommels, M. (2007). Improving quality through effective implementation of information technology in healthcare. *International Journal for Quality in Health Care, 19*(5), 259–266. doi:10.1093/intqhc/mzm031

Padarath, A., Chamberlain, C., McCoy, D., Ntuli, A., Rowson, M., & Loewenson, R. (2003). Health personnel in Southern Africa: Confronting maldistribution and brain drain. *Equinet discussion paper no. 4*. Health Systems Trust, South Africa.

Padhi, S.S. A1 & Mohapatra, P.K.J. (2010), Adoption of e-procurement in the government departments.*Electronic Government, an International Journal, 7*(1), 41-59.

Paglin, M. (1974). Public Health and Development: A New Analytical Framework. *Economica, New Series, 41*(164), 432–441. doi:10.2307/2553354

Paksuniemi, M., Sorvoja, H., Alasaarela, E., & Myllyla, R. (2006). Wireless sensor and data transmission needs and technologies for patient monitoring in the operating room and intensive care unit. In *Proceedings of the 27th Annual International IEEE EMBS05 Conference* (pp. 5182-5185).

Panayiotis, H. K., Kontogeorgisb, A., Stalidisc, G., & Kaggelidesd, K. (2010). Applying e-procurement system in the healthcare: the EPOS paradigm. *International Journal of Systems Science, 41*(3), 281–299. doi:10.1080/00207720903326878

Panayiotou, N. A., Gayialis, S. P., & Tatsiopoulos, I. P. (2004). An e-procurement system for governmental purchasing. *International Journal of Production Economics, 90*, 79–102. doi:10.1016/S0925-5273(03)00103-8

Pare, G. (2004). Investigating information systems with positivist case study research. *Communications of the Association for Information Systems, 13*, 233–264.

Paré, G., Jaana, M., & Sicotte, C. (2007). Systematic review of home telemonitoring for chronic diseases: the evidence base. *Journal of the American Medical Informatics Association*, *14*(3), 269–277. doi:10.1197/jamia.M2270

Parker, O. D., Demiris, G., Day, M., Courtney, K. L., & Porock, D. (2006). Tele-hospice support for elder caregivers of hospice patients: two case studies. *Journal of Palliative Medicine*, *9*(2), 54–59.

Patton, M. Q. (1990). *Qualitative Evaluation and Research Methods* (2nd ed.). London: Sage Publications.

Paul, L., John, I., & Pierre, C. (2003, January). Why do people use information technology, A critical review of the technology acceptance model. *Association for Information Systems*, *40*(3), 191.

Pavlovic, I., & Miklavcic, D. (2007). Web-Based Electronic Data Collection System to Support Electrochemotherapy Clinical Trial. *IEEE Transactions on Information Technology in Biomedicine*, *11*(2), 222–230. doi:10.1109/TITB.2006.879581

Pear, R. (2008a). Serious Deficiencies in Nursing Homes Are Often Missed. *New York Times*.

Pear, R. (2008b). Violations Reported at 94% of Nursing Homes. *New York Times*.

Pedersen, C. D. (2006, September 8). *MedCom - the Danish Healthcare Data Network*. Paper presented at the Meeting of the AGFA.

Pennington, T., Wilkinson, c., & Vance, J. (2004). Physical Educators Online: What is on the Minds of Teachers in the Trenches? *Physical Educator*, *61*(1), 45–56.

Pentland, A. (2004). Healthwear: Medical technology becomes wearable. *Computer*, *37*(5), 42–49. doi:10.1109/MC.2004.1297238

Perez-Lopez, F. R., & Perez-Roncero, G. R. (2006). Assessing the content and quality of information on the treatment of postmenpausal osteoporosis on the World Wide Web. *Gynecological Endocrinology*, *22*(12), 669–675. doi:10.1080/09513590601012603

Perry, M., Dowdall, A., Lines, L., & Hone, K. (2004). Multimodal and ubiquitous computing systems: supporting independent-living older users. *IEEE Transactions on Information Technology in Biomedicine*, *8*(3), 258–270. doi:10.1109/TITB.2004.835533

Peter, D. (2001). *The Nurse Shortage: Perspectives from Current Direct Care Nurses and Former Direct Care Nurses*. Washington, DC: Federation of Nurses and Health Professionals.

Peters, D., & Chao, S. (1998). The Sector-Wide Approach in Health: What Is It? Where Is It Going? *The International Journal of Health Planning and Management*, *13*, 177–190. doi:10.1002/(SICI)1099-1751(199804/06)13:2<177::AID-HPM504>3.0.CO;2-T

Pettersen B, Johnsen R (2007). Legers oppfatning av samhandlingen mellom nivåene i helsetjenesten. *Tidsskr Nor Lægeforen nr. 5, 2007; 127: 565–8.*

Pettigrew, A. (1997). What Is a Processual Analysis? *Scandinavian Journal of Management*, *13*(4), 337–348. doi:10.1016/S0956-5221(97)00020-1

Pfeffer, J., & Salancik, G. R. (1978). *The external control of organizations: a resource dependence perspective*. New York: Harper & Row.

Philipose, M., Fishkin, K. P., Perkowitz, M., Patterson, D. J., Fox, D., & Kautz, H. (2004). Inferring activities from interactions with objects. *IEEE Pervasive Computing / IEEE Computer Society [and] IEEE Communications Society*, *3*(4), 50–57. doi:10.1109/MPRV.2004.7

Pino, E., Ohno-Machado, L., Wiechmann, E., & Curtis, D. (2005). Real- Time ECG Algorithms for Ambulatory Patient Monitoring. In *Proceedings of the AMIA Annual Symposium* (pp. 604-608).

Piron, L., & Tonin, P. (2004). Motor telerehabilitation in post-stroke patients. *Medical Informatics and the Internet in Medicine*, *29*, 119–125. doi:10.1080/14639230410001723428

Pizzi, R. (2007). U.S. EHR market to approach $5 billion by 2015, Healthcare IT News, Retrieved February 4, 2008 from. www.healthcareitnews.com/story.cms?id=6332 - 31k

Polit, F. D., & Beck, T. C. (2004). *Nursing Research: Principles and Methods*. Wickford, RI: Lippincott-Raven Publishers.

Poon, E. G., Jha, A. K., Christino, M., Honour, M. M., Fernandopulle, R., & Middleton, B. (2006). Assessing the level of healthcare information technology adoption in the United States: A snapshot. *BMC Medical Informatics and Decision Making*, *6*, 1. doi:10.1186/1472-6947-6-1

Popular Mechanics. (2004, June). Robots Help Japan Care for Its Elderly. Retrieved January 30, 2009, from http://www.popularmechanics.com/science/technology_watch/1288241.html

Porn, L. N., & Patrick, K. (2002). Mobile computing acceptance grows as applications evolve. *Healthcare Financial Management*, *56*, 66–70.

Porter, M., & Tiesberg, E. (2006). *Re-defining health care delivery*. Boston: Harvard Business Press.

Poulton, B. C. (1999). User involvement in identifying health needs and shaping and evaluating services: is it being raised? *Journal of Advanced Nursing*, *30*(6), 1289–1296. doi:10.1046/j.1365-2648.1999.01224.x

Powell, P. L. (1999). Evaluation of Information Technology Investments: Business as usual. In Willcocks, L. P., & Lester, S. (Eds.), *Beyond the IT Productivity Paradox* (pp. 151–182). Chichester, England, UK: John Wiley & Sons.

Pradhan, M. R. (2003). ICTs application for better health in Nepal. [April-June.]. *Kathmandu University Medical Journal*, *2*(6), 157–163.

Presti, S., Butler, M., Leuschel, M., & Booth, C. (2006). Holistic Trust Design of E-Services. In Song, R., Korba, L., & Yee, G. (Eds.), *Trust in E-Services: Technologies, Practices and Challenges* (pp. 113–139). USA: Idea Group Publishing.

Pucheral, P., Bouganim, L., Valduriez, P., & Bobineau, C. (2001). PicoDBMS: Scaling down database techniques for the smartcard. [VLDBJ]. *Very Large Data Bases Journal*, *10*(2-3), 120–132.

Pucheral, P., & Yin, S. (2007). *System and Method of Managing Indexation of Flash Memory* (Patent by Gemalto and INRIA No. 07290567.2).

Quibria, M. G., Ahmed, S. N., Tschang, T., & Reyes-Macasaquit, M. (2003). Digital divide: determinants and policies with special reference to Asia. [October.]. *Journal of Asian Economics*, *13*(3), 285–309.

Quibria, M. G., Tschang, T., & Reyes-Macasaquit, M. (2002). New information and communication technologies and poverty. *Journal of the Asia Pacific Economy*, *7*, 11–825. doi:10.1080/1354786022000007852

Quinn, C. (2006). Low-technology Heart Failure Care in Home Health Improving Patient Outcomes. *Home Healthcare Nurse*, *24*(8), 533–540. doi:10.1097/00004045-200609000-00012

Quintana, Y., Feightner, J. W., Wathen, C. N., Sangster, L. M., & Marshall, J. N. (2001). Preventive health information on the Internet. Qualitative study of consumers' perspectives. *Canadian Family Physician Medecin de Famille Canadien*, *47*(9), 1759–1765.

Rabinovitch, I. (2007, July). Speedy EMR implementations. Technology for Doctors.

Rachlis, M. (2006). Key to sustainable healthcare system. Retrieved 21 June, 2008, from http://www.improveinchroniccare.org

Radin, P. (2006). To me, it's my life: medical communication, trust, and activism in cyberspace. *Social Science & Medicine*, *6*, 591–601. doi:10.1016/j.socscimed.2005.06.022

Raffa, L., & Esposito, G. (2006). The implementation of an e-reverse auction system in an Italian health care organization. *Journal of Public Procurement*, *6*(1-3), 46–69.

Rahimi, B., & Vimarlund, V. (2007). Methods to Evaluate Health information Systems in Healthcare Settings: A Literature Review. *J. Med. Syst.*, *31*, 397–432. Springer Science + Business Media, LLC 2007.

Raju, M. (2007). *Heart-Rate and EKG Monitor Using the MSP430FG439* [Electronic Version].

Ramanathan, S. (2004) Diffusion of e-procurement in the public sector - revisiting centralization versus decentralization debates as a twist in the tale. In Leino T, Saarinen T, Klein S (eds). *Proceedings of the Twelfth European Conference on Information Systems*, 1546-1556. Turku, Finland:Turku School of Economics and Business Administration.

Rangel-Kuoppa, R., Aviles-Cruz, C., & Mould, D. (2003). Distributed 3D rendering system in a multi-agent platform. In *Proceedings of ENC 2003* (pp. 168-175).

Rao, S. S. (2001). Integrated health care and telemedicine. [June.]. *Work Study, 50*(6), 222–229. doi:10.1108/EUM0000000006034

Rao, S., & Troshani, I. (2006). *AMC-ER Preliminary Research Report: Understanding Market and Mobile Content Selection for Distribution.* Adelaide, South Australia: Australian Mobile Content – Export Research Initiative, m.Net Corporation Ltd.

Rao, S., & Troshani, I. (2007a). *AMC-ER Challenges and Rewards: Experiences of Australian Content Exporters.* Adelaide, South Australia: Australian Mobile Content – Export Research Initiative, m.Net Corporation Ltd.

Rao, S., & Troshani, I. (2007b). *AMC-ER Initial Selection of Content, Markets, and Distribution Channels for the Australian Mobile Content – Export Research Initiative.* Adelaide, South Australia: m.Net Corporation Ltd.

Rasmussen, B., Wellard, S., & Nankervis, A. (2001). Consumer issues in navigating health care services for type I diabetes. *Journal of Clinical Nursing, 10*, 628–634. doi:10.1046/j.1365-2702.2001.00550.x

Ray, S. (2007). Development of a framework towards successful implementation of e-governance initiatives in health sector in India. [Emerald Group Publishing Limited.]. *International Journal of Health Care Quality Assurance, 20*(6), 464–483. doi:10.1108/09526860710819413

Reach, G., Zerrouki, D., Leclercq, D., & d'Ivernois, J. F. (2005). Adjusting insulin doses: from knowledge to decision. *Patient Education and Counseling, 56*(1), 98–103. doi:10.1016/j.pec.2004.01.001

Reardon, J. L., & Davidson, E. (2007). How do doctors perceive the organizing vision for electronic medical records? Preliminary findings from a study of EMR adoption in independent physician practices, Proceedings of the 40th Hawaii International Conference on Systems Science.

Redfern, S., Hannan, S., Norman, I., & Martin, F. (2002). Work satisfaction, stress, quality of care and morale of older people in a nursing home. *Health & Social Care in the Community, 10*(6), 17–35. doi:10.1046/j.1365-2524.2002.00396.x

Redmond, S. J., Lovell, N. H., Basilakis, J., & Celler, B. G. (2008, August 20-24). ECG Quality measures in telecare monitoring. In *Proceedings of the 30th Annual International IEEE EMBC08 Conference* Vancouver, BC, Canada (pp. 2869-2872).

Reilly, J., & Bischoff, J. (2008). Remote Monitoring Tested. *Technology and Health Care, 34*(9), 12–14.

Reinecke, I. (2004). *Managing Information in Health.* Melbourne National Health Information Summit.

Rhodes, R. A. W. (1986). *The National World of Local Government.* London: Allen and Unwin.

Riley, D.L. & Stewart, D.E. & Grace, S.L. (2007). Continuity of cardiac care: Cardiac rehabilitation participation and other correlated. *Int J Cardiology*, doi:10.1016.

Ritchie, J., & Lewis, J. (2003). *Qualitative Research Practice: A Guide for Social Science Students and Researchers.* London: Sage Publications.

Rodrigues, R. (2003). Deploying e-Health Solutions in Latin America and the Caribbean: Development and Policy Issues. *Forum PL11: Workshop on Telemedicine,* Geneva.

Rogers, E. M. (1995). *Diffusion of Innovations* (4th ed.). New York: The Free Press.

Rogoski, R. (2005). Wireless by Design. *Health Management Technology*, (January): 1–7.

Rogoski, R. (2003). Wireless by Design. *Health Management Technology*, 1–7.

Røstad, L., & Nytrø, O. (2008). Personalized access control for a personally controlled health record. *Proceedings of the 2nd ACM workshop on Computer security architectures* (pp. 9-16).

Rouf, E., Whittle, J., Lu, N., & Schwartz, M. D. (2007). Computers in the exam room: Differences in physician-patient interaction may be due to physician experience. *Journal of General Internal Medicine*, *22*(1), 43–48. doi:10.1007/s11606-007-0112-9

Rowe, M. (2008). *V-P Capital Health*. Alberta, Canada: Alberta Health Services.

Rowland, D. (2003). An ageing population: emergence of a new stage of life? In Khoo, S., & McDonald, P. (Eds.), *The Transformation of Australia's Population: 1970-2030* (pp. 239–265). Sydney, Australia: UNSW Press.

Russell, S. C., & Spooner, S. A. (2004). Barriers to EMR adoption in internal medicine and pediatric outpatient practices. *Tennessee Medicine*, *97*(10), 457–460.

Russell, L. B., Churl Suh, D., & Safford, M. M. (2005). Time requirements for diabetes management: too much for many? *The Journal of Family Practice*, *54*(1), 52–56.

Sachs, J. (2004). Ending Africa's Poverty Trap. *Brookings Articles on Economic Activity*, *1*, 117–240. doi:10.1353/eca.2004.0018

Sahay, S., & Walsham, G. (2006). Scaling Health Information Systems in India: Challenges and Approaches. *Information Technology for Development*, *12*(3), 185–200. doi:10.1002/itdj.20041

Salkind, N. J. (2004). Statistics for people who (think they) hate statistics. 2nd ed. London: Sage.

Samarati, P. (2001). Protecting respondents' identities in microdata release. [TKDE]. *IEEE Transactions on Knowledge and Data Engineering*, *13*(6), 1010–1027. doi:10.1109/69.971193

Samarati, P., & di Vimercati, S. D. C. (2000). Access Control: Policies, Models, and Mechanisms. In *Proceedings of the Foundations of Security Analysis and Design on Foundations of Security Analysis and Design 2000 Conference* (pp. 137-196).

Samarati, P., & Sweeney, L. (1998). Generalizing data to provide anonymity when disclosing information. In *Proceedings of the 17th ACM SIGACT-SIGMOD-SIGART PODS*, Seattle, WA (p. 188).

Sammons, M. T., & DeLeon, P. H. (2004). Whither online counseling: Conceptualizing the Challenges and promises of distance mental health service provision. In Kraus, R., Zack, J., & Stricker, G. (Eds.), *Online Counseling: A Handbook for Mental Health Professionals*. New York: Elsevier Press.

Sanchez, D., Tentori, M., & Favela, J. (2008, March-April). Activity recognition for the smart hospital. *IEEE Intelligent Systems*, *23*(2), 50–57. doi:10.1109/MIS.2008.18

Saranummi, N., & Wactlar, H. (2008). Editorial: Pervasive Healthcare. Selected papers from the pervasive healthcare 2008 conference, Tampere, Finland. *Methods of Information in Medicine*, *47*(3), 175–177.

Sargent, I. (1999). School based mental health in rural Kansas: A novel use for telepsychiatry. [abstract]. *Telemedicine Journal*, *5*(1), 52.

Sarker, S., & Wells, J. D. (2003). Understanding mobile handheld device use and adoption. *Communications of the ACM*, *46*(12), 35–40. doi:10.1145/953460.953484

SAS. (2007). Retrieved on November 20, 2007, from http://www.sas.com/industry/ pharma/cdisc/.

Sausser, G. D. (2003). Thin is in: web-based systems enhance security, clinical quality. *Healthcare Financial Management*, *57*(7), 86–88.

Sayer, A. (2000). *Realism and Social Science*. London: Sage.

Schaper, L., & Pervan, G. (2004). A model for information and communication technology acceptance and utilization by occupational therapists. http://s-cah-vishnu.infotech.monash.edu.au/dss2004/proceedings/pdf/72_Schaper_Pervan.pdf, [date accessed: 5 June, 2008].

Schepers, J., & Wetzels, M. (2007). A meta-analysis of the technology acceptance model: Investigating subjective norm and moderation effects. *Information & Management*, *44*(1), 90–103. doi:10.1016/j.im.2006.10.007

Schmier, J. K., Kane, D. W., & Halpern, M. T. (2005). Practical applications of usability theory to electronic data collection for clinical trials. *Contemporary Clinical Trials*, *26*(3), 376–385. doi:10.1016/j.cct.2005.01.012

Schware, R. (2003). Information and communications technology (ICT) agencies: functions, structures, and best operational practices. [June.]. *Information*, *5*(3), 3–7.

Scott, S. (2000) "Lived Methodology: A Situated Discussion of 'Truth and Method' in Interpretive Information Systems Research" *London School of Economics. Department of Information Systems Working Article Series 91*

Selman, T. J., Prakash, T., & Khan, K. S. (2006). Quality of Health Information for Cervical Cancer Treatment on the Internet. *BMC Women's Health*, *6*, 9. doi:10.1186/1472-6874-6-9

SeniorsSite.com. (2008). *Daily Activities*. Retrieved October 20, 2008, from http://seniors-site.com/nursingm/index.html

Serafeimidis, V., & Smithson, S. (2000). Information Systems Evaluation in Practice: a Case Study of Organizational Change. *Journal of Information Technology*, *15*(2), 93–105. doi:10.1080/026839600344294

Seror, A. (2001). The Internet, Global Healthcare Management Systems, and Sustainable Development: Future Scenarios. [August.]. *The Electronic Journal on Information Systems in Developing Countries*, *5*(1), 1–18.

Servellen, G., Fongwa, M., & Errico, E. M. (2006). Continuity of care and quality care outcomes for people experiencing chronic conditions: A literature review. *Nursing & Health Sciences*, *8*, 185–195. doi:10.1111/j.1442-2018.2006.00278.x

Shankaranarayanan, G., & Yu, C. (2006). Supporting data quality management in decision-making. *Decision Support Systems*, *42*(1), 302. doi:10.1016/j.dss.2004.12.006

Shaw, V. (2005). Health Information System Reform in South Africa: Developing an Essential Data Set. *Bulletin of the World Health Organization*, *83*(8), 632–636.

Shaw, P., Goodwin, J., Whitten, P., & Doolittle, G. (1999). Tele-Kid Care: An urban telemedicine service for an underserved pediatric population. [abstract]. *Telemedicine Journal*, *5*(1), 25.

Shekelle, P. G., Morton, S. C., & Keeler, E. B. (2006). Costs and benefits of health information technology. *Evidence Report/technology Assessment*, *132*, 1–71.

Shields, S. (2005, March 23). Culture Change in Nursing homes. *The Commonwealth Fund*.

Sidorov, J. (2006). It ain't necessarily so: The electronic health record and the unlikely prospect of reducing health care costs. *Health Affairs*, *25*(6), 1745. doi:10.1377/hlthaff.25.6.1745-a

Simon, S. J., & Simon, S. J. (2006). An examination of the financial feasibility of Electronic Medical Records (EMRs): A case study of tangible and intangible benefits. *International Journal of Electronic Healthcare*, *2*(2), 185–200.

Simpson, R. L. (2003). The patient's point of view -- IT matters. *Nursing Administration Quarterly*, *27*(3), 254–256.

Siracuse, M. V., Pharm, D., & Sowell, J. G. (2008). Doctor of Pharmacy Students' Use of Personal Digital Assistant. *American Journal of Pharmaceutical Education*, *72*(1), 1–7.

Sirvent, R., Merzky, A., Badia, R., & Kielmann, T. (2005). *Grid superscalar and SAGA: forming a high-level and platform-independent grid programming environment*. Paper presented at CoreGRID Integration WorkShop 2005.

Skinner, R. (2003). The value of information technology in healthcare. *Frontiers of Health Services Management*, *19*(3).

Skulimowski, A. M. (2006). The Challenges to the Medical Decision Making System posed by mHealth. Centre for Decision Sciences and Forecasting, Progress & Business Foundation, Institute for Prospective Technological Studies (IPTS). Retrieved 21 June, 2008, from http://ipts.jrc.ec.europa.eu/home/report/english/articles/vol81/ICT1E816.htm

Slaymaker, M., Politou, E., Power, D., & Lloyd, S. (2004). E-health security issues: the eDiaMoND perspective. In *Proceedings of the 2004 UK e-Science All Hands Meeting*.

Sloan, F., & Shayne, M. (1993). Long-Term Care, Medicaid, and the Impoverishment of the Elderly. *The Milbank Quarterly*, *70*(4), 19.

Sloane, E. B. (2006). The emerging health care IT infrastructure. *24x7, 11*(12), 42-43.

Sloane, E. B. (2009). Regulatory overview.(Networking). *24x7, 14*(4), 22-24.

Smaglik, P., Hawkins, R., Pingree, S., & Gustafson, D. (1998). The quality of interactive computer use among HIV infected individuals. *Journal of Health Communication*, *3*, 53–68. doi:10.1080/108107398127508

Smarritto, S., Mitrofanoff, M., Haddad, T., & Pavy, B. (2003). Do we need a chart of quality for websites related to cosmetic surgery? *Annales de Chirurgie Plastique et Esthetique*, *48*(4), 222–227.

Smart Card Alliance. (2005). *The Taiwan Health Care Smart Card Project.* Retrieved February 17, 2009, from http://www.smartcardalliance.org/resources/pdf/Taiwan_Health_Card_Profile.pdf

Smart Card Alliance. (2006a). *Smart Card Applications in the U.S. Healthcare Industry* (White Paper No. HC-06001). Retrieved February 17, 2009, from http://www.smartcardalliance.org/resources/hc/Smart_Card_Healthcare_Applications_FINAL.pdf

Smart Card Alliance. (2006b). *German Health Card.* Retrieved February 17, 2009, from http://www.smartcardalliance.org/resources/pdf/German_Health_Card.pdf

Smith, B. C. (1997). The Decentralization of Health Care in Developing Countries: Organisational Option. *Public Administration and Development*, *17*, 399–412. doi:10.1002/(SICI)1099-162X(199710)17:4<399::AID-PAD976>3.0.CO;2-P

Smith, M., & Madon, S. (2008). Integrated Health Information Systems in Tanzania: Experience and Challenges. *EJISDC*, *33*(1), 1–21.

Smith, D. E., Wilson, A. J., & Henry, D. A. (2005). Monitoring the Quality of Medical News Reporting: Early Experiences with Media Doctor. Medicine and the Media--Research (MJA), 183(4), 190-193.

Solovy, A. (2007). *Ten Lessons from the Top 100.* Healthcare's Most Wired, H&HN Hospitals and Health Networks.

Solow, C., Weiss, R., Bergen, B., & Sanborn, C. (1971). 24-hour psychiatric consultation via TV. *The American Journal of Psychiatry*, *127*, 120–123.

Somasundaram, R., & Damsgaard, J. (2005). Policy Recommendations for Electronic Public Procurement. *The Electronic. Journal of E-Government*, *3*, 147–156.

Soran, A., Nesbitt, L., & Mamounas, E. P. (2006). Centralized medical monitoring in phase III clinical trials: the National Surgical Adjuvant Breast and Bowel Project (NSABP) experience. *Clinical Trials*, *3*(5), 478–485. doi:10.1177/1740774506070747

Spil, T. A. M., & Schuring, R. W. (2006). *E-Health system diffusion and use.* Hershey, PA, USA: IGI Global.

Sprivulis, P., Walker, J., Johnston, D., Pan, E., Adler-Milstein, J., & Middleton, B. (2007). The economic benefits of health information exchange interoperability. *Australian Health Review*, *31*(4), 531–539. doi:10.1071/AH070531

Sproule, J. A., Tansey, C., Burns, B., & Fenelon, G. (2003). The Web: friend or foe of the hand surgeon. *Hand Surgery*, *8*(2), 181–185. doi:10.1142/S0218810403001716

Srovnal, V., & Penhaker, M. (2007). *Health Maintenance Embedded Systems in Home Care Applications.* Paper presented at ICONS 2007.

Stamm, B. H. (1999). Creating virtual community: Telehealth and self-care updated. In Stamm, B. H. (Ed.), *Secondary traumatic stress: Self-care issues for clinicians, researchers, and educators* (pp. 179–208). Lutherville, MD: Sidran Press.

Stanford, V. (2002). Using Pervasive Computing to Deliver Elder Care. *IEEE Pervasive Computing / IEEE Computer Society [and] IEEE Communications Society*, 10–13. doi:10.1109/MPRV.2002.993139

Stansfield, S. (2005). Editorial - Structuring Information and Incentives to Improve Health. *Bulletin of the World Health Organization, 83*(8), 562–563.

Starfield, B., Shi, L., & Macinko, J. (2005). Contribution of Primary Care to Health Systems and Health. *The Milbank Quarterly, 3*, 457–502. doi:10.1111/j.1468-0009.2005.00409.x

Statistical Package for the Social Sciences (SPSS). (2007). *SPSS regression models*. http:/www.spss.com/regression [date accessed: 9 April 2007].

Steg, H., et al. (2006). *Europe Is Facing a Demographic Challenge – Ambient Assisted Living Offers Solutions*. Paper presented at VDI/VDE/IT.

Steinfeld, E., & Danford, G. S. (1999). *Enabling Environments. Measuring the impact of Environment on Disability and Rehabilitation*. New York: Kluwer Academic.

Stevens, J. P. (2002). *Applied multivariate statistics for the social sciences* (4th ed.). London: Lawrence Erlbaum Associates.

Straker, N., Mostyn, P., & Marshall, C. (1976). The use of two-way TV in bringing mental health services to the inner city. *The American Journal of Psychiatry, 133*, 1202–1205.

Strandberg-Larsen, M., & Krasnik, A. (2008). *Does a public single payer system deliver integrated care? A national survey study among professional stakeholders in Denmark* (*Vol. 8*). IJIC.

Striefel, S. (2000, Summer). Telehealth uses in biofeedback and applied psychophysiology. *Biofeedback*, 28 (2). Retrieved February 4, 2004, from http://www.aapb.org/public/

Stroetmann, K., Jones, T., & Dobrev, A. (2006, May 10-12). Evaluating the economic impact of e-health applications approach and method. *E-health conference 2006*, Malaga, Spain.

Stuart, D., & Bawany, K. (2001). *Wireless Services*. United Kingdom: Gartner.

Stuart, D., & Bawany, K. (2001). *Wireless Services*. UK: Gartner.

Suomi, R. (2006). Introducing electronic patient records to hospitals: Innovation adoption paths. In Spil, T. A. M., & Schuring, R. W. (Eds.), *E-Health Systems Diffusion and Use: The Innovation, the User and the USE IT Model*. Hershey, PA: Idea Group Publishing.

Suzuki, R., Ogawa, M., Otake, S., Izutsu, T., Tobimatsu, Y., & Izumi, S. (2004). Analysis of activities of daily living in elderly people living alone: Single-subject feasibility study. *Telemedicine Journal and e-Health, 10*(2), 260–276. doi:10.1089/tmj.2004.10.260

Sweeney, L. (1998). Datafly: A system for providing anonymity in medical data. In *Proceedings of the IFIP TC11 WG11.3 11th International Conference on Database Security XI: Status and Prospects* (pp. 356-381).

Swerissen, H., & Taylor, M. J. (2008). Reforming funding for chronic illness: Medicare-CDM. *Australian Health Review, 32*(1), 76–84. doi:10.1071/AH080076

Symons, V., & Walsham, G. (1988). The evaluation of information systems: a critique. *Journal of Applied Systems Analysis, 15*, 119–132.

Tabrizi, J. S., Wilson, A. J., Coyne, E. T., & O'Rourke, P. K. (2008). Review of patient-reported type 2 diabetes service quality. *Australian Health Review, 32*(1), 23–33. doi:10.1071/AH080023

Tamura, T., Togawa, T., Ogawa, M., & Yoda, M. (1998). Fully automated health monitoring system in the home. *Medical Engineering & Physics, 20*, 573–579. doi:10.1016/S1350-4533(98)00064-2

Tapia, E., Intille, S. S., & Larson, K. (2004). Activity Recognition in the Home Using Simple and Ubiquitous Sensors. In *Pervasive Computing* (pp. 158-175).

Tarimo, E., & Fowkes, F. (1989). Strengthening the Backbone of Primary Health Care. *World Health Forum, 10*(1), 74–79.

Tavafian, S. S., Jamshidi, A., & Mohammad, A. (2007). Low back pain education and short term quality of life: a randomized trial. *BMC Muscul. Disorder*, *8*, 21.

Taylor, R. S., Watt, A., & Dalal, H. M. (2007). Home-based cardiac rehabilitation versus hospital-based rehabilitation: A cost-effectiveness analysis. *International Journal of Cardiology*, *119*, 196–201. doi:10.1016/j.ijcard.2006.07.218

Taylor, S. and Todd,P.A.(1995). Understanding information technology usage: a test of competing models, information systems Research, 6(2): 144:174.

Tazari, M. R., Furfari, F., Ramos, J. P. L., & Ferro, E. (2009). The PERSONA Service Platform for AAL Spaces. In H. Nakashima, H. Aghajan, & J.C. Augusto (Eds.), *Handbook of Ambient Intelligence and Smart Environments (AISE)*. New York: Springer.

Tech/na. (2007). ICT Integration for Equity and Excellence in Education. http://www.tech.na/download/ICTPolicy2005_15March2005.pdf [date accessed: 30th May, 2007].

Telehealth can improve quality of life. (2009). *Nursing Standard, 23*(24), 21.

Tentori, M., & Favela, J. (2008, April-June). Activity-aware computing for healthcare. *IEEE Pervasive Computing / IEEE Computer Society [and] IEEE Communications Society*, *7*(2), 51–57. doi:10.1109/MPRV.2008.24

Terry Ma, H., & Zaphiris, P. (2003). *The Usability and Content Accessibility of the E-government in the UK.* Centre for Human-Computer Interaction Design, City University, London. Available at: http://www.soi.city.ac.uk/~zaphiri/Papers/HCII2003/HCII2003-Accessibility.pdf.

Terry, K. (2005, January 21). Exclusive survey: Doctors and EHRs, Medical Economics, Retrieved 2/4/08 from http://www.memag.com/memag/article/articleDetail.jsp?id=143144

Thain, D., Tannenbaum, T., & Livny, M. (2003).*Grid Computing: Making the Global Infrastructure a Reality, chapter Condor and the grid.* New York: John Wiley & Sons.

Thakkar, M. & Davis, D. C. (2006). Risks, barriers, and benefits of EHR systems: a comparative study based on size of hospital. Perspectives in Health Information Management, August 14, 3-5.

The Financial Times. (2007, September). *Chinese military hacked into Pentagon*. Retrieved February 17, 2009, from http://www.ft.com/cms/s/0/9dba9ba2-5a3b-11dc-9bcd-0000779fd2ac.html

The International Council on Medical & Care Compunetics. (2009, January 23). *Dutch nationwide EHR postponed. Are they in good company?* Retrieved February 17, 2009, from http://articles.icmcc.org/2009/01/23/dutch-ehr-postponed-are-they-in-good-company

The Times. (2008, December 26). *Patients avoid NHS database blunders by keeping cards close to their chest.* Retrieved February 17, 2009, from http://www.timesonline.co.uk/tol/life_and_style/health/article5397883.ece

The Washington Post. (2007, July). *Consultant Breached FBI's Computers*. Retrieved February 17, 2009, from http://www.washingtonpost.com/wp-dyn/content/article/2006/07/05/AR2006070501489_pf.html

Thompson, D. I., Osheroff, J., Classen, D., & Sittig, D. F. (2007). A review of methods to estimate the benefits of electronic medical records in hospitals and the need for a national benefits database. *Journal of Healthcare Information Management*, *21*(1), 62–68.

Thompson, L. T., Dorsey, M. A., Miller, I. K., & Parrott, R. (Eds.). (2003). *Handbook of Health Communication.* Mahwah, NJ: Lawrence Earlbaum.

Tornatzky, L., & Klein, K. (1982, February). Innovation characteristics and innovation adoption-implementation: A meta-analysis of findings. *IEEE Transactions on Engineering Management*, *29*(1), 28–45.

Triantafyllidis, A., Koutkias, V., Chouvarda, I., & Maglaveras, N. (2008). An open and reconfigurable wireless sensor network for pervasive health monitoring. In *Proceedings of the Second International Conference on Pervasive Computing Technologies for Healthcare PervasiveHealth 2008* (pp. 112-115).

Troshani, I., & Rao Hill, S. (2009). Linking stakeholder salience with mobile services diffusion. *International Journal of Mobile Communications*, *7*(3), 269–289. doi:10.1504/IJMC.2009.023672

Troshani, I., & Rao, S. (2007a). The diffusion of mobile services in Australia: an evaluation using stakeholder and transaction cost economics theories. *IADIS International Journal of WWW/Internet, 5*(2), 40-57.

Tsipouras, M. G., Fotiadis, D. I., & Sideris, D. (2005). An arrhythmia classification system based on the RR-interval signal. *Artificial Intelligence in Medicine*, *33*(3), 237–250. doi:10.1016/j.artmed.2004.03.007

Turisco, F. (2000). Mobile computing is next technology frontier for health providers. *Healthcare Financial Management*, *54*, 78–82.

Turisco, F., & Case, J. (2001). *Wireless and Mobile Computing*. Health Reports, California Healthcare Foundation.

Turner, E. H. (2004). A Taxpayer-Funded Clinical Trials Registry and Results Database. *PLoS Medicine*, *1*(3), 180–182. doi:10.1371/journal.pmed.0010060

U.S. Census Bureau. (2000). *The 65 and Over Population: 2000*. Washington, DC: Author.

U.S. Department of Health and Human Services. (2003). Home Health Service. In *Code of Federal Regulations* (Sect. 484.30).

U.S. Department of Health and Human Services. (2006a). *Overview Medicaid Program: General Information*. Washington, DC: Author.

U.S. Department of Health and Human Services. (2006b). Durable medical equipment: Scope and conditions. In *Code of Federal Regulations* (Sect. 410.38).

U.S. Department of Health and Human Services. (2008). *Medical & You handbook*. Washington, DC: Author.

U.S. Government General Accountability Office. (2002). *More Can Be Done to Protect Residents from Abuse*. Washington, DC: Author.

U.S. Government General Accountability Office. (2004). *HS's efforts to promote health information technology and legal barriers to its adoption*. Washington, DC: Author

U.S. Government General Accountability Office. (2008a). *NURSING HOMES: Federal Monitoring Surveys Demonstrate Continued Understatement of Serious Care Problems and CMS Oversight Weaknesses*. Washington, DC: Author.

U.S. Government General Accountability Office. (2008b). *Inspectors Often Overlook Serious Deficiencies at U.S. Nursing Homes*. Washington, DC: Author.

United Nations Economic Commission for Africa (UNECA). (2006). National Information and Communication Infrastructure (NICI) Policies and Plans (e-strategies), Namibia. http://www.uneca.org/aisi/nici/Namibia/namibia.htm [date accessed: 1 November 2006].

United States Environmental Protection Agency. O. o. A. a. R. O., Indoor Environments Division (6604J) (1997). An Office Building Occupant's Guide to Indoor Air Quality. [Web page]. (EPA-402-K-97-003).

US Census Bureau. (2008). *Projected Population by Single Year of Age, Sex, Race, and Hispanic Origin for the United States: July 1, 2000 to July 1, 2050*. Retrieved January 27, 2009, from http://www.census.gov/population/www/projections/downloadablefiles.html

Valsiner, J. (2000). Data as Representations: Contextualizing Qualitative and Quantitative Research Strategies. *Social Sciences Information. Information Sur les Sciences Sociales*, *39*(1), 99–113. doi:10.1177/053901800039001006

Van Der Meijden, M. J., Tange, H. J., Troost, J., & Hasman, A. (2003). Determinants of success of inpatient clinical information systems: A literature review. *Journal of the American Medical Informatics Association*, *10*(3), 235–243. doi:10.1197/jamia.M1094

Van Eyk, H., & Baum, F. (2002). Learning about interagency collaboration: Trialling collaborative projects between hospitals and community health services. *Health & Social Care in the Community*, *10*(4), 262–269. doi:10.1046/j.1365-2524.2002.00369.x

Van Raak, A., Mur-Veeman, I., & Hardy, B. (2003). *Integrated Care in Europe*. Elsevier Gezondheidszorg.

Vandewalle, J-J. (2004). Smart Card Research Perspectives. *LNCS Construction and Analysis of Safe, Secure and Interoperable Smart devices.*

Vanjara, P. (2006). Application of mobile technologies in healthcare diagnostics and administration. In Lazakidou, A. (Ed.), *Handbook of Research on Informatics in Healthcare and Medicine* (pp. 113–130). Hershey, PA: Idea Group.

Vanmeerbeek, M. (2004). Exploitation of electronic medical records data in primary health care. Resistance and solutions. Study in eight Wallon health care centres. *Studies in Health Technology and Informatics*, *110*, 42–48.

Varshney, U. (2006). Using wireless technologies in healthcare. *International Journal of Mobile Communications*, *4*(3), 354–368.

Varshney, U. (2003). Pervasive healthcare. *Computer*, *36*(12), 138–140. doi:10.1109/MC.2003.1250897

Venkatesh, V., Morris, M. G., Davis, G. B., & Davis, F. (2003). User Acceptance of Information Technology: Toward A Unified View. *Management Information Systems Quarterly*, *27*(3), 425–478.

Venkatesh, V., & Davis, F. D. (2000). A theoretical extension of the technology acceptance model: Four longitudinal field studies. *Management Science*, *46*(2), 186–204. doi:10.1287/mnsc.46.2.186.11926

Verbeke, J., Nadgir, N., Ruetsch, G., & Sharapov, I. (2002). Framework for peer-to-peer distributed computing in a heterogeneous, decentralized environment. In [London: Springer-Verlag.]. *Proceedings of GRID*, *02*, 1–12.

Verberk, W. J., Kroon, A. A., & Kessels, A. G. H. (2005). Home Blood Pressure Measurement - A Systematic Review. *Journal of the American College of Cardiology*, *46*(5), 743–751. doi:10.1016/j.jacc.2005.05.058

Versel, N. (2008). Use of Mobile and Wireless Technology Jumps in Hospitals. *Digital HealthCare*, from http://www.digitalhcp.com/DigitalHealthCare_Content.aspx?id=72018

VictorianGovernment. (2007). *Diabetes Prevention and Management: A Strategic Framework for Victoria 1007-2010*. Melbourne: Victorian Government, Department of Human Services.

Virginia Department of Social Services. (2007). Assisted Living Facilities (ALF). Richmond, VA: Author.

Virone, G., Alwan, M., Dalal, S., Kell, S. W., Turner, B., & Stankovic, J. A. (2008). Behavioral Patterns of Older Adults in Assisted Living. *IEEE Transactions on Information Technology in Biomedicine*, *12*(3), 12. doi:10.1109/TITB.2007.904157

Voon, R., Celler, B. G., & Lovell, N. H. (2008). The use of an energy monitor in the management of diabetes: A pilot study. *Diabetes Technology and Therapeutics*.

Wade, E., & Asada, H. (2007, Jan.-March). Conductive fabric garment for a cable-free body area network. *IEEE Pervasive Computing / IEEE Computer Society [and] IEEE Communications Society*, *6*(1), 52–58. doi:10.1109/MPRV.2007.8

Wager, K., Lee, F. W., & White, A. W. (2002). *Life After a Disastrous Electronic Medical Record Implementation: One Clinic's Experience*. Hershey, PA: Idea Group Publishing.

Waitzkin, H. (2003). Report of the Who Commission on Macroeconomics and Health: A Summary and Critique. *Lancet*, *361*, 523–526. doi:10.1016/S0140-6736(03)12491-9

Wald, H., & Shojania, K. G. (2001). Incident reporting. In K. G. Shojania, B. W. Ducan, K. M. McDonald, & R. M. Wachter (Eds.), *Making health care safer: A critical analysis of patient safety practices* (pp. 41-47). Rockville, MD: Agency for Healthcare Research and Quality.

Walker, H., Bakker, E., Knight, L., Gough, S., & McBain, D. (2006), Sustainable procurement in the English National Health Service: learning and practice. *Paper presented at the International Purchasing and Supply Education and Research Association*.San Diego, USA.

Wallace, S. (1997). Health information in the new millennium and beyond: the role of computers and the Internet. [May.]. *Health Education*, *97*(3), 88–95. doi:10.1108/09654289710162488

Walsham, G. (1995). Interpretive Case Studies in Is Research: Nature and Method. *EJISDC*, *4*(2), 74–81.

Walsham, G. (2006). Doing Interpretive Research. *EJISDC*, *15*, 320–330.

Walsham, G. (1993). *Interpreting Information Systems in Organizations*. Chichester: John Wiley & Sons.

Walt, G., & Gilson, L. (1994). Reforming the Health Sector in Developing Countries: The Central Role of Policy Analysis. *Health Policy and Planning*, *9*(4), 353–370. doi:10.1093/heapol/9.4.353

Wang, R. Y., & Strong, D. M. (1996). Beyond accuracy: What data quality means to data consumers. *Journal of Management Information Systems: JMIS*, *12*(4), 5–33.

Wang, K., & Fung, B. C. M. (2006). Anonymizing sequential releases. In *Proceedings of the 12th ACM SIGKDD Conference*, Philadelphia.

Wang, L., Bretschneider, S., & Gant, J. (2005). Evaluating Web-Based E-Government Services with a Citizen-Centric Approach. In *Proceedings of 38th Annual Hawaii International Conference on Systems Sciences*, Big Island, Hawaii.

Warren, S., Yao, J., & Barnes, G. E. (2002). Wearable sensors and component-based design for home health care. In. *Proceedings of the Annual International Conference of IEEE Engineering in Medicine and Biology*, *3*, 1871–1872.

Waterman, J., Curtis, D., Goraczko, M., Shih, E., Sarin, P., Pino, E., et al. (2005). *Demonstration of SMART (Scalable Medical Alert Response Technology)*. Paper presented at the AMIA 2005 Annual Symposium.

Webb, A. (2001). *The Impact of the Cost of Long-Term Care on the Saving of the Elderly*. New York: International Longevity Center.

Wei, S. J., Metz, J. M., & Coyle, C. (2004). Recruitment of Patients Into an Internet-Based Clinical Trials Database: The Experience of OncoLink and the National Colorectal Cancer Research Alliance. *Journal of Clinical Oncology*, *22*(23), 4730–4736. doi:10.1200/JCO.2004.07.103

Weiler, R. M., & Pealer, L. N. (2000). The Site Legend: twelve components of a new strategy for providing website documentation. *The Journal of School Health*, *70*(4), 148–152. doi:10.1111/j.1746-1561.2000.tb06461.x

Wellard, S. J., Rennie, S., & King, R. (2008). Perceptions of people with type 2 diabetes about self-management and the efficiency of community based services. *Contemporary Nurse*, *29*(2), 218–226. doi:10.5172/conu.673.29.2.218

Wensing, M., Wollersheim, H., & Grol, R. (2006). Organisational interventions to implement improvements in patient care: a structured review of reviews. *Implementation Science; IS*, *1*, 2. doi:10.1186/1748-5908-1-2

West, D. (2000). *Assessing E-Government: The Internet, Democracy and Service Delivery by State and Federal Governments*. Brown University. Available at: www.insidepolitics.org/policyreports.html.

WFTV. (2008, August 14). *Medical Center Patient Records Posted On Internet*. Retrieved February 17, 2009, from http://www.wftv.com/news/17188045/detail.html?taf=orlc

What are the arguments for community-based mental health care? (2003). *WHO/HEN*.

Whitten, B., Cook, D. J., Shaw, P., Ermer, D., & Goodwin, J. (1998). Telekid Care: Bringing health care into schools. *Telemedicine Journal*, *4*(4), 335–343.

Whitten, P. S., & Cook, D. J. (1999). School-based telemedicine: Using technology to bring health care to inner-city children. [abstract]. *Journal of Telemedicine and Telecare*, *5*(Suppl 1), S23–S25. doi:10.1258/1357633991932423

Whitten, P., Doolittle, G., & Heilmich, S. (2001). Telehospice: using telecommunication technology for terminally ill patients. *Computer-Mediated Communications*, *6*(4), 43–47.

WHO. (2001). *Commission on Macroeconomics and Health. Macroeconomics and Health: Investing in Health for Economic Development*. Geneva: WHO.

WHO. (1978) "Declaration of Alma-Ata". in *International Conference on Primary Health Care,* Alma-Ata, USSR, 6-12 September, WHO (2000) "The World Health Report 2000" *WHO* Geneva.

Wickramasinghe, N. S., Fadlalla, A. M. A., Geisler, E., & Schaffer, J. L. (2005). A framework for assessing e-health preparedness. *International Journal of Electronic Healthcare*, *1*(3), 316–334. doi:10.1504/IJEH.2005.006478

Wickramasinghe, N. (2007). Fostering knowledge assets in healthcare with the KMI model. *International Journal of Management and Enterprise Development*, *4*(1), 52–65. doi:10.1504/IJMED.2007.011455

Wickramasinghe, N., & Goldberg, S. (2004). How M=EC2 in healthcare. *International Journal of Mobile Communications*, *2*(2), 140–156. doi:10.1504/IJMC.2004.004664

Wickramasinghe, N., & Goldberg, S. (2007a). Adaptive mapping to realisation methodology (AMR) to facilitate mobile initiatives in healthcare. *International Journal of Mobile Communications*, *5*(3), 300–318. doi:10.1504/IJMC.2007.012396

Wickramasinghe, N., Goldberg, S., & Bali, R. (2007). Enabling superior m-health project success: a tri-country validation. *International Journal of Services and Standards*, *4*(1), 97–117. doi:10.1504/IJSS.2008.016087

Wickramasinghe, N., Misra, S., Jenkins, A., & Vogel, D. R. (2006). The Competitive Forces Facing E-Health. *International Journal of Healthcare Information Systems and Informatics*, *1*(4), 68–81.

Wickramasinghe, N., & Schaffer, J. (2006). Creating knowledge driven healthcare processes with the intelligence continuum. *International Journal of Electronic Healthcare*, *2*(2), 164–174.

Wickramasinghe, N., Troshani, I., & Goldberg, S. (2009). Supporting diabetes self-management with pervasive wireless technology solutions. *International Journal of Healthcare Delivery Reform Initiatives*, *1*(4), 17–31.

Wickramasinghe, N., Troshani, I., & Goldberg, S. (2010). An investigation into the use of pervasive wireless technologies to support diabetes healthcare. In Coronato, A., & De Pietro, G. (Eds.), *Pervasive and Smart Technologies for Healthcare: Ubiquitous Methodologies and Tools* (*Vol. 114-129*). New York: IGI Global. doi:10.4018/978-1-61520-765-7.ch006

Wickramasinghe, N., Schaffer, J., & Geisler, E. (2005). Assessing e-health. In Spil, T., & Schuring, R. (Eds.), *E-Health Systems Diffusion and Use: The Innovation, The User, and The User IT Model*. Hershey, PA: Idea Group.

Wickramasinghe, N., & Goldberg, S. (2004). How M=EC2 in healthcare. *International Journal of Mobile Commerce*.

Wickramasinghe, N., & Misra, S. (2004). A wireless trust model for healthcare. *International Journal e-Healt*h.

Wickramasinghe, N., & Goldberg, S. (2003). *The wireless panacea for healthcare.* Paper presented at the 36th Hawaii International Conference on System Sciences, Hawaii, 6-10 January, IEEE.

Willcocks, L. (1992). Evaluating Information Technology Investments: Research Findings and Reappraisal. *Journal of Information Systems*, *2*(3), 243–268.

Williams, P., Nichols, D., Huntington, P., & McLean, F. (2002). Surfing for health: user evaluation of a health information website. *Health Information and Libraries Journal*, *19*(1), 98–108. doi:10.1046/j.1471-1842.2002.00374_2.x

Williams, G., Doughty, K., & Bradley, D. A. (1998). A systems approach to achieving CarerNet-an integrated and intelligent telecare system. *IEEE Transactions on Information Technology in Biomedicine*, *2*(1), 1–9. doi:10.1109/4233.678527

Williams, L. (2003). Medication-Monitoring Lawsuit: Case Study and Lessons Learned. *Nursing Homes/Long Term Care Management*, 3.

Williamson, O. E. (1985a). *The Economic Institutions of Capitalism: Firms, Markets and Relational Contracting*. New York: Free Press.

Williamson, O. E. (1991). Comparative economic organization: The analysis of discrete structural alternatives. *Administrative Science Quarterly*, *36*, 269–296. doi:10.2307/2393356

Willoughby, C., Fridsma, D., & Chatterjee, L. (2007). A standard computable clinical trial protocol: The role of the BRIDG model. *Drug Information Journal*, *41*(3), 383–392.

Wilson, L. S., Ho, P., Bengston, K. J., Dadd, M. J., Chen, C. F., Huynh, C., et al. (2001). *The CSIRO hospital without walls home telecare system*. Paper presented at the Seventh Australian and New Zealand Intelligent Information Systems Conference.

Wireless Healthcare. (2007). *Wireless Based Disease Management. Wireless Healthcare*. Royston, UK: Steinkrug Publications.

Wisnicki, H. J. (2002). Wireless networking transforms healthcare: physician's practices better able to handle workflow, increase productivity (The human connection). *Ophthalmology Times*, *27*(21), 38–41.

Wolf, A. (2003). Behind Closed Doors. *NFPA Journal*.

Wolf, D. A., & Jenkins, C. (2008). Family Care and Assisted Living. In S. M. Golant & J. Hyde (Eds.), *The Assisted Living Residence*. Baltimore, MD: Johns Hopkins University Press.

Wolfstadt, J. (2008). The effect of computerized physician order entry with clinical decision support on the rates of adverse drug events: A systematic review. *Journal of General Internal Medicine*, *23*(4), 451–458. doi:10.1007/s11606-008-0504-5

Wood, J. A., Miller, T. W., & Hargrove, D. S. (2005). Clinical supervision in rural settings: A telehealth model. *Professional Psychology, Research and Practice*, *36*(2), 173–179. doi:10.1037/0735-7028.36.2.173

Wood, J. A., O'Quin, J., & Eftink, S. (2004). A preliminary investigation of the use of videophone technology as a training tool for students working with older adults. *Journal of Teaching in Social Work*, *24*, 35–46. doi:10.1300/J067v24n03_03

Wood, J. A. & Hargrove, D. S. (2006). *Use of videoconferencing to deliver mental health services to adults with mental retardation*. Manuscript submitted for publication.

Wood, J. A. (2000). *The effectiveness of videophone technology in bringing mental healthservices to rural residents*. Unpublished master's thesis, Stephen F. Austin State University, Nacogdoches, TX.

Wood, J. A. (2006, April). *Patient and provider satisfaction with telemental health services*. Poster presented at the VA Psychology Leadership Conference, Dallas, TX.

Wootton, R. (2001). Telemedicine. *British Medical Journal*, *323*, 4. doi:10.1136/bmj.323.7303.4

World Bank. (1993). *The World Development Report 1993: Investing in Health*. New York: Oxford University Press.

World Markets Research Centre & Brown University. (2001). *Global e-government Survey 2001*. Available at: http://www.worldmarketsanalysis.com/pdf/e-govreport.pdf

Wu, J. H., Wang, S. C., & Lin, L. M. (2007). Mobile computing acceptance factors in the healthcare industry: A structural equation model. *International Journal of Medical Informatics*, *76*(1), 66–77. doi:10.1016/j.ijmedinf.2006.06.006

Wu, J. H., Wang, S. C., & Lin, L. M. (2005). *What drives mobile healthcare? An empirical evaluation of technology acceptance. 38th Hawaii International Conference on System Sciences*, Hawaii.

Wu, K., & Wu, X. (2007). *A Wireless Mobile Monitoring System for Home Healthcare and Community Medical Services*. Paper presented at the Bioinformatics and Biomedical Engineering, 2007. ICBBE 2007. The 1st International Conference on.

Wunderlich, G. S., & Kohler, P. O. (2001). *Improving the quality of long-term care: Information systems for monitoring quality.* Washington, DC: National Academy Press.

Wylde, M. A. (2008). The Future of Assisted Living: Residents' Perspectives 2006-2026. In S. M. Golant & J. Hyde (Eds.), *The Assisted Living Residence*. Baltimore, MD: Johns Hopkins University Press.

Xiao, X., & Tao, Y. (2007). m-invariance: Towards privacy preserving re-publication of dynamic datasets. In *Proceedings of the ACM SIGMOD Conference,* Beijing, China.

Xie, S., Xiao, Y., & Chen, H.-H. (in press). Nursing Home. In A. Coronato & G. De Pietro (Eds.), *Pervasive and Smart Technologies for Healthcare: Ubiquitous Methodologies and Tools*. Hershey, PA: IGI Global.

Xu, H., & Koronios, A. (2004/2005). Understanding Information Quality in E-Business. *Journal of Computer Information Systems*, *45*(2), 73–82.

Yamaguchi, A., Ogawa, M., Tamura, T., & Togawa, T. (1998). *Monitoring behavior in the home using positioning sensors.* Paper presented at the 20th Annual International Conference of the IEEE Engineering in Medicine and Biology Society.

Yamuah, L. K. (2005). ICT in the African health sector: towards healthy nations with ICT Wealth.i4d magazine: May 2005. http//:www.i4donline.net/may05/african-health.asp (date accessed: 20 June 2006).

Yang, N., Barringer, H., & Zhang, N. (2007). A Purpose-Based Access Control Model. In *Proceedings of the Symposium in Information Assurance and Security* (pp. 143-148).

Yao, C., Wang, X. S., & Jajodia, S. (2005). Checking for k-anonymity violation by views. In *Proceedings of the 31st Very Large Data Bases (VLDB) Conference,* Trondheim, Norway (pp. 910-921).

Yellowlees, P. (2005). Successfully developing a telemedicine system. *Journal of Telemedicine and Telecare*, *11*, 331–335. doi:10.1258/135763305774472024

Yin, R. K. (2003). *Case study research: Design and Methods* (3rd ed.). Thousand Oaks, CA: Sage Publications.

Yin, R. K. (2003) *Case Study Research: Design and Methods,* (Third Edition) Sage. Third Edition, London.

Yin, S., Pucheral, P., & Meng, X. (2009). *A Sequential Indexing Scheme for Flash-Based Embedded Systems*. Paper presented at the International Conference on Extending Database Technology (EDBT).

Young, T., & Irenson, C. (2003). Effectiveness of School based Telehealth Care in Rural Elementary Schools. *Pediatrics*, *112*(5), 1088–1096. doi:10.1542/peds.112.5.1088

Yu, P., Li, H., & Gagnon, M.-P. (2008). (in press). Health IT acceptance factors i n long-term care facilities: a cross-sectional survey. *International Journal of Health Informatics*. doi:.doi:10.1016/j.ijmedinf.2008.07.006

Yu, P., Li, H., & Gagnon, M.-P. (2009). Health IT acceptance factors in long-term care facilities: A cross-sectional survey. *International Journal of Medical Informatics*, *78*(4), 219–229. doi:10.1016/j.ijmedinf.2008.07.006

Zarate, C. A., Weinstock, L., Cukor, P., Morabito, C., Leahy, L., Burns, C., & Baer, L. (1997). Applicability of telemedicine for assessing patients with schizophrenia: Acceptance and reliability. *The Journal of Clinical Psychiatry*, *58*, 22–25. doi:10.4088/JCP.v58n0104

Zeithaml, V. A., Parasuraman, A., & Malhotra, A. (2000). A Conceptual Framework for Understanding e-Service Quality: Implications for Future Research and Managerial Practice. *Marketing Sciences Institute: Working Paper Series*, (115).

Zeng, X., & Parmanto, B. (2004). Web content accessibility of consumer health information Web sites for people with disabilities: a cross sectional evaluation. *Journal of Medical Internet Research*, *6*(2), e19. doi:10.2196/jmir.6.2.e19

Zhang, D. (2007). Web content adaptation for mobile handheld devices. *Communications of the ACM*, *50*(2), 75–79. doi:10.1145/1216016.1216024

Zhang, X., Parisi-Presicce, F., Sandhu, R., & Park, J. (2005). Formal model and policy specification of usage control. *ACM Transactions on Information and System Security*, *8*, 351–387. doi:10.1145/1108906.1108908

Zhenga, J., Bakkera, E., Knighta, L., Gilhespyb, H., Harlanda, C., & Walkera, H. (2006). A strategic case for e-adoption in healthcare supply chains. *International Journal of Information Management*, *26*, 290–301. doi:10.1016/j.ijinfomgt.2006.03.010

Zigbor, J. C., & Songer, T. J. (2001). External barriers to diabetes care: addressing personal and health systems issues. *Diabetes Spectrum*, *14*, 23–28. doi:10.2337/diaspect.14.1.23

Zikmund, W. (1994). *Business Research Methods* (International Ed. ed.). Orlando, FL: The Dryden Press.

Zwarenstein M, Goldman J, Reeves S (2009). Interprofessional collaboration: effects of practice-based interventions on professional practice and healthcare outcomes (Review). *Cochr Lib*, Issue 3.

About the Contributors

Matthew Guah was borne in Sanniquellie City, Nimba County, Liberia. He attended St. Mary's RC School in Sanniquellie until 1983 and spent two years at Don Bosco Polytechnic (Sinkor, Monrovia). Dr. Guah obtained BSc in Information Technology from Salford University, MSc in Technology Management from Manchester University, and PhD in Information Systems and Management Controls from Warwick Business School, (all in the UK). He migrated to Great Britain in 1994, currently holds a British passport, and has made it a home for his family while travelling and working in different parts of the world. He was deemed to have demonstrated exemplary achievement and distinguished contributions to the business community and certificated to appear in the 2008-2009 edition of *Madison Who's Who of Professionals*. Matthew Waritay Guah is Associate Professor for Business Systems at the School of Business, Claflin University in South Carolina. He previously worked in the Economics School of Erasmus University Rotterdam, The Netherlands. His research concentrate on management controls for healthcare reform; IFRS; IT impact on accounting practices; and financial accountability (Internet Fraud, Corporate Social Responsibility, ERP in auditing). Theoretical foundations: institutional theory, socio-economic, risk management, project management/escalation. Dr. Guah has served as track chair for ICIS-2009 and 2011 (healthcare IT track); VP for Accounting Information System (special-interest-group) within the Association for Information Systems (http://home.aisnet.org). He has published 3 books, 12 journals, 8 chapter contributions, and presented at more than 20 international conferences. He is editor-in-chief for the International Journal of Health Delivery Reform Initiatives. Other editorial memberships include *JCIT, SJI, JIQ, JMIS* and *IJEC*. Dr. Guah also served as visiting scholar in the Accounting Department of Hawaii University @ Manoa (Honolulu, USA) and Management School of Innsbruck University (Austria). Recent speaking engagements by invitation at research seminars include Universitá Cattolica, (Milan, Italy), Salford University (Manchester, UK), Westminster University (London, UK), and Warwick Business School (UK). He is external examiner for several universities in USA, Europe and South Africa. He came into academia with a wealth of industrial experience spanning over ten years (including Merrill Lynch, HSBC, British Airways, and United Nations).

* * *

Esko Alasaarela received MSc and PhD degrees in electrical engineering from the University of Oulu, Oulu, Finland in 1975 and 1983 respectively. His research area covers biomedical engineering including wireless technologies.He is currently CEO of Domuset Ltd and part-time Adjunct Professor (Docent) in the University of Oulu, Finland. He works also regularly as a Visiting Professor in Dongseo University, Busan, South-Korea. In addition he is a founding partner of ZEF Solutions Ltd (www.zefsolutions.com), an internet service company located in Finland and in CA, USA. Formerly he has served as Professor in the University of Oulu, Research Director in the University of Jyvaskyla and Managing Director of Moistic Ltd, HTC High Technology Center Ltd, and ZEF Solutions Ltd. Dr Alasaarela is a member of the Finnish Association of Biomedical Engineering and Physics (from 1990).

Tristan Allard is a Ph. D. Student at University of Versailles, France. He received his engineering degree from the ESILV, France, in 2006 and his M. S. degree with highest honours from the University of Versailles in 2007. His research interests encompass privacy and data distribution.

Nicolas Anciaux is a Researcher at INRIA, France. He received his Ph.D. in Computer Science from the University of Versailles in 2004. After one year at University of Twente, Netherlands, he joined the SMIS (Secured and Mobile Information Systems) at INRIA Rocquencourt. His main research area is embedded data management and privacy, in particular in the context of ambient intelligence. He has co-authored more than fifteen journal and conference papers.

Adebusoye Anifalaje is a doctoral candidate at the LSE. His thesis focuses on understanding the role of health information systems in improving public health in Nigeria. As part of an initiative to encourage interdisciplinary research between the medical and social sciences, his PhD - supervised partly at the Imperial College - is jointly funded by the ESRC and MRC. He is also involved in a comparative work on HIS in India.

Nesaar Banderker was born and bred in Cape Town, South Africa. He obtained a Bachelor of Commerce degree specializing in Information Systems and Auditing in 1997. After that, he obtained a BCom (Hons) in 2005 and is now registered for his Masters degree. He is currently a project manager working for a large international financial services company. He is married to a health professional hence his interest in health information systems. He also has two exceptionally lively boys. The 8 year old is wise in the ways of the world and is starting to ask very awkward questions. The 4 year old is wise in ways of being exceptionally entertaining, playful and naughty.

Jean-Paul Van Belle is an associate professor and Head of the Departmental of Information Systems at the University of Cape Town. Before joining UCT, he set up the Information Systems department at the University of the Western Cape. He obtained his MBA in the field of financial modelling and his doctorate in the field of enterprise modelling. Currently he is researching the adoption of technologies (including mobile technologies) in South Africa, ICTs for development and the e-readiness of SMEs and NGOs. He supervises a number of doctoral and masters students in this area. He is a family man with 3 children and a keen outdoors person.

Robert Breas is an adviser at the Dutch National IT Institute for Healthcare (Nictiz). He is project leader at the introduction programme for introducing SNOMED CT in the Netherlands. He is also the coordinator for the first work package of the epSOS project (European Patient Smart Open Services). The content of this package is to analyze and compare the national plans and/or solutions of twelve European countries. The goal of this pan-European project is to develop a working pilot for the exchange of patient summaries and ePrescription services among European countries. Robert Breas has a MSc. degree in Health Management and a MSc. degree in Informatics & Economics, both obtained at the Erasmus University of Rotterdam. His theses were respectively on the workability of an Electronic Patient Record (EPR) in a Dutch hospital and on optimizing healthcare by using Workflow Management. Recently he worked as an adviser in healthcare, with experience in the care, hospital and eHealth sector.

Luc Bouganim is a Director of Research at INRIA Rocquencourt. He obtained a PhD and the Habilitation à Diriger des Recherches, both from the University of Versailles in 1996 and 2006, respectively. He worked as an assistant professor from 1997 to 2002 when he joined INRIA. Luc co-authored more than 60 conference and journal papers, an international patent and was the recipient of 4 international awards. Since 2000, Luc is strongly engaged in research activities on ubiquitous data management and data confidentiality. He is currently the vice-head of the SMIS (Secured and Mobile Information Systems) research team.

Branko George Celler received the B.Sc. degree in computer science and physics, the B.E. (Hons) degree in electrical engineering, and the Ph.D. degree in biomedical engineering from the University of New South Wales (UNSW), Sydney, Australia, in 1969, 1972, and 1978, respectively. From 1977 to 1980, he was a Postdoctoral Fellow working at the Johns Hopkins School of Medicine in Baltimore, MD. He returned to UNSW in 1981 as a Lecturer, where he was appointed an Associate Professor in 1991 and a Professor in January 1997. Prof. Celler is a Foundation Member of the Australian College of Medical Informatics and was the Foundation Co-Director of the Centre for Health Informatics at UNSW.

Leroy Lai Yu Chan received the B.E. (Hons) degree in electrical engineering and the M.Biomed.E degree in biomedical engineering from the University of New South Wales (UNSW), Sydney, Australia, in 2001. Currently, he is pursuing the Ph.D. degree at the School of Electrical and Telecommunications Engineering at UNSW. His research focuses on smart wireless sensor networks for residential aged care management and care level classification.

Hsiao-Hwa Chen is currently a full Professor in Department of Engineering Science, National Cheng Kung University, Taiwan, and he was the founding Director of the Institute of Communications Engineering of the National Sun Yat-Sen University, Taiwan. He received BSc and MSc degrees from Zhejiang University, China, and PhD degree from University of Oulu, Finland, in 1982, 1985 and 1990, respectively, all in Electrical Engineering. He has authored or co-authored over 200 technical papers in major international journals and conferences, five books and several book chapters in the areas of communications, including the books titled "Next Generation Wireless Systems and Networks" (512 pages) and "The Next Generation CDMA Technologies" (468 pages), both published by John Wiley and Sons in 2005 and 2007, respectively. He has been an active volunteer for IEEE various technical activities for over 20 years. Currently, he is serving as the Chair of IEEE ComSoc Radio Communications Committee, and the Vice Chair of IEEE ComSoc Communications \& Information Security Technical Committee. He served or is serving as symposium chair/co-chair of many major IEEE conferences, including VTC, ICC, Globecom and WCNC, etc. He served or is serving as Associate Editor or/and Guest Editor of numerous important technical journals in communications. He is serving as the Chief Editor (Asia and Pacific) for Wiley's Wireless Communications and Mobile Computing (WCMC) Journal and Wiley's International Journal of Communication Systems, etc. He is the Editor-in-Chief of Wiley' Security and Communication Networks journal (www.interscience.wiley.com/journal/security). He is also an adjunct Professor of Zhejiang University, China, and Shanghai Jiao Tung University, China.

Dorothy Curtis is a Research Scientist at the Computer Science and Artificial Intelligence Laboratory (CSAIL) at the Massachusetts Institute of Technology in Cambridge, Massachusetts, USA. Her work focuses on physiological monitoring and indoor location systems. She has built other real-time systems, in the fields of computer networking and shipboard collision detection and avoidance and navigation. Other computer science interests include natural language processing, compilers, and object-oriented databases. She holds degrees from the Massachusetts Institute of Technology, Boston University, and Simmons College.

Antonio Coronato received the degree in information engineering at the University "Federico II" of Naples in the 1998. He is a researcher at the Institute for High Performance Computing and Networking (ICAR) of the italian National Research Council (CNR). He is grant professor of Software Engineering at the University "Federico II" of Naples and Object Oriented Programming at the Second University of Naples. He is an associate editor for the Journal of Security and Communication Networks, a member of the international editorial board for the Journal of Smart Home, the Journal of Multimedia and Ubiquitous Engineering and the Journal of Software Architecture. He is also involved in the organization of several international conferences on pervasive computing. His research interests are in the field of pervasive computing, middleware and component-based architectures and dependable computing.

Steven DeMello has over 30 years of experience in research, hospital operations, strategic planning, systems management and consulting. He is currently the Director of Health Care for the Center for Information Technology Research in the Interest of Society (CITRIS) at the University of California, Berkeley. Prior to joining CITRIS, he was Executive Director and Senior Advisor of the Health Technology Center (HealthTech), a non-profit research group and expert network based in San Francisco. Prior to HealthTech, he served as Chief Operating Officer of ezboard, Inc. a large first-generation consumer social networking company. His previous positions include serving as Senior Vice President California Healthcare System, President and COO of Alliance Home Care Management, Inc., and Principal at the global management consulting firm A.T. Kearney. He received a B.A. in economics from Claremont McKenna College, and an M.B.A. from the University of Chicago.

Giuseppe De Pietro received the degree in electronic engineering at the University "Federico II" of Naples in the 1988. He is a senior researcher at the Institute for High Performance Computing and Networking (ICAR) of the Italian National Research Council (CNR). He is grant professor of Information Systems at the Second University of Naples. He is a member of the international editorial board for the Journal of Smart Home and the Journal of Multimedia and Ubiquitous Engineering. He is also involved in the organization of several international conferences on pervasive computing. His research interests are in the field of pervasive computing, graphics and virtual reality environments, middleware and component-based architectures, software engineering. He is a member of the IEEE.

Tommaso Federici (1960, Italy) teaches Information Systems Management and Organization Theory at the Faculty of Economics of the University of Tuscia, in Viterbo, Italy, and Organization Theory at the Faculty of Sociology of the University "La Sapienza", in Rome, Italy. As author or co-author, he published papers, articles and books. His current research domains are e-procurement, as a booster to promote change in the public sector, the role of FLOSS as a support for organizational change, and the ERP introduction in the SMEs segment.

Luigi Gallo received his degree in Computer Engineering from University "Federico II" of Naples in July 2006. Since November 2006, he has been working towards a Ph.D. degree in Information Technology Engineering at the University of Naples "Parthenope", Department of Technology. Currently he is a research fellow at the National Research Council (CNR) - Institute for High-Performance Computing and Networking (ICAR). Since June 2007 he has been a member of the Advanced Medical Imaging and Computing labOratory (AMICO), developed from a cooperation agreement between the IBB and ICAR institutes of the National Research Council. His fields of interest involve Virtual Reality, CHI and Multi-Agent Systems, specifically considering healthcare application scenarios. He is a student member of ACM, ACM SIGGRAPH, ACM SIGCHI and SIGCHI-Italy.

Steve Goldberg started his 24-year information technology career at Systemhouse Ltd. At Crowntek, he developed a $30 million IT services business. During his tenure at Cybermation, he transformed the organization from mainframe to client/server solution delivery. Prior to INET, at Compugen he successfully built and managed teams to deliver enterprise e-business solutions. Mr. Goldberg has a B.A. (Economics & Computer Science) from the University of Western Ontario. He is on the Editorial Board of the International Journal of Networking and Virtual Organizations, and has many papers accepted under peer review at international conferences and published in international journals

Raj Gururajan is a Professor in Information Systems in the Faculty of Business at the University of Southern Queensland, Australia. His main area of research is user behaviour issues in using wireless technology, the management of technology and the diffusion of technology at enterprise level. Currently he is applying these interests to health settings. He has published over 100 refereed articles, won over $2 million in grant income, manages six funded projects and supervising over 10 PhD students. He also holds 3 national competitive grants (ARC) in health informatics.

Gary Hackbarth is an Assistant Professor of Management Information Systems in the College of Informatics, Department of Business Informatics', at Northern Kentucky University. He holds a Ph.D. in Management Information Systems from the Moore School of Business at the University of South Carolina. His teaching, research, and consulting areas of interest include Project Management, Health Informatics, Information System Strategy, and Organizational Memory. Gary has published in the European Journal of Information Systems, Information & Management, Database, Information Systems Management, Journal of Web-Based Learning and Teaching Technologies, Journal of Electronic Commerce Research, the Financial Times, and in both national and international conference proceedings. He is also a member of the Decision Sciences Institute and the Association for Information Systems.

Abdul Hafeez-Baig holds a PhD in the domain of healthcare and information systems from USQ and master's degrees in MIS and MBA from Griffith University, Brisbane, Australia. Since joining USQ in 2004, he has published many referred publications in the domains of health and education regarding technology management. Abdul is very conversant with wireless technology as well as emerging technologies and learning management systems. He teaches information systems concepts to both undergraduate and postgraduate students, including MBA students. Abdul also has numerous publications in academic and scholarly journals, and has a vast array of scholarly conference papers, all of which have revolved around the domain of information systems. Abdul has extensive experience in the area of information systems, especially with regards to the healthcare sector. He is particularly interested in wireless healthcare applications, systems analysis and design, adoption, the infusion and diffusion of information technology, M-learning and E-Commerce, outsourcing, networking, health care and information technology, and the re-engineering of business processes.

Rhoda C. Joseph is an Assistant Professor of Information Systems at Pennsylvania State University Harrisburg. She has earned her Ph.D. in Business from the City University of New York as well as an M.B.A from Baruch College. Her research interests include e-government, technology adoption, and IT in developing countries.

Torben Larsen is MSc Econ from Aarhus University and has a diploma in strategic management from Maryland U. He has had various consultant posts in Danish health care. Actually, he is chief consultant in the Centre of Applied HealthScience at Southern Danish University where he coordinates an international research project on integrated homecare for the European Commission. He has published a series of studies in health economics and neuroeconomics and received academic awards from the Lundbeck Foundation (1990), European Association of Medical Informatics (1996), Black SeaDiab (1998), Visiting Professor at the International Institute for Advanced Studies and Cybernetics (IIAS) since 2002.

Nigel Hamilton Lovell received the B.E. (Hons.) and Ph.D. degrees from the University of New South Wales (UNSW), Sydney, Australia. He is currently a Professor of Biomedical Engineering at the Graduate School of Biomedical Engineering, UNSW, and an Adjunct Professor in the School of Electrical Engineering and Telecommunications, UNSW. He is the author or coauthor of more than 300 refereed journals, conference proceedings, book chapters and patents. His current research interests include cardiac modeling, home telecare technologies, biological signal processing and visual prosthesis design. He has served in numerous roles on the Administrative Committee of the IEEE Engineering in Medicine and Biology Society, including Vice President for Member and Student Activities and Vice President for Conferences.

John McQuade earned his MBA at the Iowa State University College of Business. His research interests include Project Management, Health Informatics, and Business Strategy.

Dr. David Meinert is a Professor and Director of the MS CIS Program at Missouri State University. David Meinert received his doctorate in management information systems from the University of Mississippi (1990). His professional background includes software development, system integration, and project management. He has published a number of journals such as, *Information Resource Management Journal, End User Computing Management, and Journal of Marketing Theory and Practice.*

Lucila Ohno-Machado, MD, PhD, Professor and Chief of the Division of Biomedical Informatics at UCSD, holds a medical degree from the University of São Paulo in Brazil and a PhD in Medical Information Sciences and Computer Science from Stanford University where she was a research fellow in medicine from 1991 to 1996. She served as an instructor, assistant professor, and associate professor in the Department of Radiology and the Division of Health Sciences and Technology at Harvard-MIT, where she developed and taught new graduate courses in the computer science department. She is an elected fellow of the American College of Medical Informatics and of the American Institute for Medical and Biological Engineering. Besides her UCSD responsibilities, she is associate editor of the

Journal of the American Medical Informatics Association, and will also serve as associate editor of the Journal of Biomedical Informatics starting 2010. She chairs the scientific program committee for the 2009 American Medical Informatics Association Annual Symposium.

Blessing Maumbe holds a PhD in Agricultural Economics from Michigan State University, USA. His research interests cover e-government service delivery and policy development in South Africa, global food supply chain analysis, and digital rural financial service delivery in Africa. Blessing has received competitive research grants from the W.K. Kellogg Foundation, Rockefeller Foundation and the Germany Technical Agency for Development (GTZ) and has worked as consultant on Southern Africa. He was the founding Lecturer in Agribusiness at Africa University in 1993, and was later appointed its first Coordinator of Agribusiness Management studies in 2002. Blessing has taught numerous courses in Agribusiness Management, Food and Agricultural Marketing and General Economics at several Universities and colleges in South Africa, Zimbabwe, and the United States. He is currently working as an Associate Professor in the College of Business and Technology at Eastern Kentucky University (EKU), where he is responsible for the Agribusiness Management Program in the Department of Agriculture. Prior to joining EKU, he was an Associate Professor in the Faculty of Informatics and Design at Cape Peninsula University of Technology in Cape Town, South Africa.

Thomas W. Miller received his Ph.D. from the State University of New York and University of Buffalo, is a diplomate of the American Board of Professional Psychology in Clinical Psychology, and is a Fellow of the American Psychological Association, the American Psychological Society and the Royal Society of medicine. He is Professor Emeritus and Senior Research Scientist with the University of Connecticut and Professor, Department of Psychiatry, College of Medicine, University of Kentucky. His professional interest includes Telehealth applications in health care, development of laws and regulations related to practice, ethical, legal and social implications of genetics; traumatic stress disorder and stressful transitions across the life span.

Masako Miyazaki has been involved in Telehealth since 1996 and one of the founding members of Canadian Society of Telehealth. She had organized the first international congress on Multimedia and Telehealth Technologies in Edmonton in 1999 which was well attended by representatives from 22 countries. Her research and development focus on technologies to promote healthy environment, healthy food, prevention of illness, promotion of health, health community, and to enhance healthcare delivery. She was the principal investigator of the project entitled "WWPM- Wireless Wearable Physiological Monitor". This was multimillion dollar project with multidisciplinary team of scientists at the University of Alberta; Sapporo Medical University; Canadian companies and Japanese companies. She has published and presented her work at professional conferences globally over 114 times.

Ravi Nemana received a BA in the History, Philosophy and Social Studies of Science and Medicine from the University of Chicago in 1990, and an MBA with emphases in healthcare and operations from the University of California, Davis. He currently serves at the Executive Director for Services Science, Management and Engineering (SSME) at the Center for Information Technology in the Interest of Society (CITRIS) at the University of California, Berkeley, a four-campus, California State-funded Institute of Science and Innovation. He also directs the CITRIS initiative in healthcare and the CITRIS Service Lab, a unique laboratory that aims to improve service innovation. He was a founding member of the Center for Health and Technology at UC Davis, Senior Advisor and Director of IT Research at the Health Technology Center, and a co-founder of the California Regional Health Information Organization (CalRHIO). He is a member of the technical advisory board of Fluential, Inc., a firm providing speech-to-speech translation technology and services, and a board member of 360Fresh, Inc., a company that uses text-mining to improve patient safety and quality of care.

Nick Oliver received a BSc in molecular endocrinology in 1996 and qualified as a physician from Imperial College School of Medicine at St. Mary's in 1999. He passed the Membership of the Royal College of Physicians (London) in 2003. He is currently a clinical research fellow at the Imperial College, working in the Faculties of Medicine and Engineering; and at the Imperial College NHS Trust. His primary research interest is technology in diabetes and metabolic disease with clinical work in the specialty of diabetes and endocrinology. Nick is a Diabetes UK Innovator in Diabetes and is a member of the Royal College of Physicians, the Society for Endocrinology, and Diabetes UK.

Vesper T. Owei Vesper Owei received his B.S. in electrical and electronic engineering from the Ohio State University, USA, and Master's in electrical and electronic engineering and in operations research from the Georgia Institute of Technology, USA. Owei also holds a Ph.D. from Georgia Tech. He has practiced as a project, design and consulting engineer. His research work has spanned such areas as data management, data modeling, concept-based query languages, HCI, knowledge and expert systems, OLAP, information systems for disabled people, and IT for healthcare delivery. His current research interests include: ICT and society, mobile ICTs and developing countries, and HCIs and end-user issues.

Dr. Dane Peterson is a Dean's Distinguished Research Professor at Missouri State University. Dane Peterson received his doctorate in Quantitative Analysis and Applied Psychology from Southern Illinois University (1982). He has published in a number of journals such as, *International Journal of Information Management, Personnel Review, Business & Society, Business and Psychology and the Journal of Applied Psychology.*

Esteban Pino, ScD, is an assistant professor at the Electrical Engineering Department at the Universidad de Concepción in Concepción, Chile. He graduated as an electronics engineer and then obtained a MSc degree from the same institution. After a short period in the industry, he pursued doctoral studies while actively involved in the Biomedical Engineering program planning and creation in 2005. He was a research fellow at the Brigham and Women's Hospital in Boston, Massachusetts, working on ambulatory patient monitoring from 2004 to 2006. His research interests include distributed monitoring systems and biomedical signal processing.

Philippe Pucheral is Professor at the University of Versailles, currently in secondment at INRIA Rocquencourt where he is heading the SMIS (Secured and Mobile Information Systems) research team. He obtained a PhD in Computer Science from the University Paris 6 in 1991 and the Habilitation à Diriger des Recherches from the University of Versailles in 1999. He (co-) authored more than 60 conference and journal papers, 4 international patents, 4 books and was the recipient of 4 international awards (EDBT'92, VLDB'2000, e-gate'2004, SIMagine'2005). His domain of interest covers database systems, mobile and embedded databases and database security.

Andrea Resca, PhD, is Post Doc fellow at the Luiss "Guido Carli" University, Rome, Centre of Research on Information Systems (Ce.R.S.I.). After his undergraduate studies at the University of Bologna (School of Political Science), moved to South Korea where he obtained a master of arts in Korean Studies (International Area Studies).Once in Italy again, he joined the "Libera Università di Lingue e Comunicazione – IULM", Milan, as senior research fellow researching e-government until 2005. His publications range from the organisation theory discipline to information systems discipline including e-government and e-participation as his current research domains.

Meke I. Shivute Meke is a hard working and enthusiastic researcher based in Namibia. She is currently working as a Lecturer at the Polytechnic of Namibia in the Business Computing Department. She completed her Masters in Information Technology at the Cape Peninsula University of Technology in Cape Town, South Africa. Her current research interests are in ICT applications and policy development in health service delivery in Namibia. Her experience covers university undergraduate teaching, field data collection in Africa, and presentations at national and international conferences mostly in Southern Africa. Meke's future research interests lie in the area of Medical informatics and Health Information Systems.

Maricarmen D. Planas-Silva has earned her Ph.D. in Cell Biology from Baylor College of Medicine, Texas. She is currently pursuing her M.B.A. at Pennsylvania State University Harrisburg and a Clinical Research Certificate at the Pennsylvania State University College of Medicine. Her research interests include breast cancer

Thomas Stair graduated from Harvard Medical School, completed residency training in emergency medicine at Georgetown University, and served on the faculty at Georgetown for twenty years, where he was director of clinical informatics, assistant dean for continuing medical education, residency director and chair of emergency medicine. Ten years ago he returned to teach at Harvard and also sees patients in the Emergency Department of Brigham and Women's Hospital. He has edited and co-authored textbooks of emergency medicine, published articles on technology assessment, volunteered with the National Disaster Medical System and served as the President of the Society for Academic Emergency Medicine.

Romuald Thion received his Ph.D. in computer science from the University of Lyon (Institut National des Sciences Appliquées de Lyon - INSA) in 2008. His main research interests are databases, logic, access control, privacy and formal management of obligations. He is currently a postdoctoral research fellow in the LICIT (Legal Issues in Communication and Information Technologies) team at INRIA Grenoble.

Indrit Troshani, PhD MSc is a senior lecturer in Information Systems at the University of Adelaide Business School. Malaysia. His research interests include adoption and diffusion of network innovations in Business-to-Business (B2B) settings and mobile services. Dr Troshani has contributed to the body of knowledge in electronic commerce and information systems by co-authoring refereed journal and international conference publications. His work has appeared in Information Technology & People, European Journal of Innovation Management, Electronic Markets, International Journal of E-Business Research, Journal of Theoretical and Applied Electronic Commerce Research, International Journal of Mobile Communications and others.

Jennifer A. V. Wood received her Ph.D. in clinical psychology from the University of Mississippi. She completed her clinical psychology internship and post-doctoral residency at the South Texas Veterans Health Care System in San Antonio. She is currently the Acting Chief of Mental Health for the VA Texas Valley Coastal Bend Health Care System as well as an Assistant Professor with the Department of Psychiatry at the University of Texas Health Science Center at San Antonio. Her interests include research focus on the use of telecommunications technology in the delivery of rural mental health and health care.

Nilmini Wickramasinghe, PhD MBA researches and teaches within Information Systems. She is well published having written several books, over 100 refereed scholarly papers and co-edited an encyclopedia. Currently, she is the associate director of the Center for Management Medical Technology (CMMT) at Illinois Institute of Technology, USA and holds a professor position at RMIT University, Australia. In addition, she is the editor-in-chief of the international journal of networking and virtual organizations (IJNVO) and the inaugural editor-in-chief of the international journal of biomedical engineering and technology (IJBET) both published by InderScience.

Shuyan Xie studies at University of Alabama within the Health Care Management undergraduate program, and she is a candidate of the manager assistant at Veteran Affair Medical Center after graduation. Since 2008, she has worked for Professor Yang Xiao where her jobs have included writing papers on various healthcare topics, assisting in health-care organization surveys, and visiting nursing homes and different health-care providers. During her past four years, Shuyan had experience in teaching aerobic classes as a group leader--- planning, coordinating, and directing operation of the patient information system as an administrative assistant at National Maternity Hospital in Dublin, Ireland. These duties combine with her special interest in healthcare development of healthcare management in varieties. In her spare time, she likes to travel, do yoga, reading etc.

Dr. Yang Xiao worked in industry as a MAC (Medium Access Control) architect involving the IEEE 802.11 standard enhancement work before he joined Department of Computer Science at The University of Memphis in 2002. He is currently with Department of Computer Science (with tenure) at The University of Alabama. He was a voting member of IEEE 802.11 Working Group from 2001 to 2004. He is an IEEE Senior Member. He is a member of American Telemedicine Association. He currently serves as Editor-in-Chief for International Journal of Security and Networks (IJSN), International Journal of Sensor Networks (IJSNet), and International Journal of Telemedicine and Applications (IJTA). He serves as a panelist for the US National Science Foundation (NSF), Canada Foundation for Innovation (CFI)'s Telecommunications expert committee, and the American Institute of Biological Sciences (AIBS), as well as a referee/reviewer for many national and international funding agencies. He serves on TPC for more than 100 conferences such as INFOCOM, ICDCS, MOBIHOC, ICC, GLOBECOM, WCNC, etc. He serves as an associate editor for several journals, e.g., IEEE Transactions on Vehicular Technology. His research areas are security, telemedicine, robot, sensor networks, and wireless networks. He has published more than 300 papers in major journals, refereed conference proceedings, book chapters related to these research areas. Dr. Xiao's research has been supported by the US National Science Foundation (NSF), U.S. Army Research, Fleet & Industrial Supply Center San Diego (FISCSD), and The University of Alabama's Research Grants Committee. Dr. Xiao is a Guest Professor of Jilin University (2007-2012), and was an Adjunct Professor of Zhejiang University (2007-2009).

James Zhaonan Zhang received the B.E. (Hons) degree in telecommunications engineering and the M.Biomed.E degree in biomedical engineering from the University of New South Wales (UNSW), Sydney, Australia, in 2006. Currently, he is pursuing the Ph.D. degree at the School of Electrical and Telecommunications Engineering at UNSW. His research focuses on knowledge management, data fusion and decision support based on wireless sensor network technology.

Index

D

E

F

G

H

Z

Breinigsville, PA USA
16 January 2011
253151BV00003B/4/P

9 781609 601836